Complementary and Conventional Medicine

Complementary and Conventional Medicine

Edited by Jax Bailey

SYRAWOOD
PUBLISHING HOUSE

New York

Published by Syrawood Publishing House,
750 Third Avenue, 9th Floor,
New York, NY 10017, USA
www.syrawoodpublishinghouse.com

Complementary and Conventional Medicine
Edited by Jax Bailey

International Standard Book Number: 978-1-68286-479-1 (Hardback)

Cataloging-in-Publication Data

Complementary and conventional medicine / edited by Jax Bailey.
    p. cm.
Includes bibliographical references and index.
ISBN 978-1-68286-479-1
1. Alternative medicine. 2. Integrative medicine. 3. Medicine. 4. Therapeutics. I. Bailey, Jax.
R733 .C66 2017
615.5--dc23

Printed in the United States of America.

TABLE OF CONTENTS

PREFACE

This book on complementary and conventional medicine talks about the influence and effectiveness of alternative medical practices. Complementary medicine is the practice that endows both general and alternative medical treatment. Alternative medicine focuses on the pathophysiological as well as psychological condition of the patient for diagnosis. Medical practice is classified into whole medical systems and mind-body interventions. The aim of this book is to present researches that have transformed this discipline and aided its advancement. From theories to research to practical applications, case studies related to all contemporary topics of relevance to this field have been included in this book. It is an essential guide for both academicians and those who wish to pursue this discipline further.

After months of intensive research and writing, this book is the end result of all who devoted their time and efforts in the initiation and progress of this book. It will surely be a source of reference in enhancing the required knowledge of the new developments in the area. During the course of developing this book, certain measures such as accuracy, authenticity and research focused analytical studies were given preference in order to produce a comprehensive book in the area of study.

This book would not have been possible without the efforts of the authors and the publisher. I extend my sincere thanks to them. Secondly, I express my gratitude to my family and well-wishers. And most importantly, I thank my students for constantly expressing their willingness and curiosity in enhancing their knowledge in the field, which encourages me to take up further research projects for the advancement of the area.

Editor

Methanol and Butanol Extracts of *Paeonia lutea* Leaves Repress Metastasis of Squamous Cell Carcinoma

Yoshiki Mukudai,[1] Meilin Zhang,[2] Sunao Shiogama,[1] Seiji Kondo,[1] Chihiro Ito,[1] Hiromi Motohashi,[1] Kosuke Kato,[1] Miharu Fujii,[1] Satoru Shintani,[1] Hideyuki Shigemori,[3] Kazunaga Yazawa,[4] and Tatsuo Shirota[1]

[1]*Department of Oral and Maxillofacial Surgery, School of Dentistry, Showa University, 2-1-1 Kitasenzoku, Ota-ku, Tokyo 145-8515, Japan*
[2]*Graduate School of Life and Environmental Sciences, University of Tsukuba, Tsukuba, Ibaraki 305-8572, Japan*
[3]*Faculty of Life and Environmental Sciences, University of Tsukuba, Tsukuba, Ibaraki 305-8572, Japan*
[4]*Division of Health Food Science, Institute for Nanoscience and Nanotechnology, Waseda University, 2-2 Wakamatsu-cho, Shinjuku-ku, Tokyo 162-0041, Japan*

Correspondence should be addressed to Yoshiki Mukudai; mukudai@dent.showa-u.ac.jp

Academic Editor: Yew-Min Tzeng

Squamous cell carcinoma (SCC) is one of the most common cancers of the head and neck region worldwide and is generally treated surgically in combination with radiotherapy and/or chemotherapy. However, anticancer agents have numerous serious side effects, and alternative, less toxic agents that are effective as chemotherapeutics for SCC are required. The Paeoniaceae family is widely used in traditional Chinese medicine. We examined methanol and butanol extracts of *Paeonia lutea* (*P. lutea*) leaves for their potential as an anticancer agent. Both extracts decreased the proliferation of SCC cells, induced apoptotic cell death, and modulated migration, adhesion, chemotaxis, and haptotaxis in an extracellular matrix- (ECM-) dependent manner due to altered expression of several integrin subunits. Subsequently, SCC cells were subcutaneously transplanted into athymic nude mice; the extracts reduced the metastasis of SCC cells but had little effect on the volume of the primary tumor or survival or body weight of the mice. The results suggest that the extracts may hold promise for preventing cancer metastasis.

1. Introduction

Squamous cell carcinoma (SCC) is one of the most common cancers of the head and neck region worldwide, with more than sixty thousand patients diagnosed each year [1]. Commonly, SCC is treated surgically in combination with radiotherapy and/or chemotherapy. However, treatment outcome is unsatisfactory, with 20% to 50% of patients developing regional recurrence and/or distant metastasis [2]. In addition, anticancer agents often cause a variety of serious side effects; for example, *cis*-platinum (II) diammine dichloride (CDDP), which is often used for chemotherapy of SCC, causes nephrotoxicity [3], neurotoxicity [4], nausea, vomiting [5], ototoxicity [6], and xerostomia (dry mouth) [7, 8]. Hence, less toxic chemotherapeutics for SCC are required.

The Paeoniaceae family is widely used in traditional Chinese medicine. Previous studies reported that the root barks of Paeoniaceae are used as therapeutics for various diseases such as diabetes [9], Alzheimer's disease [10, 11], arthritis [12], inflammation [13], sepsis [14], brain-ischemia-reperfusion injury [15], and virus infections [16, 17]. Moreover, several studies have reported anticancer effects of Paeoniaceae family preparations [18–23].

Traditional Chinese medicine has been used to treat a variety of diseases for several thousands of years; therefore, we launched an interinstitutional collaborative project in 2010 to evaluate the therapeutic potential of herbal extracts for disorders of the head and neck region [23–26]. Here, we examined methanol and butanol extracts of *Paeonia lutea* (*P. lutea*) leaves for their potential as an anticancer agent. Our results indicate that these extracts modulate the migration and adhesion of SCC cells to the extracellular matrix (ECM) by altering integrin subunit expression *in vitro* and reduce metastasis of the cells *in vivo*; however, transplanted tumor growth and survival of the recipient animals were essentially unaffected.

2. Materials and Methods

2.1. Plant Materials and Preparation of Plant Extracts. *P. lutea* leaves were collected from Tsukuba Peony Garden (Tsukuba, Ibaraki, Japan) in October 2012. A voucher specimen (UTHS1210) was deposited at the Laboratory of Natural Products Chemistry, Graduate School of Life and Environmental Sciences, University of Tsukuba. The leaves were air dried for 2 days at room temperature (dry weight, 350 g) and then extracted with methanol (4 L) for 1 week. The extraction was repeated once. The two methanol extracts were combined and concentrated *in vacuo* at 38°C to give the methanol extract (ME, 80.1 g). The extract was partitioned with ethyl acetate three times (800 mL each) and H_2O (800 mL). The ethyl acetate was evaporated to afford ethyl acetate soluble materials (EA, 28.5 g). The H_2O layer was partitioned with butanol three times (600 mL each) to give butanol-soluble (BU, 20.5 g), butanol-insoluble (BW, 2.1 g), and H_2O-soluble materials (W, 16.5 g). Finally, aliquots of each of these materials were dissolved in phosphate-buffered saline (PBS) at a concentration of 1 mg/mL and sterilized by passage through a Millex syringe filter (Merck Millipore, Billerica, MA).

2.2. Cell Culture and Anchorage-Independent Growth Assay. SAS cells, a human oral SCC cell line [27], were cultured in high-glucose Dulbecco's Modified Eagle Medium (DMEM; Wako, Osaka, Japan) supplemented with 10% fetal bovine serum (FBS) and penicillin-streptomycin solution (Sigma-Aldrich, St. Louis, MO) at 37°C, 5% CO_2, and 100% humidity. Anchorage-independent growth assay was carried out using a commercial kit (Cytoselect 96-Well *In Vitro* Tumor Sensitivity Assay kit, Cell Biolabs, San Diego, CA) as described previously [28].

2.3. Cell Growth and Apoptosis Assays. One thousand cells were seeded into each well of a 96-well tissue culture plate. After 48 h, the cells were assayed using the tetrazolium salt 3-[4,5-dimethylthiazol-2-yl]-2,5-diphenyltetrazolium bromide (MTT) assay, as described previously [29]. The activities of caspases 3/7, 8, and 9 were measured using a Caspase-Glo (Promega, Madison, WI) and GloMax-Multi+ Detection System (Promega) according to the manufacturer's protocol. Genomic DNA fragmentation was investigated using a commercial kit (Apoladder EX; Takara, Shiga, Japan) according to the manufacturer's protocol.

2.4. Protein Preparation and Western Blotting Analysis. Total cellular protein was prepared as described previously [30].

Protein concentration was measured using Quick Start Bradford Reagent (Bio-Rad, Hercules, CA) using bovine serum albumin (BSA) as a standard. Protein aliquots were stored at −80°C until use. For Western blot analysis, 20 μg of total cellular protein was subjected to sodium dodecyl sulfate polyacrylamide electrophoresis (SDS-PAGE) on a 4% to 20% gradient gel (Bio-Rad); then the blot was transferred onto a polyvinylidene difluoride membrane (Life Technologies, Carlsbad, CA). Blocking, 1st and horseradish-peroxidase-conjugated 2nd antibody reactions and washing were conducted as previously described [28]. The chemiluminescence signals were visualized using Amersham ECL Western Blotting Detection Reagents (GE Healthcare UK Ltd., Buckinghamshire, UK) and ChimiDoc XRS Plus ImageLab System (Bio-Rad). The 1st and 2nd antibodies were purchased from common suppliers.

2.5. Adhesion, Wound Healing, and Migration Assays. The cells were grown in a monolayer culture in the presence or absence of the various *P. lutea* leaf extracts. After 3 d, the cells were assayed. Adhesion and wound healing assays were carried out using commercial kits (CytoSelect 48-Well Cell Adhesion Assay, CytoSelect 24-Well Wound Healing Assay, Cell Biolabs) according to the manufacturer's protocol. To assay migration, a chemotaxis chamber containing a membrane with 8 mm pores (Chemotaxicell, Kurabo, Osaka Japan) was coated with 50 μg/mL bovine type I collagen (Koken, Tokyo, Japan) or 50 μg/mL bovine fibronectin (Sigma-Aldrich) according to the manufacturer's protocol and was set into each well of a 24-well culture plate. After drying the Chemotaxicell membrane, 500 μL of DMEM with or without 10% FBS was added to the bottom of the well as a chemoattractant, 200 μL of DMEM containing 2×10^4 cells was added to the chamber, then the plate was incubated for 24 h at 37°C, 5% CO_2, and 100% humidity. The membranes were then washed, removed from the chamber, fixed with 4% formaldehyde (Wako, Osaka, Japan), and stained with crystal violet (Wako). The membranes were examined under an optical microscope and photographs (×400) were taken.

2.6. Animals. The care and treatment of the experimental animals complied with the Showa University Guidelines for Animal Experiments, and the experimental protocol was approved by the Animal Experimentation Committee of Showa University. The dorsal flank of four-week-old female athymic Balb/c *nu/nu* mice (CLEA Japan, Tokyo) was subcutaneously injected with a PBS-suspension of 1×10^6 SAS cells, as described previously [30]. After 1 week, tumor formation was measured (approximately 10 mm³), and the mice were divided into 6 groups (control, ME, EA, BU, BW, and W). Therefore, the 7th day after SAS cell injection was designated "day 1," thereafter. Each herbal extract was suspended in PBS at the concentration of 2 mg/mL and 100 mg/kg body weight was orally administrated using a sterilized feeding needle once every three days for 40 or 70 days. In the control group, only PBS (0.1 mL) was administrated. The body weight and diameters (large and small) of each mouse were measured and the tumor volume was determined by direct measurement and calculated using the formula [30] $\pi/6 \times$ (large diameter) $\times$ (small diameter)^2. On day 40 or 70, the mice were sacrificed, and the tumors together with the surrounding soft tissue, liver, and lungs were harvested for histochemical analysis.

2.7. Histochemistry and Immunohistochemistry. The tissue was fixed, embedded, sliced, and subjected to hematoxylin-eosin (HE) staining as described previously [31]. Immuno-histochemistry was conducted as described previously [31]. After 24 h incubation with a 1/50 dilution of primary antibody for human cytokeratin 10/13 (Santa Cruz Biotechnology, Santa Cruz, CA), the slide was incubated with Simple Stain MAX-PO (Nichirei, Tokyo, Japan) and visualized using Envision HRP/Kit (Dako, Kyoto, Japan); the manufacturer's suggested protocol for each commercial kit was used.

2.8. Statistical Analysis. Unless otherwise specified, all experiments were repeated at least *twice*, and similar results were obtained in the repeat experiments. Statistical analysis for mouse survival was determined by the log rank test. Other statistical analyses were carried out using two-tailed, unpaired Student's t-test. Data are expressed as means ± standard deviation of at least three data items. A p value < 0.05 was considered significant.

3. Results

3.1. Extracts of P. lutea Leaves Decreased Proliferation of SCC Cells in an Anchorage-Independent Manner, but No Effect Was Observed on Monolayer Cultures. We first investigated the effects of the *P. lutea* leaf extracts on the proliferation of SCC cells (Figure 1). Only 100 μg/mL EA had a significant effect on monolayer cultures ((a) and (b)). In contrast, all extracts showed a significant growth-inhibitory effect on soft agar cultures using the MTT assay (c). Importantly, phase-microscopy images (d) indicated that all the extracts decreased both the number and size of SCC cells compared to the control culture. These results suggest that extracts of *P. lutea* leaves are likely to reduce both the proliferation and malignancy of SCC cells.

3.2. Extracts of P. lutea Leaves Induce Apoptotic Cell Death of SCC Cells in Soft Agar Culture. We tested the hypothesis that the reduced MTT activity was due to apoptotic cell death by investigating the apoptotic effects of the extracts (Figure 2). Caspase activity assays (a) revealed that 10–100 mg/mL of EA significantly increased caspase 3/7 and 9 activities in a monolayer culture, whereas all the extracts strongly increased caspase activities in a soft agar culture. On the other hand, a DNA ladder assay (b) showed almost no DNA fragmentation in monolayer cultures treated with any of the extracts, whereas significant DNA fragmentation was observed in all the test soft agar cultures, in disagreement with the caspase assays. Furthermore, we examined the effects of the extracts on modulating apoptosis-related protein expressions by Western blotting analysis (c). In both monolayer and soft

agar cultures, EA and BU reduced the expression of Bcl-2, a mitochondrial antiapoptotic protein, but the expression of other proteins (p53, Bcl-X$_L$, Bax, Bad, Bid, Bak, and XIAP) was essentially unaltered. These results indicate that EA and BU might affect the mitochondrial apoptotic pathway, in an anchorage-independent manner.

3.3. Extracts of P. lutea Leaves Decreased the Adhesion of ECM. Next, we examined the effects of adhesion, migration, and invasion in an ECM-dependent manner (Figure 3). Cell adhesion assays (a) showed that EA and BU reduced the attachment of SCC cells to type I collagen (Col I) and fibronectin (FN); similar results regarding cell migration were obtained using a cell migration assay (b). Furthermore, a cell invasion assay (c) showed that EA and BA reduced SAS cell invasion of Col I and FN and that the effects were independent of a chemoattractant. Those results imply that EA and BU extracts decrease both chemotaxis and haptotaxis of SCC cells through the ECM, thereby potentially preventing the invasion and metastasis of SCC cells.

3.4. Extracts of P. lutea Leaves Decreased the Expression of Several Integrin Subunits. The adhesion, migration, and invasion of various cells, including cancer cells, rely on integrin proteins. We therefore investigated whether the extracts modulate the expression of major integrin subunits. Western blotting analysis indicated that BW and W had little effect on the expression of integrin subunits (Figure 4): the expression of α4, β3, β4, and β5 integrin subunits was attenuated by EA and BU, but expression of the other subunits was essentially unchanged. These results suggest that the altered response of SAS cells to the ECM is at least partly due to modulation of the expression of several integrin subunits.

3.5. Extracts of P. lutea Reduce Metastasis of SCC Cells. The results of the above *in vitro* experiments prompted us to investigate *in vivo* whether the extracts might be useful as a novel anticancer medicine. Each extract was orally administrated to SCC-transplanted nude mice (Figure 5). Contrary to our expectation, neither survival (a), body weight (b), nor tumor growth ((c) and (d)) was affected by the extracts compared to the control group. Furthermore, histochemical analysis (Figure 6) showed that all extracts had little effect on the primary tumor. Liver and lung tissues were examined to determine the effects of the extracts on metastasis. HE staining showed no obvious metastatic tumor cells. Immuno-histochemistry for cytokeratin 10/13, a representative marker of SCC cells, showed positive cells in the control and ME, BW, and W extracts mice, indicating micrometastasis from the primary tumor. Interestingly, however, administration of EA and BU extracts significantly reduced the number of positive cells. These results indicate that EA and BU extracts of *P. lutea* exhibit pharmacological effects to decrease hepatic and pulmonary metastasis from epidermal SCC and suggest that the extracts may hold promise as anticancer therapeutics.

(a)

(b)

(c)

(d)

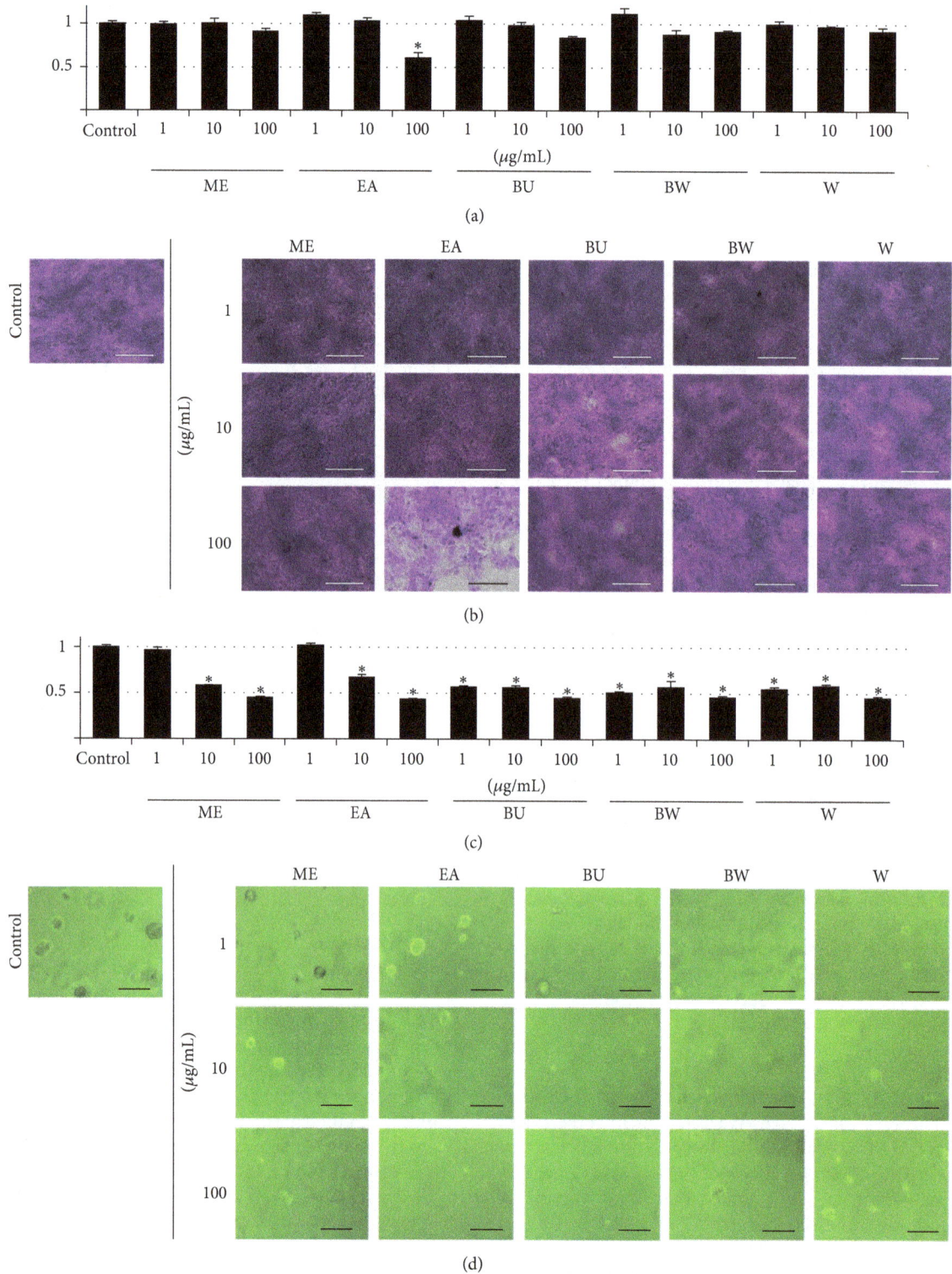

FIGURE 1: Growth-inhibitory effects of extracts of *P. lutea* leaves. SAS cells were grown in a monolayer ((a) and (b)) or on soft agar ((c) and (d)) culture. Methanol (ME), ethyl acetate (EA), butanol (BU), butanol-insoluble (BW), and water (W) extracts of *P. lutea* leaves were added to the culture medium at 0 (control) and 1, 10, or 100 μg/mL. After 7 d, the cells were subjected to MTT assay ((a) and (c)) and crystal violet staining (b) or examined under a phase-contrast microscope (d). Data in (a) and (c) are means ± standard deviations of 3 cultures; the mean of the control cultures is taken as "1." *$p < 0.05$ versus control. Bars, 100 μm (b) and 200 μm (d).

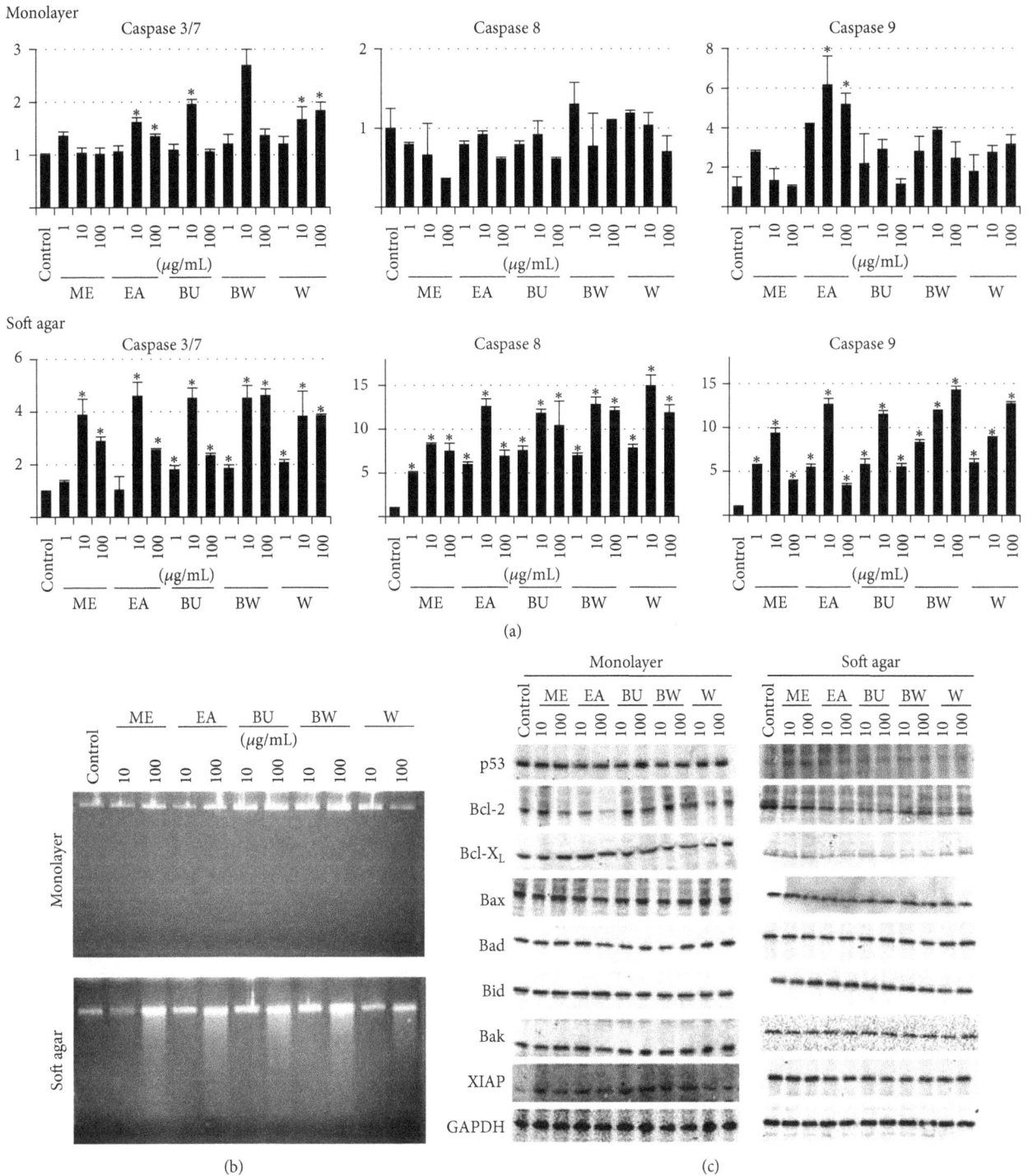

FIGURE 2: Apoptosis-induced effects of *P. lutea* leaf extracts. SAS cells were grown in a monolayer or on soft agar culture. Methanol (ME), ethyl acetate (EA), butanol (BU), butanol-insoluble (BW), and water (W) extracts of *P. lutea* leaves were added to the culture medium at 1 to 100 μg/mL ((a) and (b)), 10 to 100 μg/mL (c), or 0 μg/mL (control). After 3 d, the cells were subjected to caspase 3/7, 8, and 9 assays (a), a DNA ladder assay (b), or Western blotting analysis for apoptosis-related proteins (p53, Bcl-2, Bcl-X_L, Bax, Bad, Bid, Bak, and XIAP) using GAPDH as an internal control (c). Data in (a) are means ± standard deviations of 3 cultures; the mean of the control cultures is taken as "1." $^*p < 0.05$ versus control.

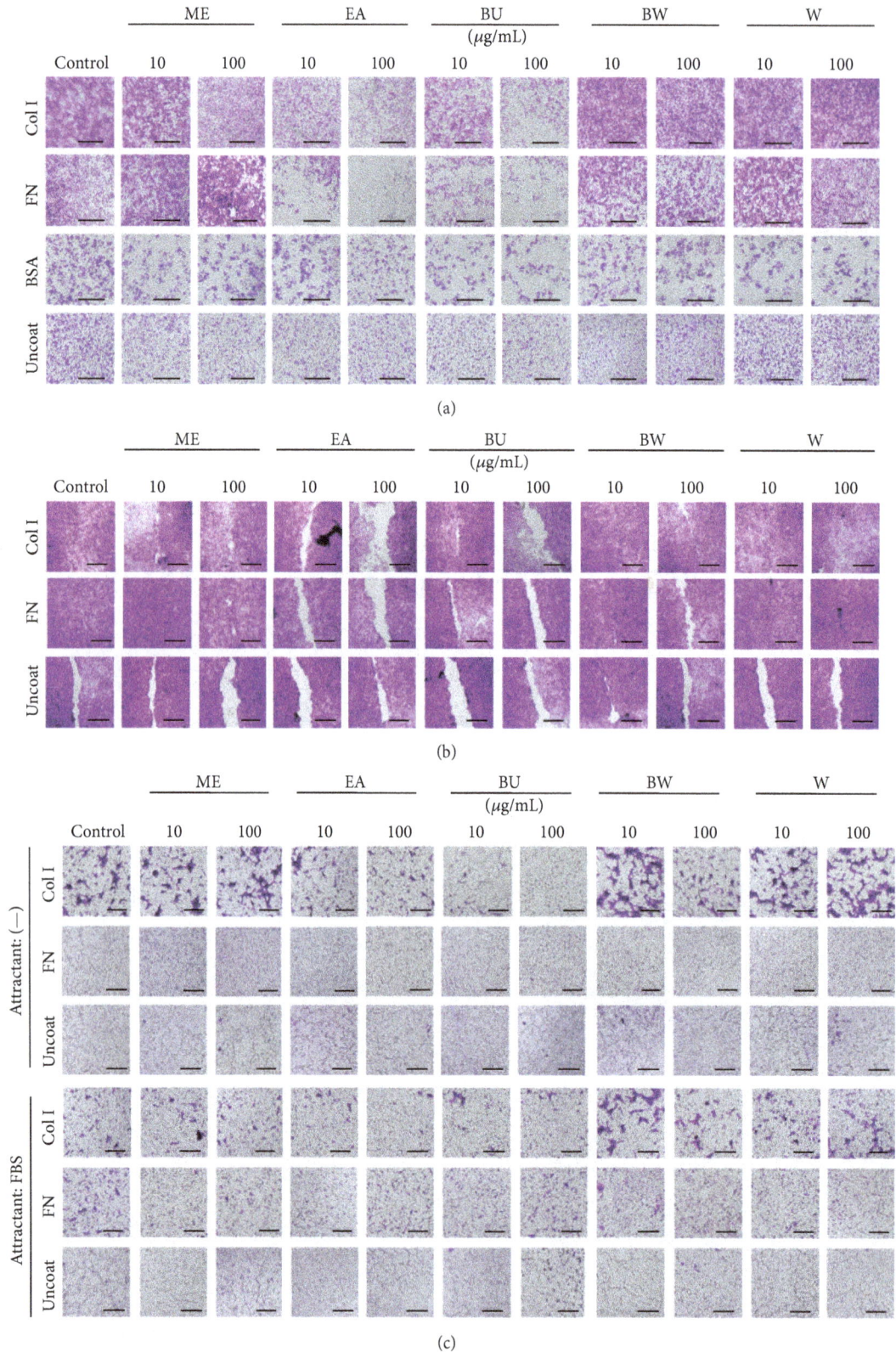

(a)

(b)

(c)

FIGURE 3: Effects of *P. lutea* leaf extracts on cell adhesion to ECMs. SAS cells were grown in a monolayer culture in the presence or absence (control) of methanol (ME), ethyl acetate (EA), butanol (BU), butanol-insoluble (BW), and water (W) extracts of *P. lutea* leaves at 10 to 100 μg/mL. After 3 d, the cells were subjected to adhesion (a), wound healing (b), and migration (c) assays for ECM (type I collagen (Col I), fibronectin (FN), and BSA) or an uncoated surface (Uncoat). 10% FBS was used as a chemoattractant or not (—) in the migration assay (c). Bars, 100 μm (a and c) and 1 mm (b).

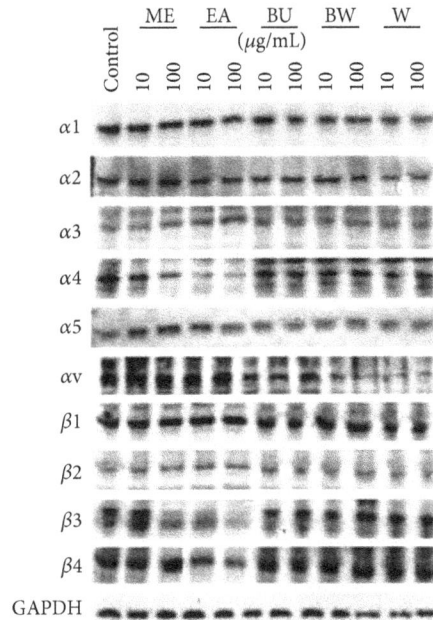

FIGURE 4: Effects of *P. lutea* leaf extracts on expression of integrin proteins. SAS cells were grown in a monolayer culture in the presence or absence (control) of methanol (ME), ethyl acetate (EA), butanol (BU), butanol-insoluble (BW), and water (W) extracts of *P. lutea* leaves at 10 to 100 μg/mL. After 3 d, total cellular proteins were purified and 20 μg aliquots were subjected to Western blotting for $\alpha 1$, $\alpha 2$, $\alpha 3$, $\alpha 4$, $\alpha 5$, αv, $\beta 1$, $\beta 2$, $\beta 3$, and $\beta 4$ integrins. GAPDH was used as an internal control.

4. Discussion

The Paeoniaceae family has been widely used in traditional Chinese medicine for thousands of years. Recent studies have revealed that extracts of *Paeoniaceae* may provide alternative anticancer therapeutics [18–23] and prompted us to investigate the extracts of *P. lutea* leaves for their anticancer potency. We first conducted *in vitro* studies to determine the effects of *P. lutea* leaf extract on proliferation (Figure 1) and apoptosis (Figure 2) of SCC cells. The extracts decreased proliferation and induced apoptotic cell death mainly by a mitochondrial signaling pathway, similar to Paeoniaceae root extracts [32]. Interestingly, the effects were more prominent in anchorage-independent cultures. Since proliferation and migration in an anchorage-independent manner reflect properties of malignant cancer cells [33], those results suggested that the extracts could be useful as an anticancer agent.

We next examined whether the extracts modulate adhesion to ECM and affect ECM-dependent migration, chemotaxis, and haptotaxis (Figure 3). EA and BU extracts significantly decreased adhesion to Col I and fibronectin. Several previous studies have reported that adhesion to ECM plays an important role in the invasion and metastasis of cancer cells [33, 34]. Thus, the present results suggest that the extracts might also decrease invasion and metastasis. Furthermore, adhesion between ECM and normal and cancer cells is supported by integrins, in particular $\alpha 5 \beta 1$ integrin, a main component of the fibronectin receptor [35]. However, Western blotting analysis for various major integrin subunits (Figure 4) showed essentially no modulation of the expression of $\alpha 5$ or $\beta 1$ subunits by the extracts, although $\alpha 4$, $\beta 3$, $\beta 4$, and $\beta 5$

integrin subunit expression was suppressed by the EA and BU extracts. Further studies, for example, on integrin-dependent signaling pathways and on other adhesion molecules, are required to resolve this discrepancy. Nevertheless, the present study demonstrated that EA and BU extracts modulate the expression of several integrin subunits, thus decreasing the invasion and metastasis of SCC cells *in vitro*.

The potential utility of the extracts for clinical use was investigated by an animal experiment and subsequent histochemical examination. A dose of 100 mg/kg body weight was chosen based on our previous studies [36–38]. The extracts were orally administered to SAS-cell-transplanted nude mice, and the survival and body weight of the mice and the volume of the primary tumor were measured (Figure 5). In contrast to the *in vivo* results, no antitumor effects were observed. HE staining and subsequent histochemical examination of the primary tumor, liver, and lung (Figure 6) showed no effect of the extracts. Cytokeratin 10/13 is highly expressed in SCC cells [39, 40], including SAS cells, and immunohistochemistry for cytokeratin 10/13 is indicative of metastasis of tumor cells in liver and lung. Mice given the extracts for 70 days showed positive cells in the organ (liver and lung). However, administration of EA and BU extracts significantly decreased the number and size of cytokeratin 10/13-positive tumor cells, suggesting that the extracts may have potency for reducing hepatic and pulmonary metastasis of epidermal SCC.

Our results demonstrate that EA and BU extracts of *P. lutea* have pharmacological effects of preventing the metastasis of SCC cells. The chemical composition, side effects, and minimum required dosage of the extracts of the extraction

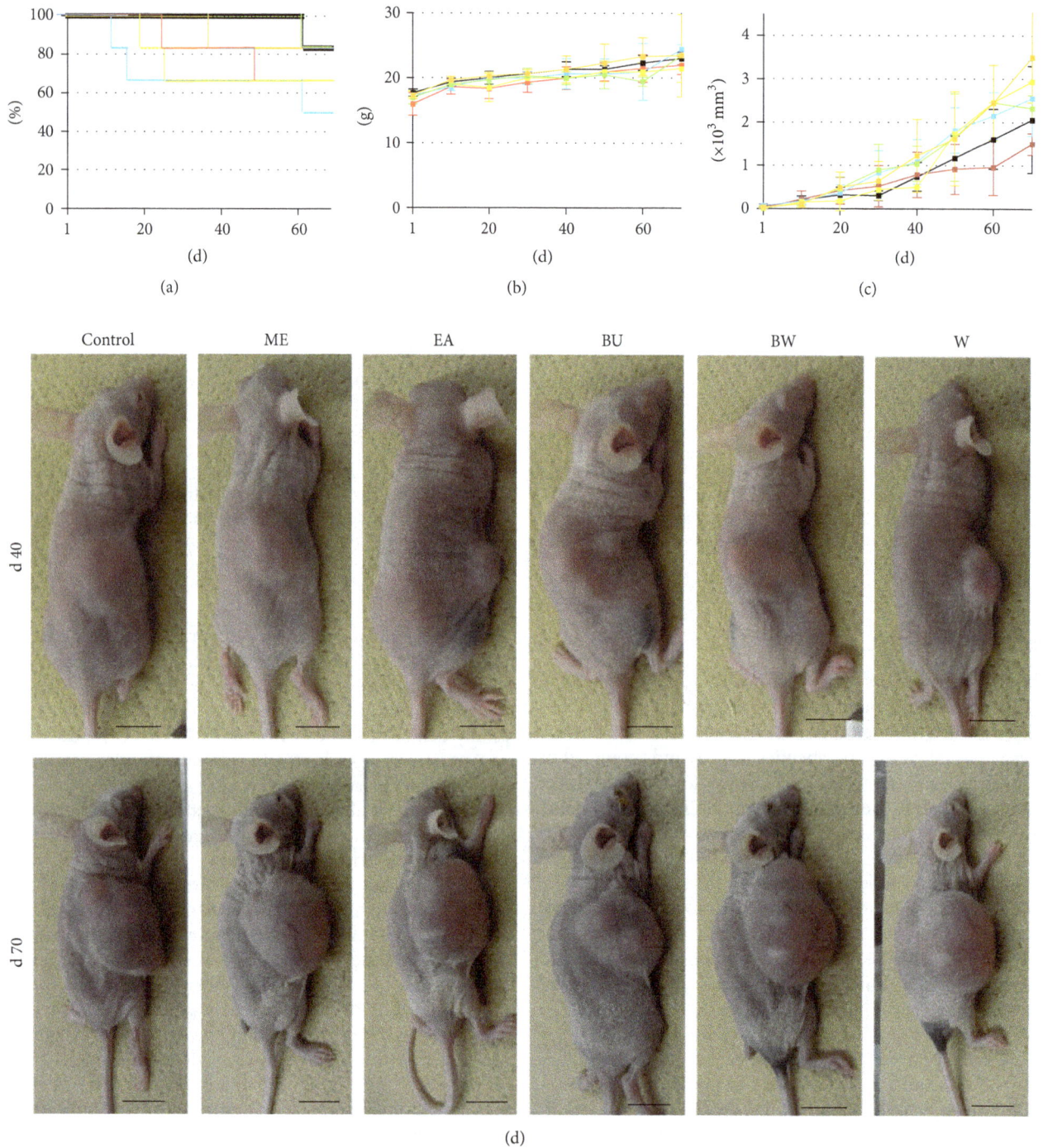

Figure 5: Effects of *P. lutea* leaf extracts on mouse survival and tumor growth in SAS-cell-xenograft nude mice. One million SAS cells were subcutaneously injected into the dorsal flank of nude mice (see Section 2). After 7 d, the mice were divided into 6 groups: vehicle (black lines in (a), (b), and (c) and control in (d)) methanol (red lines and ME), ethyl acetate (blue lines and EA), butanol (yellow lines and BU), butanol-insoluble (green lines and BW), and water (orange lines and W) extracts of *P. lutea* leaves were administrated once every three days at a concentration of 100 mg/kg body weight in PBS. Mouse survival Kaplan Meier plot in %, body weight in grams, and tumor volume in $\times 10^3$ mm^3 of each group are depicted in (a), (b), and (c), respectively; images of a representative mouse in each group were taken at d 40 and 70 (d). Bars, 1 cm.

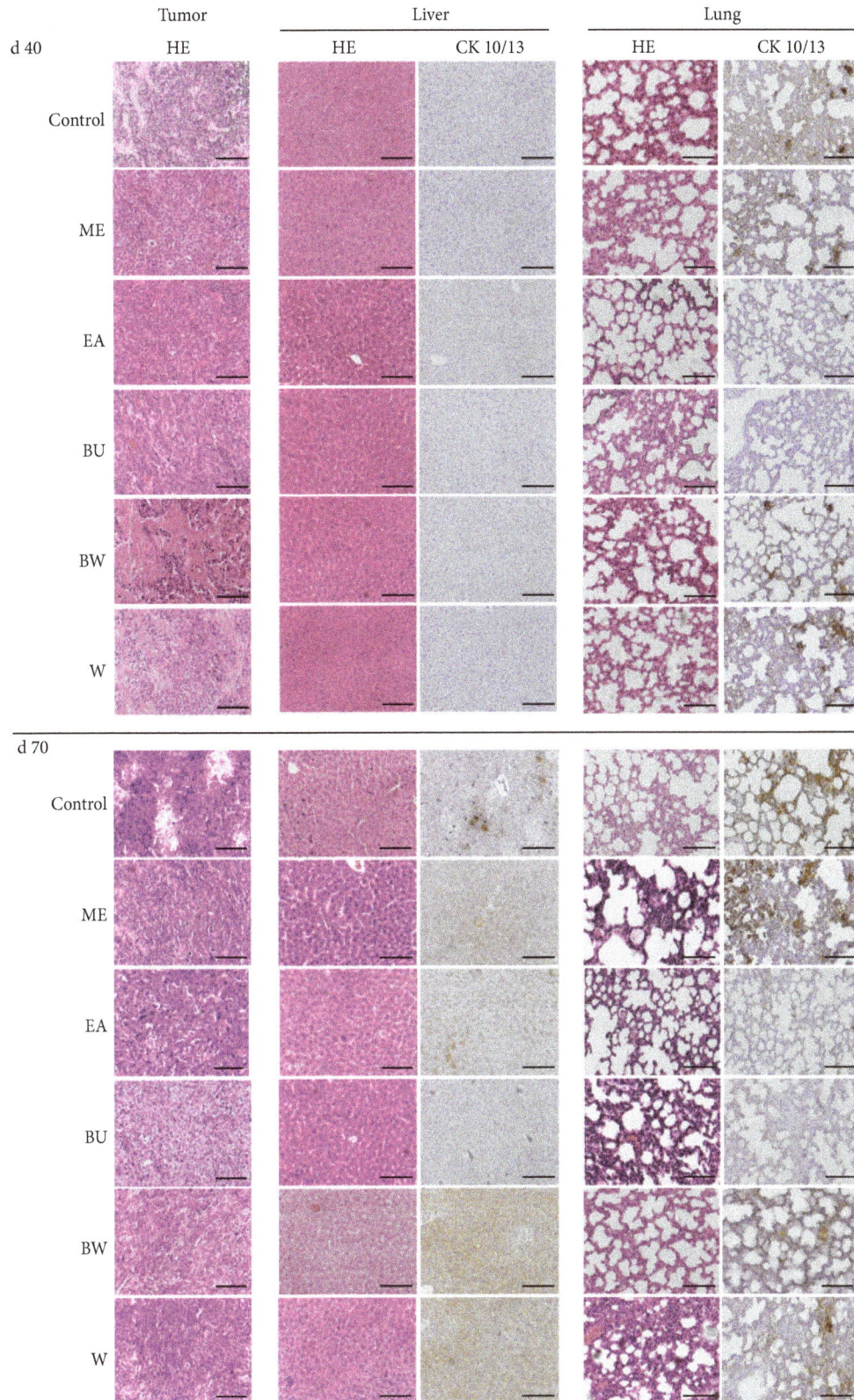

FIGURE 6: Effects of *P. lutea* leaf extracts on hepatic and pulmonary tumor-cell-metastasis in SAS-cell-xenograft nude mice. One million SAS cells were subcutaneously injected into the dorsal flank of nude mice, and vehicle (control), methanol (ME), ethyl acetate (EA), butanol (BU), butanol-insoluble (BW), and water (W) extracts of *P. lutea* leaves were administrated once every three days at 100 mg/kg body weight in PBS (see Section 2). After d 40 or 70, the mice were sacrificed, and the tumors, livers, and lungs were fixed and subjected to HE staining (HE) and immunohistochemistry for cytokeratin 10/13 (CK 10/13). Bars, 200 μm.

are currently being investigated in detail and will be reported in the near future.

Competing Interests

All authors have no competing interests.

Acknowledgments

This study was supported by Grants-in-Aid for Scientific Research (KAKENHI) from the Japan Society for the Promotion of Science (JSPS) (KAKENHI C to Yoshiki Mukudai, Seiji Kondo, and Tatsuo Shirota). The authors wish to thank all the doctors in the Department of Oral and Maxillofacial Surgery, School of Dentistry, Showa University, and Ms. Miho Yoshihara for secretarial assistance.

References

[1] J.-P. Machiels, M. Lambrecht, F.-X. Hanin et al., "Advances in the management of squamous cell carcinoma of the head and neck," *F1000Prime Reports*, vol. 6, article 44, 2014.

[2] Y.-C. Lin, H.-W. Chen, Y.-C. Kuo, Y.-F. Chang, Y.-J. Lee, and J.-J. Hwang, "Therapeutic efficacy evaluation of curcumin on human oral squamous cell carcinoma xenograft using multi-modalities of molecular imaging," *American Journal of Chinese Medicine*, vol. 38, no. 2, pp. 343–358, 2010.

[3] N. A. G. dos Santos, M. A. C. Rodrigues, N. M. Martins, and A. C. dos Santos, "Cisplatin-induced nephrotoxicity and targets of nephroprotection: an update," *Archives of Toxicology*, vol. 86, no. 8, pp. 1233–1250, 2012.

[4] S. R. McWhinney, R. M. Goldberg, and H. L. McLeod, "Platinum neurotoxicity pharmacogenetics," *Molecular Cancer Therapeutics*, vol. 8, no. 1, pp. 10–16, 2009.

[5] J. Herrstedt, "Antiemetics: an update and the MASCC guidelines applied in clinical practice," *Nature Clinical Practice Oncology*, vol. 5, no. 1, pp. 32–43, 2008.

[6] L. P. Rybak, D. Mukherjea, S. Jajoo, and V. Ramkumar, "Cisplatin ototoxicity and protection: clinical and experimental studies," *Tohoku Journal of Experimental Medicine*, vol. 219, no. 3, pp. 177–186, 2009.

[7] A. D. Rapidis, M. Trichas, E. Stavrinidis et al., "Induction chemotherapy followed by concurrent chemoradiation in advanced squamous cell carcinoma of the head and neck: final results from a phase II study with docetaxel, cisplatin and 5-fluorouracil with a four-year follow-up," *Oral Oncology*, vol. 42, no. 7, pp. 675–684, 2006.

[8] A. Psyrri, M. Kwong, S. DiStasio et al., "Cisplatin, fluorouracil, and leucovorin induction chemotherapy followed by concurrent cisplatin chemoradiotherapy for organ preservation and cure in patients with advanced head and neck cancer: long-term follow-up," *Journal of Clinical Oncology*, vol. 22, no. 15, pp. 3061–3069, 2004.

[9] C. H. Lau, C. M. Chan, Y. W. Chan et al., "Pharmacological investigations of the anti-diabetic effect of Cortex Moutan and its active component paeonol," *Phytomedicine*, vol. 14, no. 11, pp. 778–784, 2007.

[10] H. Fujiwara, M. Tabuchi, T. Yamaguchi et al., "A traditional medicinal herb Paeonia suffruticosa and its active constituent 1,2,3,4,6-penta-O-galloyl-β-d-glucopyranose have potent anti-aggregation effects on Alzheimer's amyloid β proteins in vitro

and in vivo," *Journal of Neurochemistry*, vol. 109, no. 6, pp. 1648–1657, 2009.

[11] J. Zhou, L. Zhou, D. Hou, J. Tang, J. Sun, and S. C. Bondy, "Paeonol increases levels of cortical cytochrome oxidase and vascular actin and improves behavior in a rat model of Alzheimer's disease," *Brain Research*, vol. 1388, pp. 141–147, 2011.

[12] H. S. Kim, A.-R. Kim, J. M. Lee et al., "A mixture of Trachelospermi caulis and Moutan cortex radicis extracts suppresses collagen-induced arthritis in mice by inhibiting NF-κB and AP-1," *Journal of Pharmacy and Pharmacology*, vol. 64, no. 3, pp. 420–429, 2012.

[13] T.-C. Chou, "Anti-inflammatory and analgesic effects of paeonol in carrageenan-evoked thermal hyperalgesia," *British Journal of Pharmacology*, vol. 139, no. 6, pp. 1146–1152, 2003.

[14] G. Li, C.-S. Seo, K.-S. Lee et al., "Protective constituents against sepsis in mice from the root cortex of *Paeonia suffruticosa*," *Archives of Pharmacal Research*, vol. 27, no. 11, pp. 1123–1126, 2004.

[15] C.-L. Hsieh, C.-Y. Cheng, T.-H. Tsai et al., "Paeonol reduced cerebral infarction involving the superoxide anion and microglia activation in ischemia-reperfusion injured rats," *Journal of Ethnopharmacology*, vol. 106, no. 2, pp. 208–215, 2006.

[16] C.-Y. Hsiang, C.-L. Hsieh, S.-L. Wu, L. Lu, T.-Y. Lai, and Ho, "Inhibitory effect of anti-pyretic and anti-inflammatory herbs on herpes simplex virus replication," *American Journal of Chinese Medicine*, vol. 29, no. 3-4, pp. 459–467, 2001.

[17] T. K. Au, T. L. Lam, T. B. Ng, W. P. Fong, and D. C. C. Wan, "A comparison of HIV-1 integrase inhibition by aqueous and methanol extracts of Chinese medicinal herbs," *Life Sciences*, vol. 68, no. 14, pp. 1687–1694, 2001.

[18] J.-Y. Hung, C.-J. Yang, Y.-M. Tsai, H.-W. Huang, and M.-S. Huang, "Antiproliferative activity of paeoniflorin is through cell cycle arrest and the Fas/Fas ligand-mediated apoptotic pathway in human non-small cell lung cancer A549 cells," *Clinical and Experimental Pharmacology and Physiology*, vol. 35, no. 2, pp. 141–147, 2008.

[19] H. S. Choi, H.-S. Seo, J. H. Kim, J.-Y. Um, Y. C. Shin, and S.-G. Ko, "Ethanol extract of paeonia suffruticosa Andrews (PSE) induced AGS human gastric cancer cell apoptosis via fas-dependent apoptosis and MDM2-p53 pathways," *Journal of Biomedical Science*, vol. 19, article 82, 2012.

[20] G. Xing, Z. Zhang, J. Liu, H. Hu, and N. Sugiura, "Antitumor effect of extracts from moutan cortex on DLD-1 human colon cancer cells in vitro," *Molecular Medicine Reports*, vol. 3, no. 1, pp. 57–61, 2010.

[21] S.-C. Wang, S.-W. Tang, S.-H. Lam et al., "Aqueous extract of Paeonia suffruticosa inhibits migration and metastasis of renal cell carcinoma cells via suppressing VEGFR-3 pathway," *Evidence-Based Complementary and Alternative Medicine*, vol. 2012, Article ID 409823, 9 pages, 2012.

[22] M.-Y. Lin, Y.-R. Lee, S.-Y. Chiang et al., "Cortex Moutan induces bladder cancer cell death via apoptosis and retards tumor growth in mouse bladders," *Evidence-Based Complementary and Alternative Medicine*, vol. 2013, Article ID 207279, 8 pages, 2013.

[23] C. Li, K. Yazawa, S. Kondo et al., "The root bark of Paeonia moutan is a potential anticancer agent in human oral squamous cell carcinoma cells," *Anticancer Research*, vol. 32, no. 7, pp. 2625–2630, 2012.

[24] Y. Mukudai, S. Kondo, T. Koyama et al., "Potential anti-osteoporotic effects of herbal extracts on osteoclasts, osteoblasts

and chondrocytes in vitro," *BMC Complementary and Alternative Medicine*, vol. 14, article 29, 2014.

[25] D. Sato, S. Kondo, K. Yazawa et al., "The potential anticancer activity of extracts derived from the roots of Scutellaria baicalensis on human oral squamous cell carcinoma cells," *Molecular and Clinical Oncology*, vol. 1, no. 1, pp. 105–111, 2013.

[26] Y. Mukudai, S. Kondo, S. Shiogama et al., "Root bark extracts of *Juncus effusus* and *Paeonia suffruticosa* protect salivary gland acinar cells from apoptotic cell death induced by cis-platinum (II) diammine dichloride," *Oncology Reports*, vol. 30, no. 6, pp. 2665–2671, 2013.

[27] K. Okumura, A. Konishi, M. Tanaka, M. Kanazawa, K. Kogawa, and Y. Niitsu, "Establishment of high- and low-invasion clones derived for a human tongue squamous-cell carcinoma cell line SAS," *Journal of Cancer Research and Clinical Oncology*, vol. 122, no. 4, pp. 243–248, 1996.

[28] Y. Mukudai, S. Kondo, A. Fujita, Y. Yoshihama, T. Shirota, and S. Shintani, "Tumor protein D54 is a negative regulator of extracellular matrix-dependent migration and attachment in oral squamous cell carcinoma-derived cell lines," *Cellular Oncology*, vol. 36, no. 3, pp. 233–245, 2013.

[29] H. Tsukamoto, S. Kondo, Y. Mukudai et al., "Evaluation of anticancer activities of benzo[c]phenanthridine alkaloid sanguinarine in oral squamous cell carcinoma cell line," *Anticancer Research*, vol. 31, no. 9, pp. 2841–2846, 2011.

[30] A. Yasuda, S. Kondo, T. Nagumo et al., "Anti-tumor activity of dehydroxymethylepoxyquinomicin against human oral squamous cell carcinoma cell lines in vitro and in vivo," *Oral Oncology*, vol. 47, no. 5, pp. 334–339, 2011.

[31] S. Shiogama, S. Yoshiba, D. Soga, H. Motohashi, and S. Shintani, "Aberrant expression of EZH2 is associated with pathological findings and P53 alteration," *Anticancer Research*, vol. 33, no. 10, pp. 4309–4317, 2013.

[32] D. Brenner and T. W. Mak, "Mitochondrial cell death effectors," *Current Opinion in Cell Biology*, vol. 21, no. 6, pp. 871–877, 2009.

[33] P. Paoli, E. Giannoni, and P. Chiarugi, "Anoikis molecular pathways and its role in cancer progression," *Biochimica et Biophysica Acta—Molecular Cell Research*, vol. 1833, no. 12, pp. 3481–3498, 2013.

[34] I. R. Indran, G. Tufo, S. Pervaiz, and C. Brenner, "Recent advances in apoptosis, mitochondria and drug resistance in cancer cells," *Biochimica et Biophysica Acta—Bioenergetics*, vol. 1807, no. 6, pp. 735–745, 2011.

[35] R. Rathinam and S. K. Alahari, "Important role of integrins in the cancer biology," *Cancer and Metastasis Reviews*, vol. 29, no. 1, pp. 223–237, 2010.

[36] M. Shirosaki, T. Koyama, and K. Yazawa, "Apple leaf extract as a potential candidate for suppressing postprandial elevation of the blood glucose level," *Journal of Nutritional Science and Vitaminology*, vol. 58, no. 1, pp. 63–67, 2012.

[37] M. Shirosaki, Y. Goto, S. Hirooka, H. Masuda, T. Koyama, and K. Yazawa, "Peach leaf contains multiflorin A as a potent inhibitor of glucose absorption in the small intestine in mice," *Biological and Pharmaceutical Bulletin*, vol. 35, no. 8, pp. 1264–1268, 2012.

[38] T. Koyama, C. Nakajima, S. Nishimoto, M. Takami, J.-T. Woo, and K. Yazawa, "Suppressive effects of the leaf of *Terminalia catappa* L. on osteoclast differentiation in vitro and bone weight loss in vivo," *Journal of Nutritional Science and Vitaminology*, vol. 58, no. 2, pp. 129–135, 2012.

[39] S. Soni, M. Mathur, N. K. Shukla, S. V. S. Deo, and R. Ralhan, "Stromelysin-3 expression is an early event in human oral tumorigenesis," *International Journal of Cancer*, vol. 107, no. 2, pp. 309–316, 2003.

[40] C. Qiu, H. Wu, H. He, and W. Qiu, "A cervical lymph node metastatic model of human tongue carcinoma: serial and orthotopic transplantation of histologically intact patient specimens in nude mice," *Journal of Oral and Maxillofacial Surgery*, vol. 61, no. 6, pp. 696–700, 2003.

2

Efficacy of Chinese Herbal Medicine as an Adjunctive Therapy on in-Hospital Mortality in Patients with Acute Kidney Injury: A Systematic Review and Meta-Analysis

Tuo Chen,[1,2] **Libin Zhan,**[3] **Zhiwei Fan,**[1] **Lizhi Bai,**[1] **Yi Song,**[1] **and Xiaoguang Lu**[1]

[1]*Emergency Department, Affiliated Zhongshan Hospital of Dalian University, Dalian No. 6, Jiefang Street, Zhongshan District, Dalian, Liaoning 116001, China*
[2]*Dalian Medical University, Lvshunkou District, Dalian, Liaoning 116044, China*
[3]*College of Basic Medicine, Nanjing University of Chinese Medicine, Nanjing 210000, China*

Correspondence should be addressed to Xiaoguang Lu; dllxg@126.com

Academic Editor: Kieran Cooley

Objective. We aimed to systematically assess the efficacy of Chinese herbal medicine (CHM) as an adjunctive therapy on in-hospital mortality in patients with acute kidney injury (AKI). *Methods.* We did a systematic review of articles published in any language up until Jun 23, 2015, by searching PubMed, Embase, the Cochrane Library, CBM, and CNKI. We included all RCTs that compared outcomes of patients with AKI taking CHM plus Western treatment (WT) with those taking WT alone. We applied Cochrane risk-of-bias tool to assess the methodological quality of the included trials. *Results.* Of 832 citations, 15 studies involving 966 patients met inclusion criteria. The methodological quality was assessed with unclear risk of bias. In the primary outcome of meta-analysis, pooled outcome of in-hospital mortality showed that patients randomly assigned to CHM treatment group were associated with low risk of in-hospital mortality compared with those randomly assigned to WT alone (RR = 0.41; 95% CI = 0.24 to 0.71; $P = 0.001$). *Conclusions.* CHM as an adjunctive therapy is associated with a decreased risk of in-hospital mortality compared with WT in patients with AKI. Further studies with high quality and large sample size are needed to verify our conclusions.

1. Introduction

Acute kidney injury (AKI) is a clinical syndrome characterised by a rapid reduction in kidney's excretory function with the accumulation of end products of nitrogen metabolism (urea and creatinine) or the loss of urine output. Until now, AKI is a worldwide public health problem associated with substantial morbidity and mortality [1, 2]. Epidemiologic surveys have identified that the estimated number of AKI ranges from more than 5000 cases per million people per year without dialysis-requiring AKI to 295 cases per million people per year with dialysis-requiring disease [3]. Even a small increase in serum creatinine (Scr) level is associated with higher mortality, longer time of hospital stay, and higher cost of care [4, 5].

Prominent progress has been made in the treatment of patients with severe AKI by means of renal replacement therapy (RRT) or continuous renal replacement therapy (CRRT).

Nonetheless, mortality remains unacceptably high, with multicentre studies continuing to report rates of more than 30% [6, 7]. Hence, a certain proportion of clinicians have turned to Chinese herbal medicine (CHM) as an adjunctive therapy seeking for an effective treatment by attenuating acute kidney injury and expediting recovery thus improving survival rates.

CHM accelerates kidney recovery and alleviates acute kidney injury caused by blood stasis, fluid stagnation, and qi insufficiency according to Traditional Chinese Medicine (TCM) theory. In recent studies, CHM has shown the comprehensive protection against kidney, heart, brain, intestine, liver, and lung injury in oxidative stress-related disease [8]. The mechanisms for the pharmacological action of CHM for AKI include an antioxidant activity by scavenging reactive oxygen species (ROS) and improving renal levels of superoxide dismutase (SOD) [9, 10] and an anti-inflammatory activity by reducing interleukin-6 (IL-6), interleukin-8 (IL-8), and tumor necrosis factor-alpha (TNF-α) levels [11].

Several clinical trials have been published analyzing the beneficial effects of CHM as an adjunctive therapy for AKI. However, there is no critical appraisal of the evidence on whether CHM as a complementary therapy could decrease mortality for patients with AKI. Therefore, we did a systematic review and meta-analysis to provide more reliable evidence on the effect of CHM on survival and other key outcomes.

2. Methods

2.1. Literature Search and Search Strategy. PRISMA (Preferred Reporting Items for Systematic Reviews and Meta-Analyses) was used to report a systematic review and meta-analysis of trails [12]. Two independent investigators (CT and ZLB) performed a search in PubMed, Embase, the Cochrane Central Register of Controlled Trials, and two Chinese databases including Chinese BioMedical Literature Database (CBM) and China National Knowledge Infrastructure (CNKI) for relevant randomized clinical trials published before June 23, 2015. The following keywords and corresponding titles were used in literature search: "acute kidney injury" or "acute renal failure" or "acute renal injury" or "acute renal insufficiency" or "acute kidney failure" or "acute kidney insufficiency" or "Long Bi" (Characteristic of "Long Bi" presented in Section 4.2) and "traditional herbal medicine" or "traditional Chinese herbs" or "traditional Chinese medicine" or "Chinese herbal drug" or "herbal medicine" or "alternative medicine" or "integrative medicine" and "clinical trails" or "randomized controlled trials". No restrictions were imposed on publication language and data. We manually searched references and related articles to avoid omissions. We contacted the corresponding authors of the studies for further data if needed.

2.2. Study Selection Criteria. Clinical trials regarding the efficacy of CHM as adjuvant therapy for AKI were included if they met the following criteria. (1) Types of participants: patients with AKI were enrolled by authors' criteria. (2) Types of interventions: treatment group participants received both CHM and western treatment (WT) and control group participants received the same WT alone. Other herbal or complementary medicines were not accepted as control group interventions. (3) Types of outcome measures: the primary outcome was in-hospital mortality. The secondary outcome measures included overall efficacy (defined as a three-degree measurement including "cure," "efficacy," and "invalid" based on the condition of overall symptom improvement), time of kidney recovery, and adverse events. (4) Types of studies: we included randomized controlled trials (RCTs) concerning CHM plus WT versus WT alone for patients with AKI. Case reports, pharmacokinetic studies, general reviews, animal experiments, and quasi-RCTs where allocation was obtained by use of hospital registry number or date of birth were not considered. Duplicate publications were identified and deleted.

2.3. Data Extraction. Two investigators (CT and ZLB) independently extracted the data from eligible trails based on the predefined inclusion criteria. Disagreement between two investigators was resolved by discussion with a third investigator (LXG). Detailed data from including trails were rigorously recorded, which included authors, year of publication, title of study, simple size, age, sex, CHM treatment, WT, treatment duration, in-hospital mortality, overall efficacy, time of kidney recovery, and adverse events. Outcomes reported in 1 or more articles were extracted for meta-analysis.

2.4. Risk of Bias Assessment. Study quality was evaluated as recommended in the Cochrane Handbook. Two investigators (CT and ZLB) independently rated each study on the six domains [13]: (1) adequate random sequence generation; (2) allocation concealment; (3) blinding of participants, personnel and outcome assessors; (4) incomplete outcome data; (5) selective outcome reporting; (6) other sources of bias. An assessment of "high," "unclear," or "low" risk of bias was provided for each of the above domains. We assessed a trail at high risk of bias when there was one or more domains with high risk of bias. We assessed a trail at low risk of bias when all of domains were with low risk of bias. Otherwise, we assessed a trail at unclear risk of bias. Any disagreement on the risk of bias was resolved by discussion with a third investigator (LXG).

2.5. Data Analyses. All statistical analyses were presented by Review Manager 5.3 software (Cochrane Collaboration, Oxford, UK). For dichotomous variables such as in-hospital mortality and overall efficacy, results were presented as risk ratio (RR) with 95% confidence interval (CI). For continuous variables such as time of kidney recovery, we used the mean difference (MD) with 95% CI when outcomes were measured in the same way between trials. We analyzed the heterogeneity by the Cochran Q and I^2 test. There was a considerable level of homogeneity test assessed by using the chi-squared test when the P value was less than 0.1. Meanwhile, I^2 values of 25%, 50%, and 75% correspond to low, medium, and high levels of statistical heterogeneity [14, 15]. We applied a random-effect model when $P < 0.1$ or $I^2 > 50\%$ was considered to indicate a substantial level of heterogeneity [16]. Otherwise, a fixed-effect model was used. Sensitivity analysis was performed by sequentially omitting a single study to assess the potential influence of an individual study. We applied the funnel plot to evaluate publication bias if same outcome measures (i.e., >9) were identified. $P < 0.05$ was considered to be statistically significant.

3. Results

3.1. Results of Literature Search. The search process and study selection were depicted in Figure 1. Our search identified 832 potentially relevant citations. After reading titles and abstracts of the articles, 375 studies were excluded because of duplicated publication. We excluded 425 trails due to obviously ineligible inclusion criteria. The remaining 32 trails of full-text papers were analyzed, from which 17 were excluded: 8 because CHM was used in control group, 7 because relevant CHM was applied in treatment group alone, and 2 because

Identification

Records identified through database searching
($n = 832$)

Additional records identified through other sources
($n = 0$)

Screening

Records after duplicates are removed
($n = 375$)

Records screened
($n = 457$)

Records excluded ($n = 425$)

Reviews, comments ($n = 378$)

Case reports ($n = 15$)

Animal experiments ($n = 15$)

Conference abstracts ($n = 8$)

Pharmacokinetic studies ($n = 9$)

Eligibility

Full-text articles assessed for eligibility
($n = 32$)

Full-text articles excluded, with reasons ($n = 17$)

Control group used CHM ($n = 8$)

Treating group used CHM alone ($n = 7$)

Quasi-RCTs ($n = 2$)

Studies included in qualitative synthesis
($n = 15$)

Included

Studies included in quantitative synthesis (meta-analysis)
($n = 15$)

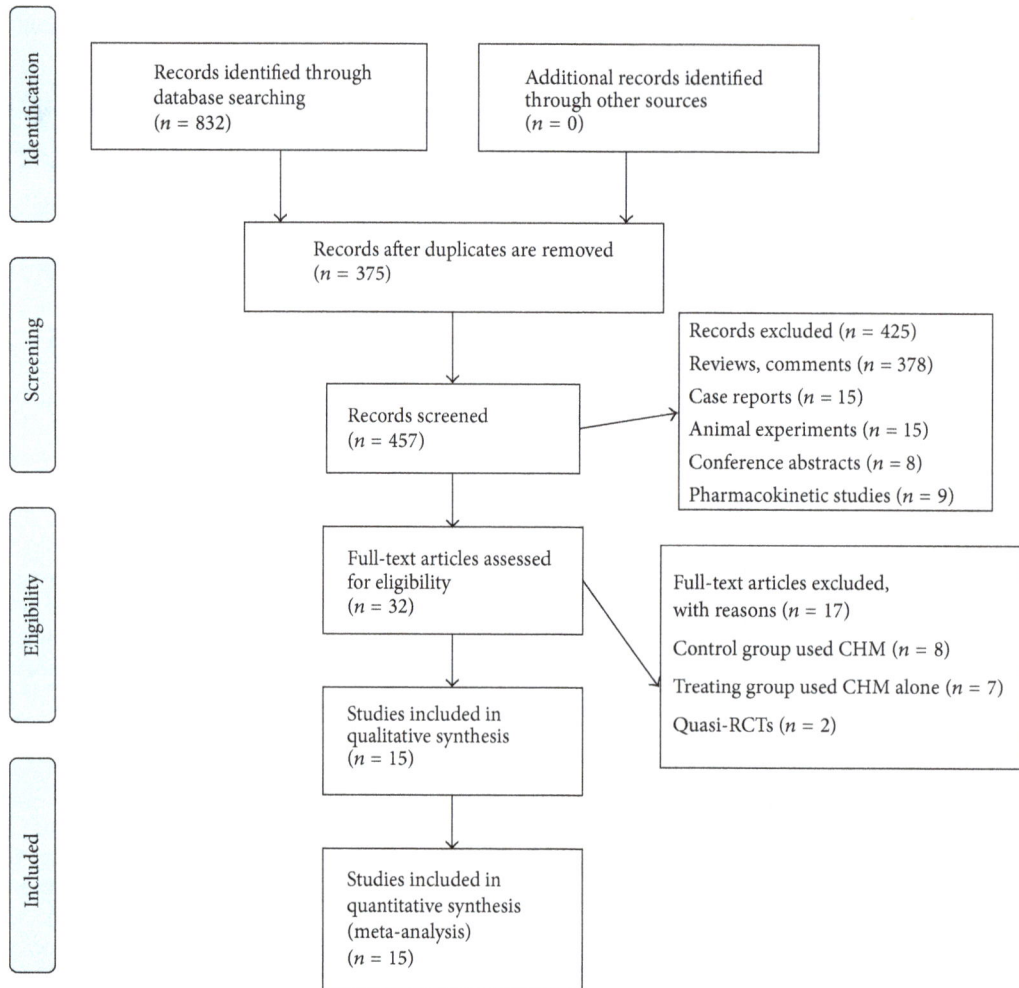

FIGURE 1: Flowchart of study identification (PRISMA 2009 Flow Diagram). For more information, visit http://www.prisma-statement.org/ [17].

patients were allocated by use of hospital registry number. 15 trails were finally retrieved in this systematic review and meta-analysis.

3.2. Study Characteristics. 15 trails (966 patients) were published in Chinese language and conducted in China between 489 patients randomly assigned to CHM combined with WT in treatment group and 477 patients randomly assigned to WT alone in control group. The included studies were conducted from 2000 to 2014. The sample size in these trails ranged from 30 to 160 participants. All of the trials were parallel arm studies. Participants' gender was reported in 15 trials, of whom 63.25% of participants were male. A variety of data were recorded in these studies, which included in-hospital mortality (12 studies) [18–29], overall efficacy (8 studies) [22–25, 28–31], and time of kidney recovery such as time to oliguria (6 studies) [20–23, 29, 32], time to Scr level recovery (4 studies) [18, 20, 29, 32], and time to Scr and BUN level recovery (4 studies) [21–24]. 12 trails observed treatment duration, ranging from 7 days to 1 month [20–22, 24–32]. Among these studies, all of articles described

the component, dosage, and frequency of CHM therapy. The main WT concerning basic treatment, RRT or CRRT, was also demonstrated. All characteristics of the included studies were summarized in Table 1.

3.3. Methodological Quality. The methodological quality of all included trails was assessed with unclear risk of bias in Figure 2. 15 included trails were described as randomized controlled trials. Only 4 trails generated adequate randomized sequence by using random number of tables [26, 27, 30, 31]. Among all studies, there was no description on the method of allocation concealment. None of included studies described the double-blind and placebo-controlled method. One trail reported the number and reasons of drop-outs [27] and the other 14 trials reported that all the enrolled patients had completed the trial. All of the 15 trials reported complete clinical outcome data. For other sources of bias, all studies declared no significant difference of enrolled patients at baseline in gender, age, and other pieces of basic information. The details of risk of bias for trails were summarized in Figure 3.

TABLE 1: Characteristics of 15 studies fulfilling the inclusion criteria.

Author (year)	Cases T/C	Age (years) range, mean	Sex M/F	Intervention Experimental group	Intervention Control group	Duration	Main outcomes
Deng and Wang 2000 [18]	80/80	NS	T: 59/21, C: 54/26	MRD (100 mL, po, bid) + basic treatment	Basic treatment	NS	In-hospital mortality, time of kidney recovery
Jiang 2012 [27]	15/15	T: 77.4, C: 78.6	T: 10/5, C: 11/4	Jishengshenqiwan pills (90–110 g, po, qd) + basic treatment + CRRT	Basic treatment + CRRT	2 weeks	In-hospital mortality
Li 2014 [31]	49/49	T: 42.2, C: 45.96	T: 28/21, C: 25/24	MRD (50 mL, po, bid) + basic treatment + RRT	Basic treatment + RRT	14 days	Overall efficacy, time of kidney recovery
Luo and Yuan 2013 [30]	20/20	T: 30–53, C: 31–59	T: 13/7, C: 11/9	MRD (200 mL, pr, qd) + basic treatment	Basic treatment	15 days	Overall efficacy
Pan et al. 2009 [24]	22/20	T: 45, C: 47	T: 13/9, C: 12/8	XBJ injection (50 mL, ivgtt, bid) + basic treatment + RRT	Basic treatment + RRT	15 days	In-hospital mortality, overall efficacy, time of kidney recovery
Ru 2013 [28]	38/38	T: 43.83, C: 42.70	T: 22/16, C: 21/17	XBJ injection (50 mL, ivgtt, bid) + basic treatment + RRT	Basic treatment + RRT	2 weeks	In-hospital mortality, overall efficacy
Sun et al. 2001 [19]	21/22	T: 38.6, C: 35.7	T: 14/7, C: 15/7	Huangqi injection (20–30 mL, ivgtt, qd) + basic treatment + RRT	Basic treatment + RRT	2 weeks	In-hospital mortality
Sun et al. 2007 [22]	34/30	T: 38.2, C: 39.1	T: 18/16, C: 17/13	Modified XBJ injection (100 mL, ivgtt, qd) + basic treatment + RRT	Basic treatment + RRT	NS	In-hospital mortality, overall efficacy, time of kidney recovery
Wang 2010 [25]	30/30	T: 54.67, C: 54.7	T: 17/13, C: 18/12	MRD (100 mL, pr, qd) + basic treatment	Basic treatment	1 week	In-hospital mortality, overall efficacy
Wen and Liu 2003 [20]	62/62	T: 17–65, C: 16–63	T: 41/21, C: 39/23	MRD (100 mL, po, qd) + basic treatment + RRT	Basic treatment + RRT	2 weeks	In-hospital mortality, overall efficacy, time of kidney recovery
Wu et al. 2014 [32]	26/22	T: 65, C: 62	T: 20/6, C: 15/7	Dongchongxiacao capsules (2-3 g, po, tid) + basic treatment	Basic treatment	2 weeks	Time of kidney recovery
Yang 2007 [23]	34/30	T: 38.2, C: 42.70	T: 18/16, C: 17/13	XBJ injection (50 mL, ivgtt, bid) + basic treatment + RRT	Basic treatment + RRT	NS	In-hospital mortality, overall efficacy, time of kidney recovery
Yu et al. 2010 [26]	25/27	T: 68.49, C: 69.37	T: 16/9, C: 19/8	Qishen Huoxue granule (10 g, po, tid) + CRRT	CRRT	14 days	In-hospital mortality
Zhang and Mao 2003 [21]	33/32	T: 38.12, C: 37.56	T: 25/8, C: 23/9	MRD (2–4 g, po, tid) + basic treatment + RRT	Basic treatment + RRT	4 weeks	In-hospital mortality, overall efficacy, time of kidney recovery
Zhu and Tang 2014 [29]	41/41	T: 49.2, C: 48.90	T: 28/13, C: 26/15	XBJ injection (50 mL, ivgtt, bid) + basic treatment + RRT	Basic treatment + RRT	7 days	In-hospital mortality, overall efficacy, time of kidney recovery

T: treatment group; C: control group; M: male; F: female; NS: no state; MRD: modified rhubarb decoction; XBJ: Xuebijing; basic treatment: remove the cause + maintain water, electrolyte, and acid-base balance + prevent infection + nutrition support; RRT: renal replacement therapy; CRRT: continuous renal replacement therapy.

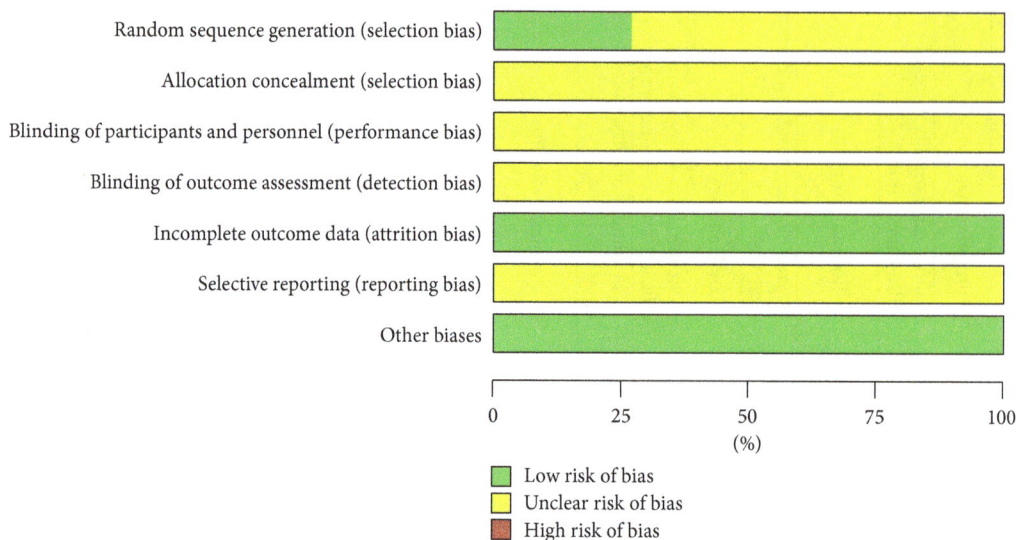

FIGURE 2: Risk of bias graph.

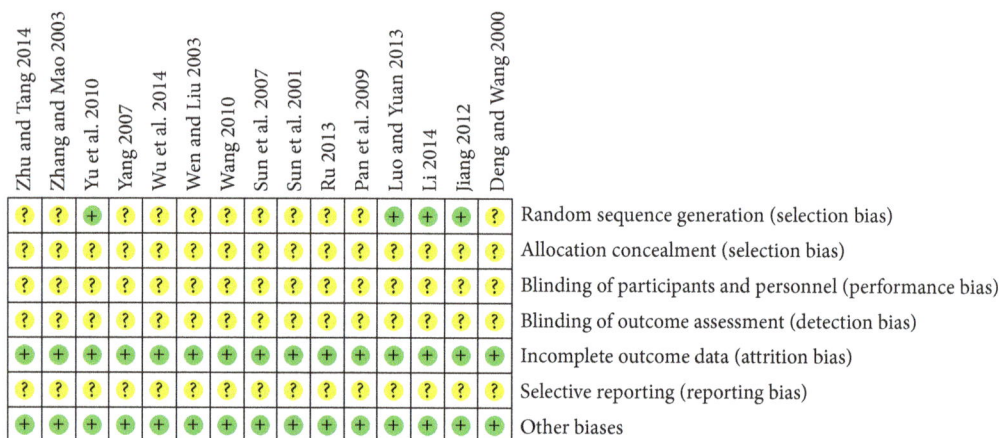

FIGURE 3: Risk of bias summary. "+": low risk of bias; "?": unclear risk of bias.

3.4. Primary Outcome

3.4.1. In-Hospital Mortality. A total of 12 trails (862 patients) provided data for in-hospital mortality [18–29]. A fixed-effects model was applied to analyze the data due to the low level of homogeneity ($P = 1.00$; $I^2 = 0\%$). Within 12 trails, as shown in Figure 4, we noted that patients randomly assigned to CHM plus WT had a statistically significant reduction in in-hospital mortality compared with those randomly assigned to WT alone (RR = 0.41; 95% CI = 0.24 to 0.71; $P = 0.001$).

3.5. Secondary Outcomes

3.5.1. Overall Efficacy. A total of 8 trails (526 patients) reported data for overall efficacy [22–25, 28–31]. The data was analyzed using a fixed-effects model based on the heterogeneity test result ($P = 0.95$; $I^2 = 0\%$). Within 8 trails, as shown in Figure 5, we noted a statistically significant improvement in overall efficacy in patients randomly assigned to CHM as an

adjuvant therapy in comparison to those randomly assigned to WT alone (RR = 1.26; 95% CI = 1.15 to 1.37; $P < 0.00001$).

3.5.2. Time of Kidney Recovery. A total of 6 trails (430 patients) described time to oliguria after treatment [20–23, 29, 32]. We applied a fixed-effects model to analyze the data according to the low level of homogeneity ($P = 0.31$; $I^2 = 16\%$). Within 6 trails, as shown in Figure 6, we noted that time to oliguria was shortened in patients assigned to CHM as an adjuvant therapy compared with those assigned to WT alone (MD = −2.26; 95% CI = −2.57 to −1.96; $P < 0.00001$).

A total of 4 trails (223 patients) reported on time to Scr and BUN level recovery [21–24]. A fixed-effects model was used to analysis the data based on the low level of homogeneity ($P = 0.48$; $I^2 = 0\%$). With in 4 trails, as shown in Figure 6, we noted a statistically significant reduction in time to Scr and BUN level recovery in patients taking CHM plus WT compared with WT alone (MD = −9.65; 95% CI = −10.69 to −8.61; $P < 0.00001$).

Study or subgroup	CHM and western treatment		Western treatment		Weight	Risk ratio M-H, fixed, 95% CI	Risk ratio M-H, fixed, 95% CI
	Events	Total	Events	Total			
Deng and Wang 2000	1	80	3	80	7.3%	0.33 [0.04, 3.14]	
Jiang 2012	3	15	4	15	9.7%	0.75 [0.20, 2.79]	
Pan et al. 2009	1	22	3	20	7.6%	0.30 [0.03, 2.68]	
Ru 2013	1	38	2	38	4.9%	0.50 [0.05, 5.28]	
Sun et al. 2001	2	21	4	22	9.5%	0.52 [0.11, 2.56]	
Sun et al. 2007	1	34	3	30	7.7%	0.29 [0.03, 2.68]	
Wang 2010	1	30	1	30	2.4%	1.00 [0.07, 15.26]	
Wen and Liu 2003	1	62	4	62	9.7%	0.25 [0.03, 2.17]	
Yang 2007	1	34	3	30	7.7%	0.29 [0.03, 2.68]	
Yu et al. 2010	3	25	8	27	18.7%	0.41 [0.12, 1.36]	
Zhang and Mao 2003	1	33	3	32	7.4%	0.32 [0.04, 2.95]	
Zhu and Tang 2014	1	41	3	41	7.3%	0.33 [0.04, 3.07]	
Total (95% CI)		435		427	100.0%	**0.41 [0.24, 0.71]**	
Total events	17		41				

Heterogeneity: $\chi^2 = 1.89$, df = 11 ($P = 1.00$); $I^2 = 0\%$
Test for overall effect: $Z = 3.24$ ($P = 0.001$)

0.01 0.1 1 10 100
Favours CHM and western treatment — Favours western treatment

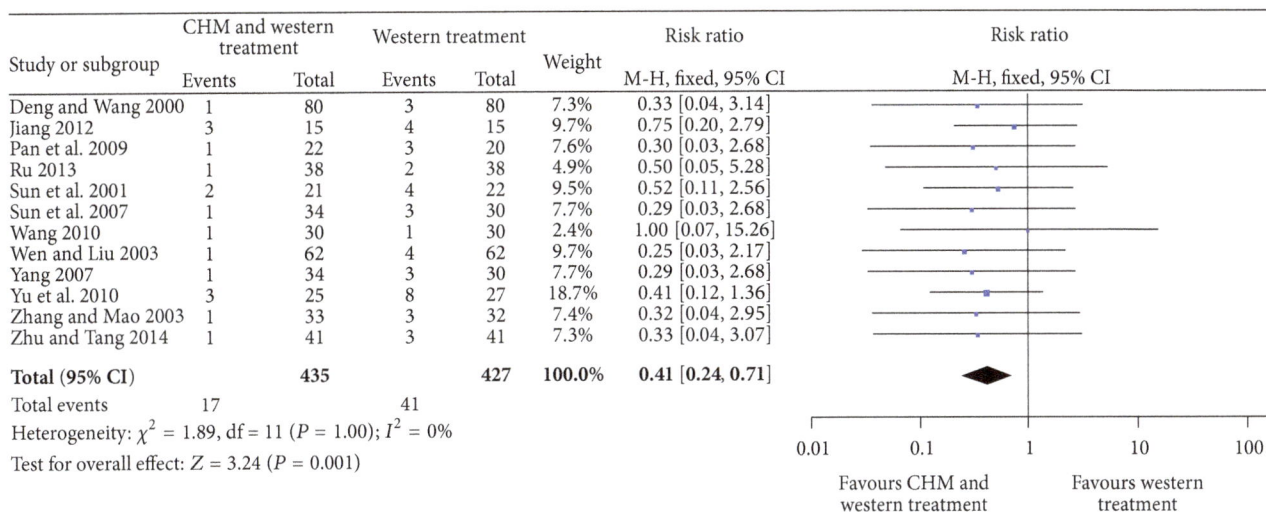

FIGURE 4: Forest plot for in-hospital mortality.

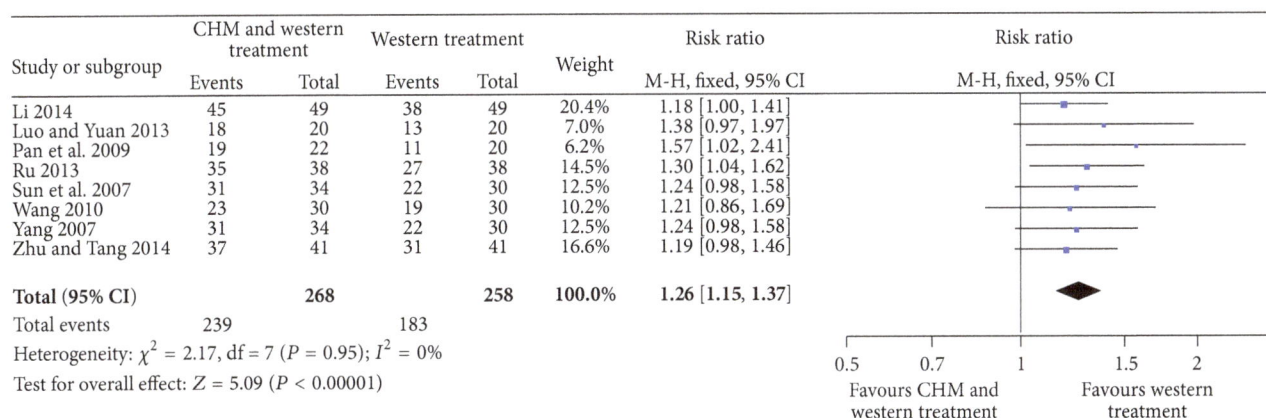

Study or subgroup	CHM and western treatment		Western treatment		Weight	Risk ratio M-H, fixed, 95% CI	Risk ratio M-H, fixed, 95% CI
	Events	Total	Events	Total			
Li 2014	45	49	38	49	20.4%	1.18 [1.00, 1.41]	
Luo and Yuan 2013	18	20	13	20	7.0%	1.38 [0.97, 1.97]	
Pan et al. 2009	19	22	11	20	6.2%	1.57 [1.02, 2.41]	
Ru 2013	35	38	27	38	14.5%	1.30 [1.04, 1.62]	
Sun et al. 2007	31	34	22	30	12.5%	1.24 [0.98, 1.58]	
Wang 2010	23	30	19	30	10.2%	1.21 [0.86, 1.69]	
Yang 2007	31	34	22	30	12.5%	1.24 [0.98, 1.58]	
Zhu and Tang 2014	37	41	31	41	16.6%	1.19 [0.98, 1.46]	
Total (95% CI)		268		258	100.0%	**1.26 [1.15, 1.37]**	
Total events	239		183				

Heterogeneity: $\chi^2 = 2.17$, df = 7 ($P = 0.95$); $I^2 = 0\%$
Test for overall effect: $Z = 5.09$ ($P < 0.00001$)

0.5 0.7 1 1.5 2
Favours CHM and western treatment — Favours western treatment

FIGURE 5: Forest plot for overall efficacy.

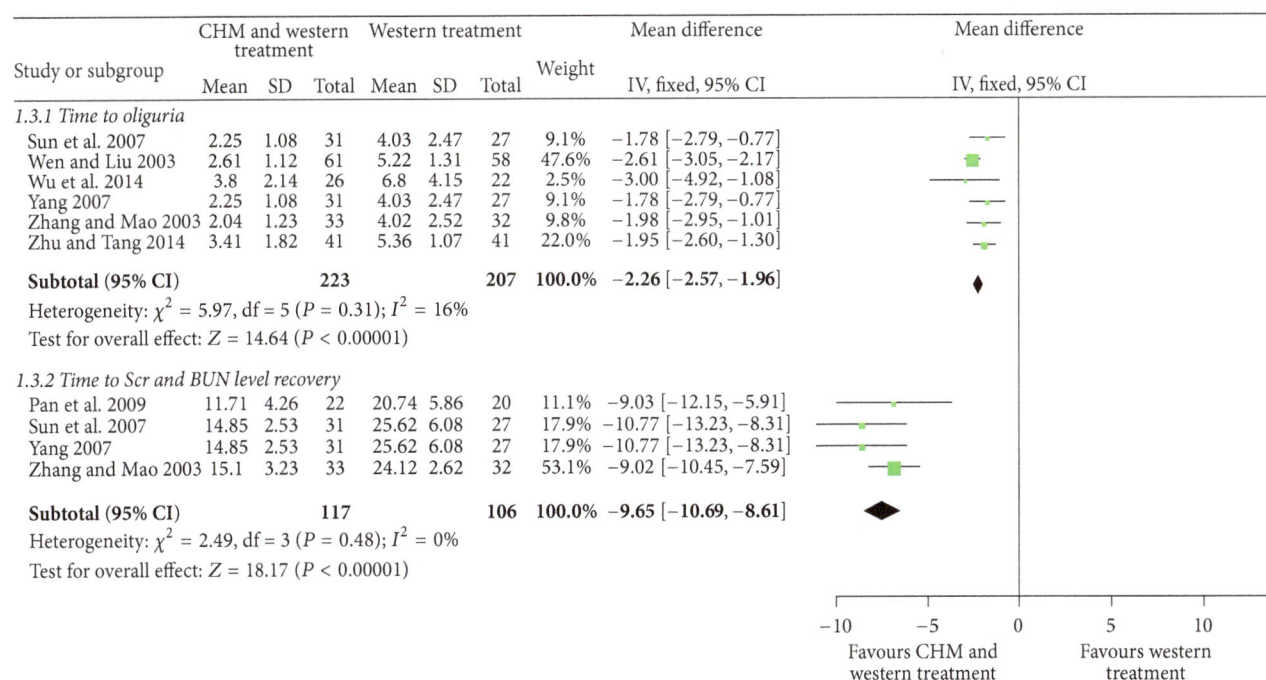

Study or subgroup	CHM and western treatment			Western treatment			Weight	Mean difference IV, fixed, 95% CI	Mean difference IV, fixed, 95% CI
	Mean	SD	Total	Mean	SD	Total			
1.3.1 Time to oliguria									
Sun et al. 2007	2.25	1.08	31	4.03	2.47	27	9.1%	−1.78 [−2.79, −0.77]	
Wen and Liu 2003	2.61	1.12	61	5.22	1.31	58	47.6%	−2.61 [−3.05, −2.17]	
Wu et al. 2014	3.8	2.14	26	6.8	4.15	22	2.5%	−3.00 [−4.92, −1.08]	
Yang 2007	2.25	1.08	31	4.03	2.47	27	9.1%	−1.78 [−2.79, −0.77]	
Zhang and Mao 2003	2.04	1.23	33	4.02	2.52	32	9.8%	−1.98 [−2.95, −1.01]	
Zhu and Tang 2014	3.41	1.82	41	5.36	1.07	41	22.0%	−1.95 [−2.60, −1.30]	
Subtotal (95% CI)			223			207	100.0%	**−2.26 [−2.57, −1.96]**	

Heterogeneity: $\chi^2 = 5.97$, df = 5 ($P = 0.31$); $I^2 = 16\%$
Test for overall effect: $Z = 14.64$ ($P < 0.00001$)

1.3.2 Time to Scr and BUN level recovery									
Pan et al. 2009	11.71	4.26	22	20.74	5.86	20	11.1%	−9.03 [−12.15, −5.91]	
Sun et al. 2007	14.85	2.53	31	25.62	6.08	27	17.9%	−10.77 [−13.23, −8.31]	
Yang 2007	14.85	2.53	31	25.62	6.08	27	17.9%	−10.77 [−13.23, −8.31]	
Zhang and Mao 2003	15.1	3.23	33	24.12	2.62	32	53.1%	−9.02 [−10.45, −7.59]	
Subtotal (95% CI)			117			106	100.0%	**−9.65 [−10.69, −8.61]**	

Heterogeneity: $\chi^2 = 2.49$, df = 3 ($P = 0.48$); $I^2 = 0\%$
Test for overall effect: $Z = 18.17$ ($P < 0.00001$)

−10 −5 0 5 10
Favours CHM and western treatment — Favours western treatment

FIGURE 6: Forest plot for time to oliguria, time to Scr and BUN level recovery.

Study or subgroup	CHM and western treatment			Western treatment			Weight	Mean difference	Mean difference
	Mean	SD	Total	Mean	SD	Total		IV, random, 95% CI	IV, random, 95% CI
Deng and Wang 2000	8.54	2.06	79	11.03	2.93	77	37.9%	−2.49 [−3.29, −1.69]	
Wen and Liu 2003	8.51	3.61	61	12.61	3.38	58	26.7%	−4.10 [−5.36, −2.84]	
Wu et al. 2014	22.4	5.2	26	27.2	6	22	7.2%	−4.80 [−8.01, −1.59]	
Zhu and Tang 2014	8.63	2.43	41	11.25	3.02	41	28.2%	−2.62 [−3.81, −1.43]	
Total (95% CI)			207			198	100.0%	−3.12 [−4.05, −2.20]	

Heterogeneity: $\tau^2 = 0.42$; $\chi^2 = 6.07$, df = 3 ($P = 0.11$); $I^2 = 51\%$
Test for overall effect: $Z = 6.62$ ($P < 0.00001$)

−10 −5 0 5 10
Favours CHM and western treatment   Favours western treatment

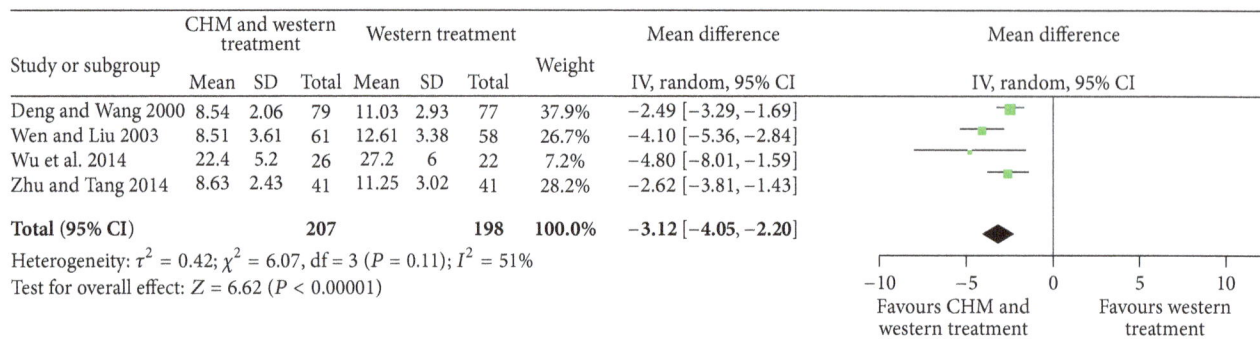

FIGURE 7: Forest plot for time to Scr level recovery.

A total of 4 trails (405 patients) reported time to Scr level recovery [18, 20, 29, 32]. Based on the medium level of homogeneity ($P = 0.11$; $I^2 = 51\%$), a random-effects model was applied to analyze the data. Within 4 trails, as shown in Figure 7, we noted that time to Scr level recovery was shortened in patients assigned to CHM combined with WT compared with those assigned to WT alone (MD = −3.12; 95% CI = −4.05 to −2.20; $P < 0.00001$).

3.5.3. *Adverse Events.* Two trails reported that there were no adverse events [25, 30], while no mention of adverse reactions was reported in the rest of 13 studies. No significant adverse effects were noted in all of included trials.

3.6. *Sensitivity Analysis.* We performed sensitivity analysis testing the robustness of our pooled results by omitting a single study. The sensitivity analysis showed that the summary RRs, MDs with 95% CI for in-hospital mortality (RR range from 0.38 to 0.43), overall efficacy (RR range from 1.24 to 1.28), time to oliguria (MD range from −2.35 to −1.95), time to Scr and BUN level recovery (MD range from −10.36 to −9.40), and time to Scr level recovery (MD range from −3.53 to −2.26) were statistically similar, which suggested that the results of this meta-analysis were robust.

3.7. *Publication Bias Assessment.* In this review, funnel plot suggested possibility of publication bias due to asymmetry (Figure 8).

4. Discussion

4.1. *Summary of Evidences.* In the present study, we reviewed 15 randomized controlled trials to evaluate the efficacy of CHM as an adjunctive therapy for patients with AKI. When we analyzed trails, the pooled results of included trials indicated a benefit of CHM as an adjunctive therapy for a significant reduction in in-hospital mortality. There was no clear evidence of a difference in this efficacy by treatment type, scheduling, trial design differences, or patient characteristics. Moreover, the pooled data with AKI has shown that combined therapy significantly improved overall efficacy. On the other hand, we found that the adjunctive use of CHM with WT had significantly shortened time of kidney recovery. These two effects further confirmed the efficacy of CHM as an

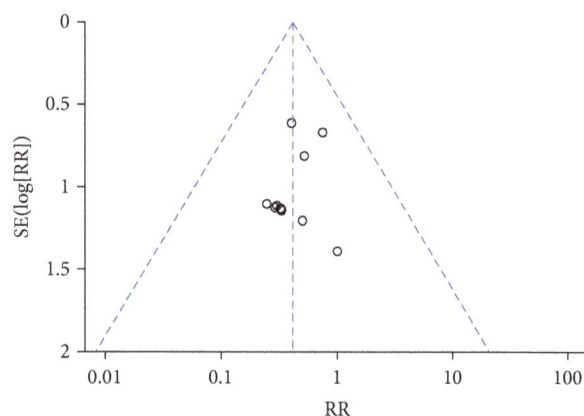

FIGURE 8: Funnel plot for in-hospital mortality.

adjunctive therapy for AKI possibly related to reducing in-hospital mortality.

4.2. *Strength of Chinese Herbal Medicine for Acute Kidney Injury Treatment.* The principles of WT for preventing acute kidney injury are to remove or treat the trigger, to maintain homoeostasis, and to set up extracorporeal renal replacement therapy. After fluid resuscitation and removal of nephrotoxins, CHM as a specific drug-based intervention has been significantly and meaningfully indicated to be nephroprotective. According to Traditional Chinese Medicine (TCM), AKI belongs to the scope of "Long Bi." In TCM theory, "Long Bi" is caused by blood stasis, fluid stagnation, and qi insufficiency, which is characterised by oliguric syndrome or enuretic syndrome. The principles behind treating these syndromes were through removing blood stasis, reducing fluid retention, and tonifying qi.

In the present study, 5 studies applied the prescription of Xuebijing (XBJ) injection or modified XBJ injection [22–24, 29, 30]. XBJ injection is a representative Chinese patent medicine with the function of removing blood stasis, which is derived from Xuefu Zhuyu decoction recorded in the medical classic Yi Lin Gai Cuo by the Chinese clinician Qingren Wang approximately 200 years ago [33]. Pharmacological studies have indicated that mechanisms of protective effects of XBJ injection against kidney injury may be related to its anti-inflammation effects by decreasing circulating inflammatory cytokines and inhibition of endothelial injury [34, 35]. There were 6 studies which used modified rhubarb decoction (MRD), which had the function of reducing fluid retention [18, 20, 21, 25, 30, 31]. Several experimental researches have shown that MRD or rhubarb extract provides nephroprotection by suppressing the accumulation of end products of nitrogen metabolism, ameliorating tubular epithelial apoptosis, scavenging-free radicals, and augmenting capacity of antioxidant enzymes [36–39]. Astragalus injection or modified astragalus granule in 2 studies has an active function of tonifying qi [19, 26]. In the modern pharmacology research, astragalus provided protection through decreasing the level of malondialdehyde and inhibiting the decline of SOD activity against renal injury [40, 41]. In summary, based on TCM theory and pharmacology research, CHM as an adjunctive therapy for AKI has potentially prominent nephroprotection.

4.3. Limitations. Before accepting the above positive findings, the following limitations should also be noted. First, all of included trails were assessed at unclear risk of bias. So many factors that were noted to be unclear may have affected the results. Only 26% (4/15) trails described the details of randomization procedure and allocation concealment was not found in any of the trials. None of included studies described the methods of placebo-controlled and double-blind. None of the studies formally described follow-up and explicitly explained the reasons for the failures at follow-up. Although the authors did not find any related information about adverse effects during the treatment period, it needs more research about whether potential long-term adverse effects are existent in the future.

Second, our funnel plot analysis showed a potential publication bias due to all of included trails published in Chinese, which showed that it is necessary for these types of treatment to be publish in the English resource and to be drawing more attention.

Third, a combination of several herbs was applied in some studies included, and researches about active ingredients of CHM compound in AKI treatment have not been established yet. Therefore, further exploration of the mechanisms of herbal combinations in the treatment of patients with AKI will be required.

Moreover, information about quality control for the development of the herbal manufacture or for the combinations of the herbal products lacks mention, which is one of the obstacles to bring CHM to the world. We hope that more trials should provide complete information about standardization including quality control, compositions, and detailed scheme in the future. Many limitations were existent, whereas we had decreased bias via the process by our methods of studying identification, data selection, statistical analysis, and sensitivity. These efforts should improve reliability and stability of the meta-analysis.

5. Conclusion

The preliminary meta-analysis review proved that CHM as an adjunctive therapy for AKI is associated with low risk of in-hospital mortality. As the results of potential publication bias and the methodological drawbacks in the included studies, more rigorously designed, randomized double-blind, placebo-controlled trials with larger numbers of participants are needed to verify our conclusions.

Competing Interests

No competing interests were declared.

Authors' Contributions

Xiaoguang Lu constructed the study, verified data extraction and analyses, and revised the paper. Tuo Chen and Libin Zhan participated in data extraction, performed the statistical analysis, and drafted the paper. Zhiwei Fan, Lizhi Bai, and Yi Song participated in search strategies development, study selection, data extraction, data analysis, and drafting the paper. All the authors read and approved the final paper.

Acknowledgments

The study was supported by two funds from National Natural Science Foundation of China (NSFC) (no. 81173397, no. 81473512).

References

[1] G. M. Chertow, E. Burdick, M. Honour, J. V. Bonventre, and D. W. Bates, "Acute kidney injury, mortality, length of stay, and costs in hospitalized patients," *Journal of the American Society of Nephrology*, vol. 16, no. 11, pp. 3365–3370, 2005.

[2] R. Bellomo, J. A. Kellum, and C. Ronco, "Acute kidney injury," *The Lancet*, vol. 380, no. 9843, pp. 756–766, 2012.

[3] C.-Y. Hsu, C. E. McCulloch, D. Fan, J. D. Ordoñez, G. M. Chertow, and A. S. Go, "Community-based incidence of acute renal failure," *Kidney International*, vol. 72, no. 2, pp. 208–212, 2007.

[4] A. Lassnigg, D. Schmidlin, M. Mouhieddine et al., "Minimal changes of serum creatinine predict prognosis in patients after cardiothoracic surgery: a prospective cohort study," *Journal of the American Society of Nephrology*, vol. 15, no. 6, pp. 1597–1605, 2004.

[5] B. G. Loef, A. H. Epema, T. D. Smilde et al., "Immediate postoperative renal function deterioration in cardiac surgical patients predicts in-hospital mortality and long-term survival," *Journal of the American Society of Nephrology*, vol. 16, no. 1, pp. 195–200, 2005.

[6] S. Uchino, J. A. Kellum, R. Bellomo et al., "Acute renal failure in critically ill patients: a multinational, multicenter study," *Journal of the American Medical Association*, vol. 294, no. 7, pp. 813–818, 2005.

[7] C. Vinsonneau, C. Camus, A. Combes et al., "Continuous venovenous haemodiafiltration versus intermittent haemodialysis for acute renal failure in patients with multiple-organ dysfunction syndrome: a multicentre randomised trial," *The Lancet*, vol. 368, no. 9533, pp. 379–385, 2006.

[8] M. Shahzad, A. Shabbir, K. Wojcikowski, H. Wohlmuth, and G. C. Gobe, "The antioxidant effects of Radix Astragali (*Astragalus membranaceus* and related species) in protecting tissues from injury and disease," *Current Drug Targets*, In press.

[9] L. Feng, Y. Xiong, F. Cheng, L. Zhang, S. Li, and Y. Li, "Effect of ligustrazine on ischemia-reperfusion injury in murine kidney," *Transplantation Proceedings*, vol. 36, no. 7, pp. 1949–1951, 2004.

[10] Z. Lan, K. S. Bi, and X. H. Chen, "Ligustrazine attenuates elevated levels of indoxyl sulfate, kidney injury molecule-1 and clusterin in rats exposed to cadmium," *Food and Chemical Toxicology*, vol. 63, pp. 62–68, 2014.

[11] G. Chen, Y. Fu, and X. Wu, "Protective effect of salvia miltiorrhiza extract against renal ischemia-reperfusion-induced injury in rats," *Molecules*, vol. 17, no. 2, pp. 1191–1202, 2012.

[12] D. Moher, L. Shamseer, M. Clarke et al., "Preferred reporting items for systematic review and meta-analysis protocols (PRISMA-P) 2015 statement," *Systematic Reviews*, vol. 4, article 1, 2015.

[13] J. P. Higgins, D. G. Altman, P. C. Gotzsche et al., "The Cochrane Collaboration's tool for assessing risk of bias in randomised trials," *British Medical Journal*, vol. 343, Article ID d5928, 2011.

[14] J. P. T. Higgins and S. G. Thompson, "Quantifying heterogeneity in a meta-analysis," *Statistics in Medicine*, vol. 21, no. 11, pp. 1539–1558, 2002.

[15] J. P. T. Higgins, S. G. Thompson, J. J. Deeks, and D. G. Altman, "Measuring inconsistency in meta-analyses," *BMJ*, vol. 327, no. 7414, pp. 557–560, 2003.

[16] J. Wetterslev, K. Thorlund, J. Brok, and C. Gluud, "Estimating required information size by quantifying diversity in random-effects model meta-analyses," *BMC Medical Research Methodology*, vol. 9, article 86, 2009.

[17] D. Moher, A. Liberati, J. Tetzlaff, and D. G. Altman, "Preferred reporting items for systematic reviews and meta-analyses: the PRISMA statement," *PLoS Medicine*, vol. 6, no. 7, Article ID e1000097, 2009.

[18] Y. T. Deng and M. Y. Wang, "Effect of Western treatment combined with Traditional Chinese Medicine for acute kidney injury with hemorrhagic fever with," *Clinical Focus*, vol. 15, no. 11, pp. 521–522, 2000.

[19] X. Z. Sun, J. G. Chen, and M. Liu, "Effect of Huangqi injection combined with Western treatment for acute kidney injury with hemorrhagic fever," *Chinese Journal of Integrated Traditional and Western Nephrology*, vol. 2, no. 9, pp. 546–547, 2001.

[20] L. R. Wen and Y. Liu, "Effect of Traditional Chinese Medicine combined with Western treatment for acute kidney injury with hemorrhagic fever," *Journal of Emergency in Traditional Chinese Medicine*, vol. 12, no. 3, pp. 214–246, 2003.

[21] X. C. Zhang and X. C. Mao, "Effect of Traditional Chinese Medicine combined with Western treatment for acute kidney injury with hemorrhagic fever," *Journal of Emergency in Traditional Chinese Medicine*, vol. 12, no. 6, pp. 541–547, 2003.

[22] Y. Y. Sun, L. Min, Z. J. Li et al., "Effect of "Shennong 33"injection combined with Western treatment on 34 cases of acute kidney injury," *Chinese Journal of Integrated Traditional and Western Nephrology*, vol. 8, no. 6, pp. 361–362, 2007.

[23] Y. Yang, "Effect of Xuebijing injection combined with Western treatment on 34 cases of acute kidney injury," *Chinese Journal of Critical Care Medicine*, vol. 27, no. 3, pp. 281–282, 2007.

[24] Y. T. Pan, J. G. Xu, and M. Xu, "Effect of Xuebijin injection combined with Western treatment for acute kidney injury with systemic inflammatory response," *Chinese Journal of Integrated Traditional and Western Nephrology*, vol. 10, no. 11, pp. 999–1000, 2009.

[25] X. Y. Wang, *Clinical research of treatment of Jishenning 1 for acute renal failure on acid-base imbalance and electrolyte disturbance [M.S. thesis]*, Heilongjiang University of Chinese Medicine, Harbin, China, 2010.

[26] Y. B. Yu, H. Z. Zhuang, C. Liu et al., "Effect of qishen huoxue granule for auxiliary treatment of critical cases of acute kidney injury," *Chinese Journal of Integrated Traditional and Western Medicine*, vol. 30, no. 8, pp. 819–822, 2010.

[27] R. Y. Jiang, *Clinical efficacy of Jishengshenqiwan pill on elderly patients with acute renal failure [M.S. thesis]*, Shandong University Of Chinese Medicine, Jinan, China, 2012.

[28] Y. H. Ru, "Effect of Xuebijin injection combined with Western treatment on 38 cases of acute kidney injury," *Journal of Clinical Rational Drug Use*, vol. 6, no. 7, pp. 86–87, 2013.

[29] Z. G. Zhu and K. Tang, "Effect of Xuebijing injection combined with Western treatment for acute kidney injury," *Henan Traditional Chinese Medicine*, vol. 3, no. 2, pp. 351–352, 2014.

[30] Y. D. Luo and C. Y. Yuan, "Effect of Traditional Chinese Medicine colon dialysis combined with Western treatment on 20 cases of acute kidney injury," *Gui Zhou Medical Journal*, vol. 37, no. 7, pp. 598–599, 2013.

[31] Y. F. Li, "Effect of Traditional Chinese Medicine combined with Western medicine for acute kidney injury," *Journal of Emergency in Traditional Chinese Medicine*, vol. 23, no. 10, pp. 1910–1911, 2014.

[32] H. R. Wu, Y. Cai, S. C. Zeng et al., "Effects of cordyceps sinenses on acute cerebral infarction complicated with acute renal failure: analyses of 48 cases," *Journal of Hainan Medical College*, vol. 20, no. 1, pp. 44–46, 2014.

[33] M. M. Shoja, R. S. Tubbs, G. Shokouhi, and M. Loukas, "Wang Qingren and the 19th century Chinese doctrine of the bloodless heart," *International Journal of Cardiology*, vol. 145, no. 2, pp. 305–306, 2010.

[34] J.-F. Ma, L.-Z. Xuan, W. Wu, and D.-M. Zhu, "Effect of Xuebijing injection on rabbits ischemia/reperfusion injury induced by femoral arterial disease," *Chinese Critical Care Medicine*, vol. 24, no. 4, pp. 233–236, 2012.

[35] Q. Xu, J. Liu, X. Guo et al., "Xuebijing injection reduces organ injuries and improves survival by attenuating inflammatory responses and endothelial injury in heatstroke mice," *BMC Complementary and Alternative Medicine*, vol. 15, article 4, 2015.

[36] G. Hu, J. Liu, Y.-Z. Zhen et al., "Rhein lysinate increases the median survival time of SAMP10 mice: protective role in the kidney," *Acta Pharmacologica Sinica*, vol. 34, no. 4, pp. 515–521, 2013.

[37] M. I. Waly, B. H. Ali, I. Al-Lawati, and A. Nemmar, "Protective effects of emodin against cisplatin-induced oxidative stress in cultured human kidney (HEK 293) cells," *Journal of Applied Toxicology*, vol. 33, no. 7, pp. 626–630, 2013.

[38] L.-N. Zeng, Z.-J. Ma, Y.-L. Zhao et al., "The protective and toxic effects of rhubarb tannins and anthraquinones in treating hexavalent chromium-injured rats: the Yin/Yang actions of rhubarb," *Journal of Hazardous Materials*, vol. 246-247, pp. 1–9, 2013.

[39] Y. Tu, W. Sun, Y.-G. Wan et al., "Dahuang Fuzi Decoction ameliorates tubular epithelial apoptosis and renal damage via inhibiting TGF-β1-JNK signaling pathway activation in vivo," *Journal of Ethnopharmacology*, vol. 156, pp. 115–124, 2014.

[40] B.-W. Sheng, X.-F. Chen, J. Zhao, D.-L. He, and X.-Y. Nan, "Astragalus membranaceus reduces free radical-mediated

injury to renal tubules in rabbits receiving high-energy shock waves," *Chinese Medical Journal*, vol. 118, no. 1, pp. 43–49, 2005.

[41] X. Li, D. He, L. Zhang, X. Cheng, B. Sheng, and Y. Luo, "A novel antioxidant agent, astragalosides, prevents shock wave-induced renal oxidative injury in rabbits," *Urological Research*, vol. 34, no. 4, pp. 277–282, 2006.

3

Du-Huo-Ji-Sheng-Tang Attenuates Inflammation of TNF-Tg Mice Related to Promoting Lymphatic Drainage Function

Yan Chen,[1] Jinlong Li,[1] Qiang Li,[1] Tengteng Wang,[1] Lianping Xing,[2,3] Hao Xu,[1] Yongjun Wang,[1] Qi Shi,[1] Quan Zhou,[1] and Qianqian Liang[1]

[1]*Department of Orthopaedics, Longhua Hospital, Shanghai University of Traditional Chinese Medicine, Shanghai 200032, China*
[2]*Department of Pathology and Laboratory Medicine, University of Rochester Medical Center, 601 Elmwood Avenue, Rochester, NY 14642, USA*
[3]*Center for Musculoskeletal Research, University of Rochester Medical Center, 601 Elmwood Avenue, Rochester, NY 14642, USA*

Correspondence should be addressed to Qianqian Liang; liangqianqiantcm@126.com

Academic Editor: José L. Ríos

To investigate whether Du-Huo-Ji-Sheng-Tang (DHJST) attenuate inflammation of RA related to lymphatic drainage function in vivo, we treated eight 3-month-old TNF-Tg mice with DHJST (12 g/kg) or the same volume of physiological saline once every day for 12 weeks, and 3-month-old WT littermates were used as negative control. After twelve weeks, we performed NIR-ICG imaging and found that DHJST increased the ICG clearance at the footpad and the pulse of efferent lymphatic vessel between popliteal lymph node and footpad. Histology staining at ankle joints showed that DHJST decreases synovial inflammation, bone erosion, cartilage erosion, and TRAP+ osteoclast area in TNF-Tg mice. Immunohistochemical staining by using anti-Lyve-1 and anti-podoplanin antibody showed that DHJST stimulated lymphangiogenesis in ankle joints of TNF-Tg mice. And zebrafish study suggested that DHJST promoted the formation of lymphatic thoracic duct. In conclusion, DHJST inhibits inflammation severity and promotes lymphangiogenesis and lymphatic drainage function of TNF-Tg mice.

1. Introduction

Rheumatoid arthritis (RA) is a chronic autoimmune disease, characterized by progressive destruction of cartilage and bone, infiltration of inflammatory cells in joints, and presence of proliferative synovitis, usually compromising both the quality and duration of life. The pathology of this disease is complex, including the activation and infiltration of various populations of immune cells, which release inflammatory mediators into the synovial membrane of affected joints. The lymphatic system has vital functions in draining interstitial fluid from tissues into the blood and immune surveillance. Several clinical and laboratory observations indicate that inflammatory arthritis is associated with changes in lymphatic vessel. In 2001, it was reported that lymph drained from RA patients' joints contains high concentrations of cytokines and chemokines [1]. In addition, increased lymphatic vessel formation appears in synovial specimens from RA patients [2]. Consistent with these clinical reports, we previously found that joint specimens from TNF transgenic (Tg) mice [3], a mouse model of chronic inflammatory arthritis, have increased lymphatic vessel formation [4, 5]. By using indocyanine green near-infrared (ICG-NIR) lymphatic imaging and other outcome measures, in the past, we demonstrated that inhibition of lymphatic drainage via intraperitoneal injection VEGFR-3 neutralizing antibody increases the severity of joint inflammation [3, 4, 6–9], while stimulation of lymphatic drainage via injection of VEGF-C adenovirus at ankle joint decreases joint inflammation and tissue damage in TNF-Tg mice [10]. These findings illustrate that sufficient lymphatic drainage is favorable for the treatment of RA. Treatment targeting joint lymphatic drainage function contributes to the improvement of chronic inflammatory arthritis [11].

Currently, anti-inflammatory and reducing sequelae are main treatment in modern medicine for RA, although recombinant protein and monoclonal antibody drugs have emerged to bring hopes for millions of RA patients, those effects remain to be further followed up. TNF inhibitors etanercept, infliximab, and adalimumab alpha and other drugs could effectively reduce swelling and pain of RA patients, but there are still many patients who do not have any response at the initial treatment of TNF inhibitors, or failure in the second times of treatment, and about 10% of the patients discontinued per year. Looking for safe and effective treatment has become a major problem in the research of RA.

Du-Huo-Ji-Sheng-Tang (DHJST), a Chinese patent medicine, which is composed of radix Angelicae Pubescentis, Herba Taxilli, Radix Acanthopanacis Bidentatae, Herba Asari, Radix Gentianae Macrophyllae, Cortex Cinnamomi, *Eucommia*, Rhizoma Chuanxiong, Radix Saposhnikoviae, Radix Saposhnikoviae, liquorice, angelica, peony, *Rehmannia*, Ginseng, and poria, has been widely used for the treatment of rheumatoid arthritis (RA) in China [12]. It can improve clinical symptoms and knee function of patients [13]. But the mechanism deserves further research. Our preliminary screening identified DHJST stimulate lymphatic vessel growth of transgenic zebrafish. Those results suggested that DHJST has good effect on lymphatic vascular system. Our hypothesis is that DHJST attenuate inflammation severity of RA through promoting lymphatic drainage function. Thus, the aim of this study is to investigate whether DHJST could attenuate inflammation and promote lymphatic drainage function of TNF-Tg mice.

2. Experimental

2.1. Animals. zThe 3647 lines of TNF transgenic (TNF-Tg) mice were kindly provided by Dr. G. Kollias (Institute of Immunology, Alexander Fleming Biomedical Sciences Research Center, Vari, Greece) and were backcrossed with C57BL/6 mice to be maintained as heterozygotes; therefore, nontransgenic littermates are used as aged-matched wild type (WT) controls. This line of TNF-Tg mice carries one copy of the human TNF transgene and develops a disease that closely resembles RA, which is characterized by spontaneous, chronic, progressive inflammatory erosive joint disease [14]. TNF-Tg mice have normal ankle joints when they are 1 month old; they develop mild ankle joint inflammation and bone erosion at 3 months old, which become more severe at 5 months old or older [15, 16]. Three-month-old TNF-Tg mice (mild ankle joint inflammation and bone erosion) and WT littermates were used.

The transgenic zebrafish line (fli1:egfp; gata1:DsRed), in which endothelial cells express eGFP and blood cells express DsRed [17], was kindly provided by Simon Ming Yuen Lee (Institute of Chinese Medical Sciences, Macau). It was maintained in a controlled environment described in the Zebrafish Handbook [18]. Embryos were generated by natural pairwise mating, when the fish were 3–12 months old and were raised in embryo water (13.7 mM NaCl; 540 μM KCl; pH 7.4; 25 μM Na$_2$HPO$_4$; 44 μM KH$_2$PO$_4$; 300 μM CaCl$_2$; 100 μM MgSO$_4$; 420 μM NaHCO$_3$; pH 7.4).

All animal procedures were followed by the Guiding Principles for the Care and Use of Laboratory Animals of National Science and Technology Committee of China.

TABLE 1: Prescription of Du-Huo-Ji-Sheng-Tang (DHJST).

Latin name	Amount (g)
Radix angelicae pubescentis	9 g
Taxillus sutchuenensis (Lecomte) danser	6 g
Radix Acanthopanacis Bidentatae	6 g
Asarum sieboldii Miq.	6 g
Radix Gentianae Macrophyllae	6 g
Cortex Cinnamomi cassia	6 g
Sclerotium poriae cocos	6 g
Eucommia ulmoides	6 g
Radix ledebouriellae divaricatae	6 g
Ligusticum chuanxiong Hort.	6 g
Panax ginseng C. A. Mey.	6 g
Glycyrrhiza uralensis Fisch.	6 g
Cynanchum otophyllum	6 g
Rehmannia glutinosa (Gaertn.) Libosch. ex Fisch. et Mey.	6 g

2.2. Indocyanine Green Near-Infrared (ICG-NIR) Lymphatic Imaging. ICG-NIR lymphatic imaging was performed by using Fluobeam 800 imaging system (United States) according to the method previously described [6, 15, 19–21]. Indocyanine green (Acorn) solution (0.1 μg/mL, 10 μL) was injected intradermally into the mouse footpad using a 30-gauge needle, after removing fur from legs with hair removal lotion. Under an infrared laser, the dynamics of ICG fluorescence over the entire leg was visualized. ICG fluorescence at the whole leg was recorded for 1 hour immediately after ICG injection and again for 5 minutes at 24 hours after ICG injection. Sequential images were analyzed for the ICG intensity of the injection site and collecting lymphatic vessels efferent ankle joint using Image J software to quantify (1) % clearance, which is an assessment of ICG washout through the lymphatics and is quantified as the percent difference of ICG signal intensity between the two ICG-NIR images from the ROI of the injection site at 1 hour after ICG injection and 24 hours later and (2) lymphatic pulse, which is the ICG pulses that pass the region of interest (ROI) of the draining lymphatic vessel afferent to PLN within 500 seconds, as we described previously [6, 15, 19–23].

2.3. Plant Material and Preparation. Herbs in DHJST (Table 1), provided by Shanghai Huayu Chinese Herbs Co. Ltd., China, were accredited by a pharmacognosist according to standard protocols, prepared by Longhua Hospital affiliated to Shanghai University of Traditional Chinese Medicine. The drugs were extracted according to standard methods of Chinese Pharmacopoeia (China Pharmacopoeia and Committee, 2000). The Ginseng was soaked in 12 times the volume of water for 40 mins and boiled for 40 mins, the drug solution was filtered, and the filter residue was boiled in 8 times the volume of water for another 40 mins and the solution was filtered again. Both filtrates of Ginseng were mixed to get decoction 1. The remaining 13 crude drugs except Cortex Cinnamomi were soaked in 12 times the volume of water for 40 mins and boiled for 40 mins (Cortex Cinnamomi was added at 35 mins), the drug solution was filtered, and the filter residue was boiled in 8 times volume of water for another 40 mins and the solution was filtered again. Both filtrates of the remaining 13 crude drugs were mixed to get decoction 2. Decoction 1 and decoction 2 were mixed and concentrated to 77 mL under reduced pressure, the concentration of Du-Huo-Ji-Sheng-Tang for 1.2 kg/L, and then stored at $-20°C$ until use.

DHJST samples were diluted with 4 times the water. The standard compounds of 0.125 mg ferulic acid and 2×10^{-3} mg osthole were mixed and dissolved in 1 mL of methanol. The standard compounds of 1.7 mg gentiopicroside and 0.7 mg paeoniflorin were mixed and dissolved in 1 mL of methanol. All the above 4 kinds of standard compounds were purchased from the National Institute for Food and Drug Control (Beijing, China). Methanol (HPLC grade, Merck KGaA, Darmstadt, Germany) and deionized water purified using the Milli-Q Reagent Water System (Millipore, Bedford, MA, USA) were used for HPLC analysis. All final solutions were passed through a $0.22 \mu m$ membrane prior to use. An aliquot of $10 \mu L$ of each sample solution was injected into the HPLC system for analysis.

The high-performance liquid chromatography equipment was an Agilent 1260 series system consisting of a G1322A degasser, a G1311A quaternary pump, a G1311A autosampler, a G1316A column temperature controller, and a G1315B DAD detector (Palo Alto, CA, USA). A Waters XBridge C18 column (250 mm × 4.6 mm i.d., $5 \mu m$) was used and maintained at 30°C. The mobile phase was 0.1% formic acid aqueous solution (A) and methanol (B) with a gradient program as follows: 0~125 min, linear gradient 10→15% B; 125~185 min, linear gradient 15→21% B; 185~250 min, 21% B; 250~450 min, linear gradient 21→44% B; 450~480 min, 44% B; 480~510 min, linear gradient 44→70% B; 510~530 min, 70% B and the postrun (10 min) at a flow-rate of 0.5 mL/min. Monitoring was performed at 325 nm and 274 nm. Overlaid chromatograms indicate that ferulic acid, gentiopicroside, paeoniflorin and osthole existed in DHJST (Appendices 1 and 2 of the Supplementary Material (see Supplementary Material available online at http://dx.doi.org/10.1155/2016/7067691)). Only samples that were confirmed by HPLC to meet the pharmacopoeial specifications were used in the present study.

2.4. Treatment.

Eight 3-month-old TNF-Tg mice were given Du-Huo-Ji-Sheng-Tang (12 g/kg) or same volume physiological saline by gavage once every day for 12 weeks. Eight 3-month-old WT littermates that accepted same volume physiological saline were used as negative control. At the twelfth week, all mice were subjected to NIR-ICG imaging again. After that, ankle joints were harvested for histology staining and analysis.

Healthy zebrafish embryos were picked out at 48 hours after fecundation (hpf) and were distributed into a 12-well microplate with 10 fishes per well. Following this, the embryos were pretreated with the $30 \mu M$ VEGFR-3 kinase inhibitor (MAZ51, Calbiochem, La Jolla, CA, cat. #676492, lot. #D00152431) for 6 hrs. The medium was then replaced with different concentrations (10–100 μg/mL) of DHJST for 48 hrs. Embryos treated with 0.2% DMSO served as a

vehicle control and were equivalent to not treatment. Each group had more than 9-10 fishes. The effect of DHJST on lymphangiogenesis was quantified by measuring the length of lymphatic thoracic duct at 10 somites of the trunk region, spanning from somite boundary 7 or 8 to 18 of each zebrafish. The photos were taken under Confocal Fluorescence Imaging Microscope (Leica TCS-SP5, Germany).

2.5. Histology.

Ankle joints were fixed in 10% phosphate-buffered formalin at room temperature for 48 hours, decalcified in 10% EDTA for 21 days, and embedded in paraffin. A total of 30 consecutive sections from one ankle joint were collected and at least $4 \mu m$ consecutive sections were cut and mounted on common slides and were collected and divided into 3 levels. Each level was $40 \mu m$ from the previous level. One section from each of the 3 levels was assessed for hematoxylin and eosin (H&E), Alcian blue/orange G (ABHO) staining or tartrate resistant acid phosphatase (TRAP) staining, and histomorphometry analysis. The inflammatory area and bone area were analyzed by using HE-stained sections, cartilage area at ankle joint was measured on ABHO-stained sections, and TRAP positive area expressed as a % of the total tissue area was measured on TRAP-stained sections. The data are presented as the mean from 3 levels cut from each joint sample.

2.6. Immunohistochemistry.

Double immunofluorescence staining was performed on paraffin sections of ankle joints as described previously [24, 25]. Briefly, after antigen retrieval with 20 μg/mL proteinase K, sections were blocked in 5% BSA-PBST for 30 min and then incubated with hamster monoclonal anti-mouse podoplanin (Abcam Inc., Cambridge, MA; cat. #ab11936; clone: 8.1.1, 1 : 1,000) and rabbit anti-mouse lymphatic vessel endothelial hyaluronan receptor 1 (LYVE-1, Abcam Inc., Cambridge, MA, USA; cat. #ab14917; lot. #GR126653-4, 1 : 1,000) in 1% BSA-PBST at 4°C overnight. Secondary antibodies, Alexa Fluor 546-goat-anti-hamster (Invitrogen-Molecular Probes, Eugene, OR; cat. #A21111, 1 : 400), and Alexa 488-conjugated goat against rabbit secondary antibody (Molecular Probes, Eugene, OR, USA; cat. #A11001; lot. #99E2-1, 1 : 400) were used to incubate sections for 2 hours after extensive washing. After mounting, the double immunofluorescence stained slides were scanned using an Olympus VS-110 whole-slide imaging system and analyzed using Olympus VS-110 software version 2.3.

We outlined regions of interest (ROIs), from the distal of tibia to the distal of talus, which included articular capsules, adjacent soft tissues, and articular cartilage and bones. The total tissue area of the ROI and the area and numbers of lymphatic vessels within the entire ROI were determined automatically with Olympus VS-110 software. The total tissue area ranged from 3.5 to 3.508 mm^2, and the area of lymphatic vessels was calculated by dividing the lymphatic area by the total tissue area. Podoplanin+/LYVE-1+ vessels were defined as lymphatic vessels according to published literature [26–30].

2.7. Statistical Analysis.

Data were expressed as means ± standard deviation. Statistical analyses were performed using

(a)

(b)

(c)

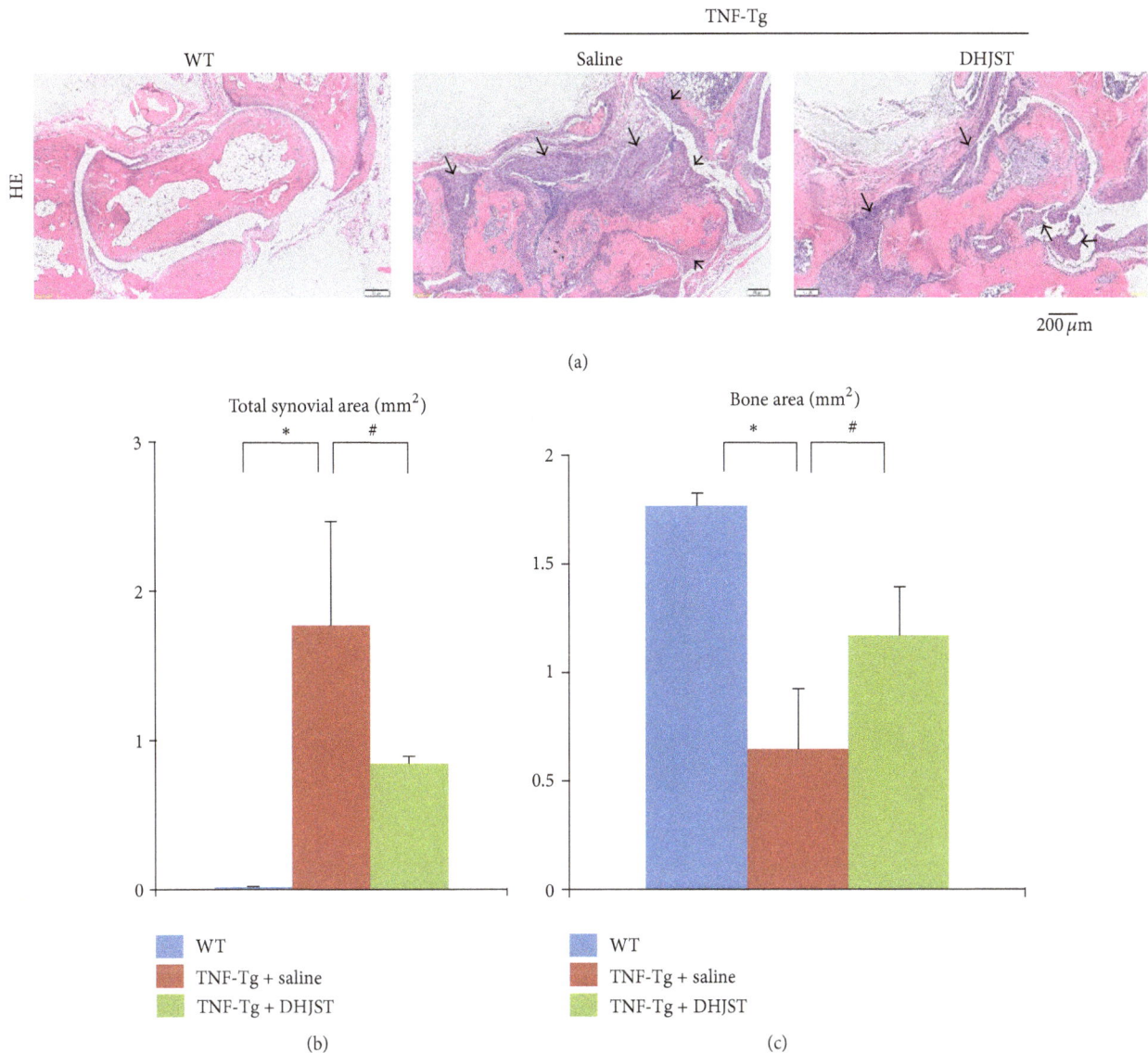

FIGURE 1: Du-Huo-Ji-Sheng-Tang reduces inflammation and bone erosion in TNF-Tg mice. Three-month-old TNF-Tg mice were treated with Du-Huo-Ji-Sheng-Tang (12 g/kg/gavage, daily ×12 weeks) or saline. Ankle joints were harvested and subjected to histologic analysis. WT mice were included as control. (a) Representative HE-stained sections show decreased inflammation and bone loss in the Du-Huo-Ji-Sheng-Tang-treated joints. Bar, 200 μm, black arrow indicates inflammatory synovial tissue. Quantitation of bone area (b) and inflammatory synovial area (c). Values are the mean ± SD of 6–8 legs per group. $^{*}p < 0.05$ versus WT; $^{#}p < 0.05$ versus TNF-Tg + saline.

SPSS 18.0 software. One-way ANOVA test followed by Bonferroni posttest was used for multiple group comparisons. Statistically significant differences were considered when $p < 0.05$.

3. Results

3.1. DHJST Decreases Severity of Arthritis in TNF-Tg Mice. To investigate the effect of DHJST on arthritis, TNF-Tg mice were given DHJST by gavage daily for 12 weeks. We quantified synovial inflammation and bone erosion in HE staining sections of ankle joints, cartilage damage in ABHO staining sections, and osteoclast invasion in TRAP

staining section. Synovial volume in ankle joint of WT mice is $0.015 \pm 0.0044\,\text{mm}^2$, while severely increased synovial inflammation volume was observed in saline treated TNF-Tg mice ($1.767 \pm 0.69\,\text{mm}^2$). Impressively, DHJST treatment significantly reduced inflammatory synovial volume of TNF-Tg mice, versus saline treated control (Figures 1(a) and 1(b)). In addition, significantly reduced bone area was observed in saline treated TNF-Tg mice, versus WT littermates. However DHJST treatment restored the bone volume of TNF-Tg mice, compared with saline treated group (Figures 1(a) and 1(c)). Besides that, the cartilage area is also significantly reduced in saline treated TNF-Tg mice versus WT mice. Compared with saline treated TNF-Tg mice, DHJST significantly increased

(a)

(b)

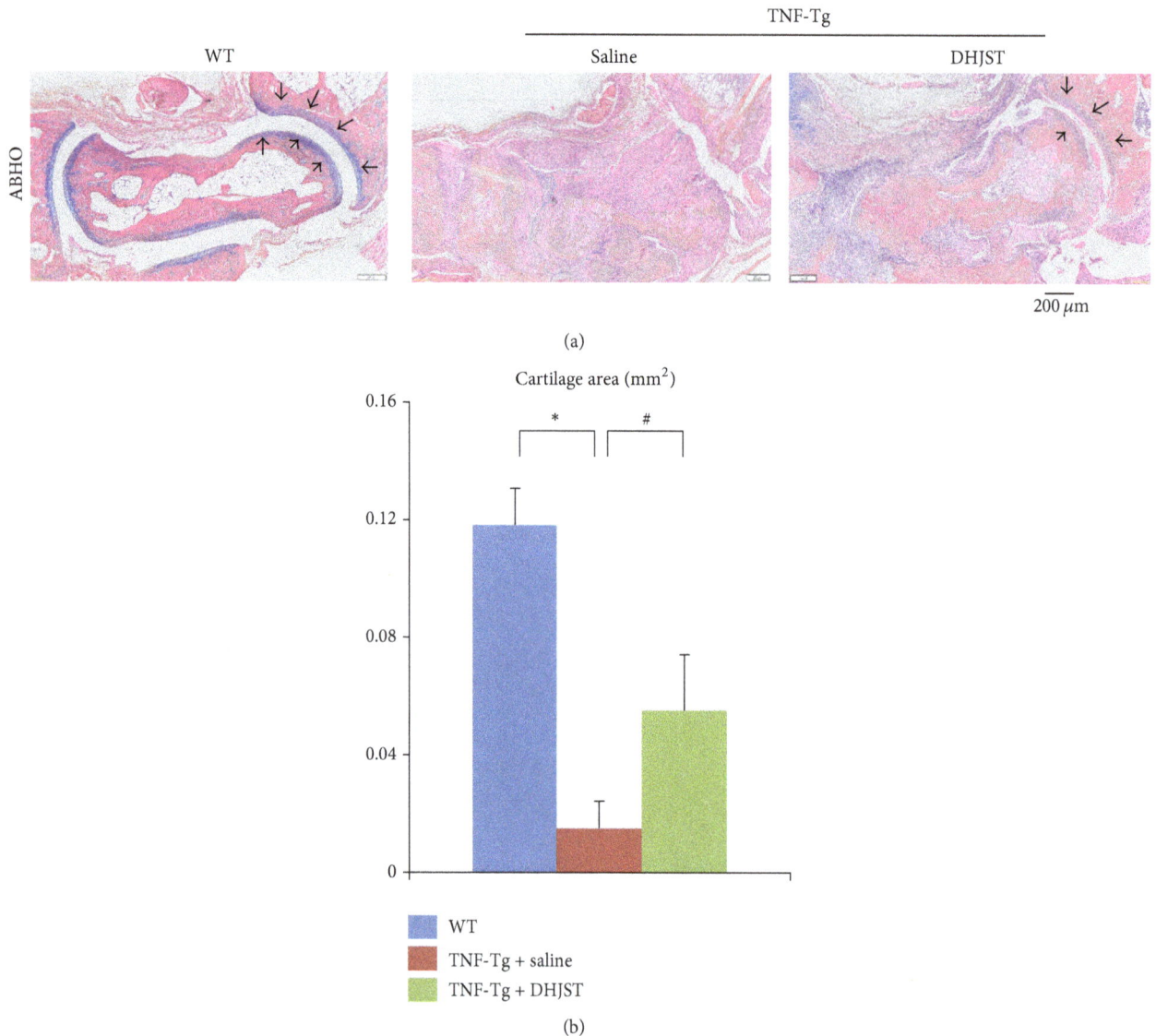

FIGURE 2: Du-Huo-Ji-Sheng-Tang reduces cartilage erosion in TNF-Tg mice. (a) Representative ABHO-stained sections show loss of cartilage at ankle joint of saline treated TNF-Tg mice and reduced cartilage erosion in the Du-Huo-Ji-Sheng-Tang-treated joints. Bar, $200\,\mu$m, Alcian blue positive staining (black arrow) indicates cartilage at ankle joint. Quantitation of cartilage area (b). Values are the mean $\pm$ SD of 6–8 legs per group. $^*p < 0.05$ versus WT; $^\#p < 0.05$ versus TNF-Tg + saline.

cartilage area of TNF-Tg mice (Figures 2(a) and 2(b)). Furthermore, severely increased osteoclast area was observed in ankle joints of saline treated TNF-Tg mice, which was significantly reduced by DHJST treatment (Figures 3(a) and 3(b)).

3.2. DHJST Promotes Lymphatic Drainage Function in TNF-Tg Mice. Consistent with previous study [3, 10, 20, 22, 23], lymphatic drainage function (including clearance and pulse) was impaired in TNF-Tg mice. But DHJST increased the ICG clearance at the footpad and the pulse of efferent lymphatic vessel between popliteal lymph node and footpad of TNF-Tg mice (Figures 4(a)–4(d)).

3.3. DHJST Promotes Lymphangiogenesis in Ankle Joint of TNF-Tg Mice. Previously we reported that TNF-Tg mice develop ankle synovitis and significantly increased numbers of LYVE-1+ lymphatic vessels [4]. To investigate the effect of DHJST on lymphatic formation at ankle joint of TNF-Tg mice and avoid nonspecific staining, we performed double immunofluorescence staining with anti-LYVE-1 and anti-podoplanin antibodies to visualize lymphatic vessel endothelial cells. We found a similar increase of podoplanin+/LYVE-1+ lymphatic vessels in saline treated TNF-Tg mice, compared with WT littermates. Interestingly, we observed that DHJST treatment significantly increased podoplanin+/LYVE-1+ lymphatic vessels of TNF-Tg mice (Figures 5(a) and 5(b)).

(a)

(b)

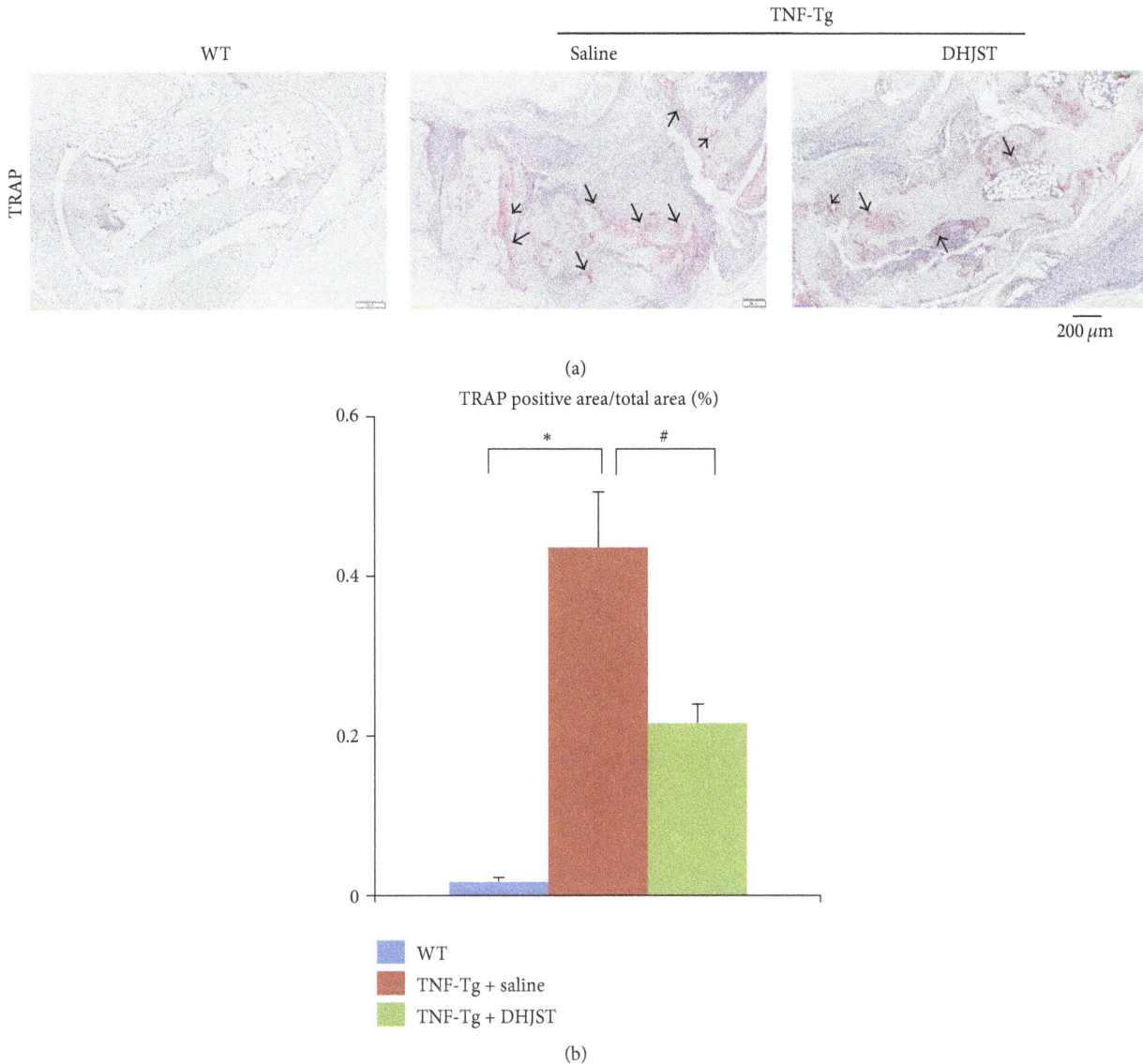

FIGURE 3: Du-Huo-Ji-Sheng-Tang reduces TRAP+ osteoclast in TNF-Tg mice. (a) Representative TRAP-stained sections show decreased TRAP+ osteoclast number in the Du-Huo-Ji-Sheng-Tang-treated joints. Bar, $200\,\mu m$, arrow indicates TRAP+ osteoclast. Quantitation of TRAP+ osteoclast area (b). Values are the mean ± SD of 6–8 legs per group. $^{*}p < 0.05$ versus WT; $^{\#}p < 0.05$ versus TNF-Tg + saline.

3.4. DHJST Promotes Lymphangiogenesis in Zebrafish. In order to determine the effect of DHJST on lymphatic vessel, we used zebrafish screening system. In zebrafish, by 5 days after fertilization, the lymphatic thoracic duct (TD) is fully developed [21]. Thus we added VEGFR-3 specific inhibitor for 6 hours 48 hpf and then changed the medium with different doses of DHJST (10, 30, and 100 μg/mL) for 48 hours. In our study, we found that MAZ51 severely impaired the number and length of TD formation, but DHJST treatment for 48 hours increased the number and length of TD formation in dose dependent manner (Figures 6(a)–6(c)).

4. Discussion

The objective of this study was to assess the effects of Du-Huo-Ji-Sheng-Tang on the inflammatory severity at ankle joints of TNF-Tg mice. These mice were chosen as a rheumatoid arthritis animal model because this transgenic (Tg) mouse overexpresses human TNF-alpha and develops erosive polyarthritis with many characteristics observed in rheumatoid arthritis patients, which has already been widely used for dissecting the molecular mechanisms of the pathogenic process and evaluating the efficacy of novel therapeutic strategies for rheumatoid arthritis [31]. In our current study, we found that DHJST reduced the inflammation severity, increased bone volume, and decreased TRAP+ osteoclast invasion of TNF-Tg mice. This result suggests that DHJST is an effective treatment on the inflammation severity of RA.

Our previous studies suggested that sufficient lymphatic drainage was essential for RA, and therapeutic approaches targeting joint lymphatic function showed promise for

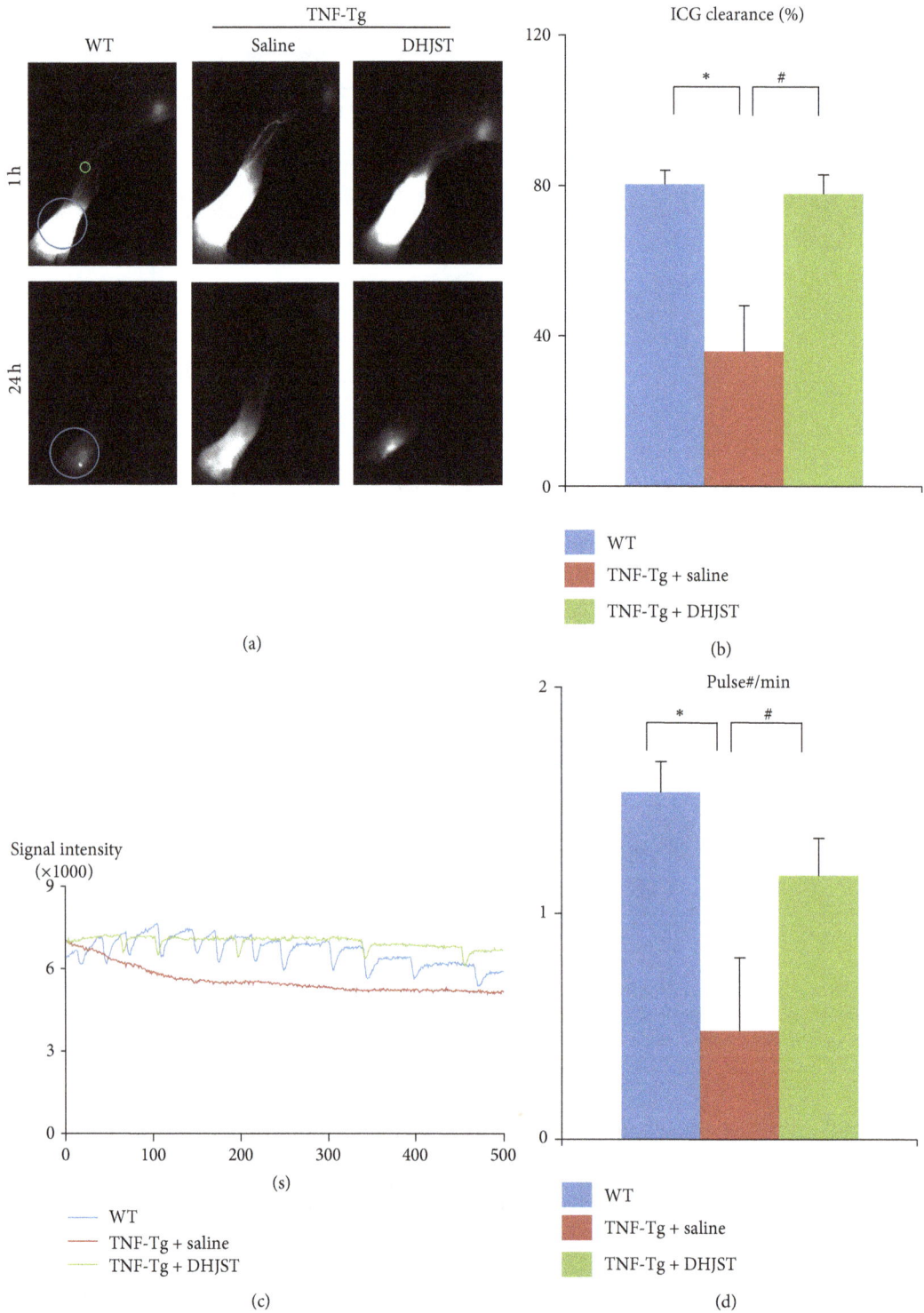

(a)

(b)

(c)

(d)

FIGURE 4: Impaired lymphatic function of TNF-Tg mice was rescued by Du-Huo-Ji-Sheng-Tang. Three-month-old TNF-Tg mice were treated with Du-Huo-Ji-Sheng-Tang or saline for 12 weeks and were subjected to ICG-NIR imagining. (a) Representative ICG images show that Du-Huo-Ji-Sheng-Tang increased ICG removal from ankle area. (b) Quantitation of % ICG clearance. Values are mean ± SD of 8–18 legs. (c) Lymphatic pulses were measured at a region of interest. Histogram shows that Du-Huo-Ji-Sheng-Tang restored lymphatic pulses in TNF-Tg mice. (d) Quantitation of lymphatic pulses/min. Values are mean ± SD of 7–18 legs from 4–9 mice. $^*p < 0.05$ versus WT mice, $^\#p < 0.05$ versus saline treated TNF-Tg group.

(a)

(b)

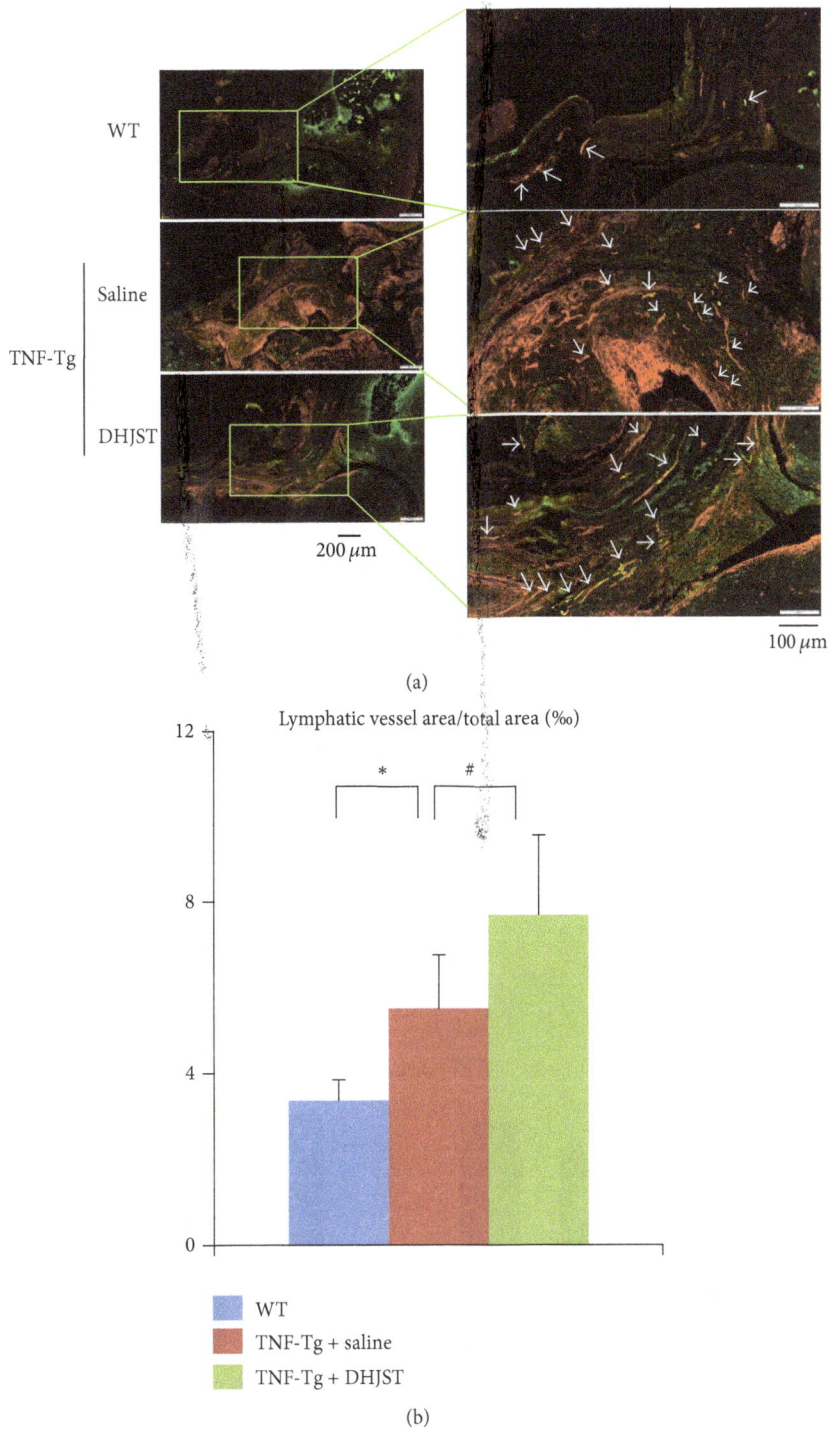

FIGURE 5: DHJST increases lymphangiogenesis in ankle joints of TNF-Tg mice. (a) Three-month DHJST or saline treatment, ankle joints were harvested and subjected to double immunofluorescence staining with anti-LYVE-1 and anti-podoplanin antibodies. Representative LYVE-1 (green) and podoplanin (red) stained ankle sections show that LYVE-1+/podoplanin+ lymphatic vessels (white arrows) are present at synovium and soft tissue surrounding the ankle joints of WT and TNF-Tg mice. (b) Quantitation of LYVE-1+/podoplanin+ lymphatic vessel area inside the areas of ankle joint. Values are the means ± SD of 5-6 legs per group. $^{*}p < 0.05$ versus WT group, $^{\#}p < 0.05$ versus saline treated TNF-Tg group.

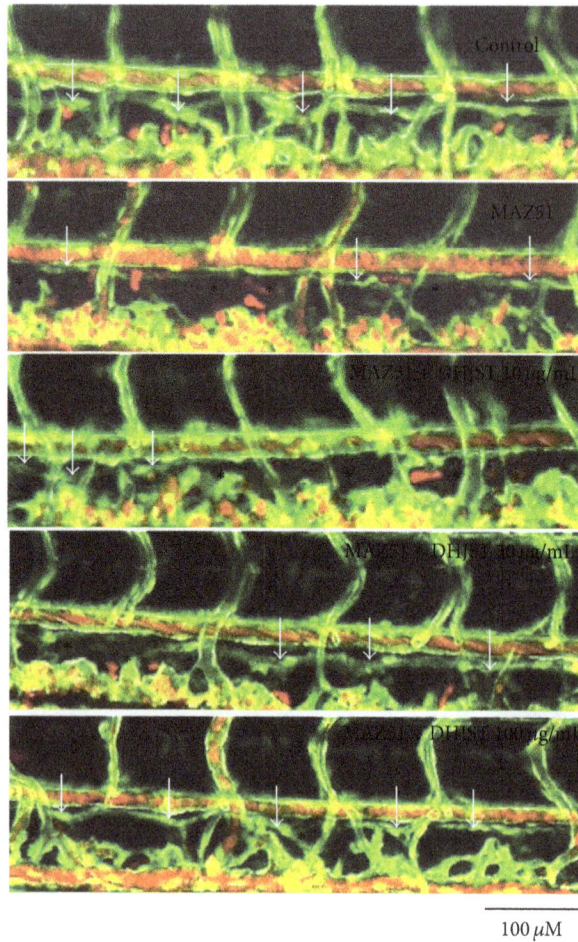

(a)

(b)

(c)

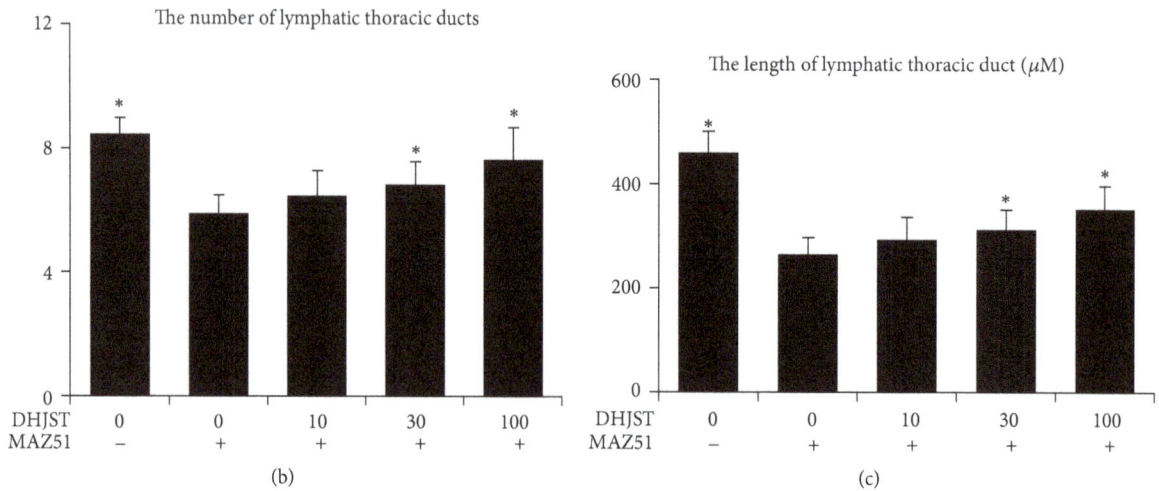

FIGURE 6: Impaired lymphatic thoracic duct formation induced by VEGFR-3 kinase inhibitor (MAZ51) was rescued by Du-Huo-Ji-Sheng-Tang in dose dependent manner. Two dpf zebrafish (fli1:egfp; gata1:DsRed) were treated with 30 μM MAZ51 for 6 hours and then changed to be treated with different doses of Du-Huo-Ji-Sheng-Tang (10–100 μg/mL) for 48 hours. Embryos treated with 0.2% DMSO served as a vehicle control. (a) Representative confocal images show that Du-Huo-Ji-Sheng-Tang increased lymphatic thoracic duct formation of zebrafish, white arrow indicates lymphatic thoracic duct, and white star indicates lack of lymphatic vessel. (b) Quantitation of the number of lymphatic thoracic ducts. (c) Quantitation of the length of lymphatic thoracic duct. Values are mean ± SD of 9–11 zebrafishes. $^{*}p < 0.05$ versus MAZ51.

chronic inflammatory arthritis [11]. In order to investigate the lymphatic drainage function, our group previously established NIR-ICG lymphatic draining function imaging system [6, 15, 19–21]. Based on this imaging system, we found that DHJST could effectively promote the ICG clearance and pulse of efferent lymphatic vessel between footpad and popliteal lymph node, which suggested that DHJST was an effective drug for lymphatic drainage function. Consistent with our study, it was reported that DHJST has a good therapeutic effect on lymphedema syndrome [32].

It has been widely accepted that inflammation stimulates lymphangiogenesis as a compensatory mechanism to augment the clearance of inflammatory products [10]. We found that increased podoplanin+/LYVE-1+ lymphatics vessels in synovium of TNF-Tg mice are insufficient to be fully effective and that DHJST can rectify these deficiencies. Thus functional improvement of lymphatic vessels within the inflammatory sites and surrounding tissues is another therapeutic alternative to inflammation-induced edema and tissue damage.

Zebrafish has become a popular animal model in the fields of drug screening and has been widely used for assessment of efficacy and toxicity of any types of drugs, especially for multi-ingredient drugs, herbs, and exacts [33]. In current study, it is the first time for us to use zebrafish to determine the effect of drugs and herbs on lymphatic vessel. We used TG (gata1:DsRed; fli1:EGFP) zebrafish, in which the blood flow is visible in red (gata1:DsRed) and the lymphatic vessel and blood vessels are visible in green. Thus we could identify the green lymphatic vessel from blood vessel, which has red blood cells in the vessel. By using zebrafish we found that DHJST could accelerate lymphangiogenesis at the trunk of zebrafish after VEGFR3 inhibitor impairment. This result indicated that DHJST has good therapeutic effect on lymphatic vessel after impairment, and this may account for the good effect of DHJST on the lymphatic drainage function.

DHJST is one of Chinese patent medicines (CPMs), which is widely used for the treatment of rheumatoid arthritis (RA) [12] and osteoarthritis [34–36]. It was reported that DHJST inhibited sodium nitroprussiate-induced apoptosis [37] and promoted proliferation of chondrocytes [38–40]. Duhuo attenuated adjuvant-induced hind paw inflammation and hyperalgesia in rats [41]. Previous quality control study of DHJST suggested that this drug comprises osthole, gentiopicroside, loganic acid, and paeoniflorin [42, 43]. Osthole exhibited anti-inflammation [44, 45] and anti-bone-resorption effect [46] and stimulated osteoblast differentiation and bone formation by activation of beta-catenin-BMP signaling [47]. Gentiopicroside exhibits analgesic activities in the mice [48]. Loganic acid decreased proinflammatory cytokines in hypercholesterolemic rabbits [49]. Paeoniflorin is able to suppress inflammation in experimental arthritis by inhibiting abnormal proliferation of lymphocytes and synoviocytes and the production of proinflammatory cytokines and chemokines, nitric oxide, VEGF, and GM-CSF by synoviocytes [50, 51]. Ferulic acid, isolated from Rhizoma Chuanxiong and Dang-Gui [52] and Panax Notoginseng Saponins extracts from Ginseng, has antioxidative and anti-inflammatory effects [53, 54]. All the above study indicates that DHJST has anti-inflammatory actions, consistent with the result in current study that DHJST inhibits inflammation of TNF-Tg mice. But in our study, we firstly found that the promoting effect of DHJST on lymphatic drainage function is associated with reduced inflammation. And this improvement effect might be an important way for DHJST to attenuate inflammation of TNF-Tg mice.

5. Conclusion

DHJST inhibits inflammation severity and promotes lymphatic drainage function of TNF-Tg mice. DHJST is a promising medicine for RA and the mechanism is associated with lymphangiogenesis and lymphatic drainage function.

Competing Interests

The authors do not have commercial or other associations that might have competing interests.

Authors' Contributions

Yan Chen, Jinlong Li, and Qiang Li contributed equally to this paper.

Acknowledgments

This work was sponsored by research grants from National Natural Science Foundation (81403417 to Qianqian Liang, 81173278 to Quan Zhou, 81330085 to Qi Shi, 81220108027 to Yongjun Wang and Lianping Xing, and 81403418 to Hao Xu) and special funding from the National Outstanding Doctoral Dissertation (201276 to Qianqian Liang), Ministry of Education, "Innovative Research Team" (IRT1270 to Yongjun Wang), and Shanghai University of Traditional Chinese Medicine "085 Project" (085ZY1204 to Yongjun Wang).

References

[1] W. L. Olszewski, J. Pazdur, E. Kubasiewicz, M. Zaleska, C. J. Cooke, and N. E. Miller, "Lymph draining from foot joints in rheumatoid arthritis provides insight into local cytokine and chemokine production and transport to lymph nodes," *Arthritis and Rheumatism*, vol. 44, no. 3, pp. 541–549, 2001.

[2] K. Wauke, M. Nagashima, T. Ishiwata, G. Asano, and S. Yoshino, "Expression and localization of vascular endothelial growth factor-C in rheumatoid arthritis synovial tissue," *The Journal of Rheumatology*, vol. 29, no. 1, pp. 34–38, 2002.

[3] Q. Zhou, R. Wood, E. M. Schwarz, Y.-J. Wang, and L. Xing, "Near-infrared lymphatic imaging demonstrates the dynamics of lymph flow and lymphangiogenesis during the acute versus chronic phases of arthritis in mice," *Arthritis and Rheumatism*, vol. 62, no. 7, pp. 1881–1889, 2010.

[4] Q. Zhang, Y. Lu, S. T. Proulx et al., "Increased lymphangiogenesis in joints of mice with inflammatory arthritis," *Arthritis Research & Therapy*, vol. 9, no. 6, article R118, 2007.

[5] K. Polzer, D. Baeten, A. Soleiman et al., "Tumour necrosis factor blockade increases lymphangiogenesis in murine and human

arthritic joints," *Annals of the Rheumatic Diseases*, vol. 67, no. 11, pp. 1610–1616, 2008.

[6] S. T. Proulx, E. Kwok, Z. You et al., "Longitudinal assessment of synovial, lymph node, and bone volumes in inflammatory arthritis in mice by in vivo magnetic resonance imaging and microfocal computed tomography," *Arthritis and Rheumatism*, vol. 56, no. 12, pp. 4024–4037, 2007.

[7] P. Baluk, T. Tammela, E. Ator et al., "Pathogenesis of persistent lymphatic vessel hyperplasia in chronic airway inflammation," *The Journal of Clinical Investigation*, vol. 115, no. 2, pp. 247–257, 2005.

[8] M. J. Flister, A. Wilber, K. L. Hall et al., "Inflammation induces lymphangiogenesis through up-regulation of VEGFR-3 mediated by NF-κB and Prox1," *Blood*, vol. 115, no. 2, pp. 418–429, 2010.

[9] M. Jeltsch, A. Kaipainen, V. Joukov et al., "Hyperplasia of lymphatic vessels in VEGF-C transgenic mice," *Science*, vol. 276, no. 5317, pp. 1423–1425, 1997.

[10] Q. Zhou, R. Guo, R. Wood et al., "Vascular endothelial growth factor C attenuates joint damage in chronic inflammatory arthritis by accelerating local lymphatic drainage in mice," *Arthritis and Rheumatism*, vol. 63, no. 8, pp. 2318–2328, 2011.

[11] J. Buckland, "Experimental arthritis: targeting joint lymphatic function," *Nature Reviews Rheumatology*, vol. 7, no. 7, article 376, 2011.

[12] J. Zhao, Q. Zha, M. Jiang, H. Cao, and A. Lu, "Expert consensus on the treatment of rheumatoid arthritis with chinese patent medicines," *Journal of Alternative and Complementary Medicine*, vol. 19, no. 2, pp. 111–118, 2013.

[13] L. C. Qin, "A randomized controlled observation on the combination of duhuojisheng decoction and 99Tc-MDP in the treatment of rheumatoid arthritis," *Journal of Practical Traditional Chinese Internal Medicine*, vol. 27, no. 1, pp. 50–51, 2013.

[14] J. Keffer, L. Probert, H. Cazlaris et al., "Transgenic mice expressing human tumour necrosis factor: a predictive genetic model of arthritis," *The EMBO Journal*, vol. 10, no. 13, pp. 4025–4031, 1991.

[15] R. Guo, Q. Zhou, S. T. Proulx et al., "Inhibition of lymphangiogenesis and lymphatic drainage via vascular endothelial growth factor receptor 3 blockade increases the severity of inflammation in a mouse model of chronic inflammatory arthritis," *Arthritis and Rheumatism*, vol. 60, no. 9, pp. 2666–2676, 2009.

[16] P. Li, E. M. Schwarz, R. J. O'Keefe et al., "Systemic tumor necrosis factor alpha mediates an increase in peripheral CD11bhigh osteoclast precursors in tumor necrosis factor alpha-transgenic mice," *Arthritis and Rheumatism*, vol. 50, no. 1, pp. 265–276, 2004.

[17] M. Omae, N. Takada, S. Yamamoto, H. Nakajima, and T. N. Sato, "Identification of inter-organ vascular network: vessels bridging between organs," *PLoS ONE*, vol. 8, no. 6, Article ID e65720, 2013.

[18] M. Westerfield, *The Zebrafish Book. A Guide for the Laboratory Use of Zebrafish (Danio Rerio)*, University of Oregon Press, Eugene, Ore, USA, 3rd edition, 1995.

[19] S. T. Proulx, E. Kwok, Z. You et al., "MRI and quantification of draining lymph node function in inflammatory arthritis," *Annals of the New York Academy of Sciences*, vol. 1117, pp. 106–123, 2007.

[20] J. Li, Y. Ju, E. M. Bouta et al., "Efficacy of B cell depletion therapy for murine joint arthritis flare is associated with increased lymphatic flow," *Arthritis and Rheumatism*, vol. 65, no. 1, pp. 130–138, 2013.

[21] Y. Luo, W. Chen, H. Zhou et al., "Cryptotanshinone inhibits lymphatic endothelial cell tube formation by suppressing VEGFR-3/ERK and small GTPase pathways," *Cancer Prevention Research*, vol. 4, no. 12, pp. 2083–2091, 2011.

[22] E. M. Bouta, R. W. Wood, E. B. Brown, H. Rahimi, C. T. Ritchlin, and E. M. Schwarz, "In vivo quantification of lymph viscosity and pressure in lymphatic vessels and draining lymph nodes of arthritic joints in mice," *The Journal of Physiology*, vol. 592, no. 6, pp. 1213–1223, 2014.

[23] E. M. Bouta, R. W. Wood, S. W. Perry et al., "Measuring intranodal pressure and lymph viscosity to elucidate mechanisms of arthritic flare and therapeutic outcomes," *Annals of the New York Academy of Sciences*, vol. 1240, no. 1, pp. 47–52, 2011.

[24] J. X. Shi, Q. Q. Liang, Y. J. Wang, R. A. Mooney, B. F. Boyce, and L. Xing, "Use of a whole-slide imaging system to assess the presence and alteration of lymphatic vessels in joint sections of arthritic mice," *Biotechnic & Histochemistry*, vol. 88, no. 8, pp. 428–439, 2013.

[25] J. Shi, Q. Liang, M. Zuscik et al., "Distribution and alteration of lymphatic vessels in knee joints of normal and osteoarthritic mice," *Arthritis and Rheumatology*, vol. 66, no. 3, pp. 657–666, 2014.

[26] R. Bianchi, A. Teijeira, S. T. Proulx et al., "A transgenic Prox1-Cre-tdTomato reporter mouse for lymphatic vessel research," *PLoS ONE*, vol. 10, no. 4, Article ID e0122976, 2015.

[27] X. Wu, Z. Yu, and N. Liu, "Comparison of approaches for microscopic imaging of skin lymphatic vessels," *Scanning*, vol. 34, no. 3, pp. 174–180, 2012.

[28] P. Baluk and D. M. McDonald, "Markers for microscopic imaging of lymphangiogenesis and angiogenesis," *Annals of the New York Academy of Sciences*, vol. 1131, pp. 1–12, 2008.

[29] S. Loukovaara, E. Gucciardo, P. Repo, P. Lohi, P. Salven, and K. Lehti, "A case of abnormal lymphatic-like differentiation and endothelial progenitor cell activation in neovascularization associated with hemi-retinal vein occlusion," *Case Reports in Ophthalmology*, vol. 6, no. 2, pp. 228–238, 2015.

[30] A. Kaser-Eichberger, F. Schrödl, A. Trost et al., "Topography of lymphatic markers in human iris and ciliary body," *Investigative Opthalmology & Visual Science*, vol. 56, no. 8, pp. 4943–4953, 2015.

[31] P. Li and E. M. Schwarz, "The TNF-α transgenic mouse model of inflammatory arthritis," *Springer Seminars in Immunopathology*, vol. 25, no. 1, pp. 19–33, 2003.

[32] X.-H. Yang, H. Liu, J.-H. Chai, and X.-C. Zhao, "Observation on 27 elderly women in britain with lymphedema syndrome treated by acupuncture combined with medicine," *Chinese Acupuncture & Moxibustion*, vol. 29, no. 12, pp. 998–1000, 2009.

[33] L. L. Tian and G. F. Zhu, "Application of zebra fishes in studies on traditional Chinese medicines," *Zhongguo Zhong Yao Za Zhi*, vol. 40, no. 5, pp. 822–827, 2015.

[34] J.-N. Lai, H.-J. Chen, C.-C. Chen, J.-H. Lin, J.-S. Hwang, and J.-D. Wang, "Duhuo jisheng tang for treating osteoarthritis of the knee: a prospective clinical observation," *Chinese Medicine*, vol. 2, article 4, 2007.

[35] L. G. Ameye and W. S. S. Chee, "Osteoarthritis and nutrition. From nutraceuticals to functional foods: a systematic review of the scientific evidence," *Arthritis Research & Therapy*, vol. 8, no. 4, article R127, 2006.

[36] S. Teekachunhatean, P. Kunanusorn, N. Rojanasthien et al., "Chinese herbal recipe versus diclofenac in symptomatic treatment of osteoarthritis of the knee: a randomized controlled trial [ISRCTN70292892]," *BMC Complementary and Alternative Medicine*, vol. 4, article 19, 2004.

[37] F. Liu, G. Liu, W. Liang et al., "Duhuo Jisheng decoction treatment inhibits the sodium nitroprussiate-induced apoptosis of chondrocytes through the mitochondrial-dependent signaling pathway," *International Journal of Molecular Medicine*, vol. 34, no. 6, pp. 1573–1580, 2014.

[38] J. S. Chen, X. H. Li, H. T. Li et al., "Effect of water extracts from duhuo jisheng decoction on expression of chondrocyte G1 phase regulator mRNA," *Zhongguo Zhongyao Zazhi*, vol. 38, no. 22, pp. 3949–3952, 2013.

[39] G. Wu, W. Chen, H. Fan et al., "Duhuo Jisheng Decoction promotes chondrocyte proliferation through accelerated G1/S transition in osteoarthritis," *International Journal of Molecular Medicine*, vol. 32, no. 5, pp. 1001–1010, 2013.

[40] G. Wu, H. Fan, Y. Huang, C. Zheng, J. Ye, and X. Liu, "Duhuo Jisheng Decoctioncontaining serum promotes proliferation of interleukin1βinduced chondrocytes through the p16cyclin D1/CDK4Rb pathway," *Molecular Medicine Reports*, vol. 10, no. 5, pp. 2525–2534, 2014.

[41] F. Wei, S. Zou, A. Young, R. Dubner, and K. Ren, "Effects of four herbal extracts on adjuvant-induced inflammation and hyperalgesia in rats," *Journal of Alternative and Complementary Medicine*, vol. 5, no. 5, pp. 429–436, 1999.

[42] X. F. Cao and L. Zhou, "HPLC determination of osthole in Duhuojisheng pills," *China Practical Medicine*, vol. 5, no. 9, pp. 36–37, 2010.

[43] L. Wu, A. Wang, H. Geng, J. Tian, and H. Liu, "Determination of paeoniflorin in Duhuojisheng mixture by HPLC-ELSD," *China Pharmacist*, vol. 8, no. 2, pp. 122–123, 2005.

[44] S.-J. Wu, "Osthole attenuates inflammatory responses and regulates the expression of inflammatory mediators in HepG2 cells grown in differentiated medium from 3T3-L1 preadipocytes," *Journal of Medicinal Food*, vol. 18, no. 9, pp. 972–979, 2015.

[45] X. L. Wang, X. Shang, Y. Cui, X. Zhao, Y. Zhang, and M. Xie, "Osthole inhibits inflammatory cytokine release through PPARalpha/gamma-mediated mechanisms in LPS-stimulated 3T3-L1 adipocytes," *Immunopharmacology and Immunotoxicology*, vol. 37, no. 2, pp. 185–192, 2015.

[46] Y. K. Zhai, Y. L. Pan, Y. B. Niu et al., "The importance of the prenyl group in the activities of osthole in enhancing bone formation and inhibiting bone resorption *in vitro*," *International Journal of Endocrinology*, vol. 2014, Article ID 921954, 16 pages, 2014.

[47] D.-Z. Tang, W. Hou, Q. Zhou et al., "Osthole stimulates osteoblast differentiation and bone formation by activation of β-catenin–BMP signaling," *Journal of Bone and Mineral Research*, vol. 25, no. 6, pp. 1234–1245, 2010.

[48] L. Chen, J.-C. Liu, X.-N. Zhang et al., "Down-regulation of NR2B receptors partially contributes to analgesic effects of Gentiopicroside in persistent inflammatory pain," *Neuropharmacology*, vol. 54, no. 8, pp. 1175–1181, 2008.

[49] T. Sozański, A. Z. Kucharska, A. Szumny et al., "The protective effect of the *Cornus mas* fruits (cornelian cherry) on hypertriglyceridemia and atherosclerosis through PPARα activation in hypercholesterolemic rabbits," *Phytomedicine*, vol. 21, no. 13, pp. 1774–1784, 2014.

[50] Y.-Q. Zheng, W. Wei, L. Zhu, and J.-X. Liu, "Effects and mechanisms of Paeoniflorin, a bioactive glucoside from paeony

root, on adjuvant arthritis in rats," *Inflammation Research*, vol. 56, no. 5, pp. 182–188, 2007.

[51] W. Zhang and S.-M. Dai, "Mechanisms involved in the therapeutic effects of *Paeonia lactiflora* Pallas in rheumatoid arthritis," *International Immunopharmacology*, vol. 14, no. 1, pp. 27–31, 2012.

[52] S. Wang, Z. Gao, X. Chen et al., "The anticoagulant ability of ferulic acid and its applications for improving the blood compatibility of silk fibroin," *Biomedical Materials*, vol. 3, no. 4, Article ID 044106, 2008.

[53] J.-H. Zhang, J.-P. Wang, and H.-J. Wang, "Clinical study on effect of total panax notoginseng saponins on immune related inner environment imbalance in rheumatoid arthritis patients," *Chinese Journal of Integrated Traditional and Western Medicine*, vol. 27, no. 7, pp. 589–592, 2007.

[54] S.-H. Park, S.-K. Kim, I.-H. Shin, H.-G. Kim, and J.-Y. Choe, "Effects of AIF on knee osteoarthritis patients: double-blind, randomized placebo-controlled study," *The Korean Journal of Physiology & Pharmacology*, vol. 13, no. 1, pp. 33–37, 2009.

4

A *Fomitopsis pinicola Jeseng* Formulation Has an Antiobesity Effect and Protects against Hepatic Steatosis in Mice with High-Fat Diet-Induced Obesity

Hoe-Yune Jung,[1,2,3] Yosep Ji,[4] Na-Ri Kim,[1] Do-Young Kim,[1] Kyong-Tai Kim,[2] and Bo-Hwa Choi[1]

[1]*Pohang Center for Evaluation of Biomaterials, Pohang Technopark, Pohang 37668, Republic of Korea*
[2]*Department of Life Science, Division of Integrative Biosciences and Biotechnology, POSTECH, Pohang 37673, Republic of Korea*
[3]*R&D Center, NovMetaPharma Co., Ltd., Pohang 37668, Republic of Korea*
[4]*School of Life Science, Handong Global University, Pohang 37554, Republic of Korea*

Correspondence should be addressed to Bo-Hwa Choi; bhchoi@pohangtp.org

Academic Editor: Menaka C. Thounaojam

This study investigated the antiobesity effect of an extract of the Fomitopsis pinicola Jeseng-containing formulation (FAVA), which is a combination of four natural components: *Fomitopsis pinicola Jeseng*; *Acanthopanax senticosus*; *Viscum album coloratum*; and *Allium tuberosum*. High-fat diet- (HFD-) fed male C57BL/6J mice were treated with FAVA (200 mg/kg/day) for 12 weeks to monitor the antiobesity effect and amelioration of nonalcoholic fatty liver diseases (NAFLD). Body and white adipose tissue (WAT) weights were reduced in FAVA-treated mice, and a histological examination showed an amelioration of fatty liver in FAVA-treated mice without decreasing food consumption. Additionally, FAVA reduced serum lipid profiles, leptin, and insulin levels compared with the HFD control group. The FAVA extract suppressed lipogenic mRNA expression levels from WAT concomitantly with the cholesterol biosynthesis level in the liver. These results demonstrate the inhibitory effects of FAVA on obesity and NAFLD in the diet-induced obese (DIO) mouse model. Therefore, FAVA may be an effective therapeutic candidate for treating obesity and fatty liver caused by a high-fat diet.

1. Introduction

There is increasing consensus that obesity may be the main cause of various metabolic disorders. Obesity is caused by the combined effects of excess energy intake and reduced energy expenditure. It is one of the fastest growing disorders worldwide and is associated with various clinical symptoms in developed countries [1], such as hyperlipidemia, insulin resistance, and nonalcoholic fatty liver diseases (NAFLD) [2]. It is well known that excessive fat consumption is implicated in the development of obesity in mice [3], and long-term feeding with a high-fat diet (HFD) can induce obesity together with hyperlipidemia, insulin resistance, and NAFLD [4]. Hyperlipidemia is associated with high levels of lipids and lipoproteins in the blood and causes atherosclerosis and acute pancreatitis [5]. Although NAFLD is the second leading

cause of death in the general population [6, 7], there is no pharmacological agent known to reverse NAFLD. Recently, effective medical interventions have been focused on the modification of risk factors, such as diet and weight reduction [8].

Adipose tissue, an important repository for energy storage, regulates energy homeostasis. Adipogenesis, a differentiation process of adipocytes, involves changes in gene expression and cellular morphology. Adipocyte hypertrophy results from an excessive accumulation of lipids from the intake of inordinate energy sources such as HFD. During adipogenesis, peroxisome proliferator-activated receptor-γ (PPAR-γ) and CCAAT/enhancer-binding protein-α (C/EBP-α) play key roles as major transcriptional factors [9]. Expression of PPAR-γ, a transcription factor of the nuclear-receptor superfamily, and C/EBP-α, a member of the C/EBP family of basic leucine zipper class of transcription factors, increases during 3T3-L1 cell differentiation [10]. Lipin is also a central regulator of adipose tissue development. Mammalian lipin proteins have been shown to control gene expression and to enzymatically convert phosphatidate into diacylglycerol, an essential precursor in triacylglycerol and phospholipid synthesis [11]. Previous studies have established that lipin-1 is required at an early step in adipocyte differentiation for the induction of the adipogenic gene transcription program, including the key regulator PPAR-γ [12].

Acetoacetyl-CoA synthetase (AACS) regulation is related to cholesterol and lipid homeostasis [13]. Sterol response element binding protein-2 (SREBP-2) may play an essential role in the transcriptional regulation of AACS. SREBP-2 is a leucine zipper transcription factor that controls a rate-limiting enzyme in cholesterol synthesis, HMG-CoA reductase (HMGCR), when the factor binds sterol response element [14, 15].

The effects of *Acanthopanax senticosus, Allium tuberosum,* and *Viscum album coloratum* have been studied for inhibition of fatty acid synthase and prevention of obesity, as well as reducing hepatic steatosis [16–18]. *Fomitopsis pinicola Jeseng* has been reported for antihyperglycemic effect in diabetic rats [19]. In addition, it has been reported that β-glucan-rich extract, a major component of *Fomitopsis pinicola Jeseng*, effectively reduces adiposity [19, 20]. However, to our knowledge, no reports are available on the effect of *Fomitopsis pinicola Jeseng* on obesity.

In this study, we investigated the effect of FAVA in a high-fat diet-induced mouse model. The FAVA is a combination of herbal extracts (i.e., *Fomitopsis pinicola Jeseng, Acanthopanax senticosus, Allium tuberosum,* and *Viscum album coloratum*) at a ratio of 5 : 3 : 1 : 1. This study investigated the effect of a mixture containing dietary components on metabolic disorders including obesity, hyperlipidemia, and NAFLD using a high-fat diet-induced obesity mouse model and the molecular mechanism level of adipogenesis and cholesterol biosynthesis. Our results indicate the great potential of FAVA as a potential metabolic regulator of adipogenesis and cholesterol biosynthesis and as a potential therapeutic agent for preventing or treating obesity and NAFLD.

2. Materials and Methods

2.1. Preparation of FAVA. The oriental, medicinal, and herbal mixture used in this experiment (FAVA) was prepared as described previously [21–23]. Briefly, *Acanthopanax senticosus* and *Allium tuberosum* were extracted with 80% methanol while water extracted *Fomitopsis pinicola Jeseng* and *Viscum album coloratum* were purchased from commercial vendor (Mistle Biotech Co., Ltd., Korea). Each extraction of FAVA was resuspended in distilled water (DW) in a ratio of 50%, 30%, 10%, and 10%, respectively, and prepared in appropriate diluent for further *in vivo* study.

2.2. Animals and Diets. Lean, male C57BL/6J mice (7 weeks old) were purchased from Charles River Laboratories Japan, Inc. (Yokohama, Japan). All animal experiments were approved by the Ethics Review Committee of the Pohang

Center for the Evaluation of Biomaterials, Republic of Korea. All mice were housed for 1 week under a 12/12-h light/dark cycle in a temperature- ($22 \pm 1°C$) and humidity- ($55 \pm 5\%$) controlled room and fed standard laboratory chow and water *ad libitum* while FAVA, orlistat, and saline supplementation were performed using oral gavage once a day. To induce obesity, the mice were fed a HFD (Rodent Diet D12492, Research Diet, New Brunswick, NJ, USA) consisting of 60% kcal fat. Control mice were fed a low-fat chow diet (Rodent Diet D12450B, Research Diet, New Brunswick, NJ, USA) consisting of 10% kcal fat. Experimental mice were given FAVA or orlistat as a positive control (Chongqing Zein Pharmaceutical Co., Ltd., Chongqing, China). The mice were randomly divided into four groups ($n = 8$ per group) that were fed a low-fat chow diet (CHOW), a high-fat diet (HFD), HFD plus FAVA (200 mg/kg/day), or HFD plus orlistat (60 mg/kg/day). Animals were fed via oral feeding needles for 12 weeks, and the CHOW and HFD group received an equivalent volume of saline. Body weight was measured once a week, and food intake was measured three times per week during the course of the study. At the conclusion of the *in vivo* experiment, the mice were sacrificed by cervical vertebral dislocation, and the epididymal, mesenteric, and subcutaneous fat pads and liver were collected and weighed. The epididymal fat pad samples were stored at $-80°C$ until analysis.

2.3. Serum Analysis. Serum was collected by cardiac puncture, stored for 20 minutes at room temperature for coagulation, and then separated by centrifugation at 2,000 ×g for 20 minutes. The serum was stored at $-70°C$ until analysis. The levels of triglycerides, total cholesterol, high-density lipoprotein (HDL) cholesterol, low-density lipoprotein (LDL) cholesterol, glucose, alanine transaminase (ALT), aspartate transaminase (AST), BUN, and creatinine in serum were measured by using an automated biochemical analyzer (BS-390, Mindray Bio-Medical Electronics Co., Ltd., China).

2.4. Measurement of Leptin and Insulin. The leptin and insulin concentrations in serum were determined by a mouse enzyme-linked immunosorbent assay (ELISA) kit (Morinaga Institute of Biological Science, Yokohama, Japan). The preparation of serum samples is described above.

2.5. Abdominal Computed Tomography Analysis. Experiments of micro-computed tomography (micro-CT) were performed with an animal positron emission tomography (PET)/CT/single photon emission computed tomography (SPECT) system (Inveon, Siemens, USA) prior to the sacrifice of animals under 1.5–2% isoflurane in O_2 anesthesia. Computed tomography pictures were further analyzed using Siemens Inveon software to calculate the three-dimensional volume of the fat mass between lumbar vertebrae one to five.

2.6. Liver Histology. Liver tissues were immediately isolated after sacrifice. For hematoxylin and eosin (H&E) staining, the tissues were fixed in 10% formalin, processed, and embedded in paraffin prior to sectioning (10 μm) and staining. The liver

TABLE 1: Primers used in the reverse transcriptase-polymerase chain reaction analysis.

Gene name	Accession number		Sequence
Lipin-1	NM_172950	Forward	5′-TCA GAC ACT TTC AGT AAC TTC AC-3′
		Reverse	5′-TAT CAG CCT TCC CAG CAG-3′
C/EBP-α	NM_007678	Forward	5′-CGT CTA AGA TGA GGG AGT C-3′
		Reverse	5′-GGC ACA AGG TTA CTT CCT-3′
PPAR-γ	NM_001127330	Forward	5′-GAA AGA CAA CGG ACA AAT CAC-3′
		Reverse	5′-GAA ACT GGC ACC CTT GAA-3′
AACS	NM_030210	Forward	5′-AAG CCC AGA GTT ACG AGT AT-3′
		Reverse	5′-ACA CAG GAA TAG AGG AGT TCT-3′
HMGCR	NM_008255	Forward	5′-AGA ATA ATG TGC TAA GTA GTG CTA A-3′
		Reverse	5′-GCC TCT CTG AAC AAA GAC TC-3′
SREBP-2	NM_033218	Forward	5′-GCG ACC AGG AAG AAG AGA-3′
		Reverse	5′-ACA AAT CCC ACA GAG TCC A-3′
β-actin	NM_007393	Forward	5′-GGG AAG GTG ACA GCA TTG-3′
		Reverse	5′-ATG AAG TAT TAA GGC GGA AGA TT-3′

C/EBP-α: CCAAT/enhancer-binding protein-α; PPAR-γ: peroxisome proliferator-activated receptor-γ; AACS: acetoacetyl-CoA synthetase; HMGCR: HMG-CoA reductase; and SREBP-2: sterol regulatory element binding protein-2.

samples of 3 mice from each group (CHOW, HFD, HFD + FAVA, and HFD + ORLISTAT) were measured. Briefly, the following criteria were used for scoring hepatic steatosis: grade 0 (no fatty liver) and grade 1 (mild fatty liver), if hepatocytes occupied <33% of the hepatic parenchyma [24].

2.7. RNA Preparation and Real-Time PCR. Total RNA was extracted by ReliaPrep RNA Tissue Miniprep System (Promega) according to the manufacturer's instructions. RNA integrity was assessed by an automated microfluidics-based system (Bioanalyzer 2100, Agilent, Palo Alto, CA, USA). First-strand cDNA was synthesized with the iScript cDNA Synthesis Kit (Bio-Rad, Hercules, CA, USA), and real-time PCR was performed using an iCycler iQ Real-Time Detection System (Bio-Rad). PCR reactions were conducted with iQ SYBR Green Supermix (Bio-Rad). Real-time PCR analysis was performed using an iCycler iQ Real-Time Detection System (Bio-Rad). Amplification of real-time PCR was performed according to the protocols of Jung et al. [25]. The reaction was performed at 95°C for 3 min, followed by 39 cycles of amplification (95°C for 10 s, 58°C for 10 s, and 72°C for 30 s). A melting curve was produced to confirm a single gene-specific peak and detect primer/dimer formation by heating the samples from 65 to 95°C in 0.5°C increments with a dwell time at each temperature of 10 s, while continuously monitoring fluorescence. The mRNA levels of specific genes were normalized to those of β-actin. The primers used are listed in Table 1.

2.8. Statistical Analyses. The data (mean ± SE) were analyzed using GraphPad Prism (version 5.04, GraphPad Software, USA). Unpaired two-tailed Student's t-tests were used to evaluate differences between means as indicated and p values < 0.05 were considered significant.

3. Results

3.1. Effects of FAVA on Body Weight, Dietary Intake, and Fat Mass in White Adipose Tissue in HFD-Fed Mice. The effects of FAVA on body weights are shown in Figure 1(a). During the 12-week experiment, body weight was measured weekly, and food intake was measured every other day. After 9 weeks, the body weight of the mice in the HFD group was significantly higher than that of the mice in the CHOW group ($p < 0.0005$). The FAVA-treated group showed a significant decrease in body weight compared with the HFD group. At the end of the experiment, the body weight of the mice fed FAVA was 9.7 ± 2.0% lower ($p < 0.05$) than that of the mice in the HFD group, whereas HF diet plus orlistat-fed mice weighed almost the same as the mice that were fed FAVA (Figure 1(a)). These effects of FAVA on body weight were not due to decreased food intake, because the amount of kcal consumed per mouse over a 24-h period remained unchanged (Figure 1(b)). These data indicate that FAVA might have antiobesity effects *in vivo*, without affecting food intake. To investigate whether body weight loss was caused by decreased adiposity, the animals were sacrificed, and the epididymal fat pad, the mesenteric fat pad, and the subcutaneous fat pad were dissected and weighed. FAVA supplementation significantly suppressed the increase of fat mass in all white adipose tissues, including mesenteric, sub-cutaneous, and epididymal adipose tissue (Figures 1(c)–1(e)).

3.2. Effect of FAVA on Adiposity in HFD-Fed Mice. We performed micro-CT imaging to assess the effect of FAVA on adiposity. CT imaging showed a significant reduction in body fat profiles with FAVA treatment (Figure 2(a)). There was a significant reduction in fat volume (Figure 2(b)) and total body fat percentage in FAVA-fed groups compared with the HFD group (Figures 2(b) and 2(c)).

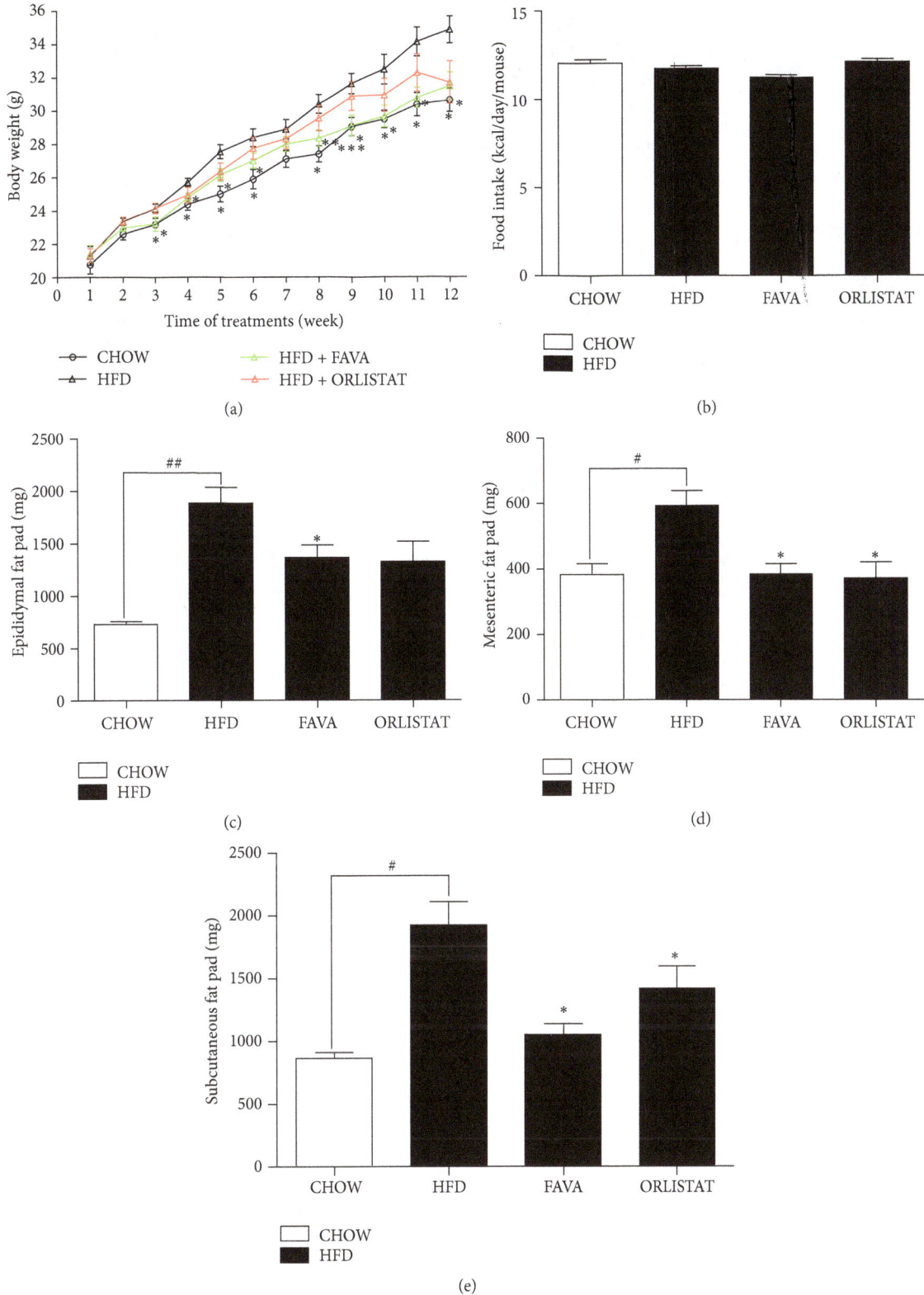

FIGURE 1: Effect of FAVA on body weight, food intake, and white fat pad in mice fed a high-fat diet for 12 weeks. (a) Changes in body weight gain at each treatment period are shown: (circle) CHOW: chow diet; (black triangle) HFD: high-fat diet; (red triangle) HFD + ORLISTAT: high-fat diet plus orlistat 60 mg/kg; and (green triangle) HFD + FAVA: high-fat diet plus FAVA 200 mg/kg. (b) Average food intake expressed as kcal/mouse/day. ((c)–(e)) Epididymal fat pad (c), mesenteric fat pad (d), and subcutaneous fat pad (e) weights expressed. The values represent the mean ± standard error of mean (SEM) ($^{\#}p < 0.05$ and $^{\#\#}p < 0.005$ versus the CHOW group; $^{*}p < 0.05$, $^{**}p < 0.005$, and $^{***}p < 0.0005$ versus the HFD group, $n = 8$ per group).

(a)

(b)

(c)

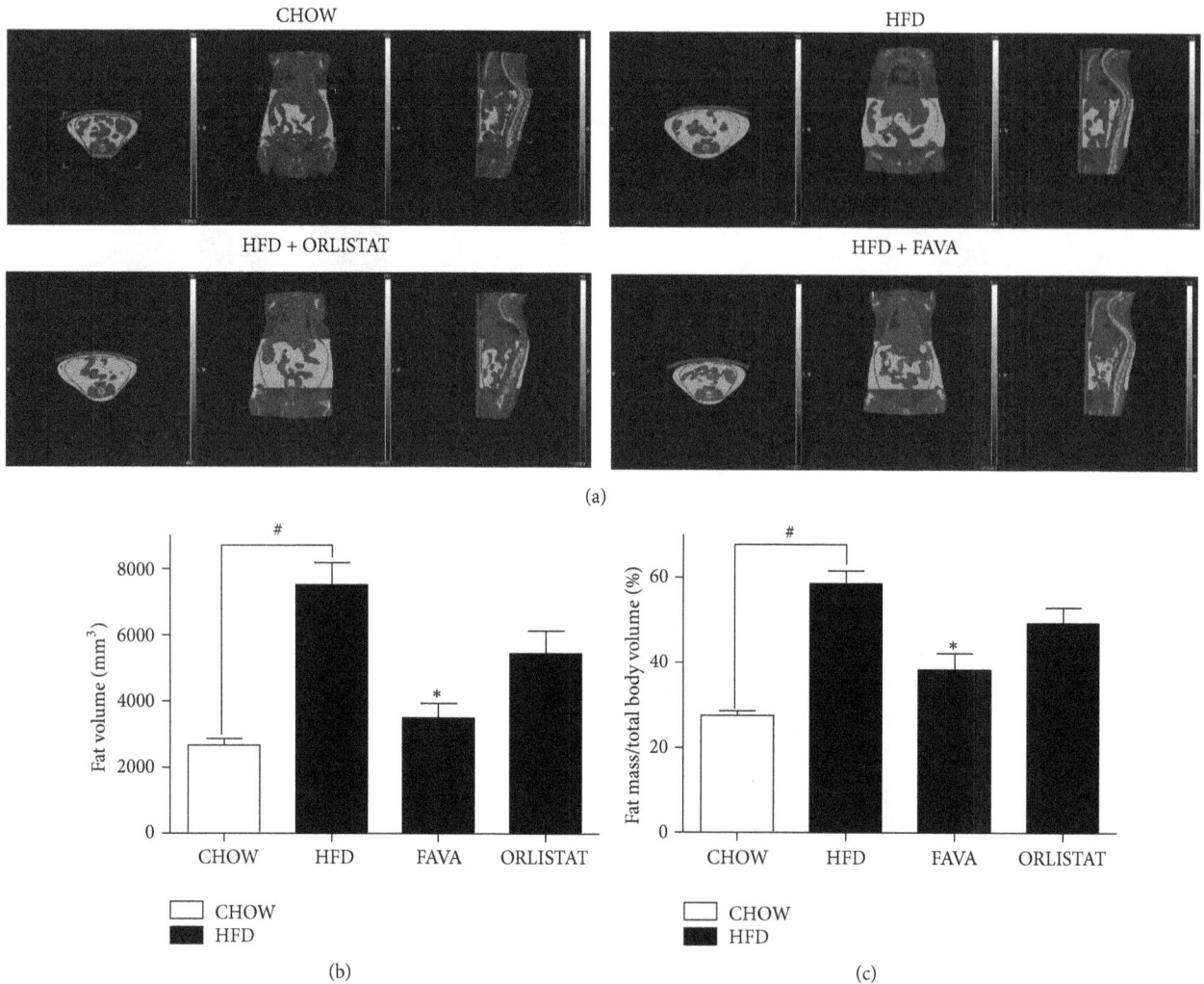

FIGURE 2: Effect of FAVA on high-fat diet-induced adiposity. (a) Micro-computed tomography (micro-CT) pictures were analyzed using Siemens Inveon software to calculate the three-dimensional volume of the fat mass between vertebrae number one to five of mice fed a chow diet (CHOW), high-fat diet (HFD), HFD with 60 mg/kg/day orlistat (ORLISTAT), or HFD with 200 mg/kg/day FAVA (FAVA). (b) Fat volumes (mm^3) in mice are shown. (c) Fat pad mass expressed as percentage of total body weight. The values represent the mean ± SEM ($^{\#}p < 0.05$ versus the CHOW group; $^{*}p < 0.05$ versus the HFD group, $n = 3$).

3.3. Effects of FAVA on Serum Insulin, Leptin, and Lipid Profiles in the Serum of HFD-Fed Mice.

The changes in the blood plasma parameters are shown in Figures 3(a)–3(e). As shown in Figures 3(a) and 3(b), HFD-induced obese mice showed significantly higher levels of serum insulin and leptin, whereas the FAVA group showed significantly decreased levels of serum insulin and leptin by 60.9 ± 8.1% and 40.4 ± 3.0%, respectively. Concomitant reductions of serum insulin and leptin levels were monitored in the orlistat group in a similar manner. Additionally, the FAVA group showed lower levels of serum total cholesterol and the ratio of LDL cholesterol/total cholesterol than those of the HFD group.

3.4. Effects of FAVA on mRNA Levels of Transcriptional Factors in Epididymal Fat Pad.

Because FAVA extract reduced fat mass in all white adipose tissues and serum insulin levels (Figures 1 and 3), we evaluated the effect of FAVA on the expression of various adipogenic and lipogenic genes [26]. PPARγ and C/EBPα are known to have roles in insulin sensitivity, lipogenesis, and lipolysis [27]. Lipin-1 is also thought to regulate the transcription of genes involved in adipocyte differentiation and fat synthesis and storage [28]. To investigate the antiadipogenic mechanism, the effects of FAVA on mRNA expression levels of PPARγ, C/EBPα, and lipin-1 were determined in the epididymal fat pad. The expression of both adipogenic genes, PPARγ and C/EBPα, was significantly decreased by FAVA (Figures 4(b) and 4(c)). Additionally, FAVA significantly suppressed lipin-1 expression by 95.6 ± 0.5% compared with that of the HFD group and was greater than that of the orlistat group as a positive control.

3.5. Effects of FAVA on Hepatic Histology of HFD-Fed C57BL/6 Mice and mRNA Levels of Cholesterol Biosynthesis in Liver.

A common characteristic among people with obesity is

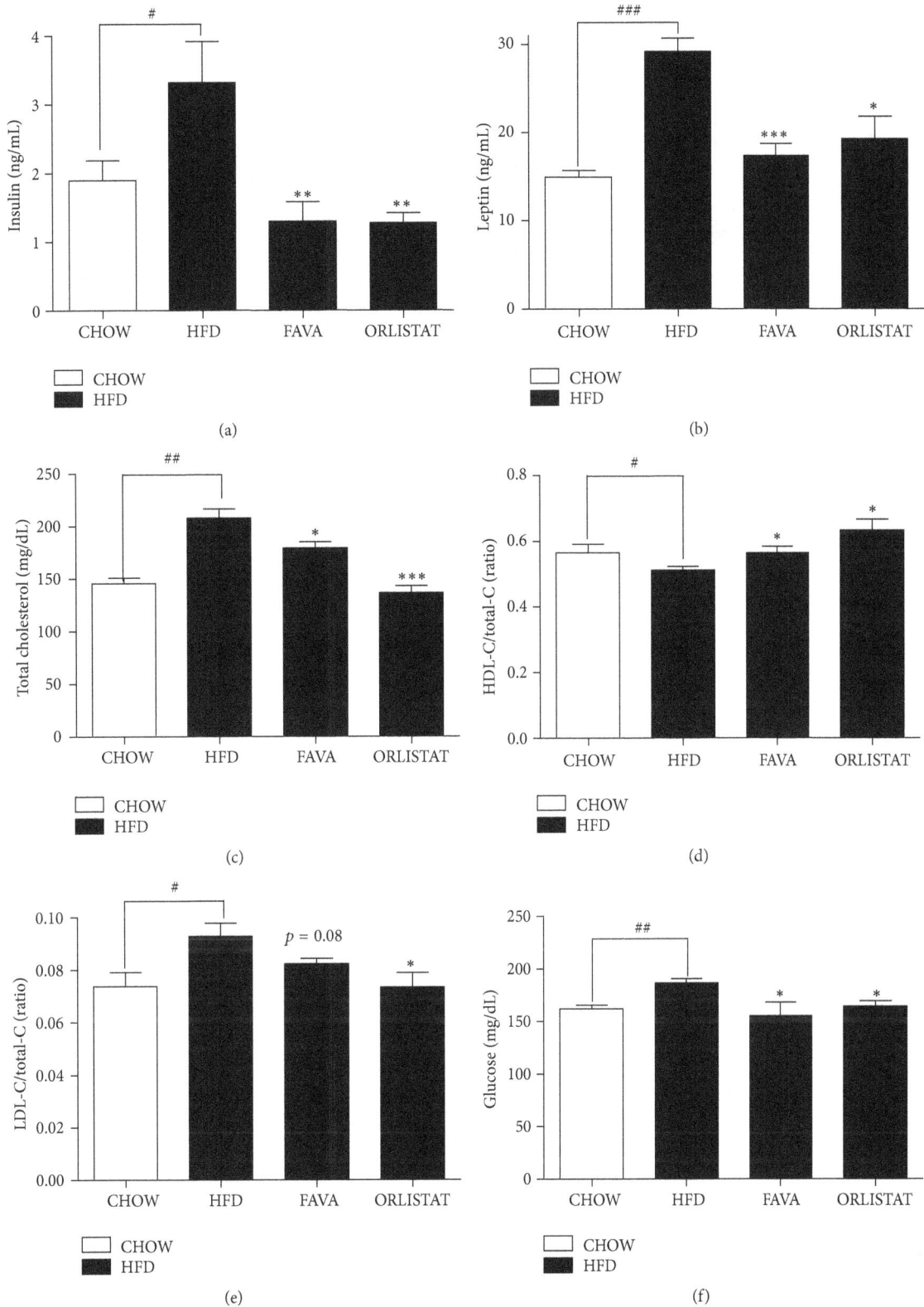

FIGURE 3: Effect of FAVA on serum insulin, leptin, and lipid profiles in mice fed a high-fat diet. Changes in insulin (a), leptin (b), total cholesterol (c), the ratio of HDL cholesterol/total cholesterol (d), and the ratio of LDL cholesterol/total cholesterol (e) of the mice were measured. The values represent the mean ± SEM ($^{#}p < 0.05$, $^{##}p < 0.005$, and $^{###}p < 0.0005$ versus the CHOW group; $^{*}p < 0.05$, $^{**}p < 0.005$, and $^{***}p < 0.0005$ versus the HFD group, $n = 5\sim7$ per group).

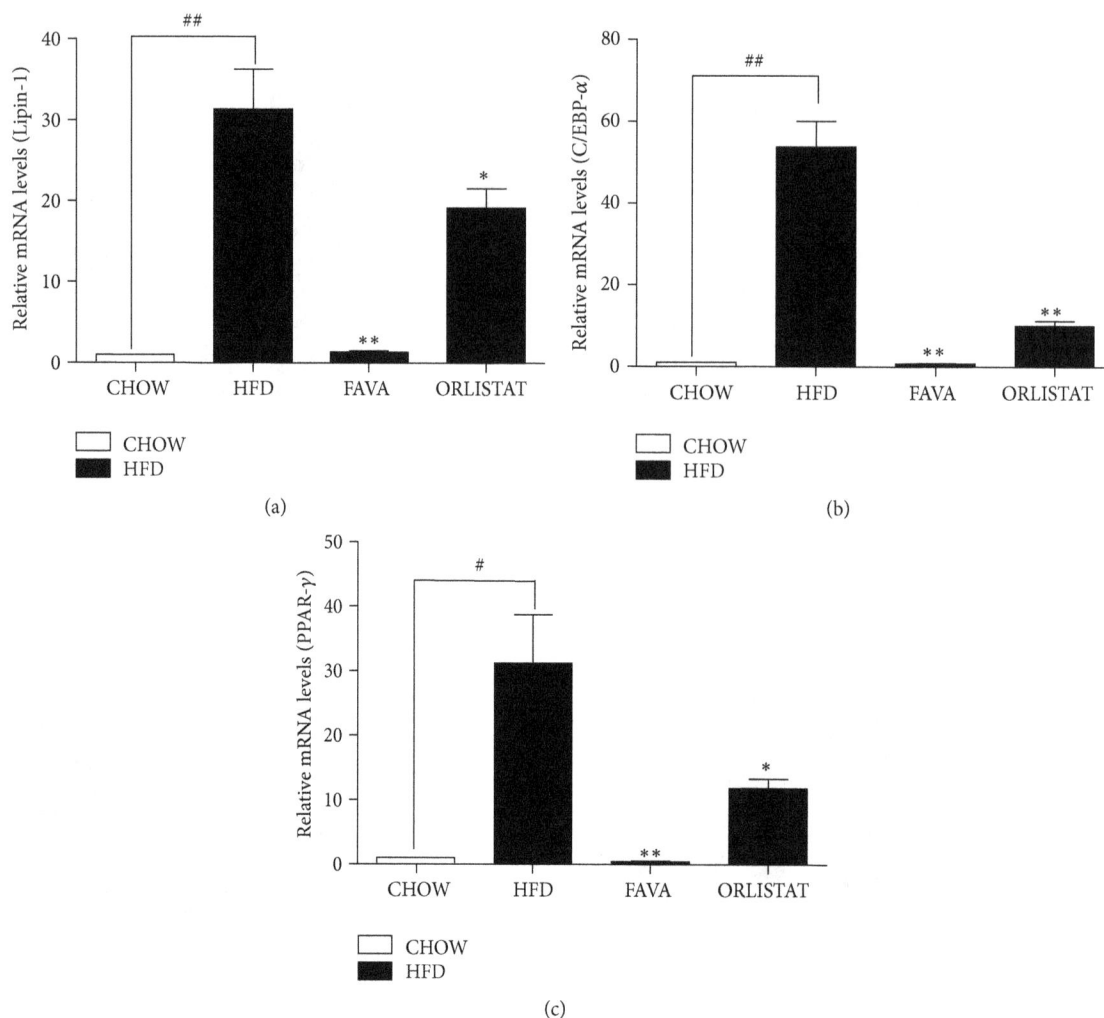

(a)

(b)

(c)

Figure 4: mRNA expressions of transcription factors in the epididymal fat pad of animals treated with HFD or HFD + ORLISTAT (high-fat diet plus orlistat 60 mg/kg) or FAVA (high-fat diet plus FAVA 200 mg/kg) or chow as quantified by real-time PCR. The graphs represent mRNA expression of transcription factors Lipin-1 (a), ACC and C/EBP-α (b), and PPAR-γ. The data represent the mean $\pm$ SEM ($^{\#}p < 0.05$ and $^{\#\#}p < 0.005$ versus the CHOW group; $^{*}p < 0.05$ and $^{**}p < 0.005$ versus the HFD group, $n = 5$).

the development of fatty liver [29, 30]. Therefore, we also analyzed the effect of FAVA on fatty liver development. Histological evaluation is regarded as the "gold standard" for assessing the presence and severity of NAFLD [31]. We histologically evaluated liver sections to determine the extent to which FAVA attenuated hepatic steatosis development. As shown in Figure 5(a), mild fatty liver was observed in mice that were fed a high-fat diet without FAVA. However, a marked reduction in the degree of steatosis was shown in livers from high-fat diet mice treated with FAVA. Moreover, FAVA treatment also decreased total serum cholesterol in mice to 13.7 $\pm$ 3.4% (Figure 3(c)). Therefore, we investigated whether SREBP-2, AACS, and HMGCR RNA in the mouse liver were induced by FAVA. Total RNA was prepared from mouse livers, and SREBP-2, AACS, and HMGCR mRNA levels were quantified using real-time PCR. SREBP-2, AACS, and HMGCR mRNA levels were dramatically suppressed in the mice that were fed FAVA (Figures 5(b) and 5(c)).

4. Discussion

Our study is the first to demonstrate that FAVA prevents weight gain in HFD-induced obesity in C57Bl/6 mice. Our results showed that body weight gain in groups fed a diet supplemented with FAVA was reduced compared with control HFD mice (Figure 1(a)). Epididymal, mesenteric, and subcutaneous fat pads in C57BL/6 mice were significantly reduced by FAVA supplementation (Figures 1(c)–1(e)). There was a significant reduction in subcutaneous and abdominal fat mass in FAVA-fed groups compared with the HFD group (Figures 2(a)–2(c)). Subcutaneous fat and abdominal fat are the major types of white adipose tissue. Abdominal obesity is associated with an increased risk of cardiovascular diseases and insulin resistance [32]. This study also provides evidence that dietary supplementation of FAVA protects against hepatic steatosis development (Figure 5(a)). We have considered the possibility that the effect of FAVA

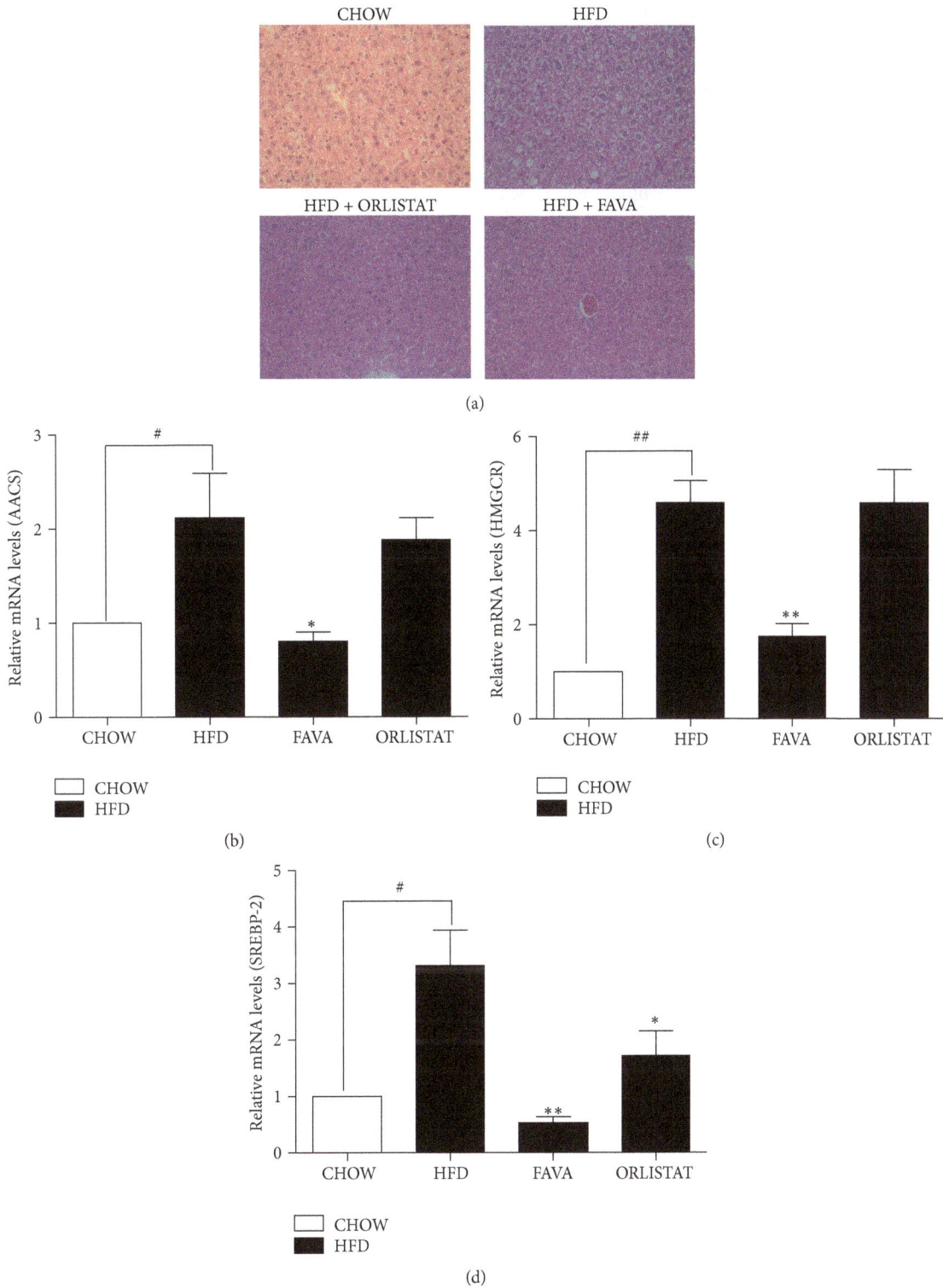

(a)

(b)

(c)

(d)

FIGURE 5: Effect of FAVA on hepatic steatosis and mRNA expressions of cholesterol biosynthesis in the liver of mice. (a) Hematoxylin and eosin staining of liver from mice fed chow diet (CHOW), high-fat diet (HFD), or high-fat diet supplemented with orlistat at 60 mg/kg/day (HFD + ORLISTAT) or high-fat diet supplemented with FAVA at 200 mg/kg/day (HFD + FAVA) (40x magnification). ((b)–(d)) The graphs represent mRNA expression of cholesterol synthesis factors AACS (b), HMGCR (c), and SREBP2 (d), which was analyzed by real-time PCR. The data represent the mean ± SEM ($^{\#}p < 0.05$ and $^{\#\#}p < 0.005$ versus the CHOW group; $^{*}p < 0.05$ and $^{**}p < 0.005$ versus the HFD group, $n = 5$).

may be mediated through food intake because decreased food intake would be expected to significantly affect body weight, which influences hepatic steatosis. In this study, however, there was no difference in food intake-induced increase of body weight between the FAVA-fed and non-FAVA-fed groups (Figure 1(b)). This result suggests that FAVA directly protected against obesity and hepatic steatosis independent of food intake.

Obesity is most likely to cause hyperlipidemia, which is considered the leading cardiovascular risk. The hallmark of dyslipidemia in obesity is hypertriglyceridemia in combination with the preponderance of high LDL and low HDL cholesterol [33]. This study shows that, in high-fat diet-fed mice, FAVA supplementation significantly reduced serum levels of cholesterol and the ratio of LDL cholesterol/total cholesterol (Figures 3(c) and 3(d)). Furthermore, insulin levels were increased in the HFD group and were decreased significantly by FAVA supplementation (Figure 3(a)). In the case of prediabetes, increases of blood glucose stimulate the secretion of insulin and subsequently induce hyperinsulinemia to a normal blood glucose range. Hyperinsulinemia, which is a biomarker of insulin resistance, is frequently accompanied by obesity [34]. Leptin is a fat-derived hormone that plays an important role in appetite control and energy expenditure [35]. It has been reported that the concentration of serum leptin is associated with general adiposity and reflects the body fat content [36]. In this report, it was demonstrated that FAVA treatment suppressed the plasma leptin level in mice fed with HFD (Figure 3(b)). Moreover, the weight of adipose tissues strongly correlated with the plasma leptin level. These results confirm that FAVA treatment exerted an antiobesity effect in the diet-induced obesity C57BL/6 mouse model.

PPAR-γ, a transcription factor predominantly expressed in adipose tissue, plays an essential role in adipocyte differentiation, lipid storage, and glucose homeostasis [37]. Additionally, adipogenesis is highly regulated by two primary adipogenic transcription factors, PPAR-γ and C/EBPs [38]. Among those factors, PPAR-γ is well known as the key regulator of adipogenic transcription [10]. PPAR-γ is also known to bind to the C/EBP-α promoter region that induces the expression of C/EBP-α [39]. C/EBP-α is a promising candidate transcription factor for directly controlling adipocyte differentiation [40]. We found that FAVA significantly downregulated PPAR-γ and C/EBP-α mRNA levels in the epididymal fat pad. This effect might be explained in two ways: FAVA either inhibited PPAR-γ and C/EBP-α or suppressed the upstream molecules. Lipin-1 is also required in adipocyte differentiation for the induction of the adipogenic gene transcription [12]. We found that FAVA could inhibit adipocyte differentiation through the suppression of lipin-1.

Acetoacetyl-CoA synthetase (AACS) can facilitate the incorporation of ketones into lipogenesis [13]. Hasegawa et al. [13] demonstrated that the AACS gene, which encodes the ketone body-utilizing enzyme, is transcriptionally regulated by SREBP-2 and the knockdown of SREBP-2 induced downregulation of AACS and HMGCR gene expression. Additionally, ketone body metabolism via AACS plays an essential role in cholesterol homeostasis. In this study, we

showed that the treatment of mice with FAVA resulted in a decrease of SREBP2, AACS, and HMGCR mRNA levels. Therefore, our results suggest that FAVA improves obesity, hyperlipidemia, and NAFLD and that FAVA treatment might be a promising adjuvant therapy in the management of these metabolic disorders.

5. Conclusions

FAVA had a marked inhibitory effect on the development of obesity and NAFLD in a high-fat diet-induced obesity mouse model. Inhibiting transcription factors and adipocyte-specific lipogenic genes and decreasing cholesterol synthesis are two possible mechanisms for the antiobesity effect of FAVA. This study suggests that FAVA might be a potential dietary supplement for preventing obesity and NAFLD.

Competing Interests

The authors declare that they have no competing interests.

Acknowledgments

The work was supported by Current Subsidies of Pohang city.

References

[1] B. M. Spiegelman and J. S. Flier, "Obesity and the regulation of energy balance," *Cell*, vol. 104, no. 4, pp. 531–543, 2001.

[2] C. Couillard, P. Mauriège, P. Imbeault et al., "Hyperleptinemia is more closely associated with adipose cell hypertrophy than with adipose tissue hyperplasia," *International Journal of Obesity*, vol. 24, no. 6, pp. 782–788, 2000.

[3] M. Rebuffé-Scrive, R. Surwit, M. Feinglos, C. Kuhn, and J. Rodin, "Regional fat distribution and metabolism in a new mouse model (C57BL/6J) of non-insulin-dependent diabetes mellitus," *Metabolism*, vol. 42, no. 11, pp. 1405–1409, 1993.

[4] R. S. Surwit, C. M. Kuhn, C. Cochrane, J. A. McCubbin, and M. N. Feinglos, "Diet-induced type II diabetes in C57BL/6J mice," *Diabetes*, vol. 37, no. 9, pp. 1163–1167, 1988.

[5] N. Ewald, P. D. Hardt, and H.-U. Kloer, "Severe hypertriglyceridemia and pancreatitis: presentation and management," *Current Opinion in Lipidology*, vol. 20, no. 6, pp. 497–504, 2009.

[6] Z. M. Younossi, A. M. Diehl, and J. P. Ong, "Nonalcoholic fatty liver disease: an agenda for clinical research," *Hepatology*, vol. 35, no. 4, pp. 746–752, 2002.

[7] A. Franzese, P. Vajro, A. Argenziano et al., "Liver involvement in obese children: ultrasonography and liver enzyme levels at diagnosis and during follow-up in an Italian population," *Digestive Diseases and Sciences*, vol. 42, no. 7, pp. 1428–1432, 1997.

[8] J. Medina, L. I. Fernández-Salazar, L. García-Buey, and R. Moreno-Otero, "Approach to the pathogenesis and treatment of nonalcoholic steatohepatitis," *Diabetes Care*, vol. 27, no. 8, pp. 2057–2066, 2004.

[9] R. F. Morrison and S. R. Farmer, "Insights into the transcriptional control of adipocyte differentiation," *Journal of Cellular Biochemistry*, vol. 76, supplement 33, pp. 59–67, 1999.

[10] E. D. Rosen, C. J. Walkey, P. Puigserver, and B. M. Spiegelman, "Transcriptional regulation of adipogenesis," *Genes and Development*, vol. 14, no. 11, pp. 1293–1307, 2000.

[11] R. Ugrankar, Y. Liu, J. Provaznik, S. Schmitt, and M. Lehmann, "Lipin is a central regulator of adipose tissue development and function in *Drosophila melanogaster*," *Molecular and Cellular Biology*, vol. 31, no. 8, pp. 1646–1656, 2011.

[12] P. Zhang, K. Takeuchi, L. S. Csaki, and K. Reue, "Lipin-1 phosphatidic phosphatase activity modulates phosphatidate levels to promote peroxisome proliferator-activated receptor γ (PPARγ) gene expression during adipogenesis," *Journal of Biological Chemistry*, vol. 287, no. 5, pp. 3485–3494, 2012.

[13] S. Hasegawa, K. Noda, A. Maeda, M. Matsuoka, M. Yamasaki, and T. Fukui, "Acetoacetyl-CoA synthetase, a ketone body-utilizing enzyme, is controlled by SREBP-2 and affects serum cholesterol levels," *Molecular Genetics and Metabolism*, vol. 107, no. 3, pp. 553–560, 2012.

[14] S. M. Vallett, H. B. Sanchez, J. M. Rosenfeld, and T. F. Osborne, "A direct role for sterol regulatory element binding protein in activation of 3-hydroxy-3-methylglutaryl coenzyme A reductase gene," *The Journal of Biological Chemistry*, vol. 271, no. 21, pp. 12247–12253, 1996.

[15] X. Hua, C. Yokoyama, J. Wu et al., "SREBP-2, a second basic-helix–loop–helix–leucine zipper protein that stimulates transcription by binding to a sterol regulatory element," *Proceedings of the National Academy of Sciences of the United States of America*, vol. 90, no. 24, pp. 11603–11607, 1993.

[16] Y.-S. Cha, S.-J. Rhee, and Y.-R. Heo, "*Acanthopanax senticosus* extract prepared from cultured cells decreases adiposity and obesity indices in C57BL/6J mice fed a high fat diet," *Journal of Medicinal Food*, vol. 7, no. 4, pp. 422–429, 2004.

[17] W. X. Tian, X. F. Ma, S. Y. Zhang, Y. H. Sun, and B. H. Li, "Fatty acid synthase inhibitors from plants and their potential application in the prevention of metabolic syndrome," *Clinical Oncology and Cancer Research*, vol. 8, no. 1, pp. 1–9, 2011.

[18] H.-Y. Jung, Y.-H. Kim, I.-B. Kim et al., "The Korean mistletoe (*Viscum album coloratum*) extract has an antiobesity effect and protects against hepatic steatosis in mice with high-fat diet-induced obesity," *Evidence-Based Complementary and Alternative Medicine*, vol. 2013, Article ID 168207, 9 pages, 2013.

[19] S.-I. Lee, J.-S. Kim, S.-H. Oh, K.-Y. Park, H.-G. Lee, and S.-D. Kim, "Antihyperglycemic effect of *Fomitopsis pinicola* extracts in streptozotocin-induced diabetic rats," *Journal of Medicinal Food*, vol. 11, no. 3, pp. 518–524, 2008.

[20] Y. Zhang, L. Xia, W. Pang et al., "A novel soluble β-1,3-d-glucan Salecan reduces adiposity and improves glucose tolerance in high-fat diet-fed mice," *British Journal of Nutrition*, vol. 109, no. 2, pp. 254–262, 2013.

[21] M. Sung, H. Y. Jung, J. Choi, S. Lee, B. Choi, and S. S. Park, "Preparation of functional healthy drinks by *Acanthopanax senticosus* extracts," *Journal of Life Science*, vol. 24, no. 9, pp. 959–966, 2014.

[22] J.-M. Gu and S.-S. Park, "Optimization of endoglucanase production from *Fomitopsis pinicola* mycelia," *Korean Journal of Microbiology and Biotechnology*, vol. 41, no. 2, pp. 145–152, 2013.

[23] M. Lee, B. Ryu, M. Kim, Y. Lee, and G. Moon, "Protective effect of dietary buchu (Chinese chives) against oxidative damage from aging and ultraviolet irradiation in ICR mice skin," *Nutraceuticals and Food*, vol. 7, no. 3, pp. 238–244, 2002.

[24] R. S. Bruno, C. E. Dugan, J. A. Smyth, D. A. DiNatale, and S. I. Koo, "Green tea extract protects leptin-deficient, spontaneously obese mice from hepatic steatosis and injury," *The Journal of Nutrition*, vol. 138, no. 2, pp. 323–331, 2008.

[25] H.-Y. Jung, J.-C. Shin, S.-M. Park, N.-R. Kim, W. Kwak, and B.-H. Choi, "*Pinus densiflora* extract protects human skin

fibroblasts against UVB-induced photoaging by inhibiting the expression of MMPs and increasing type I procollagen expression," *Toxicology Reports*, vol. 1, pp. 658–666, 2014.

[26] L. Fajas, "Adipogenesis: a cross-talk between cell proliferation and cell differentiation," *Annals of Medicine*, vol. 35, no. 2, pp. 79–85, 2003.

[27] C. E. Lowe, S. O'Rahilly, and J. J. Rochford, "Adipogenesis at a glance," *Journal of Cell Science*, vol. 124, no. 16, pp. 2681–2686, 2011.

[28] K. A. Fawcett, N. Grimsey, R. J. F. Loos et al., "Evaluating the role of LPIN1 variation in insulin resistance, body weight, and human lipodystrophy in U.K. populations," *Diabetes*, vol. 57, no. 9, pp. 2527–2533, 2008.

[29] Y.-X. Wang, C.-H. Lee, S. Tiep et al., "Peroxisome-proliferator-activated receptor delta activates fat metabolism to prevent obesity," *Cell*, vol. 113, no. 2, pp. 159–170, 2003.

[30] J. E. Schaffer, "Lipotoxicity: when tissues overeat," *Current Opinion in Lipidology*, vol. 14, no. 3, pp. 281–287, 2003.

[31] E. M. Brunt, "Pathology of nonalcoholic steatohepatitis," *Hepatology Research*, vol. 33, no. 2, pp. 68–71, 2005.

[32] A. Wronska and Z. Kmiec, "Structural and biochemical characteristics of various white adipose tissue depots," *Acta Physiologica*, vol. 205, no. 2, pp. 194–208, 2012.

[33] B. Klop, J. W. F. Elte, and M. C. Cabezas, "Dyslipidemia in obesity: mechanisms and potential targets," *Nutrients*, vol. 5, no. 4, pp. 1218–1240, 2013.

[34] A. G. Tabák, C. Herder, W. Rathmann, E. J. Brunner, and M. Kivimäki, "Prediabetes: a high-risk state for diabetes development," *The Lancet*, vol. 379, no. 9833, pp. 2279–2290, 2012.

[35] A. M. Brennan and C. S. Mantzoros, "Drug insight: the role of leptin in human physiology and pathophysiology—emerging clinical applications," *Nature Clinical Practice Endocrinology & Metabolism*, vol. 2, no. 6, pp. 318–327, 2006.

[36] H. Staiger and H.-U. Häring, "Adipocytokines: fat-derived humoral mediators of metabolic homeostasis," *Experimental and Clinical Endocrinology and Diabetes*, vol. 113, no. 2, pp. 67–79, 2005.

[37] Y.-Y. Sung, T. Yoon, W.-K. Yang, S. J. Kim, D.-S. Kim, and H. K. Kim, "The antiobesity effect of *Polygonum aviculare* L. Ethanol extract in high-fat diet-induced obese mice," *Evidence-Based Complementary and Alternative Medicine*, vol. 2013, Article ID 626397, 11 pages, 2013.

[38] A. Soukas, N. D. Socci, B. D. Saatkamp, S. Novelli, and J. M. Friedman, "Distinct transcriptional profiles of adipogenesis in vivo and in vitro," *The Journal of Biological Chemistry*, vol. 276, no. 36, pp. 34167–34174, 2001.

[39] E. D. Rosen, C.-H. Hsu, X. Wang et al., "C/EBPα induces adipogenesis through PPARγ: a unified pathway," *Genes and Development*, vol. 16, no. 1, pp. 22–26, 2002.

[40] Z. Wu, Y. Xie, N. L. R. Bucher, and S. R. Farmer, "Conditional ectopic expression of C/EBPβ in NIH-3T3 cells induces PPARγ and stimulates adipogenesis," *Genes and Development*, vol. 9, no. 19, pp. 2350–2363, 1995.

5

The Genus *Phyllanthus*: An Ethnopharmacological, Phytochemical, and Pharmacological Review

Xin Mao,[1,2] **Ling-Fang Wu,**[1] **Hong-Ling Guo,**[3] **Wen-Jing Chen,**[1] **Ya-Ping Cui,**[1]
Qi Qi,[1] **Shi Li,**[1] **Wen-Yi Liang,**[1] **Guang-Hui Yang,**[1] **Yan-Yan Shao,**[1] **Dan Zhu,**[1]
Gai-Mei She,[1] **Yun You,**[2,4] **and Lan-Zhen Zhang**[1]

[1]*School of Chinese Materia Medica, Beijing University of Chinese Medicine, Beijing 100102, China*
[2]*Institute of Chinese Materia Medica, China Academy of Chinese Medical Sciences, Beijing 100700, China*
[3]*Institute of Zoology, Chinese Academy of Sciences, Beijing 100101, China*
[4]*Key laboratory of Chinese Internal Medicine, Beijing University of Chinese Medicine, Beijing 100700, China*

Correspondence should be addressed to Yun You; youyunrice@126.com and Lan-Zhen Zhang; zhanglanzhen01@126.com

Academic Editor: Gloria Brusotti

The plants of the genus *Phyllanthus* (Euphorbiaceae) have been used as traditional medicinal materials for a long time in China, India, Brazil, and the Southeast Asian countries. They can be used for the treatment of digestive disease, jaundice, and renal calculus. This review discusses the ethnopharmacological, phytochemical, and pharmacological studies of *Phyllanthus* over the past few decades. More than 510 compounds have been isolated, the majority of which are lignins, triterpenoids, flavonoids, and tannins. The researches of their remarkable antiviral, antioxidant, antidiabetic, and anticancer activities have become hot topics. More pharmacological screenings and phytochemical investigations are required to support the traditional uses and develop leading compounds.

1. Introduction

Phyllanthus (Euphorbiaceae) is a large genus and widely distributed in tropical and subtropical zones like tropical Africa, tropical America, Asia, and Oceania. This genus, consisting of more than 700 species, can be classified into 11 subgenuses [1, 2]. The most popular 24 species are chiefly belonging to subgenus *Kirganelia*, *Cicca*, and *Phyllanthus* and they are traditionally used by different nationalities.

Genus *Phyllanthus* has been employed as herbal drugs for a long time in China, India, Brazil, and Southeast Asian countries. The most abundant species are used in India and have a beneficial role in Ayurveda for the treatment of digestive, genitourinary, respiratory, and skin diseases [3, 4]. In China, herbs and their prescriptions are used to treat hepatitis B, hypertension, dropsy, and sore throat [2]. These herbal drugs are employed by local inhabitants of Thailand, Latin America (especially Brazil), and Africa to cure jaundice, renal calculus, and malaria, respectively [5–7].

By virtue of the wide uses of *Phyllanthus* as anti-HIV, anticancer, and anti-HBV agents, there has been considerable interest in the investigations of this genus in recent years and the researches about pharmacology and chemistry had been finished in a deep going way. This report reviews the ethnopharmacological, phytochemical, and pharmacological investigations of *Phyllanthus* over the past few decades. More than three hundred articles were selected from the data taken from SciFinder Scholar database by searching the keyword "*Phyllanthus*".

2. Ethnopharmacological Uses

The traditional application experiences of these herbs may have reference value for the treatment of recent diseases. Botanical data, folk name, and medicinal properties of twenty-four *Phyllanthus* species are depicted in Table 1. In Asia, seventeen plants are considered to have bitter and astringent taste. They are regarded as stomachic, diuretic, febrifuge,

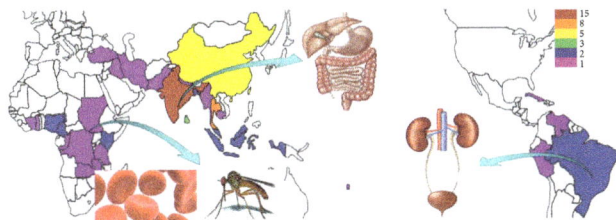

FIGURE 1: Traditional use of genus *Phyllanthus* in different countries. Different color represents the number of plants traditionally used in different countries: red, orange, yellow, green, blue, and purple represent fifteen, eight, five, three, two, and one kinds of plants under use, respectively. In Asia, *Phyllanthus* are used to treat digestive system disease, in south America, *Phyllanthus* are used to treat urinary system disease, and in Africa, *Phyllanthus* are used to treat malaria and wound.

deobstruent, and antiseptic agents and effective remedies for hepatopathy, hypertensive, diabetes, and jaundice. In Africa, six herbs are widely employed by many tribes for the treatment of malaria wound and tetanus. Six species are used extensively in Latin America for the treatment of urination disorder and diabetes. The distribution and the main uses of *Phyllanthus* are pictured in Figure 1.

2.1. Asia.
In Asia, the clinical use of genus *Phyllanthus* is very prevalent. The fruit of *P. emblica* has a long history of use in India and is called "amla" or "Indian gooseberry." As a tonic in Indian Ayurveda, it is often used for liver diseases [3, 4]. This fruit is known as "yuganzi" in China. It has sweet and slightly astringent taste and is used for clearing heat from throat and moistening lung for arresting cough in Traditional Chinese Medicine (TCM). In Tibetan medicine this herb is used to treat blood and bile disease, and its preparations are clinically applicable to hypertension and anuria [2]. In Thailand, it is named "makham pom" and is employed to treat gastrointestinal chronic diseases. *P. emblica* is commonly used together with *Terminalia chebula* and *T. belerica* and called "Triphala." "Triphala" is used as a clinical treatment protocol of gastropathy in India and as a remedy for pestilence and fatigue in China [62].

In India, fifteen species of genus *Phyllanthus* are widely used by indigenous medicine. These plants have bitter and astringent taste and are considered as stomachic, diuretic, febrifuge, deobstruent, antiseptic, and effective remedies for hepatopathy. Some herbs such as *P. niruri*, *P. amarus*, *P. fraternus*, *P. debilis*, and *P. maderaspatensis* share the same name "bhuiamlki" [29]. The fruits of "bhuiamlki" are employed by Ayurveda to cure jaundice. *P. simplex*, *P. reticulatus*, and *P. acidus* are therapy of urinary disease and have the names of "bhuiaveli," "pancoli," and "harfarauri," respectively. The leaves of *P. polyphyllus*, called "sirunelli," are used for liver disease. Additionally, the rest of these herbs can be employed as remedies for diabetes, jaundice, wound, fever, and inflammation.

In China, five herbs are commonly used by TCM, Tibetan medicine, Dai People, and Yi People [2]. They have bitter and

sweet taste and are usually used as prescriptions. The whole plant of *P. urinaria*, known as "yexiazhu," can clear heat-toxin and remove dampness and is employed to treat jaundice, enteritis, diarrhea, and dropsy. Besides, the TCM prescription, named "yexiazhu capsule," performs a beneficial role in curing hepatitis B. Other herbs such as *P. reticulatus*, *P. niruri*, and *P. simplex* are beneficial to the treatment of ophthalmopathy, urinary infection, inflammation, and rheumatism.

In Thailand, eight herbs of this genus are widely used by residents. *P. amarus*, *P. urinaria*, and *P. virgatus* share the name "look tai bai," all of which are used for treating gonorrhea, jaundice, diabetic, and liver disease. *P. acidus* has three names: "otaheiti gooseberry," "star gooseberry," and "mayom," and it can be used as remedy for hypertensive, constipation, skin disease, and fever. The rest of herbal drugs including *P. taxodiifolius*, *P. niruri*, and *P. reticulatus* are employed for the treatment of urination disorder and malaria.

2.2. Africa.
Many African tribes employ six plants of genus *Phyllanthus* to treat malaria, fever, and wound. *P. muellerianus* is the most popular herbal drugs of this genus in Africa. It is named "mbolongo" in Cameroon. In Ghana and Cameroon, the stem bark is used for the therapy of wound and tetanus. In Nigeria, Zambia, and Ivory Coast the leaves and root are applied as a fever remedy. In Kenya, the root of *P. polyanthus* is used to cure sexually transmitted diseases. What is more, the whole plants of *P. muellerianus* and *P. reticulatus* can be used for the treatment of malaria.

2.3. Latin America.
About six herb species of this genus are used in many countries in Latin America. In Brazil, *P. tenellus* is popularly known as "quebra-pedras" whose leaves can be used as diuretic. *P. amarus* is named "chanca piedra" in Peru and the leaves are employed for diabetic and jaundice therapy or as sedative and astringent. *P. sellowianus* is called "sarandi blanco" in South America and used widely in folk for the treatment of urination disorder and diabetes.

In summary, *P. emblica*, *P. reticulatus*, and *P. niruri* are the top three species widely used around the world. *P. niruri* is probably the most widespread herb of *Phyllanthus*, which is named "chanka piedra," "bhuiamlki," "zhuzicao," "dukung anak," "quebra-pedra," and "chanca piedra." Its whole plant can treat inflammation, lithiasis, fever, malaria, hepatitis, and gonorrhea [7, 18, 19, 21, 22].

3. Chemical Constituents

More than 510 compounds have been isolated from *Phyllanthus*, the majority of which are lignins, triterpenoids, flavonoids, and tannins. The compositions isolated from each species and their biological activities are partially summarized in Table 2. Lignins and tannins exhibit various activities and are considered to be the biological active compounds of this genus. Corilagin, geraniin, and gallic acid are three most prevalent compounds in this genus, and the pharmacological researches mainly focus on phyllanthin, niranthin, and geraniin.

TABLE 1: The traditional use of *Phyllanthus*.

Species	Region	Local name	Plant part used	Traditional use	Reference
	Bangladesh		Fruit	Constipation, urinary diseases	[8]
	Burma		Juice/bark	Constipation, hemostasis, keratitis	[8]
	Cambodia		Leaves	Muscle pain, fever	[8]
	China	Yuganzi	Fruit	Digestive disease, hypertension, fever, respiratory inflammation	[8]
	Fiji		Fruit	Tonic	[8]
	India	Amla, Indian gooseberry	Fruit	Diabetes, chronic diarrhea, inflammation, fever, liver diseases, stomach ulcers, metabolic disorders, skin disorders, beauty care	[3, 4]
P. emblica	Indonesia		Leaves/fruit	Diarrhea, abdominal pain, stomach Disease, gallbladder disease, bleeding	[8]
	Iran		Fruit	Parasitic	[8]
	Iraq		Fruit	Bleeding, gastrointestinal system disorder	[8]
	Nepal		Stem/fruit/seed	Urination disorder, constipation, bleeding, diarrhea, ophthalmopathy, asthma, bronchitis	[8]
	Pakistan		Fruit	Diarrhea, preterm, skin diseases, gonorrhea, ophthalmopathy, anemia, hair care	[8, 9]
	Sri Lanka		Fruit/whole plant	Constipation, indigestion, keratitis	[8]
	Thailand	Makham pom	Juice/bark	Diarrhea, leukorrhagia, cough, parasitosis, gastrointestinal chronic diseases, hair treatment and nourishment, skin care	[8, 10, 11]
	Turkey		Fruit	Diarrhea, dysentery, hemostasis, gastroenteritis	[8]
	Bangladesh		Whole plant	Edema, constipation, helminthiasis, dysentery, diarrhea, pain	[12]
	China	Huangguo yexiazhu zhuzicao		Inflammation, rheumatism	[13]
	India	Pancoli, karineli	Leaves/bark	Urination disorder, fever, smallpox, colic, constipation, diabetes	[12, 14, 15]
	Kenya			Malaria	[7]
P. reticulatus	Malaysia		Leaves	Smallpox, syphilis, asthma, diarrhea, bleeding from gums, diabetes, urination disorder, sores, burn, suppuration, chafe, venereal sores	[16, 17]
	Sri Lanka		Bark/fruit	Enteritis, urination disorder	[15]
	Sudan			Urination disorder, fever	[15]
	Tanzania		Whole plant/leaves	Dysmenorrhea, gonorrhea, urination disorder, intestinal hemorrhage and anemia, muscle spasms, diarrhea with anal bleeding, promoting fertility, sores	[12, 15]
	Thailand			Urination disorder, asthma, anemia, fever, thirst, astringent, inflammation	[16]
	Brazil	Quebra-pedra	Whole plant	Kidney calculi	[18]
	China	zhuzicao	Whole plant	Hepatitis, dysentery, enteritis, urinary infection	[19]
	Congo		Whole plant	Malaria	[20]
P. niruri	India	Chanka piedra, bhuiamlki	Fruit/whole plant	Bronchitis, anaemia, leprosy, asthma, kidney calculi, ulcer, wound, sore, scabies, ring worm, jaundice, gonorrhea, menstruation, diabetes	[18, 21–23]
	Indonesia		Whole plant	Viral infection, hepatitis	[22]
	Latin America	Chanca piedra	Whole plant	Gallstone, kidney calculi, fever, excess uric acid	[6, 18, 24]
	Malaysia	Dukong anak	Whole plant	Diarrhoea, kidney disorder, gonorrhea, cough	[22]
	Thailand		Aerial parts	Anorexia, malaria	[18]
	Africa			Malaria	[25]
	Cameroon	Mbolongo	Stem bark	Wound, tetanus	[26]
P. muellerianus	Ghana			Wound	[27]
	Ivory Coast		Leaves	Fever	[26]
	Nigeria		Root	Fever	[26]
	Zambia		leaves	Fever	[26]

TABLE 1: Continued.

Species	Region	Local name	Plant part used	Traditional use	Reference
P. amarus	Africa		Whole plant	Urinary concretions, dysentery, jaundice, diarrhoea	[28]
	India	Bhuiamlki	Whole plant	Gastropathy, diarrhoea, dysentery, intermittent fevers, ophthalmopathy, scabies, ulcers, wound, malaria, jaundice, diabetes, asthma, hepatitis, tuberculosis, urinary diseases, bodyache, immunomodulatory	[29–34]
	Nigeria		Leaves	Diabetes mellitus, obesity, hyperlipidemia, malaria	[35, 36]
	Peru	Chanca piedra	Leaves	Diabetes, jaundice, kidney diseases, urination disorder, sedative, astringent, tonic	[37]
	Thailand	Look tai bai		Gonorrhea, jaundice, diabetes, liver diseases	[5]
P. urinaria	China	Yexiazhu	Whole plant	Kidney calculi, painful disorder, jaundice, enteritis, diarrhea, dropsy, inflammation	[38–41]
	India			Inflammation, diarrheal, kidney calculi, painful disorder	[38, 39]
	Thailand	Look tai bai		Inflammation, diarrheal, gonorrhea, jaundice, diabetes	[5, 38]
P. acidus	India	Harfarauri	Fruit/leaves/roots	Jaundice, constipation, vomiting, biliousness, urinary concretions, piles, fever, smallpox, rheumatism, asthma, hepatic disease, diabetes, gonorrhea, ophthalmopathy, amnesia, psoriasis	[42, 43]
	Thailand	Otaheiti gooseberry, star gooseberry, mayom	Leaves/bark/root	Constipation, alcoholic addicts, hypertension, fever, dermatitis, menstruation fever	[44–46]
P. debilis	India	Bhuiamlki		Swelling, intestinal worms, fever, wound, inflammation, rheumatism	[34]
	Sri Lanka			Diabetes	[47]
P. simplex	India	Bhuiaveli, uchchiyusirika	Leaves/whole plant	Ophthalmopathy, gonorrhea, jaundice, mammary abscess, pruritus, diarrhea, hepatitis, urinary infection	[48, 49]
	China	Huang zhuzicao		Ophthalmopathy, diarrhea, hepatitis, urinary infection	[49]
P. discoideus	Cameroon			Insomnia, epilepsy	[50]
P. fraternus	India	Bhuiamlki	Whole plant	Constipation, jaundice, hepatic disorder, kidney disorders, bacterial infection	[29, 51, 52]
P. hookeri	India			Diabetes, wound, fever, inflammation, snake bite, bacterial infection	[34]
P. kozhikodianus	India			Dysentery, jaundice, ulcer, itching, bacterial infection	[34]
P. maderaspatensis	India	Bhuiamlki	Whole plant	Headache, constipation, diarrhea, edematous, dysentery, fever, ulcer, burn, jaundice, bacterial infection, immunomodulatory	[34, 52]
P. nozeranii	India			Spasmodic, piles, headache, boils, indigestion, viral and bacterial infection	[34]
P. orbicularis	Cuba			Jaundice, diabetes, kidney calculi, ulcer, rheumatism, fever	[53, 54]
P. piscatorum	Venezuela		Aerial parts	Wound, fungal infection	[55]
P. polyanthus	Kenya		Root	Sexually transmitted diseases	[56]
P. polyphyllus	India	Sirunelli	Leaves	Liver disease	[57]
P. rheedii	India		Whole plant	Diabetes	[58]
P. sellowianus	South America	Sarandi blanco	Stems/leaves	Urination disorder, diabetes	[59]
P. taxodiifolius	Thailand		Leaves/twigs	Urination disorder	[60]
P. tenellus	Brazil	Erva pombinha, quebra-pedra	Leaves	Urination disorder, kidney calculi	[61]
P. virgatus	Thailand	Look tai bai		Gonorrhea, jaundice, diabetes, liver disease	[5]

TABLE 2: The compounds isolated from the genus *Phyllanthus* and part of pharmacological effects.

Number	Compounds	Species	Pharmacological effects	References
1	(20S)-3α-Acetoxy-24-methylenedammaran-20-ol	*P. polyanthus*		[56]
2	(20S)-3β-Acetoxy-24-methylenedammaran-20-ol	*P. polyanthus*		[56]
3	Ocotillol-II	*P. flexuosus*		[63]
4	Phyllanthenol	*P. niruri*		[64]
5	Phyllanthenone	*P. niruri*		[64]
6	Phyllantheol	*P. niruri*		[64]
7	(+)-Songbodichapetalin	*P. songboiensis*		[65]
8	Acutissimatriterpene A	*P. acutissima*		[66]
9	Acutissimatriterpene B	*P. acutissima*		[66]
10	Acutissimatriterpene C	*P. acutissima*		[66]
11	Acutissimatriterpene D	*P. acutissima*		[66]
12	Acutissimatriterpene E	*P. acutissima*		[66]
13	Flexuosoids A	*P. flexuosus*		[67]
14	Flexuosoids B	*P. flexuosus*		[67]
15	δ-Amyrin acetate	*P. polyanthus*		[56]
16	12(13)-Dehydro-3α-acetoxyolean-28-oic acid	*P. pulcher*		[68]
17	3'-O-Acetyl-3-O-α-L-arabinosyl-23-hydroxyolean-12-en-28-oic acid	*P. polyphyllus*		[69]
18	3α-Acetoxyl-25-hydroxyolean-12-en-28-oic acid	*P. pulcher*	Antitumor	[68]
19	4'-O-Acetyl-3-O-α-L-arabinosyl-23-hydroxyolean-12-en-28-oic acid	*P. polyphyllus*		[69]
20	Olean-12-en-3β,15α,24-triol	*P. flexuosus*	Antitumor	[70, 71]
21	Olean-12-en-3β,15α-diol	*P. flexuosus*	Antitumor	[70, 71]
22	Olean-12-en-3β,24-diol	*P. flexuosus*		[70]
23	Olean-18-en-3α-ol	*P. fraternus*		[72]
24	Oleana-11:13(18)-dien-3β-ol	*P. flexuosus*		[70]
25	Oleana-11:13(18)-dien-3β,24-diol	*P. flexuosus*		[70]
26	Oleana-9(11):12-dien-3β-ol	*P. flexuosus*		[70]
27	Oleanolic acid	*P. urinaria*		[73]
28	Phyllanoside	*P. amarus*		[74]
29	Phyllenolide A	*P. myrtifolius*		[75]
30	Phyllenolide B	*P. myrtifolius*		[75]
31	Phyllenolide C	*P. myrtifolius*		[75]
32	Taraxerol	*P. columnaris*		[76]
33	Taraxerone	*P. reticulatus*		[77]
33	Taraxerone	*P. columnaris*		[76]
34	Taraxeryl acetate	*P. reticulatus*		[77]
35	α-Amyrin	*P. singampattiana*		[78]
36	β-Amyrin	*P. urinaria*		[79]
36	β-Amyrin	*P. flexuosus*		[80]
36	β-Amyrin	*P. acidus*		[81]
37	11β-Hydroxy-D:A-friedoolean-1-en-3-one	*P. flexuosus*		[82]
38	1β,22β-Dihydroxyfriedelin	*P. muellerianus*		[83]
39	21α-Hydroxyfriedel-4(23)-en-3-one	*P. reticulatus*		[84]
40	21α-Hydroxyfriedelan-3-one	*P. reticulatus*		[84]
41	22β-Hydroxyfriedel-1-ene	*P. muellerianus*		[83]
42	26-Nor-D:A-friedoolean-14-en-3-one	*P. watsonii*		[85]
43	26-Nor-D:A-friedoolean-14-en-3β-ol	*P. watsonii*		[85]
43	Friedelin	*P. columnaris*		[86]

TABLE 2: Continued.

Number	Compounds	Species	Pharmacological effects	References
44	3,20-Dioxo-dinorfriedelane	P. emblica		[87]
45	Epifriedelinol	P. reticulatus		[77]
45	Epifriedelinol	P. singampattiana		[78]
46	Friedelan-3β-ol	P. reticulatus		[84]
47	Friedelin	P. niruri		[88]
47	Friedelin	P. reticulatus		[84]
47	Friedelin	P. flexuosus		[80]
47	Friedelin	P. watsonii		[85]
47	Friedelin	P. wightianus		[89]
47	Friedelin	P. singampattiana		[78]
48	Polpunonic acid	P. oxyphyllus		[90]
49	Trichadenic acid B	P. flexuosus		[91]
50	3-Friedelanone	P. muellerianus		[92]
51	Betulin	P. reticulatus		[77]
51	Betulin	P. flexuosus	Antitumor	[70, 71]
52	Betulinic acid	P. reticulatus		[84]
53	Glochidiol	P. urinaria		[73]
53	Glochidiol	P. sellowianus		[93]
54	Glochidone	P. virgatus		[94]
54	Glochidone	P. sellowianus		[95]
54	Glochidone	P. watsonii		[85]
54	Glochidone	P. taxodiifolius	Antitumor	[60, 96]
54	Glochidone	P. pulcher	Antitumor	[68]
54	Glochidone	P. flexuosus		[80]
55	Glochidonol	P. reticulatus		[84]
55	Glochidonol	P. sellowianus		[93]
55	Glochidonol	P. watsonii		[85]
55	Glochidonol	P. pulcher	Antitumor	[68]
56	Lup-20(29)-en-3β,15α-diol	P. flexuosus	Antitumor	[63, 71]
57	Lup-20(29)-en-3β,24-diol	P. flexuosus	Antitumor	[70, 71]
58	Lup-20(29)-en-3β-ol	P. urinaria		[97]
59	Lup-20(29)-ene-3β,24-diol	P. flexuosus		[98]
60	Lup-20(29)-ene-1β,3β-diol	P. sellowianus		[93]
60	Lup-20(29)-ene-1β,3β-diol	P. watsonii		[85]
61	Lupanyl acetate	P. urinaria		[99]
61	Lupanyl acetate	P. watsonii		[85]
61	Lupanyl acetate	P. columnaris		[86]
61	Lupanyl acetate	P. pulcher		[68]
62	Lupenone	P. polyanthus		[56]
63	Lupenyl palmitate	P. watsonii		[85]
64	Lupeol	P. emblica		[100]
64	Lupeol	P. urinaria		[79]
64	Lupeol	P. reticulatus		[17]
64	Lupeol	P. flexuosus	Antitumor	[71, 80]
64	Lupeol	P. oxyphyllus		[90]
64	Lupeol	P. watsonii		[85]
64	Lupeol	P. taxodiifolius	Antitumor	[60, 96]

TABLE 2: Continued.

Number	Compounds	Species	Pharmacological effects	References
64	Lupeol	*P. wightianus*		[89]
64	Lupeol	*P. columnaris*		[86]
65	Lupeol acetate	*P. reticulatus*		[17]
66	29-Nor-3,4-seco-friedelan-4(23),20(30)-dien-3-oic acid	*P. oxyphyllus*		[90]
67	3,7,11,15,19,23-Hexamethyl-2Z,6Z,10Z,14E,18E,22E-tetracosahexen-1-ol	*P. niruri*		[101]
68	Phyllanthol	*P. sellowianus*		[102]
68	Phyllanthol	*P. polyanthus*		[56]
68	Phyllanthol	*P. acidus*		[81]
69	Phyllanthone	*P. polyanthus*		[56]
70	4′-Hydroxyphyllaemblicin B	*P. emblica*		[103]
71	5-Hydroxy-6,9-epoxyguaiane	*P. oxyphyllus*		[90]
72	5-O-Acetyl-6,9-epoxyguaiane	*P. oxyphyllus*		[90]
73	Cloven-2β,9α-diol	*P. urinaria*		[73]
74	Descinnamoylphyllanthocindiol	*P. acuminatus*		[104]
75	Didesacetylphyllanthostatin 3	*P. acuminatus*		[104]
76	Dihydrophaseic acid-4′-O-β-D-glucopyranoside	*P. reticulatus*		[105]
77	Englerins A	*P. engleri*	Antitumor	[106]
78	Englerins B	*P. engleri*		[106]
79	Glochicoccin D	*P. emblica*		[107]
80	Jaslanceoside B	*P. cochinchinensis*		[108]
81	Jasminoside	*P. cochinchinensis*		[108]
82	Phyllaemblic acid	*P. emblica*		[109]
83	Phyllaemblic acid B	*P. emblica*		[110]
84	Phyllaemblic acid C	*P. emblica*		[110]
85	Phyllaemblicin A	*P. emblica*		[109]
86	Phyllaemblicin B	*P. emblica*	Antiviral and antitumor	[109, 111, 112]
87	Phyllaemblicin C	*P. emblica*	Antitumor and antiviral	[109, 111, 113]
88	Phyllaemblicin D	*P. emblica*		[110]
89	Phyllaemblicin E	*P. emblica*		[103]
90	Phyllaemblicin F	*P. emblica*		[103]
91	Phyllaemblicin G1	*P. emblica*		[107]
92	Phyllaemblicin G2	*P. emblica*		[107]
93	Phyllaemblicin G3	*P. emblica*		[107]
94	Phyllaemblicin G4	*P. emblica*		[107]
95	Phyllaemblicin G5	*P. emblica*		[107]
96	Phyllaemblicin G6	*P. emblica*	Antiviral	[107]
97	Phyllaemblicin G7	*P. emblica*		[107]
98	Phyllaemblicin G8	*P. emblica*		[107]
99	Phyllaemblinol	*P. emblica*		[114]
100	Phyllanthocin	*P. brasiliensis*		[115]
101	Phyllanthoside	*P. acuminatus*	Antitumor	[116]
101	Phyllanthoside	*P. veuminatus*	Antitumor	[117]
101	Phyllanthoside	*P. brasiliensis*	Antitumor	[115]
102	Phyllanthostatin 1	*P. acuminatus*	Antitumor	[116]
102	Phyllanthostatin 1	*P. veuminatus*	Antitumor	[117]
103	Phyllanthostatin 2	*P. acuminatus*	Antitumor	[117]

TABLE 2: Continued.

Number	Compounds	Species	Pharmacological effects	References
103	Phyllanthostatin 2	*P. veuminatus*	Antitumor	[117]
104	Phyllanthostatin 3	*P. acuminatus*	Antitumor	[117]
104	Phyllanthostatin 3	*P. veuminatus*	Antitumor	[117]
105	Phyllanthostatin 6	*P. acuminatus*	Antitumor	[104]
106	Phyllanthusol A	*P. acidus*	Antitumor	[46]
107	Phyllanthusol B	*P. acidus*	Antitumor	[46]
108	β-Caryophyllene	*P. emblica*		[113]
109	β-Bourbonene	*P. emblica*		[113]
110	19-Hydroxyspruceanol 19-O-β-D-glucopyranoside	*P. reticulatus*		[118]
111	Cleistanthol	*P. urinaria*		[73]
111	Cleistanthol	*P. reticulatus*		[13]
111	Cleistanthol	*P. flexuosus*	Antitumor	[119]
111	Cleistanthol	*P. oxyphyllus*		[90]
112	Ent-3β-Hydroxykaur-l6-ene	*P. flexuosus*		[80]
113	Orthosiphol G	*P. niruri*		[120]
114	Orthosiphol I	*P. niruri*		[120]
115	Phyllanflexoid A	*P. flexuosus*	Antitumor	[119]
116	Phyllanflexoid B	*P. flexuosus*	Antitumor	[119]
117	Phyllanflexoid C	*P. flexuosus*		[119]
118	Phyllanterpenyl ester	*P. fraternus*		[121]
119	Spruceanol	*P. urinaria*		[73]
119	Spruceanol	*P. reticulatus*		[13]
119	Spruceanol	*P. oxyphyllus*		[90]
119	Spruceanol	*P. songboiensis*		[65]
120	*trans*-Phytol	*P. niruri*		[122]
121	(3S,5R,6S,9R)-Megastigmane-3,9-diol 3-O-α-L-arabinofuranosyl-(1 → 6)-β-D-glucopyranoside	*P. reticulatus*		[13]
122	(6R)-Menthiafolic acid	*P. urinaria*		[73]
123	7-Megastigmen-3-ol-9-one 3-O-α-L-arabinofuranosyl-(1 → 6)-β-D-glucopyranoside	*P. reticulatus*		[13]
124	Turpenionoside A	*P. reticulatus*		[118]
125	Turpenionoside B	*P. reticulatus*		[118]
126	7-O-[(2,3,4-Tri-O-acetyl)-α-L-arabinopyranosyl]diphyllin	*P. poilanei*	Antitumor	[123]
127	Arabelline	*P. flexuosus*		[67]
128	Acutissimalignans A	*P. songboiensis*		[65]
128	Acutissimalignans A	*P. acutissima*		[66]
129	Cleistanthin A	*P. taxodiifolius*	Antitumor	[96, 124]
130	Cleistanthin A acetate	*P. taxodiifolius*	Antitumor	[96, 124]
131	Cleistanthin A Me ether	*P. taxodiifolius*	Antitumor	[96, 124]
132	Cleistanthin B	*P. poilanei*		[123]
133	Cleistanthoside A	*P. taxodiifolius*		[96]
134	Cleistanthoside A tetraacetate	*P. taxodiifolius*	Antitumor	[96, 124]
135	Dextrobursehernin	*P. urinaria*		[125]
136	Diphyllin	*P. poilanei*		[123]
136	Diphyllin	*P. polyphyllus*	Anti-inflammatory	[126]
137	Hypophyllanthin	*P. niruri*	Hepatoprotection and hypotensive	[127–129]

TABLE 2: Continued.

Number	Compounds	Species	Pharmacological effects	References
137	Hypophyllanthin	P. urinaria	Hypotensive	[125, 130]
137	Hypophyllanthin	P. virgatus		[131]
137	Hypophyllanthin	P. amarus	Antitumor and anti-CYP3A4	[132–134]
137	Hypophyllanthin	P. debilis		[135]
138	Isolariciresinol	P. emblica		[114]
139	Isolintetralin	P. niruri		[136]
139	Isolintetralin	P. urinaria		[125]
139	Isolintetralin	P. virgatus		[131]
140	Justicidin A	P. myrtifolius		[131]
141	Iusticidin B	P. myrtifolius		[137]
141	Iusticidin B	P. polyphyllus	Anti-inflammatory	[126]
141	Iusticidin B	P. anisolobus		[138]
141	Iusticidin B	P. piscatorum	Antifungal, antitumor, and antiparasitic	[139]
142	Lintetralin	P. niruri		[128]
142	Lintetralin	P. urinaria		[125]
143	(+)-Lyoniresinol	P. reticulatus		[13]
144	(+)-Lyoniresiol	P. urinaria		[73]
145	Mananthoside I	P. reticulatus		[118]
146	Neonirtetralin	P. niruri		[140]
146	Neonirtetralin	P. urinaria		[141]
147	Nirtetralin	P. niruri	Antiviral and hypotensive	[127, 128, 142]
147	Nirtetralin	P. urinaria		[125]
147	Nirtetralin	P. virgatus	Antiviral	[131, 143]
147	Nirtetralin	P. amarus	Anti-inflammatory and antitumor	[132, 144, 145]
148	Nirtetralin A	P. niruri	Antiviral	[142]
149	Nirtetralin B	P. niruri	Antiviral	[142, 146]
150	Phyllamyricin A	P. myrtifolius		[137]
151	Phyllamyricin B	P. myrtifolius		[137]
152	Phyllamyricin C	P. myrtifolius		[137]
152	Phyllamyricin C	P. polyphyllus	Anti-inflammatory	[126]
153	Phyllamyricin D	P. myrtifolius		[147]
154	Phyllamyricin E	P. myrtifolius		[147]
155	Phyllamyricin F	P. myrtifolius		[147]
156	Phyllamyricoside A	P. myrtifolius	Anti-HIV	[147]
157	Phyllamyricoside B	P. myrtifolius		[147]
158	Phyllamyricoside C	P. myrtifolius		[147]
159	Phyllanthostatin A	P. acuminatus		[148]
159	Phyllanthostatin A	P. anisolobus		[138]
160	Phyllanthuoside C	P. cochinchinensis		[149]
161	Phyllanthusmin A	P. poilanei		[123]
161	Phyllanthusmin A	P. oligospermus	Antitumor	[150]
162	Phyllanthusmin B	P. reticulatus		[13]

TABLE 2: Continued.

Number	Compounds	Species	Pharmacological effects	References
162	Phyllanthusmin B	*P. poilanei*		[123]
162	Phyllanthusmin B	*P. oligospermus*		[150]
163	Phyllanthusmin C	*P. reticulatus*		[13]
163	Phyllanthusmin C	*P. flexuosus*		[67]
163	Phyllanthusmin C	*P. poilanei*	Antitumor	[123]
163	Phyllanthusmin C	*P. oligospermus*		[150]
164	Phyllanthusmin D	*P. poilanei*		[123]
165	Phyllanthusmin E	*P. poilanei*		[123]
166	Phyllanthusmin D′	*P. flexuosus*		[67]
167	Phyllanthusmin E′	*P. flexuosus*		[67]
168	Phyllanthusmin F	*P. flexuosus*		[67]
169	Phyltetralin	*P. niruri*		[128]
169	Phyltetralin	*P. urinaria*	Anti-inflammatory	[125, 151]
169	Phyltetralin	*P. virgatus*		[131]
169	Phyltetralin	*P. amarus*	Anti-inflammatory	[145]
170	Piscatorin	*P. piscatorum*	Antitumor	[139]
171	Reticulatuside A	*P. reticulatus*		[13]
172	Reticulatuside B	*P. reticulatus*		[13]
173	Retrojusticidin B	*P. myrtifolius*	Anti-HIV	[137, 152]
174	Seco-4-hydroxylintetralin	*P. niruri*		[153]
175	Taxodiifoloside	*P. taxodiifolius*	Antitumor	[124]
176	Urinatetralin	*P. niruri*		[154]
176	Urinatetralin	*P. urinaria*		[125]
177	2,3-Desmethoxy seco-isolintetralin	*P. niruri*		[155]
178	2,3-Desmethoxy seco-isolintetralin diacetate	*P. niruri*		[155]
179	4-(3,4-Dimethoxy-phenyl)-1-(7-methoxy-benzo[1,3]dioxol-5-yl)-2,3-bis-methoxymethyl-butan-1-ol	*P. amarus*		[132]
180	5-Demethoxy niranthin	*P. urinaria*		[125]
180	5-Demethoxy niranthin	*P. amarus*		[132]
181	7′-Hydroxy-3′,4′,5,9,9′-pentamethoxy-3,4-methylene dioxy lignan	*P. urinaria*	Antitumor	[156]
182	Demethylenedioxyniranthin	*P. niruri*		[155]
183	Dihydrocubebin	*P. niruri*		[155]
183	Dihydrocubebin	*P. urinaria*		[73]
184	Hydroxyniranthin	*P. niruri*		[153]
185	Linnanthin	*P. niruri*		[155]
186	Niranthin	*P. niruri*		[157]
186	Niranthin	*P. urinaria*		[125]
186	Niranthin	*P. virgatus*	Antiviral	[131, 143]
186	Niranthin	*P. amarus*	Anti-inflammatory, antiparasitic, antihyperalgesic, and antitumor	[132, 144, 158, 159]
187	Nirphyllin	*P. niruri*		[160]
188	Phyllanthin	*P. niruri*	Hepatoprotection, hypotensive, and antihyperuricemic	[127, 157, 161, 162]
188	Phyllanthin	*P. urinaria*	Immunomodulatory and hypotensive	[125, 130, 163]

TABLE 2: Continued.

Number	Compounds	Species	Pharmacological effects	References
188	Phyllanthin	P. amarus	Cell-protection, hepatoprotection, antitumor, and anti-CYP3A4	[134, 144, 164, 165]
188	Phyllanthin	P. fraternus		[72]
188	Phyllanthin	P. debilis		[135]
189	Seco-isolariciresinol	P. oxyphyllus		[90]
190	Seco-isolariciresinol trimethyl ether	P. niruri		[153]
191	(+)-8-(3,4-(Methylenedioxy)benzyl)-8′-(3′,4′-dimethoxybenzyl)-butyrolactone	P. virgatus		[131]
192	(+)-Secoisolariciresinol	P. songboiensis		[65]
193	(+)-Songbosin	P. songboiensis		[65]
194	2S,3S-Bursehernin	P. urinaria		[166]
195	3-(3,4-Dimethoxy-benzyl)-4-(7-methoxy-benzo[1,3]dioxol-5-yl-methyl)-dihydrofuran-2-one	P. amarus		[132]
196	Acutissimalignans B	P. acutissima		[66]
197	Bursehernin	P. amarus		[132]
198	Cubebin dimethyl ether	P. niruri		[154]
199	Dibenzylbutyrolactone	P. niruri		[153]
200	Heliobuphthalmin lactone	P. urinaria		[125]
200	Heliobuphthalmin lactone	P. amarus		[132]
201	Hinokinin	P. niruri		[136]
201	Hinokinin	P. virgatus	Antiviral	[131, 143]
202	(7 R,7′R,8S,8′S)-Icariol A2	P. urinaria		[73]
203	Phyllnirurin	P. niruri		[160]
204	Urinaligran	P. urinaria		[125]
205	Virgatusin	P. urinaria		[125]
205	Virgatusin	P. virgatus		[131]
205	Virgatusin	P. amarus		[132]
206	(+)-Diasyringaresinol	P. flexuosus		[67]
207	(−)-Episyringaresinol	P. urinaria		[73]
207	(−)-Episyringaresinol	P. songboiensis		[65]
208	(−)-Lirioresinol-B	P. virgatus		[94]
209	4-Ketopinoresinol	P. emblica		[114]
210	4-Oxopinoresinol	P. urinaria		[73]
211	Lirioresinol A	P. emblica		[114]
212	Medioresinol	P. emblica		[114]
213	Pinoresinol	P. oxyphyllus		[90]
213	Pinoresinol	P. songboiensis		[65]
214	Syringaresinol	P. emblica		[114]
214	Syringaresinol	P. urinaria		[73]
214	Syringaresinol	P. reticulatus		[13]
215	Virgatyne	P. virgatus		[94]
216	4,9,9′-Trihydroxy-3,4′-dimethoxy-8-O-3′-neolignan	P. emblica		[114]
217	Caffeic acid	P. urinaria		[167]
217	Caffeic acid	P. sellowianus		[168]
217	Caffeic acid	P. muellerianus		[169]

TABLE 2: Continued.

Number	Compounds	Species	Pharmacological effects	References
217	Caffeic acid	*P. simplex*		[170]
218	Cinnamic acid	*P. emblica*	Antioxidant	[171]
219	Coniferyl aldehyde	*P. emblica*		[114]
220	Evofolin B	*P. urinaria*		[73]
221	Ferulic acid	*P. urinaria*		[172]
221	Ferulic acid	*P. simplex*		[170]
222	Methyl caffeate	*P. emblica*		[114]
223	Phyllanthuoside A	*P. cochinchinensis*	Antitumor	[149]
224	Phyllanthuoside B	*P. cochinchinensis*		[149]
225	Debelalactone	*P. debilis*	Hepatoprotection	[173]
226	Isofraxidin	*P. sellowianus*		[174]
227	Scopoletin	*P. sellowianus*		[174]
228	1,2,4,6-Tetra-O-galloyl-β-D-glucose	*P. emblica*	Antiviral	[175]
228	1,2,4,6-Tetra-O-galloyl-β-D-glucose	*P. niruri*	Antiviral	[176, 177]
229	1,3,4,6-Tetra-O-galloyl-β-D-glucose	*P. virgatus*		[94]
230	1,4,6-Tri-O-galloyl-β-D-glucose	*P. virgatus*		[94]
231	1,6-Di-O-galloyl-β-D-glucose	*P. virgatus*		[94]
232	1,2-Di-O-galloyl-3,6-(R)-hexa-hydroxydiphenoyl-β-D-glucose	*P. niruri*		[176]
233	Amariin	*P. amarus*	Hepatoprotection, radioprotective, and antioxidant	[178–181]
234	Amariinic acid	*P. amarus*		[182]
235	Amarulone	*P. amarus*		[183]
236	Carpinusnin	*P. emblica*		[184]
237	Chebulagic acid	*P. emblica*	Antioxidant and antitumor	[111, 184, 185]
237	Chebulagic acid	*P. myrtifolius*		[186]
238	Chebulanin	*P. emblica*	Antioxidant	[184, 185]
239	Corilagin	*P. emblica*	Antioxidant and antitumor	[111, 184, 187]
239	Corilagin	*P. niruri*	Antihyperalgesic and anti-inflammatory	[6, 176, 188]
239	Corilagin	*P. urinaria*	Antiviral and antiplatelet	[189–191]
239	Corilagin	*P. reticulatus*		[192]
239	Corilagin	*P. virgatus*		[94]
239	Corilagin	*P. amarus*	Antidiabetic, radioprotective, and anti-HIV	[179, 181, 193, 194]
239	Corilagin	*P. myrtifolius*		[186]
239	Corilagin	*P. muellerianus*		[169]
239	Corilagin	*P. debilis*	Antioxidant	[195]
239	Corilagin	*P. matsumurae*		[196]
239	Corilagin	*P. wightianus*		[89]
239	Corilagin	*P. ussuriensis*	Antioxidant	[197, 198]
240	Excoecarianin	*P. urinaria*	Antiviral	[199]
241	Furosin	*P. emblica*	Antioxidant	[184, 187]
241	Furosin	*P. virgatus*		[94]
241	Furosin	*P. sellowianus*	Antihyperalgesic	[200]

TABLE 2: Continued.

Number	Compounds	Species	Pharmacological effects	References
241	Furosin	P. muellerianus	Wound healing	[169]
241	Furosin	P. debilis	Antioxidant	[195]
242	Geraniin	P. emblica	Antioxidant and antitumor	[111, 185, 201]
242	Geraniin	P. niruri	Antiviral	[177]
242	Geraniin	P. urinaria	Immunomodulatory, antioxidant, and hypotensive	[41, 163]
242	Geraniin	P. virgatus	Antiviral	[94, 143]
242	Geraniin	P. amarus	Hepatoprotection, radioprotective, and anti-HIV	[179–181, 194]
242	Geraniin	P. myrtifolius		[186]
242	Geraniin	P. sellowianus	Antihyperalgesic	[200]
242	Geraniin	P. muellerianus	Wound healing and antimalarial	[169, 202]
242	Geraniin	P. debilis	Antioxidant	[195]
242	Geraniin	P. matsumurae		[196]
242	Geraniin	P. wightianus		[89]
242	Geraniin	P. ussuriensis		[197]
242	Geraniin	P. caroliniensis		[203]
243	Geraniinic acid B	P. amarus		[182]
244	Hippomanin A	P. urinaria	Antiviral	[204]
245	Isocorilagin	P. emblica	Antioxidant and antitumor	[185, 201, 205]
245	Isocorilagin	P. niruri	Cholinesterase inhibition	[206, 207]
246	Isomallotusinin	P. emblica	Antioxidant	[185]
247	Isostrictinin	P. emblica		[208]
247	Isostrictinin	P. urinaria		[209]
248	Mallonin	P. emblica		[184]
249	Mallotusinin	P. emblica	Antioxidant	[210]
249	Mallotusinin	P. myrtifolius		[186]
250	Neochebulagic acid	P. emblica		[184]
251	Phyllanemblinin A	P. emblica		[184]
251	Phyllanemblinin A	P. flexuosus		[211]
252	Phyllanemblinin B	P. emblica		[184]
252	Phyllanemblinin B	P. flexuosus		[211]
253	Phyllanemblinin C	P. emblica		[184]
253	Phyllanemblinin C	P. flexuosus		[211]
254	Phyllanemblinin D	P. emblica		[184]
254	Phyllanemblinin D	P. flexuosus		[211]
255	Phyllanemblinin E	P. emblica		[184]
255	Phyllanemblinin E	P. flexuosus		[211]
256	Phyllanemblinin F	P. emblica		[184]
257	Phyllanthunin	P. emblica		[212]
258	PhyllanthusiinC	P. myrtifolius		[186]
259	PhyllanthusiinD	P. niruri		[176]

TABLE 2: Continued.

Number	Compounds	Species	Pharmacological effects	References
259	PhyllanthusiinD	*P. amarus*	Radioprotective and antioxidant	[178, 181]
260	Phyllanthusiin G	*P. urinaria*		[213]
261	Phyllanthusiin U	*P. urinaria*		[167]
262	Pinocembrin-7-O-[3″-O-galloyl-4″,6″-(S)-hexahydroxydiphenoyl]-β-D-glucose	*P. tenellus*		[214]
263	Pinocembrin-7-O-[4″,6″-(S)-hexahydroxydiphenoyl]-β-D-glucose	*P. tenellus*		[214]
264	Punicafolin	*P. emblica*		[184]
265	Putranjivain A	*P. emblica*		[184]
266	Putranjivain B	*P. emblica*		[185]
267	Repandusinic acid	*P. amarus*	Antioxidant	[178, 182]
268	Terchebin	*P. niruri*		[176]
269	Tercatain	*P. emblica*		[184]
270	Virganin	*P. virgatus*		[94]
271	Dimeric procyanidins mono-gallates	*P. orbicularis*	Antiviral	[53]
272	Dimeric procyanidins-3,3′-di-O-gallates	*P. orbicularis*	Antiviral	[53]
273	Epicatechin-(4β → 8)-epigallocatechin	*P. emblica*		[184]
274	Oligomeric procyanidins	*P. orbicularis*	Antiviral	[53]
275	Oligomeric procyanidins mono-gallates	*P. orbicularis*	Antiviral	[53]
276	Phyllemtannin	*P. emblica*	Antitumor	[111]
277	Prodelphinidin B1	*P. emblica*		[184]
277	Prodelphinidin B1	*P. niruri*		[215]
277	Prodelphinidin B1	*P. sellowianus*		[216]
277	Prodelphinidin B1	*P. orbicularis*		[215]
277	Prodelphinidin B1	*P. matsumurae*		[217]
278	Prodelphinidin B2	*P. emblica*		[184]
278	Prodelphinidin B2	*P. orbicularis*	Antioxidant	[53, 54]
278	Prodelphinidin B2	*P. simplex*		[170]
278	Prodelphinidin B2	*P. matsumurae*		[218]
279	Prodelphinidin B-2,3′-O-gallate	*P. emblica*		[184]
280	5,7-Dihydroxy-4′-methoxyflavonol	*P. virgatus*		[94]
281	5,3′-Dihydroxy-6,7,4′-trimethoxyflavone	*P. niruri*		[207]
282	Astragalin	*P. urinaria*		[141]
282	Astragalin	*P. virgatus*		[94]
282	Astragalin	*P. muellerianus*		[169]
283	Avicularin	*P. emblica*		[219]
284	Galangin 3-O-β-D-glucoside 8-sulfonate	*P. virgatus*		[94]
285	Isoquercitrin	*P. emblica*		[201]
285	Isoquercitrin	*P. urinaria*		[220]
285	Isoquercitrin	*P. reticulatus*		[192]
285	Isoquercitrin	*P. virgatus*		[94]
285	Isoquercitrin	*P. muellerianus*		[169]
286	Kaempferol	*P. emblica*	Antioxidant	[201]
286	Kaempferol	*P. niruri*		[79]
286	Kaempferol	*P. virgatus*		[94]
286	Kaempferol	*P. cochinchinensis*		[149]
287	Kaempferol-3-O-α-L-(6″-ethyl)-rhamnopyranoside	*P. emblica*		[221]
288	Kaempferol-3-O-α-L-(6″-methyl)-rhamnopyranoside	*P. emblica*		[221]

TABLE 2: Continued.

Number	Compounds	Species	Pharmacological effects	References
289	Kaempferol-3-O-β-D-glucopyranoside	P. emblica	Antioxidant	[201]
290	Kaempferol 8-sulfonate	P. virgatus		[94]
291	Myricitrin	P. virgatus		[94]
292	Quercetin	P. emblica	Antioxidant	[171]
292	Quercetin	P. urinaria		[215]
292	Quercetin	P. virgatus		[94]
292	Quercetin	P. caroliniensis	Anti-inflammatory	[203]
293	Quercetin 3-O-α-L-(2,4-di-O-acetyl) rhamnopyranoside-7-O-α-L-rhamnopyranoside	P. urinaria		[222]
294	Quercetin 3-O-α-L-(3,4-di-O-acetyl) rhamnopyranoside-7-O-α-L-rhamnopyranoside	P. urinaria		[222]
295	Quercetin 3-O-α-L-rhamnopyranoside	P. urinaria		[222]
296	Quercetin-3-O-β-D-glucopyranoside	P. emblica	Antioxidant	[201]
297	Quercetin-3-O-β-D-glucopyranosyl$(1 \rightarrow 4)$-α-rhamnopyranoside	P. niruri		[79]
298	Quercetin-3-O-β-D-glucosyl-$(1 \rightarrow 6)$-β-D-glucoside	P. virgatus		[94]
299	Quercetin 3-O-β-D-glucopyranosyl-$(2 \rightarrow 1)$-O-β-D-xylopyranoside	P. niruri		[223]
300	Quercetin pentaacetate	P. orbicularis		[54]
301	Quercitrin	P. niruri	Antinociceptive	[215, 224]
301	Quercitrin	P. urinaria	Anti-inflammatory	[151, 215]
301	Quercitrin	P. virgatus		[94]
301	Quercitrin	P. sellowianus		[95]
301	Quercitrin	P. muellerianus		[169]
301	Quercitrin	P. orbicularis		[54]
301	Quercitrin	P. ussuriensis		[225]
302	Rhamnocitrin	P. urinaria	Anti-inflammatory	[151]
302	Rhamnocitrin	P. amarus		[179]
302	Rhamnocitrin	P. cochinchinensis		[149]
302	Rhamnocitrin	P. simplex		[170]
303	Rutin	P. niruri	Anti-inflammatory	[224]
303	Rutin	P. urinaria	Anti-inflammatory	[151, 215]
303	Rutin	P. reticulatus		[192]
303	Rutin	P. virgatus		[94]
303	Rutin	P. amarus	Radioprotective and antioxidant	[178, 181]
303	Rutin	P. debilis	Antioxidant	[195]
304	Rutin decaacetate	P. orbicularis		[54]
305	Schaftoside	P. cochinchinensis		[149]
306	Sodium galangin-8-sulfonate	P. virgatus		[94]
307	Sodium galangin-3-O-β-glucoside-8-sulfonate	P. virgatus		[94]
308	Sodium kaempferol-8-sulfonate	P. virgatus		[94]
309	Vicenin-2	P. cochinchinensis		[149]
310	4'-Methoxyscutellarein	P. urinaria		[226]
311	Apigenin	P. amarus		[74]
311	Apigenin	P. orbicularis	Antioxidant	[54]
312	Apigenin-7-O-(6''-butyryl-β-glucopyranoside)	P. emblica		[227]
312	Apigenin-7-O-(6''-butyryl-β-glucopyranoside)	P. niruri		[215]
312	Apigenin-7-O-(6''-butyryl-β-glucopyranoside)	P. urinaria		[215]
313	Demethoxysudachitin (4',5,7-trihydroxy-6,8-dimethoxyflavone)	P. atropurpureus		[228]

TABLE 2: Continued.

Number	Compounds	Species	Pharmacological effects	References
314	Galangin 8-sulfonate	*P. virgatus*		[94]
315	Luteolin	*P. amarus*		[74]
315	Luteolin	*P. singampattiana*		[78]
316	Niruriflavone	*P. niruri*	Antioxidant	[206]
317	Urinariaflavone	*P. urinaria*		[141]
318	2-(4-Hydroxyphenyl)-8-(3-methylbut-2-enyl)-chroman-4-one	*P. niruri*		[23]
319	7-Hydroxyflavanone	*P. sellowianus*		[168]
320	8-(3-Methyl-but-2-enyl)-2-phenyl chroman-4-one	*P. niruri*	Antiparasitic	[23]
321	Nirurin	*P. niruri*		[229]
322	Nirurinetin	*P. niruri*		[229]
323	(S)-Eriodictyol 7-O-(6″-O-(E)-β-coumaroyl)-β-D-glucopyranoside	*P. emblica*		[230]
324	(S)-Eriodictyol 7-O-(6″-O-galloyl)-β-D-glucopyranoside	*P. emblica*		[230]
325	(+)-Catechin	*P. niruri*		[176]
325	(+)-Catechin	*P. orbicularis*		[53]
326	(−)-Epiafzelechin	*P. emblica*		[184]
327	(−)-Epicatechin	*P. emblica*		[184]
327	(−)-Epicatechin	*P. niruri*		[176]
327	(−)-Epicatechin	*P. cochinchinensis*		[149]
327	(−)-Epicatechin	*P. orbicularis*		[53]
328	(−)-Epigallocatechin	*P. emblica*		[184]
328	(−)-Epigallocatechin	*P. niruri*		[176]
328	(−)-Epigallocatechin	*P. reticulatus*		[118]
329	(+)-Gallocatechin	*P. emblica*		[184]
329	(+)-Gallocatechin	*P. niruri*		[176]
330	8-(2-Pyrrolidinone-5-yl)-(−)-epicatechin	*P. cochinchinensis*		[149]
331	5,7-Dimethoxy-3,4′-dihydroxy-3′,8-di-C-prenylflavanone	*P. niruri*		[231]
332	5,6,8,4′-Tetrahydroxy isoflavone	*P. atropurpureus*		[228]
333	6-Hydroxy-7,8,2′,3′,4′-pentamethoxyisoflavone	*P. niruri*		[207]
334	(−)-β-Sitosterol-3-O-β-D-(6-O-palmitoyl) glucopyranoside	*P. songboiensis*		[65]
335	(3β,22E)-Stigmasta-5,22-diene-3,25-diol	*P. urinaria*		[73]
336	24-Isopropylcholesterol	*P. niruri*		[157]
337	5α,6β-Dihydroxysitosterol	*P. emblica*		[232]
338	5α,6β,7α-Trihydroxysitosterol	*P. emblica*		[232]
339	6′-(Stigmast-5-en-3-O-β-D-glucopyranosidyl) hexadecanoate	*P. emblica*		[232]
340	6′-(Stigmast-5-en-7-one-3-O-β-D-glucopyranosidyl) hexadecanoate	*P. emblica*		[232]
341	7-Ketositosterol	*P. emblica*		[232]
342	7α-Hydroxysitosterol	*P. emblica*		[232]
343	7α-Acetoxysitosterol	*P. emblica*		[232]
344	7β-Ethoxysiterol	*P. emblica*		[232]
345	Amarosterol A	*P. amarus*		[233]
346	Amarosterol B	*P. amarus*		[233]
347	Campesterol	*P. sellowianus*		[216]
348	Daucosterol	*P. emblica*		[232]
348	Daucosterol	*P. urinaria*		[220]
348	Daucosterol	*P. amarus*		[74]
349	Fraternusterol	*P. fraternus*		[234]

TABLE 2: Continued.

Number	Compounds	Species	Pharmacological effects	References
350	Phyllanthosecosteryl ester	P. fraternus		[234]
351	Phyllanthosterol	P. fraternus		[234]
352	Phyllanthostigmasterol	P. fraternus		[234]
353	Stigmast-4-en-3-one	P. emblica		[232]
354	Stigmast-4-en-3,6-dione	P. emblica		[232]
355	Stigmast-4-en-6β-ol-3-one	P. emblica		[232]
356	Stigmast-4-ene-3β,6α-diol	P. emblica		[232]
357	Stigmast-4,5-en-3-one	P. oxyphyllus		[90]
358	Stigmast-5-en-3-ol, oleate	P. amarus		[74]
359	Stigmasterol	P. urinaria		[97]
359	Stigmasterol	P. sellowianus		[216]
359	Stigmasterol	P. columnaris		[76]
360	Stigmasterol 3-O-β-D-glucoside	P. urinaria		[97]
361	β-Daucosterol	P. emblica	Antioxidant	[171, 212]
362	β-Sitosterol	P. emblica		[100]
362	β-Sitosterol	P. niruri		[157]
362	β-Sitosterol	P. urinaria		[220]
362	β-Sitosterol	P. reticulatus		[77]
362	β-Sitosterol	P. sellowianus		[216]
362	β-Sitosterol	P. muellerianus		[92]
362	β-Sitosterol	P. oxyphyllus		[90]
362	β-Sitosterol	P. fraternus		[72]
362	β-Sitosterol	P. debilis		[135]
362	β-Sitosterol	P. singampattiana		[78]
363	β-Sitosterol-3-O-β-D-glucopyranoside	P. urinaria		[151]
364	14,15-Dihydroallosecurinin-15β-ol	P. discoideus		[148]
365	4-Hydroxysecurinine	P. niruri		[235]
366	4-Methoxydihydronorsecurinine	P. niruri		[235]
367	β-Sitosterol-3-β-D-glucopyranoside	P. singampattiana		[78]
368	4-Methoxynorsecurinine	P. niruri		[236]
369	4-Methoxytetrahydrosecurinine	P. niruri		[235]
370	Allosecurinine	P. niruri		[235]
370	Allosecurinine	P. glaucus		[237]
371	Dihydrosecurinine	P. niruri		[235]
372	Ent-norsecurinine	P. niruri		[238]
373	Epibubbialine	P. niruri		[239]
373	Epibubbialine	P. amarus		[240]
374	Isobubbialine	P. niruri		[215]
374	Isobubbialine	P. urinaria		[215]
374	Isobubbialine	P. amarus		[240]
375	Methyl (2S)-1-[2-(furan-2-yl)-2-oxoethyl]-5-oxopyrrolidine-2-carboxylate	P. emblica		[114]
376	Nirurine	P. niruri		[241]
377	Niruroidine	P. niruroides		[242]
378	Nitidine	P. sellowianus		[243]
379	Norsecurinine	P. niruri		[235]

TABLE 2: Continued.

Number	Compounds	Species	Pharmacological effects	References
379	Norsecurinine	*P. amarus*	Antifungal	[240, 244]
379	Norsecurinine	*P. simplex*		[245]
379	Norsecurinine	*P. discoides*		[246]
380	Phyllanthine	*P. niruri*		[236]
380	Phyllanthine	*P. amarus*		[240]
381	Securinine	*P. niruri*		[235]
381	Securinine	*P. amarus*		[240]
381	Securinine	*P. glaucus*		[237]
382	Securinol A	*P. niruri*		[235]
383	Securinol B	*P. niruri*		[235]
384	Simplexine	*P. simplex*		[245]
385	Tetrahydrosecurinine	*P. niruri*		[235]
386	Virosecurinine	*P. discoides*		[247]
387	1,12-Diazacyclodocosane-2,11-dione	*P. niruri*		[248]
388	3-(3-Methylbut-2-en-1-yl) isoguanine	*P. reticulatus*		[118]
389	5-Hydroxy-isoquinoline	*P. emblica*		[249]
390	E,E-2,4-Octadienamide	*P. fraternus*	Antimalarial	[250]
391	E,Z-2,4-Decadienamide	*P. fraternus*	Antimalarial	[250]
392	Indole-3-carboxaldehyde	*P. virgatus*		[94]
393	Indole-3-carboxylic acid	*P. virgatus*		[131]
394	Phyllanthimide	*P. sellowianus*		[251]
395	Phyllurine	*P. urinaria*		[252]
396	(−)-Epicatechin 3-O-gallate	*P. niruri*		[176]
396	(−)-Epicatechin 3-O-gallate	*P. orbicularis*	Antiviral	[53]
397	(−)-Epigallocatechin 3-O-gallate	*P. emblica*		[111]
397	(−)-Epigallocatechin 3-O-gallate	*P. niruri*		[176]
398	(5R*R*)-4,6-Dimethoxycarbonyl-5-[2′,3′,4′-trihydroxy-6′-(methoxycarbonyl) phenyl]-5,6-dihydro-2H-pyran-2-one	*P. reticulatus*		[16]
399	1-O-Galloyl-6-O-luteoyl-α-D-glucose	*P. niruri*	Antimalarial	[223]
400	1-O-Galloyl-β-D-glucose	*P. emblica*	Antidiabetic and antitumor	[111, 253, 254]
400	1-O-Galloyl-β-D-glucose	*P. virgatus*		[94]
401	2-(2-Methylbutyryl)phloroglucinol 1-O-(6″-O-β-D-apiofuranosyl)-β-D-glucopyranoside	*P. emblica*		[230]
402	2,3,4,5,6-Pentahydroxybenzoic acid	*P. urinaria*		[255]
403	2,3,5,6-Tetrahydroxybenzyl acetate	*P. niruri*		[256]
404	2,6-Dimethoxy-4-(2-hydroxyethyl)phenol 1-O-β-D-glucopyranoside	*P. emblica*		[110]
405	2-Carboxylmethylphenol 1-O-β-D-glucopyranoside	*P. emblica*		[110]
406	3″-Hydroxy robustaside A (6′-(3″,4″-dihydroxy cinnamoyl) arbutin)	*P. atropurpureus*		[228]
407	3,3′-Di-O-methylellagic acid	*P. reticulatus*		[105]
408	3,4,3′-Tri-O-methylellagic acid	*P. urinaria*		[172]
408	3,4,3′-Tri-O-methylellagic acid	*P. reticulatus*		[16]
409	3,4,8,9,10-Pentahydroxy-dibenzo[b,d] pyran-6-one	*P. emblica*		[114]
410	3,4-di-O-Methylellagic acid	*P. reticulatus*		[105]
411	3,5-Dicaffeoylquinic acid	*P. muellerianus*		[169]
412	3,5-Dihydroxy-4-methoxybenzoic acid	*P. urinaria*		[73]

TABLE 2: Continued.

Number	Compounds	Species	Pharmacological effects	References
413	3-Ethylgallic acid	P. emblica		[208]
414	3-O-Methylellagic acid 4'-O-α-L-rhamnopyranoside	P. reticulatus		[105]
415	4,4'-Di-O-methylellagic acid	P. reticulatus		[105]
416	4-Hydroxy-3-methoxybenzaldehyde	P. emblica		[114]
417	4-Hydroxy-3-methoxy-benzoic acid	P. amarus		[74]
418	4-O-Caffeoylquinic acid	P. niruri		[257]
419	4-O-Methylellagic acid-3'-α-rhamnoside	P. emblica		[87]
420	4-O-Methylgallic acid	P. polyphyllus	Anti-inflammatory	[126]
421	8,9-Epoxy brevifolin	P. simplex	Hepatoprotective	[258]
422	Bergenin	P. flexuosus		[80]
422	Bergenin	P. wightianus		[89]
423	Brevifolin	P. urinaria		[259]
423	Brevifolin	P. virgatus		[94]
423	Brevifolin	P. simplex	Hepatoprotective	[260]
424	Brevifolin carboxylic acid	P. niruri		[261]
424	Brevifolin carboxylic acid	P. urinaria		[209]
424	Brevifolin carboxylic acid	P. amarus	Antidiabetic	[193]
424	Brevifolin carboxylic acid	P. matsumurae		[196]
425	Caffeoylmalic acid	P. muellerianus		[169]
426	Chebulic acid	P. emblica		[253]
427	Chlorogenic acid	P. sellowianus		[168]
427	Chlorogenic acid	P. muellerianus		[169]
428	Dehydrochebulic acid trimethyl ester	P. urinaria		[73]
429	Di [3,4,5-trihydroxy-phenyl] ether	P. atropurpureus		[228]
430	Ellagic acid	P. emblica	Antioxidant	[100, 210]
430	Ellagic acid	P. niruri	Antidiabetic	[202, 261]
430	Ellagic acid	P. urinaria	Antitumor	[220, 262]
430	Ellagic acid	P. reticulatus		[192]
430	Ellagic acid	P. matsumurae		[196]
430	Ellagic acid	P. wightianus		[89]
431	Ethyl brevifolin carboxylate	P. niruri		[261]
431	Ethyl brevifolin carboxylate	P. urinaria		[189]
432	Ethyl gallate	P. emblica	Antitussive	[212, 263]
432	Ethyl gallate	P. myrtifolius		[186]
433	Flavogallonic acid bislactone	P. emblica		[184]
434	Gallic acid	P. emblica	Antiulcer and antioxidant	[210, 264]
434	Gallic acid	P. niruri	Anti-inflammatory	[202, 224]
434	Gallic acid	P. urinaria		[220]
434	Gallic acid	P. virgatus		[94]
434	Gallic acid	P. amarus	Antijaundice	[265]
434	Gallic acid	P. myrtifolius		[186]
434	Gallic acid	P. muellerianus		[169]
434	Gallic acid	P. debilis	Antioxidant	[195]
434	Gallic acid	P. simplex		[170]
434	Gallic acid	P. matsumurae		[196]

TABLE 2: Continued.

Number	Compounds	Species	Pharmacological effects	References
434	Gallic acid	*P. wightianus*		[89]
434	Gallic acid	*P. ussuriensis*		[225]
435	Gallic acid 3-O-(6′-O-galloyl)-β-D-glucoside	*P. emblica*		[184]
436	Gallic acid 3-O-β-D-glucoside	*P. emblica*		[184]
437	Gallic acid 4-methyl ether	*P. cochinchinensis*		[149]
438	Gallic acid ethyl ester	*P. urinaria*	Antihyperalgesic	[266]
438	Gallic acid ethyl ester	*P. sellowianus*		[95]
438	Gallic acid ethyl ester	*P. caroliniensis*	Anti-inflammatory	[203]
439	Koaburaside	*P. cochinchinensis*		[149]
440	L-Malic acid 2-O-gallate	*P. emblica*	Antitumor	[111, 253]
441	Methyl-4-hydroxybenzoate	*P. emblica*		[114]
442	Methyl brevifolin carboxylate	*P. niruri*	Hypotensive and antiplatelet	[206, 267, 268]
442	Methyl brevifolin carboxylate	*P. urinaria*	Antioxidant and anti-inflammatory	[151, 269]
442	Methyl brevifolin carboxylate	*P. reticulatus*		[192]
442	Methyl brevifolin carboxylate	*P. virgatus*		[94]
443	Methyl ester dehydrochebulic acid	*P. urinaria*		[269]
444	Methyl gallate	*P. emblica*	Antioxidant and antitussive	[187, 263]
444	Methyl gallate	*P. urinaria*	Antioxidant and anti-inflammatory	[151]
444	Methyl gallate	*P. reticulatus*		[192]
444	Methyl gallate	*P. virgatus*		[94]
444	Methyl gallate	*P. myrtifolius*		[186]
444	Methyl gallate	*P. muellerianus*		[169]
444	Methyl gallate	*P. ussuriensis*		[197]
445	Mucic acid 1,4-lactone 2-O-gallate	*P. emblica*		[253]
446	Mucic acid 1,4-lactone 3,5-di-O-gallate	*P. emblica*		[253]
447	Mucic acid 1,4-lactone 3-O-gallate	*P. emblica*	Antioxidant	[185, 253]
448	Mucic acid 1,4-lactone 5-O-gallate	*P. emblica*		[253]
449	Mucic acid 1,4-lactone 6-methyl ester 2-O-gallate	*P. emblica*		[253]
450	Mucic acid 1,4-lactone 6-methyl ester 5-O-gallate	*P. emblica*		[253]
451	Mucic acid 1-methyl ester 2-O-gallate	*P. emblica*		[253]
452	Mucic acid 2-O-gallate	*P. emblica*	Antitumor	[111, 253]
453	Mucic acid 3-O-gallate	*P. emblica*		[270]
454	Mucic acid 6-methyl ester 2-O-gallate	*P. emblica*		[253]
455	Mucic acid di-methyl ester 2-O-gallate	*P. emblica*		[253]
456	p-Hydroxybenzaldehyde	*P. urinaria*		[73]
457	Phloroglucinol	*P. ussuriensis*		[225]
458	Phyllangin	*P. niruri*		[256]
459	Phyllanthusin F	*P. urinaria*		[271]
460	Potassium brevifolin carboxylate	*P. virgatus*		[94]
461	Protocatechuic acid	*P. urinaria*		[189]
461	Protocatechuic acid	*P. matsumurae*		[196]
462	Pyrogallol	*P. emblica*	Antitumor and anti-inflammatory	[249, 272]
462	Pyrogallol	*P. urinaria*		[167]

TABLE 2: Continued.

Number	Compounds	Species	Pharmacological effects	References
463	Robustaside A	P. atropurpureus	Antitumor	[228]
464	Shikimic acid	P. myrtifolius		[186]
465	Syringaldehyde	P. emblica		[114]
466	Tri-Me dehydrochebulic acid	P. urinaria		[220]
467	Trimethyl-3,4-dehydrochebulate	P. urinaria	Antioxidant and anti-inflammatory	[151]
468	Vanillic acid	P. emblica		[114]
469	(−)-7′-Hydroxydivanillyltetrahydrofuran	P. songboiensis		[65]
470	(+)-Cucurbic acid	P. urinaria		[73]
471	(+)-Methyl cucurbate	P. urinaria		[73]
472	(E)-3-(5′-Hydroperoxy-2,2′-dihydroxy[1,1′-biphenyl]-4-yl)-2-propenoic acid	P. urinaria		[255]
473	1′S-11-Dehydroxy penicillide	P. emblica		[114]
474	2R-Diethyl malate	P. emblica		[114]
475	3,6′-Di-O-benzoyl-2′-O-acetylsucrose	P. cochinchinensis		[108]
476	3,6′-Di-O-benzoyl-3′-O-acetylsucrose	P. cochinchinensis		[108]
477	3,6′-Di-O-benzoyl-4′-O-acetylsucrose	P. cochinchinensis		[108]
478	3,6′-Di-O-benzoylsucrose	P. cochinchinensis		[108]
479	3,4-Dimethoxyphenyl-β-D-glucopyranoside	P. cochinchinensis		[149]
480	3,4-Dihydroxyphenylpropanol 3-O-β-D-glucopyranoside	P. reticulatus		[118]
481	3,4,5-Trimethoxy-phenyl-β-D-glucopyranoside	P. cochinchinensis		[149]
482	3-O-Benzoyl-6′-O-(E)-cinnamoylsucrose	P. cochinchinensis		[108]
483	4,4,8-Trimethoxy chroman	P. amarus		[273]
484	5-Hydroxymethyl-2-furaldehyde	P. urinaria		[73]
485	4-Hydroxysesamin	P. niruri		[274]
486	5-Hydroxymethylfurfural	P. emblica	Antioxidant	[171]
487	Aquilegiolide	P. anisolobus		[138]
487	Aquilegiolide	P. klotzschianus		[275]
488	Bis(2-ethylicosyl)phthalate	P. muellerianus		[92]
489	Bis(2-ethyloctyl)phthalate	P. muellerianus		[92]
490	Di-O-methylcrenatin	P. cochinchinensis		[149]
491	Byzantionoside B	P. multiflorus		[276]
492	Carthamoside B5	P. reticulatus		[118]
493	Dendranthemoside B	P. urinaria		[141]
494	Hovetrichoside A	P. reticulatus		[118]
495	Isotachioside	P. reticulatus		[118]
496	Menisdaurilide	P. anisolobus		[138]
496	Menisdaurilide	P. klotzschianus		[275]
497	Methyl (1 R,2R,2′Z)-2-(5′-hydroxy-pent-2′-enyl)-3-oxocyclopentaneacetate	P. urinaria		[73]
498	Mucic acid	P. emblica		[277]
499	Mucic acid 1-methyl ester-6-ethyl ester	P. emblica		[114]
500	Penicillide	P. emblica		[114]
501	Phthalic acid bis(2,5-dimethylhexyl) ester	P. urinaria		[99]
502	Phyllanthoid A	P. cochinchinensis	Antitumor	[278]
503	Phyllanthoid B	P. cochinchinensis		[278]
504	Phyllanthurinolactone	P. urinaria		[279]
505	Phyllanthusone	P. fraternus		[121]

TABLE 2: Continued.

Number	Compounds	Species	Pharmacological effects	References
506	Phyllester	*P. niruri*		[157]
507	Purpactin A	*P. emblica*		[114]
508	Roseoside	*P. multiflorus*		[276]
509	Succinic acid	*P. niruri*		[280]
510	Terephthalic acid mono-[2-(4-carboxy-phenoxycarbonyl)-vinyl] ester	*P. urinaria*		[255]
511	Vanilloloside	*P. cochinchinensis*		[149]
512	Xanthoxyline	*P. sellowianus*		[281]

3.1. Terpenoids. Terpenoids are the most prevalent chemical class of the genus. About 125 compounds including 69 triterpenoids (1–69), 40 sesquiterpenes (70–109), 11 diterpenoids (110–120), and 5 monoterpenes (121–125) are mainly identified from *P. flexuosus*, *P. reticulatus*, *P. watsonii*, *P. emblica*, *P. acuminatus*, and *P. veuminatus*. Compounds 1–14 are tetracyclic triterpenoids, and compounds 15–69 are pentacyclic triterpenoids. In pentacyclic triterpenoids, compounds 15–36, compounds 37–49, and compounds 50–65 are oleanane type, friedelane type, and lupine type, respectively. Glochidone and lupeol are representatives of lupine type triterpenoids, which were suggested to have antitumor activities and mainly isolated from *Phyllanthus* species [68, 80, 96].

3.2. Phenylpropanoids. Phenylpropanoids (126–227) have typical C6–C3 constituents, which chiefly involve three groups including lignins, simple phenylpropanoids, and coumarins. 90 lignins (126–215) have been isolated from genus *Phyllanthus* since 1944. Compounds 126–176 are arylnaphthalene type lignins with a ring caused by the link of C-6 and C-7'. Compounds 177–190 are dibenzylbutane type lignins with two simple phenylpropanoids bounded by C-8 and C-8'. Phyllanthin, which had been studied to the most extent, was considered to be correlated with anti-inflammatory, immunomodulatory, antitumor, and hypotensive activities [127, 144, 163]. Pharmacokinetic studies of retrojusticidin B, a potential anti-HIV compound, had been done. The oral bioavailabilities dissolved in Tween 80 and in corn oil were found to be 22.1 and 33.1%, respectively [152].

3.3. Tannins. Tannins were progressively reported from the genus *Phyllanthus* since 1992. Hydrolyzable tannins (228–270) are characterized by the presence of one or more galloyl, hexahydroxydiphenoyl (HHDP), and HHDP metabolites attached to a glucopyranose core, which are mainly isolated from *P. emblica*, *P. amarus*, *P. niruri*, and *P. urinaria*. Compounds 271–279 are condensed tannins, which are the condensation of flavan-3-ols and linked by C-C. A great many condensed tannins were proved to have antiviral activity [53]. Ellagitannins (232–270) are the largest group of hydrolyzable tannins. Corilagin and geraniin are most extensively obtained from this genus and are characteristic compounds of ellagitannins, which exhibited multiple activities such as antioxidant, anti-HIV, antitumor, and antihyperalgesic activities [6, 111, 188, 195, 196, 199, 201, 202].

3.4. Flavonoids. Compounds 281–334 are flavonoids, which mainly contain flavonols (280–309), flavones (310–317), flavonones (318–324), flavan-3-ols (325–330), flavanonols (331), and isoflavone (332-333). Flavan-3-ols are the basic constitution of condensed tannins. Flavonols such as quercetin, quercitrin, and rutin demonstrated anti-inflammatory and antioxidant activities [151, 171, 178, 195, 203, 224].

3.5. Sterols. Until now, thirty sterols (334–363) from *Phyllanthus* have been reported. All the sterols are phytosterols with a side chain (C8–C10) substitution at C-17, and half of which were isolated from *P. emblica*.

3.6. Alkaloids. Thirty-two alkaloids (364–395) have been found in genus *Phyllanthus*, most of which are securinine and securinine-related compounds and mainly distributed in *P. niruri*. Compounds 390-391 isolated from *P. fraternus* are amide type alkaloids and exhibited antimalarial potential [250].

3.7. Phenols and Others. Compounds 396–468 belong to phenols, which have one and several phenolic hydroxyl groups. Thirty other constitutions (469–512) have been isolated. Mucic acid (compounds 445–455) and its derivatives (compounds 498-499) can only be found in *P. emblica* among this genus.

4. Biological Activity

The remarkable traditional uses of genus *Phyllanthus* lead to the various researches of biological activities, such as antiviral, antioxidant, antidiabetic, anticancer, and immunomodulatory activities. In this section, biological activity researches of the extracts of the plants are highlighted.

4.1. Antiviral Activity. Various *Phyllanthus* plants were reported to have strong antiviral potential such as anti-HIV, anti-HCV, anti-HSV, and anti-HCMV. The aqueous extract of *P. emblica* reduced viral load of HIV significantly at the dose of 400 μg/mL [282]. DNA-polymerase and ribonuclease H (RNase H) activities of HIV-1 reverse transcriptase were inhibited by aqueous extract of *P. sellowianus* with IC_{50} values of 2.4 ± 0.8 μg/mL and 5.9 ± 1.4 μg/mL, respectively [283]. Moreover, methanol extract of *P. reticulatus* strongly inhibited the activity of RNase H by 99% at the dose of $50 \mu g/mL$ [284].

HCV-infected HuH7 cells were used to test the anti-HCV activities of methanolic fraction of *P. amarus*. The fraction was proved to suppress the replication of HCV monocistronic replicon RNA and HCV H77S viral RNA without toxic effect in host cells. Inhibiting HCV-NS3 protease enzyme and NS5B enzyme may be the main mechanism [285]. Aqueous extract of *P. orbicularis* revealed inhibition activity against the replication of HCMV, HSV-1, and HSV-2 as well as BHV-1 with EC_{50} values of 57.7, 28.8, 25.7, and $21.27 \mu g/mL$, respectively. The selectivity indexes (SI) were ranged from 8.7 to 37.6 [286, 287].

Friend murine leukemia virus (FMuLv) induced erythroleukemia in BALB/c mice was relieved by metabolic extract of *P. amarus*. The extract inhibited leukemic cells from infiltrating into the sinusoidal space, decreased the morbidity of anemia, and improved survival rate of leukemia animals. Besides, the extract induced the upregulation of p53 and p45NFE2 and downregulation of Bcl-2 in the spleen [288].

4.2. Antioxidant Activity.
Methanolic and aqueous parts of this genus have remarkable antioxidant activity, which may be correlated with the hydroxyl rich compositions. *P. acidus*, *P. polyphyllus*, and *P. fraternus* showed remarkable hepatoprotective activity against liver toxicity which was induced by acetaminophen, carbon tetrachloride, bromobenzene, and thioacetamide [42, 289–291]. The biochemical parameters as well as antioxidants levels were restored by these parts at the dose of 300 mg/kg. What is more, mitochondrial dysfunction in liver, induced by bromobenzene, was relieved by prior oral administration of aqueous part of *P. fraternus* at the dose of 100 mg/kg [51, 291].

Antimycin A governed mitochondrial protein degeneration, lipid peroxidation and mitochondrial DNA damage, and H_2O_2 induced membrane damage of Hep3B cells were considerably mitigated by aqueous fraction of *P. amarus* [164]. Mutagenesis induced by PhIP and 4-ABP and DNA damage induced by γ-ray and UVB were protected by aqueous fraction of *P. orbicularis* [292–294].

Methanol extract of *P. debilis* showed strong antioxidant activity when tested by various antioxidant assays including total antioxidant, free radical scavenging, superoxide anion radical scavenging, hydrogen peroxide scavenging, and nitric oxide scavenging assays. Besides, further study demonstrated that total phenolic was correlated with antioxidant activity [52]. In addition, hydromethanolic extract of *P. virgatus* exhibited substantially antioxidant capacity in both DPPH scavenging ($IC_{50} = 30.4 \mu g/mL$) and linoleic acid oxidation inhibiting (84%) method [5].

4.3. Antidiabetic Activity.
Twelve herb drugs such as *P. emblica*, *P. reticulatus*, *P. niruri*, *P. amarus*, *P. urinaria*, *P. acidus*, *P. debilis*, *P. virgatus*, *P. sellowianus*, *P. rheedii*, *P. orbicularis*, and *P. hookeri* are traditionally employed for diabetes in many countries. Recent researches about the hypoglycemic effect of *Phyllanthus* plants were abundant. Streptozotocin- and alloxan-induced diabetic rats were employed for the evaluation of antidiabetic potential of *P. emblica*, *P. niruri*,

P. reticulatus, *P. sellowianus*, *P. virgatus*, and *P. simplex* [4, 295–299]. After oral administration of these (aqueous, methanol, and ethanol) extracts for 21–45 days, the concentration of blood glucose was significantly reduced, and the effects of *P. sellowianus* and *P. simplex* were similar to the glibenclamide group (10 mg/kg). In addition, methanol fraction of *P. virgatus* considerably inhibited the activity of α-amylase in the noncompetitive pattern with IC_{50} of $33.20 \pm 0.556 \mu g/mL$ [300].

After oral aqueous extract of *P. niruri* for 28 days, the levels of LPO and MDA were decreased while the concentrations of SOD, CAT, and GPx were increased. After being pretreated with the aqueous fraction of *P. sellowianus*, hemorheological parameters were ameliorated and red blood cells (RBCs) showed large globular aggregates and agglutination [301].

4.4. Anticancer Activity.
Different extracts of the plants have been assessed for anticancer effects and the related mechanisms. Cancer cell lines such as NCI-H1703, MDA-MB-231, HeLa, 143B, PC-3, MCF-7, HepG2, A549, SKOV3, and HT-29 were considerably inhibited by *P. emblica*, *P. urinaria*, *P. polyphyllus*, *P. watsonii*, and *P. pulcher* [57, 68, 302–309]. In addition, *P. emblica* showed no toxicity to normal cells (MRC5). The extracts inhibited growth of cells through fragmentation of DNA and dysfunction of mitochondrial including upregulated mitochondrial fission 1 protein and downregulated optic atrophy type 1 and mitofusin 1 [304]. Moreover, the extracts suppressed the ability of cell invasion, migration, and adhesion. Further researches demonstrated that the fractions induced apoptosis, invasion, and migration through increasing the expression of caspase-3, caspase-7, caspase-8, and p-JNK and decreasing the expression of ERK, p-ERK1/2, JNK, MMP-2, MMP-9, Wnt, NF-κB, Myc/Max, and hypoxia [302, 303, 307].

Ehrlich ascites carcinoma tumor model was used to evaluate the antitumor activity of *P. polyphyllus*. Oral administration of methanol fraction at the dose of 200 mg/kg could significantly reduce the solid tumor volume. Hematological parameters, protein, packed cellular volume (PCV), and antioxidant enzymes such as LPO, GPx, GST, SOD, and CAT were greatly regulated [57].

4.5. Immunomodulatory Activity.
Ethanol extracts of *P. urinaria* and *P. amarus* were demonstrated to have inhibitory effects on the chemotaxis of neutrophils and monocytes with IC_{50} lower than $2.92 \mu g/mL$. In addition, phagocytic activity and CD18 expression of neutrophils and monocytes were downregulated [163].

Oral administration of *P. reticulatus* extract at the dose of 100 mg/kg demonstrated a significant increase in phagocytic activity, the percentage of neutrophil adhesion, and white blood cell in albino mice [310].

4.6. Analgesic Activity.
The extracts of *P. corcovadensis*, *P. niruri*, and *P. tenellus* showed significant reduction in writhing response induced by acetic acid, with ID_{50} values of 30, 19, and >30 mg/kg, respectively. The late phase of formalin-induced pain could be relieved by *P. tenellus* with ID_{50} of 100 mg/kg and both phases of formalin-induced pain could

be reduced by *P. corcovadensis* and *P. niruri* with ID_{50} values of 100 and 52 mg/kg, respectively. The analgesic effects could not be antagonized by naloxone [311]. In addition, intraperitoneally given hydroalcoholic extracts of *P. amarus*, *P. orbicularis*, and *P. fraternus* produced a marked analgesic activity by inhibiting acetic acid-induced abdominal constriction, capsaicin-induced neurogenic pain, and late phase of formalin-induced paw licking [312]. The ethanol and aqueous extracts of *P. emblica* succeeded in inhibiting acetic acid-induced writhing response but failed in the tail-immersion test [313].

4.7. Anti-Inflammatory Activity. In recent years, different inflammatory models such as Freund's complete adjuvant induced arthritis, carrageenin induced paw edema, and cotton pellet induced granuloma were employed to evaluate the anti-inflammatory effect of *Phyllanthus*. After receiving the aqueous extract of *P. amarus*, indexes of arthritis, joint diameter, and paw volume were decreased and thresholds of mechanical hyperalgesia and nociceptive were increased [314]. The ethanol fraction of *P. simplex* ameliorated the parameters of paw edema and granuloma and substantially inhibited nitric oxide (NO) production [315].

4.8. Antispasmodic Activity. Isolated rabbit jejunum and guinea-pig ileum were employed for the *in vitro* tests for the antispasmodic effects of *P. emblica*. Carbachol and K^+ induced contractions of rabbit jejunum were released by the extract with IC_{50} values of 0.09 mg/mL and 1.38 mg/mL. The pretreatment of guinea-pig ileum with the extract at 0.3 mg/mL caused a rightward parallel shift in the concentration-response curves of acetylcholine without suppression of the maximum contractile response. Dual blockade of muscarinic receptors and Ca^{2+} channels can explain its antispasmodic activity [316].

4.9. Hypotensive and Hypolipidemic Activity. Aqueous extract of the leaves of *P. amarus* was found to restrain both force and rate of myocardial contraction and to inhibit the intrinsic myogenic contraction of isolated rat portal vein [317]. Aqueous part of *P. reticulatus* was effective in releasing total cholesterol, lipid profile, and oxidative stress in hypercholesterolemic albino rats after oral administrated for 45 days at 250 mg/kg [14].

4.10. Wound Healing. Extracts of *P. emblica* and *P. niruri* were demonstrated to have wound healing effect. Topical application with *P. emblica* could promote the proliferation of cells and cross-link of collagen in the full thickness excision wound [318]. Oral administration of *P. emblica* at the dose of 60 mg/kg showed healing effect against NSAID-induced gastric ulcer through upregulating the concentration of IL-10 and downregulating the levels of TNF-α and IL-1β [319]. After treatment with *P. niruri* at the dose of 200 mg/kg, 98.8% of wound could be recovered in the excision and incision wound models on the 16th day [320].

4.11. Antimalarial Activity. Malaria is a prevalent disease in many tropical and subtropical countries and folks of these places especially African people employed *Phyllanthus* as

antimalarial agency. *Plasmodium falciparum* was suppressed by ethyl acetate fraction of *P. acidus* with IC_{50} of 9.37 μg/mL, and the SI equals 4.88 for HEp-2 cells and 11.75 for Vero cells [321]. What is more, chloroquine-resistant *P. falciparum* could be exhibited by *P. amarus* and *P. muellerianus* with IC_{50} values of 11.7 and 9.4 μg/mL, respectively. *P. amarus* presented protection effect on human RBCs damage caused by the virus [322]. The SI of *P. muellerianus* was higher than 5.3 for L-6 and MRC-5 cell lines [25, 202].

4.12. Antidepressant Activity. The aqueous extract of *P. emblica* (200 mg/kg) significantly decreased immobility period in both tail suspension test and forced swim test by decreasing the levels of MAO-A and GABA [323]. In the plus-maze, Hebb-Williams maze, and passive avoidance apparatus test, preparation of *P. emblica* produced a dose-dependent upgrade in scores. The preparation was also proved to reverse the amnesia induced by diazepam and scopolamine and to reduce the cholinesterase activity and total cholesterol level in brain [324, 325].

4.13. Others. The essential oil fraction of *P. muellerianus* exhibited strong antibacterial activity against *Clostridium sporogenes*, *Streptococcus mutans*, and *S. pyogenes* with MIC values ranging from 13.5 to 126 μg/mL [326]. Methanol extract of *P. acuminatus* (100 mg/mL) showed stronger antifungal than Dithane M-45 (10 000-ppm solution) against *Pythium ultimum* [327].

Aqueous extract of *P. acidus* was proved to regulate electrolyte transport in cystic fibrosis airways by increasing the intracellular levels of cAMP and Ca^{2+}, stimulating basolateral K^+ channels, and activating and redistributing cellular localization of cystic fibrosis transmembrane conductance regulator [328].

Eight hours after being treated with the aqueous extract of *P. sellowianus* at a dose of 400 mg/kg, urine output of test animals was decreased from 2.59 to 3.69 mL/100 g [329].

5. Clinical Studies

The extracts of *P. niruri* were proved to have immunomodulatory effect and played a crucial role in treating pulmonary tuberculosis and vaginal candidiasis as well as varicella. In patients with pulmonary tuberculosis, after oral administration of *P. niruri* 50 mg/mL for 2–6 months, the level of IL-10 was decreased and the levels of plasma IFN-γ and TNF-α were significantly increased. After 1-month treatment, the increase of the ratio of $CD4^+/CD8^+$ was observed. In the vaginal candidiasis patients, after receiving *P. niruri* 100 mg/mL for 1–3 months, the levels of IFN-γ and IL-12 were elevated. As for varicella patients, the number of papules and the number crusts were decreased after treatment with the extract at the dose of 5 mg/mL [330].

Clinical studies of *P. niruri* in Brazil had been finished, from which the *P. niruri* showed beneficial effects on the treatment of urolithiasis. After 3-month treatment, calculi elimination was increased. Furthermore, urinary calcium excretion and residual stone fragments after lithotripsy were decreased. Toxic effects on kidney, cardiovascular, and nervous systems were not found [331].

In China, the clinical study of *P. urinaria* in treating chronic hepatitis B with 140 patients was well established. The results indicated that, after treatment with *P. urinaria* capsule for 3 months or 2 years, especially in the long term, the recovery rate in the index of HBV-DNA and HBeAg was 88.2% and 52.5%, respectively. Once the treatment stopped, the recurrence rate was 10.4% to 13.4% [332].

6. Toxicity Studies

After given aqueous leaf extract of *P. niruri* at the dose of 2000 mg/mL, no acute toxicity was observed at the levels of bilirubin, ALT, AST, total protein, albumin, globulin, ALP, GGT, urea, creatinine, full blood count, and hemoglobin [333]. After being treated with ethanol extract of *P. niruri* over a period of 90 days at doses of 30 and 300 mg/kg, the rats showed no genotoxic effect at the test of PCE/NCE ratio [334]. Reproductive toxicity of *P. niruri* was tested using estrogen values, progesterone values, and testosterone levels. The estrogen and progesterone levels increased more than 1.5-fold above the control group after receiving 50 and 500 mg/kg aqueous leaf extract for 90 days, which reminded us of the cytotoxic of male antifertility properties [335].

Nephrotoxicity including interstitial oedema and tubular necrosis were detected after receiving 400 and 800 mg/kg of aqueous extract from *P. amarus* for 30 days [336]. The test animals were given 800 and 1600 mg/kg of the aqueous extract of *P. amarus* for 10 days, and significant pathological changes were found in the liver, kidney, and testis. The frequency of MNPCE, sperm abnormalities, total white blood cell, and lymphocyte counts were significantly increased, which suggested the genetic and systemic toxicity of *P. amarus* [337]. In addition, aqueous, methanolic, and hydromethanolic extracts of *P. amarus* (400 mg/kg) reduced locomotor activity and showed CNS depressant effect [338].

The LD_{50} of ethanolic extract from *P. fraternus* was 1125 mg/kg in the toxicity test. When the rats received the extract at doses of 400 mg/kg for 7 days, no toxicity was detected in liver and kidney [339]. Hydroethanolic extract *P. fraternus* showed the quick onset and long duration of reduction of locomotor activity at the dose of 400 mg/kg [338].

7. Conclusion

514 compounds have been isolated from different species of *Phyllanthus*, including 126 terpenoids, 102 phenylpropanoids, 73 phenols, 54 flavonoids, 53 tannins, 33 sterols, 31 alkaloids, and a number of other compositions. Their wide range of biological activities such as antiviral, antioxidant, antidiabetic, anticancer, anti-inflammatory, hypolipidemic, immunomodulatory, and antidepressant activities are tested using polar solvents (water, methanol, and ethanol) extracts. These extracts are considered rich in phenols, flavonoids, and tannins, which may exhibit antioxidant activity in different degree due to their hydroxyl [340]. Consequently, most bioactivities of *Phyllanthus* may be correlated with the hydroxyl rich compounds.

In recent years, the traditional uses of *Phyllanthus* had been partly confirmed, and more evidences such as pharmacological researches and clinical studies are urgently needed to be taken. Further studies of phytochemical discovery and subsequent screenings are necessary to be taken to extend the use of *Phyllanthus* and to develop leading compound.

Competing Interests

The authors declare that they have no competing interests.

Acknowledgments

This project was supported by the National Natural Science Foundation of China (81274187 and 81274006) and Transformation and industrialization of Science and Technology Achievements, "New Drug AIKEXIN Development Research for the Treatment of AIDS."

References

[1] D. W. Unander, G. L. Webster, and B. S. Blumberg, "Usage and bioassays in *Phyllanthus* (Euphorbiaceae). IV. Clustering of antiviral uses and other effects," *Journal of Ethnopharmacology*, vol. 45, no. 1, pp. 1–18, 1995.

[2] Q. Xia, *A pharmacognostic and ethnopharmacological studies of Chinese phyllanthus [Ph.D. thesis]*, Peking Union Medical College, Beijing, China, 1997.

[3] M. D. Adil, P. Kaiser, N. K. Satti, A. M. Zargar, R. A. Vishwakarma, and S. A. Tasduq, "Effect of *Emblica officinalis* (fruit) against UVB-induced photo-aging in human skin fibroblasts," *Journal of Ethnopharmacology*, vol. 132, no. 1, pp. 109–114, 2010.

[4] P. Nain, V. Saini, S. Sharma, and J. Nain, "Antidiabetic and antioxidant potential of Emblica officinalis Gaertn. leaves extract in streptozotocin-induced type-2 diabetes mellitus (T2DM) rats," *Journal of Ethnopharmacology*, vol. 142, no. 1, pp. 65–71, 2012.

[5] K. Poompachee and N. Chudapongse, "Comparison of the antioxidant and cytotoxic activities of *Phyllanthus virgatus* and *Phyllanthus amarus* extracts," *Medical Principles and Practice*, vol. 21, no. 1, pp. 24–29, 2011.

[6] J. Moreira, L. C. Klein-Júnior, V. Cechinel Filho, and F. de Campos Buzzi, "Anti-hyperalgesic activity of corilagin, a tannin isolated from *Phyllanthus niruri* L. (Euphorbiaceae)," *Journal of Ethnopharmacology*, vol. 146, no. 1, pp. 318–323, 2013.

[7] E. Omulokoli, B. Khan, and S. C. Chhabra, "Antiplasmodial activity of four Kenyan medicinal plants," *Journal of Ethnopharmacology*, vol. 56, no. 2, pp. 133–137, 1997.

[8] Q. Xia, P. Xiao, L. Wang, and J. Kong, "Ethnopharmacology of *Phyllanthus emblica* L," *Zhongguo Zhongyao Zazhi*, vol. 22, no. 9, pp. 515–525, 1997.

[9] M. Ishtiaq, W. Hanif, M. A. Khan, M. Ashraf, and A. M. Butt, "An ethnomedicinal survey and documentation of important medicinal folklore food phytonims of flora of Samahni valley, (Azad Kashmir) Pakistan," *Pakistan Journal of Biological Sciences*, vol. 10, no. 13, pp. 2241–2256, 2007.

[10] N. Kumar, W. Rungseevijitprapa, N.-A. Narkkhong, M. Suttajit, and C. Chaiyasut, "5α-reductase inhibition and hair growth promotion of some Thai plants traditionally used for hair treatment," *Journal of Ethnopharmacology*, vol. 139, no. 3, pp. 765–771, 2012.

[11] P. Mayachiew and S. Devahastin, "Antimicrobial and antioxidant activities of Indian gooseberry and galangal extracts," *LWT—Food Science and Technology*, vol. 41, no. 7, pp. 1153–1159, 2008.

[12] M. Rahmatullah, K. C. Ghosh, A. A. Mamun et al., "A pharmacological study on antinociceptive and anti-hyperglycemic effects of methanol extract of leaves of *Phyllanthus reticulatus* Poir. In Swiss albino mice," *Advances in Natural and Applied Sciences*, vol. 4, no. 3, pp. 229–232, 2010.

[13] J.-X. Ma, M.-S. Lan, S.-J. Qu et al., "Arylnaphthalene lignan glycosides and other constituents from *Phyllanthus reticulatus*," *Journal of Asian Natural Products Research*, vol. 14, no. 11, pp. 1073–1077, 2012.

[14] V. Maruthappan and K. S. Shree, "Effects of *Phyllanthus reticulatus* on lipid profile and oxidative stress in hypercholesterolemic albino rats," *Indian Journal of Pharmacology*, vol. 42, no. 6, pp. 388–391, 2010.

[15] S. Sharma and S. Kumar, "*Phyllanthus reticulatus* Poir.—an important medicinal plant: a review of its phytochemistry, traditional uses and pharmacological properties," *International Journal of Pharmaceutical Sciences and Research*, vol. 4, no. 7, pp. 2528–2534, 2013.

[16] N. Pojchaijongdee, U. Sotanaphun, S. Limsirichaikul, and O. Poobrasert, "Geraniinic acid derivative from the leaves of *Phyllanthus reticulatus*," *Pharmaceutical Biology*, vol. 48, no. 7, pp. 740–744, 2010.

[17] A. K. Jamal, W. A. Yaacob, and L. B. Din, "A chemical study on *Phyllanthus reticulatus*," *Journal of Physical Science*, vol. 19, no. 2, pp. 45–50, 2008.

[18] O. Ifeoma, O. Samuel, A. M. Itohan, and S. O. Adeola, "Isolation, fractionation and evaluation of the antiplasmodial properties of Phyllanthus niruri resident in its chloroform fraction," *Asian Pacific Journal of Tropical Medicine*, vol. 6, no. 3, pp. 169–175, 2013.

[19] X. R. Li, W. Zhou, and W. X. Wei, "Chemical component and bioactivities of *Phyllanthus niruri* L," *Tianran Chanwu Yanjiu Yu Kaifa*, vol. 19, no. 5, pp. 890–896, 2007.

[20] L. Tona, N. P. Ngimbi, M. Tsakala et al., "Antimalarial activity of 20 crude extracts from nine African medicinal plants used in Kinshasa, Congo," *Journal of Ethnopharmacology*, vol. 68, no. 1-3, pp. 193–203, 1999.

[21] K. Narendra, J. Swathi, K. Sowjanya, and A. Satya, "*Phyllanthus niruri*: a review on its ethno botanical, phytochemical and pharmacological profile," *Journal of Pharmacy Research*, vol. 5, no. 9, pp. 4681–4691, 2012.

[22] G. Bagalkotkar, S. R. Sagineedu, M. S. Saad, and J. Stanslas, "Phytochemicals from *Phyllanthus niruri* Linn. and their pharmacological properties: a review," *Journal of Pharmacy and Pharmacology*, vol. 58, no. 12, pp. 1559–1570, 2006.

[23] N. A. Shakil, Pankaj, J. Kumar, R. K. Pandey, and D. B. Saxena, "Nematicidal prenylated flavanones from *Phyllanthus niruri*," *Phytochemistry*, vol. 69, no. 3, pp. 759–764, 2008.

[24] V. Murugaiyah and K.-L. Chan, "Mechanisms of antihyperuricemic effect of *Phyllanthus niruri* and its lignan constituents," *Journal of Ethnopharmacology*, vol. 124, no. 2, pp. 233–239, 2009.

[25] G. N. Zirihi, L. Mambu, F. Guédé-Guina, B. Bodo, and P. Grellier, "In vitro antiplasmodial activity and cytotoxicity of 33 West African plants used for treatment of malaria," *Journal of Ethnopharmacology*, vol. 98, no. 3, pp. 281–285, 2005.

[26] S. Das, S. Das, and B. De, "In vitro inhibition of key enzymes related to diabetes by the aqueous extracts of some fruits of West Bengal, India," *Current Nutrition and Food Science*, vol. 8, no. 1, pp. 19–24, 2012.

[27] C. Agyare, A. Asase, M. Lechtenberg, M. Niehues, A. Deters, and A. Hensel, "An ethnopharmacological survey and in vitro confirmation of ethnopharmacological use of medicinal plants used for wound healing in Bosomtwi-Atwima-Kwanwoma area, Ghana," *Journal of Ethnopharmacology*, vol. 125, no. 3, pp. 393–403, 2009.

[28] A. O. Eweka and A. Enogieru, "Effects of oral administration of *Phyllanthus amarus* leaf extract on the kidneys of adult wistar rats- a histological study," *African Journal of Traditional, Complementary and Alternative Medicines*, vol. 8, no. 3, pp. 307–311, 2011.

[29] S. Khatoon, V. Rai, A. K. S. Rawat, and S. Mehrotra, "Comparative pharmacognostic studies of three *Phyllanthus* species," *Journal of Ethnopharmacology*, vol. 104, no. 1-2, pp. 79–86, 2006.

[30] P. Keluskar and S. Ingle, "Ethnopharmacology guided screening of traditional Indian herbs for selective inhibition of *Plasmodium* specific lactate dehydrogenase," *Journal of Ethnopharmacology*, vol. 144, no. 1, pp. 201–207, 2012.

[31] J. R. Patel, P. Tripathi, V. Sharma, N. S. Chauhan, and V. K. Dixit, "*Phyllanthus amarus*: ethnomedicinal uses, phytochemistry and pharmacology: a review," *Journal of Ethnopharmacology*, vol. 138, no. 2, pp. 286–313, 2011.

[32] J. R. Xavier, R. Gnanam, M. P. Murugan, and A. Pappachan, "Clonal propagation of *Phyllanthus amarus*: a hepatoprotector," *Pharmacognosy Magazine*, vol. 8, no. 29, pp. 78–82, 2012.

[33] I. G. Tamil, B. Dineshkumar, M. Nandhakumar, M. Senthilkumar, and A. Mitra, "In vitro study on α-amylase inhibitory activity of an Indian medicinal plant, *Phyllanthus amarus*," *Indian Journal of Pharmacology*, vol. 42, no. 5, pp. 280–282, 2010.

[34] A. Komuraiah, K. Bolla, K. N. Rao, A. Ragan, V. S. Rajum, and M. A. Singara Charya, "Antibacterial studies and phytochemical constituents of South Indian *Phyllanthus* species," *African Journal of Biotechnology*, vol. 8, no. 19, pp. 4991–4995, 2009.

[35] A. A. Adeneye, "The leaf and seed aqueous extract of *Phyllanthus amarus* improves insulin resistance diabetes in experimental animal studies," *Journal of Ethnopharmacology*, vol. 144, no. 3, pp. 705–711, 2012.

[36] E. O. Ajaiyeoba, C. O. Falade, O. I. Fawole et al., "Efficacy of herbal remedies used by herbalists in Oyo State Nigeria for treatment of *Plasmodium falciparum* infections—a survey and an observation," *African Journal of Medicine and Medical Sciences*, vol. 33, no. 2, pp. 115–119, 2004.

[37] P. Kloucek, Z. Polesny, B. Svobodova, E. Vlkova, and L. Kokoska, "Antibacterial screening of some Peruvian medicinal plants used in Callería District," *Journal of Ethnopharmacology*, vol. 99, no. 2, pp. 309–312, 2005.

[38] N. Chudapongse, M. Kamkhunthod, and K. Poompachee, "Effects of *Phyllanthus urinaria* extract on HepG2 cell viability and oxidative phosphorylation by isolated rat liver mitochondria," *Journal of Ethnopharmacology*, vol. 130, no. 2, pp. 315–319, 2010.

[39] S.-T. Huang, R.-C. Yang, L.-J. Yang, P.-N. Lee, and J.-H. S. Pang, "*Phyllanthus urinaria* triggers the apoptosis and Bcl-2 downregulation in Lewis lung carcinoma cells," *Life Sciences*, vol. 72, no. 15, pp. 1705–1716, 2003.

[40] M. Xu, Z.-J. Zha, X.-L. Qin, X.-L. Zhang, C.-R. Yang, and Y.-J. Zhang, "Phenolic antioxidants from the whole plant of *Phyllanthus urinaria*," *Chemistry & Biodiversity*, vol. 4, no. 9, pp. 2246–2252, 2007.

[41] S.-Y. Lin, C.-C. Wang, Y.-L. Lu, W.-C. Wu, and W.-C. Hou, "Antioxidant, anti-semicarbazide-sensitive amine oxidase, and anti-hypertensive activities of geraniin isolated from *Phyllanthus urinaria*," *Food and Chemical Toxicology*, vol. 46, no. 7, pp. 2485–2492, 2008.

[42] N. K. Jain and A. K. Singhai, "Protective effects of *Phyllanthus acidus* (L.) Skeels leaf extracts on acetaminophen and thioacetamide induced hepatic injuries in Wistar rats," *Asian Pacific Journal of Tropical Medicine*, vol. 4, no. 6, pp. 470–474, 2011.

[43] R. Chakraborty, D. Biplab, N. Devanna, and S. Sen, "Anti-inflammatory, antinociceptive and antioxidant activities of *Phyllanthus acidus* L. extracts," *Asian Pacific Journal of Tropical Biomedicine*, vol. 2, no. 2, pp. S953–S961, 2012.

[44] Y. Leeya, M. J. Mulvany, E. F. Queiroz, A. Marston, K. Hostettmann, and C. Jansakul, "Hypotensive activity of an n-butanol extract and their purified compounds from leaves of *Phyllanthus acidus* (L.) Skeels in rats," *European Journal of Pharmacology*, vol. 649, no. 1–3, pp. 301–313, 2010.

[45] D. G. Durham, R. G. Reid, J. Wangboonskul, and S. Daodee, "Extraction of Phyllanthusols A and B from *Phyllanthus acidus* and analysis by capillary electrophoresis," *Phytochemical Analysis*, vol. 13, no. 6, pp. 358–362, 2002.

[46] N. Vongvanich, P. Kittakoop, J. Kramyu, M. Tanticharoen, and Y. Thebtaranonth, "Phyllanthusols A and B, cytotoxic norbisabolane glycosides from *Phyllanthus acidus* skeels," *Journal of Organic Chemistry*, vol. 65, no. 17, pp. 5420–5423, 2000.

[47] K. K. Wanniarachchi, L. D. C. Peiris, and W. D. Ratnasooriya, "Antihyperglycemic and hypoglycemic activities of *Phyllanthus debilis* aqueous plant extract in mice," *Pharmaceutical Biology*, vol. 47, no. 3, pp. 260–265, 2009.

[48] S. Kumar, N. Sachdeva, M. Amir, A. Kumar, and S. K. Singh, "Free radical scavenging effect of *Phyllanthus simplex*: in vitro and in vivo study," *Saudi Pharmaceutical Journal*, vol. 15, no. 1, pp. 55–59, 2007.

[49] S. Han, Y. Zhang, and J. R. Wang, "Chemical composition in the leaves of *Phyllanthus simplex* Retz," *Medicinal Plant*, vol. 3, no. 3, pp. 21–22, 2012.

[50] E. Bum Ngo, M. M. Pelanken, N. Njikam et al., "The decoction of leaves of *Phyllanthus discoideus* possesses anticonvulsant and sedative properties in mice," *International Journal of Pharmacology*, vol. 5, no. 2, pp. 168–172, 2009.

[51] V. Ramakrishna, S. Gopi, and O. H. Setty, "Protective effect of *Phyllanthus fraternus* against bromobenzene-induced mitochondrial dysfunction in rat kidney," *Chinese Journal of Natural Medicines*, vol. 10, no. 5, pp. 328–333, 2012.

[52] A. Kumaran and R. Joel Karunakaran, "In vitro antioxidant activities of methanol extracts of five *Phyllanthus* species from India," *LWT-Food Science and Technology*, vol. 40, no. 2, pp. 344–352, 2007.

[53] Á. L. Álvarez, K. P. Dalton, I. Nicieza et al., "Bioactivity-guided fractionation of *Phyllanthus orbicularis* and identification of the principal anti HSV-2 compounds," *Phytotherapy Research*, vol. 26, no. 10, pp. 1513–1520, 2012.

[54] Y. I. G. Gaitén, M. M. Martínez, A. B. Alarcón et al., "Anti-inflammatory and antioxidant activity of a methanolic extract of *Phyllanthus orbicularis* and its derived flavonols," *Journal of Essential Oil Research*, vol. 23, no. 5, pp. 50–53, 2011.

[55] J. Gertsch, Niomawë, K. Gertsch-Roost, and O. Sticher, "*Phyllanthus piscatorum*, ethnopharmacological studies on a women's medicinal plant of the Yanomamï Amerindians," *Journal of Ethnopharmacology*, vol. 91, no. 2-3, pp. 181–188, 2004.

[56] V. J. Ndlebe, N. R. Crouch, and D. A. Mulholland, "Triterpenoids from the African tree *Phyllanthus polyanthus*," *Phytochemistry Letters*, vol. 1, no. 1, pp. 11–17, 2008.

[57] B. Rajkapoor, M. Sankari, M. Sumithra et al., "Antitumor and cytotoxic effects of *Phyllanthus polyphyllus* on ehrlich ascites carcinoma and human cancer cell lines," *Bioscience, Biotechnology and Biochemistry*, vol. 71, no. 9, pp. 2177–2183, 2007.

[58] V. Sivajothi, A. Dey, B. Jayakar, and B. Rajkapoor, "Antihyperglycemic, antihyperlipidemic and antioxidant effect of *Phyllanthus rheedii* on streptozotocin induced diabetic rats," *Iranian Journal of Pharmaceutical Research*, vol. 7, no. 1, pp. 53–59, 2008.

[59] O. Hnatyszyn, J. Miño, S. Gorzalczany, G. Ferraro, J. Coussio, and C. Acevedo, "Antidiabetic activity of *Phyllanthus sellowianus* in streptozotocin-induced diabetic rats," *Phytomedicine*, vol. 4, no. 3, pp. 251–253, 1997.

[60] P. Sakkrom, W. Pompimon, P. Meepowpan, N. Nuntasaen, and C. Loetchutinat, "The effect of *Phyllanthus taxodiifolius* beille extracts and its triterpenoids studying on cellular energetic stage of cancer cells," *American Journal of Pharmacology and Toxicology*, vol. 5, no. 3, pp. 139–144, 2010.

[61] L. J. M. Santiago, R. P. Louro, and D. E. De Oliveira, "Compartmentation of phenolic compounds and phenylalanine ammonia-lyase in leaves of *Phyllanthus tenellus* roxb. and their induction by copper sulphate," *Annals of Botany*, vol. 86, no. 5, pp. 1023–1032, 2000.

[62] M. S. Baliga, "Triphala, ayurvedic formulation for treating and preventing cancer: a review," *Journal of Alternative and Complementary Medicine*, vol. 16, no. 12, pp. 1301–1308, 2010.

[63] R. Tanaka, K. Masuda, and S. Matsunaga, "Lup-20(29)-en-3β,15α-diol and ocotillol-II from the stem bark of *Phyllanthus flexuosus*," *Phytochemistry*, vol. 32, no. 2, pp. 472–474, 1993.

[64] B. Singh, P. K. Agrawal, and R. S. Thakur, "Euphane triterpenoids from *Phyllanthus niruri*," *Indian Journal of Chemistry Section B-Organic Chemistry Including Medicinal Chemistry*, vol. 28, no. 4, pp. 319–321, 1989.

[65] Y. L. Ren, C. H. Yuan, Y. C. Deng et al., "Cytotoxic and natural killer cell stimulatory constituents of *Phyllanthus songboiensis*," *Phytochemistry*, vol. 111, pp. 132–140, 2015.

[66] P. Tuchinda, J. Kornsakulkarn, M. Pohmakotr et al., "Dichapetalin-type triterpenoids and lignans from the aerial parts of *Phyllanthus acutissima*," *Journal of Natural Products*, vol. 71, no. 4, pp. 655–663, 2008.

[67] J. Zhao, Y. Wang, H. Zhu et al., "Highly oxygenated limonoids and lignans from *Phyllanthus flexuosus*," *Natural Products and Bioprospecting*, vol. 4, no. 4, pp. 233–242, 2014.

[68] G. Bagalkotkar, T. S. Chuan, S. I. Khalivulla et al., "Isolation and cytotoxicity of triterpenes from the roots of *Phyllanthus pulcher* Wall. ex Müll. Arg. (Euphorbiaceae)," *African Journal of Pharmacy and Pharmacology*, vol. 5, no. 2, pp. 183–188, 2011.

[69] J. Youkwan, P. Srisomphot, and S. Sutthivaiyakit, "Bioactive constituents of the leaves of *Phyllanthus polyphyllus* var. siamensis," *Journal of Natural Products*, vol. 68, no. 7, pp. 1006–1009, 2005.

[70] R. Tanaka, M. Tabuse, and S. Matsunaga, "Triterpenes from the stem bark of *Phyllanthus flexuosus*," *Phytochemistry*, vol. 27, no. 11, pp. 3563–3567, 1988.

[71] S.-I. Wada, A. Iida, and R. Tanaka, "Screening of triterpenoids isolated from *Phyllanthus flexuosus* for DNA topoisomerase inhibitory activity," *Journal of Natural Products*, vol. 64, no. 12, pp. 1545–1547, 2001.

[72] Habib-Ur-Rehman, Atta-Ur-Rehman, M. I. Chodhary, and A. R. Raza, "Studies on the chemical constituents of *Phyllanthus fraternus*," *Journal of the Chemical Society of Pakistan*, vol. 26, no. 1, pp. 77–81, 2004.

[73] Z. Hu, Y. Lai, J. Zhang et al., "Phytochemical and chemotaxonomic studies on *Phyllanthus urinaria*," *Biochemical Systematics and Ecology*, vol. 56, pp. 60–64, 2014.

[74] W. Sun, "Chemical constituents of *Phyllanthus amarus*," *Chinese Traditional and Herbal Drugs*, vol. 43, no. 1, pp. 23–26, 2012.

[75] S.-S. Lee, P. H. Kishore, and C.-H. Chen, "Three novel triterpenoid dienolides from *Phyllanthus myrtifolius*," *Helvetica Chimica Acta*, vol. 85, no. 8, pp. 2403–2408, 2002.

[76] A. K. Jamal, W. A. Yaacob, and L. B. Din, "Triterpenes from the root bark of *Phyllanthus columnaris*," *Australian Journal of Basic and Applied Sciences*, vol. 3, no. 2, pp. 1428–1431, 2009.

[77] K. C. Joshi, P. Singh, and A. Mehra, "Crystalline components of the roots of *Phyllanthus reticulatus*," *Journal of the Indian Chemical Society*, vol. 58, no. 1, pp. 102–103, 1981.

[78] N. Ramesh, M. B. Viswanathan, V. T. Selvi, and P. Lakshmanaperumalsamy, "Antimicrobial and phytochemical studies on the leaves of *Phyllanthus singampattiana* (Sebastine & A.N. Henry) Kumari & Chandrabose from India," *Medicinal Chemistry Research*, vol. 13, no. 6-7, pp. 348–360, 2004.

[79] T. Agarwal and J. S. Tiwari, "A note on the flavanoid and other constituents of *Phyllanthus* genus," *Journal of the Indian Chemical Society*, vol. 68, no. 8, pp. 479–480, 1991.

[80] R. Tanaka and S. Matsunaga, "Triterpene dienols and other constituents from the bark of *Phyllanthus flexuosus*," *Phytochemistry*, vol. 27, no. 7, pp. 2273–2277, 1988.

[81] P. Sengupta and J. Mukhopad, "Terpenoids and related compounds 7. Triterpenoids of *Phyllanthus acidus* skeels," *Phytochemistry*, vol. 5, no. 3, pp. 531–534, 1966.

[82] R. Tanaka, Y. In, T. Ishida, and S. Matsunaga, "11β-hydroxy-D: a-friedoolean-1-en-3-one from the stem bark of *Phyllanthus flexuosus*," *Journal of Natural Products*, vol. 57, no. 11, pp. 1523–1528, 1994.

[83] G. A. Adesida, P. Girgis, and D. A. H. Taylor, "Friedelin derivatives from *Phyllanthus muellerianus*," *Phytochemistry*, vol. 11, no. 2, pp. 851–852, 1972.

[84] W.-H. Hui, M.-M. Li, and K.-M. Wong, "A new compound, 21α-hydroxyfriedel-4(23)-en-3-one and other triterpenoids from *Phyllanthus reticulatus*," *Phytochemistry*, vol. 15, no. 5, pp. 797–798, 1976.

[85] S. Matsunaga, R. Tanaka, Y. Takaoka et al., "26-Nor-D:A-friedooleanane triterpenes from *Phyllanthus watsonii*," *Phytochemistry*, vol. 32, no. 1, pp. 165–170, 1992.

[86] J. A. Nasser, W. A. Yaacob, and L. B. Din, "Studies on the chemical constituents of bark roots of *Phyllanthus columnaris*," *Asian Journal of Chemistry*, vol. 21, no. 9, pp. 7067–7071, 2009.

[87] Q. Zhao, R. J. Liang, Y. J. Zhang, A. H. Hong, Y. F. Wang, and Y. Z. Cen, "Chemical constituents in roots of *Phyllanthus emblica*," *Zhongcaoyao*, vol. 44, no. 2, pp. 133–136, 2013.

[88] W. X. Wei, Y. J. Pan, H. Zhang, and Y. Z. Chen, "Structures in crystal and in solution of friedelin isolated from *Phyllanthus niruri* linn," *Tianran Chanwu Yanjiu Yu Kaifa*, vol. 16, no. 3, pp. 201–203, 2004.

[89] O. S. Priya, M. B. G. Viswanathan, K. Balakrishna, and M. Venkatesan, "Chemical constituents and in vitro antioxidant activity of *Phyllanthus wightianus*," *Natural Product Research*, vol. 25, no. 10, pp. 949–958, 2011.

[90] S. Sutthivaiyakit, N. N. Nakorn, W. Kraus, and P. Sutthivaiyakit, "A novel 29-nor-3,4-seco-friedelane triterpene and a new guaiane sesquiterpene from the roots of *Phyllanthus oxyphyllus*," *Tetrahedron*, vol. 59, no. 50, pp. 9991–9995, 2003.

[91] R. Tanaka, S. Matsunaga, and T. Ishida, "Revised structure of trichadenic acid B, a stem bark constituent of *Phyllanthus flexuosus*," *Tetrahedron Letters*, vol. 29, no. 37, pp. 4751–4754, 1988.

[92] M. Saleem, M. Nazir, N. Akhtar et al., "New phthalates from *Phyllanthus muellerianus* (Euphorbiaceae)," *Journal of Asian Natural Products Research*, vol. 11, no. 11, pp. 974–977, 2009.

[93] V. Cechinel-Filho, A. R. S. Santos, J. B. Calixto, F. Delle-Monache, O. G. Miguel, and R. Yunes, "Triterpenes from *Phyllanthus sellowianus* roots," *Planta Medica*, vol. 64, no. 2, p. 194, 1998.

[94] Y.-L. Huang, C.-C. Chen, F.-L. Hsu, and C.-F. Chen, "Tannins, flavonol sulfonates, and a norlignan from *Phyllanthus virgatus*," *Journal of Natural Products*, vol. 61, no. 10, pp. 1194–1197, 1998.

[95] O. G. Miguel, V. Cechinel Filho, R. Niero et al., "Constituents of *Phyllanthus sellowianus*," *Fitoterapia*, vol. 66, no. 3, p. 275, 1995.

[96] R. M. Serra, "Investigation of quinine in *Phyllanthus niruri* L," *Anales de la Universidad de Santo Domingo*, vol. 8, pp. 295–297, 1944.

[97] R. S. Li, S. Y. Wang, and W. H. Zhang, "Studies on the chemical components of common leaf-flower (*Phyllanthus urinaria*)," *Zhongcaoyao*, vol. 26, no. 5, pp. 231–232, 1995.

[98] R. Tanaka, Y. Kinouchi, S.-I. Wada, and H. Tokuda, "Potential anti-tumor promoting activity of lupane-type triterpenoids from the stem Bark of *Glochidion zeylanicum* and *Phyllanthus flexuosus*," *Planta Medica*, vol. 70, no. 12, pp. 1234–1236, 2004.

[99] K. S. Satyan, A. Prakash, R. P. Singh, and R. S. Srivastava, "Phthalic acid bis-ester and other phytoconstituents of *Phyllanthus urinaria*," *Planta Medica*, vol. 61, no. 3, pp. 293–294, 1995.

[100] W. H. Hui and M. Sung, "An examination of the Euphorbiaceae of Hong Kong. II. The occurrence of epitaraxerol and other triterpenoids," *Australian Journal of Chemistry*, vol. 21, no. 8, pp. 2137–2140, 1968.

[101] B. Singh, P. K. Agrawal, and R. S. Thakur, "An acyclic triterpene from *Phyllanthus niruri*," *Phytochemistry*, vol. 28, no. 7, pp. 1980–1981, 1989.

[102] O. Hnatyszyn and G. Ferraro, "Phyllanthol from *Phyllanthus sellowianus* (Euphorbiaceae)," *Planta Medica*, vol. 51, no. 5, pp. 467–467, 1985.

[103] X. Liu, M. Zhao, W. Luo, B. Yang, and Y. Jiang, "Identification of volatile components in *Phyllanthus emblica* L. and their antimicrobial activity," *Journal of Medicinal Food*, vol. 12, no. 2, pp. 423–428, 2009.

[104] G. R. Pettit, D. E. Schaufelberger, R. A. Nieman, C. Dufresne, and J. A. Saenz-Renauld, "Antineoplastic agents, 177. Isolation and structure of phyllanthostatin 6," *Journal of Natural Products*, vol. 53, no. 6, pp. 1406–1413, 1990.

[105] M. S. Lan, J. X. Ma, C. H. Tan et al., "Chemical constituents from *Phyllanthus reticulatus* var. Glaber," *Zhongcaoyao*, vol. 42, no. 9, pp. 1712–1714, 2011.

[106] R. Ratnayake, D. Covell, T. T. Ransom, K. R. Gustafson, and J. A. Beutler, "Englerin a, a selective inhibitor of renal cancer cell growth, from *Phyllanthus engleri*," *Organic Letters*, vol. 11, no. 1, pp. 57–60, 2009.

[107] J.-J. Lv, Y.-F. Wang, J.-M. Zhang et al., "Anti-hepatitis B virus activities and absolute configurations of sesquiterpenoid glycosides from *Phyllanthus emblica*," *Organic and Biomolecular Chemistry*, vol. 12, no. 43, pp. 8764–8774, 2014.

[108] J. Q. Zhao, Y. M. Wang, D. Wang, C. R. Yang, M. Xu, and Y. J. Zhang, "Five new sucrose esters from the whole plants of *Phyllanthus cochinchinensis*," *Natural Products and Bioprospecting*, vol. 3, no. 2, pp. 61–65, 2013.

[109] Y.-J. Zhang, T. Tanaka, Y. Iwamoto, C.-R. Yang, and I. Kouno, "Novel norsesquiterpenoids from the roots of *Phyllanthus emblica*," *Journal of Natural Products*, vol. 63, no. 11, pp. 1507–1510, 2000.

[110] Y.-J. Zhang, T. Tanaka, Y. Iwamoto, C.-R. Yang, and I. Kouno, "Novel sesquiterpenoids from the roots of *Phyllanthus emblica*," *Journal of Natural Products*, vol. 64, no. 7, pp. 870–873, 2001.

[111] Y.-J. Zhang, T. Nagao, T. Tanaka, C.-R. Yang, H. Okabe, and I. Kouno, "Antiproliferative activity of the main constituents from *Phyllanthus emblica*," *Biological and Pharmaceutical Bulletin*, vol. 27, no. 2, pp. 251–255, 2004.

[112] Y.-F. Wang, X.-Y. Wang, Z. Ren et al., "Phyllaemblicin B inhibits Coxsackie virus B3 induced apoptosis and myocarditis," *Antiviral Research*, vol. 84, no. 2, pp. 150–158, 2009.

[113] Q. Liu, Y.-F. Wang, R.-J. Chen et al., "Anti-coxsackie virus B3 norsesquiterpenoids from the roots of *Phyllanthus emblica*," *Journal of Natural Products*, vol. 72, no. 5, pp. 969–972, 2009.

[114] Y. Zhang, L. Zhao, X. Guo et al., "Chemical constituents from *Phyllanthus emblica* and the cytoprotective effects on H_2O_2-induced PC12 cell injuries," *Archives of Pharmacal Research*, 2014.

[115] S. M. Kupchan, E. J. LaVoie, A. R. Branfman, B. Y. Fei, W. M. Bright, and R. F. Bryan, "Tumor inhibitors. 120. Phyllanthocin, a novel bisabolane aglycone from the antileukemic glycoside, phyllanthoside," *Journal of the American Chemical Society*, vol. 99, no. 9, pp. 3199–3201, 1977.

[116] G. R. Pettit, G. M. Cragg, D. Gust, P. Brown, and J. M. Schmidt, "The structures of phyllanthostatin 1 and phyllanthoside from the central american tree *Phyllanthus acuminatus* vahl," *Canadian Journal of Chemistry*, vol. 60, no. 7, pp. 939–941, 1982.

[117] G. R. Pettit, G. M. Cragg, D. Gust, and P. Brown, "The isolation and structure of phyllanthostatins 2 and 3," *Canadian Journal of Chemistry*, vol. 60, no. 4, pp. 544–546, 1982.

[118] M.-S. Lan, J.-X. Ma, C.-H. Tan, S. Wei, and D.-Y. Zhu, "Chemical constituents of *Phyllanthus reticulatus*," *Helvetica Chimica Acta*, vol. 93, no. 11, pp. 2276–2280, 2010.

[119] J.-Q. Zhao, J.-J. Lv, Y.-M. Wang et al., "Phyllanflexoid C: first example of phenylacetylene-bearing 18-nor-diterpenoid glycoside from the roots of *Phyllanthus flexuosus*," *Tetrahedron Letters*, vol. 54, no. 35, pp. 4670–4674, 2013.

[120] M. A. Hossain and S. M. Salehuddin, "Diterpenes from the leaves of *Phyllanthus niruri*," *Indian Journal of Natural Products*, vol. 22, no. 2, pp. 18–20, 2006.

[121] J. Gupta and M. Ali, "Isolation of rare phytoconstituents from *Phyllanthus fraternus* roots," *Journal of Medicinal and Aromatic Plant Sciences*, vol. 21, pp. 352–357, 1999.

[122] B. Singh, P. K. Agrawal, and R. S. Thakur, "Studies on medicinal-plants 33. Isolation of trans-phytol from *Phyllanthus niruri*," *Planta Medica*, vol. 57, no. 1, p. 98, 1991.

[123] Y. L. Ren, D. D. Lantvit, Y. C. Deng et al., "Potent cytotoxic arylnaphthalene lignan lactones from *Phyllanthus poilanei*," *Journal of Natural Products*, vol. 77, no. 6, pp. 1494–1504, 2014.

[124] P. Tuchinda, A. Kumkao, M. Pohmakotr, S. Sophasan, T. Santisuk, and V. Reutrakul, "Cytotoxic arylnaphthalide lignan glycosides from the aerial parts of *Phyllanthus taxodiifolius*," *Planta Medica*, vol. 72, no. 1, pp. 60–62, 2006.

[125] C.-C. Chang, Y.-C. Lien, K. C. S. C. Liu, and S.-S. Lee, "Lignans from *Phyllanthus urinaria*," *Phytochemistry*, vol. 63, no. 7, pp. 825–833, 2003.

[126] Y. K. Rao, S.-H. Fang, and Y.-M. Tzeng, "Anti-inflammatory activities of constituents isolated from *Phyllanthus polyphyllus*," *Journal of Ethnopharmacology*, vol. 103, no. 2, pp. 181–186, 2006.

[127] R. A. Hussain, J. K. Dickey, M. P. Rosser et al., "A novel class of non-peptidic endothelin antagonists isolated from the medicinal herb *Phyllanthus niruri*," *Journal of Natural Products*, vol. 58, no. 10, pp. 1515–1520, 1995.

[128] P. A. Ganeshpure, G. E. Schneiders, and R. Stevenson, "Structure and synthesis of hypophyllanthin, nirtetralin, phyltetralin and lintetralin," *Tetrahedron Letters*, vol. 22, no. 5, pp. 393–396, 1981.

[129] K. V. Syamasundar, B. Singh, R. Singh Thakur, A. Husain, K. Yoshinobu, and H. Hiroshi, "Antihepatotoxic principles of *Phyllanthus niruri* herbs," *Journal of Ethnopharmacology*, vol. 14, no. 1, pp. 41–44, 1985.

[130] M. Inchoo, H. Chirdchupunseree, P. Pramyothin, and S. Jianmongkol, "Endothelium-independent effects of phyllanthin and hypophyllanthin on vascular tension," *Fitoterapia*, vol. 82, no. 8, pp. 1231–1236, 2011.

[131] Y.-L. Huang, C.-C. Chen, F.-L. Hsu, and C.-F. Chen, "A new lignan from *Phyllanthus virgatus*," *Journal of Natural Products*, vol. 59, no. 5, pp. 520–521, 1996.

[132] M. Singh, N. Tiwari, K. Shanker, R. K. Verma, A. K. Gupta, and M. M. Gupta, "Two new lignans from *Phyllanthus amarus*," *Journal of Asian Natural Products Research*, vol. 11, no. 6, pp. 562–568, 2009.

[133] A. Islam, T. Selvan, U. K. Mazumder, M. Gupta, and S. Ghosal, "Antitumour effect of phyllanthin and hypophyllanthin from *Phyllanthus amarus* against Ehrlich ascites carcinoma in mice," *Pharmacologyonline*, vol. 2, pp. 796–807, 2008.

[134] T. Taesotikul, W. Dumrongsakulchai, N. Wattanachai et al., "Inhibitory effects of *Phyllanthus amarus* and its major lignans on human microsomal cytochrome P450 activities: evidence for CYP3A4 mechanism-based Inhibition," *Drug Metabolism and Pharmacokinetics*, vol. 26, no. 2, pp. 154–161, 2011.

[135] K. S. Chandrashekar, D. Satyanarayana, A. B. Joshi, and E. V. S. Subrahmanyam, "Phytochemical studies of *Phyllanthus debilis*," *Natural Product Sciences*, vol. 10, no. 3, pp. 101–103, 2004.

[136] Y. L. Huang, C. C. Chen, and J. C. Ou, "Isolintetralin: a new lignan from *Phyllanthus niruri*," *Planta Medica*, vol. 58, no. 5, pp. 473–474, 1992.

[137] M.-T. Lin, S.-S. Lee, and K. C. S. Chen Liu, "Phyllamyricins A-C, three novel lignans from *Phyllanthus myrtifolius*," *Journal of Natural Products*, vol. 58, no. 2, pp. 244–249, 1995.

[138] T. L. Bachmann, F. Ghia, and K. B. G. Torssell, "Lignans and lactones from *Phyllanthus anisolobus*," *Phytochemistry*, vol. 33, no. 1, pp. 189–191, 1993.

[139] J. Gertsch, R. T. Tobler, R. Brun, O. Sticher, and J. Heilmann, "Antifungal, antiprotozoal, cytotoxic and piscicidal properties of justicidin B and a new arylnaphthalide lignan from *Phyllanthus piscatorum*," *Planta Medica*, vol. 69, no. 5, pp. 420–424, 2003.

[140] W.-X. Wei, X.-G. Gong, O. Ishrud, and Y.-J. Pan, "New lignan isolated from *Phyllanthus niruri* Linn. structure elucidation by NMR spectroscopy," *Bulletin of the Korean Chemical Society*, vol. 23, no. 6, pp. 896–898, 2002.

[141] N. V. Thanh, P. T. T. Huong, N. H. Nam et al., "A new flavone sulfonic acid from *Phyllanthus urinaria*," *Phytochemistry Letters*, vol. 7, no. 1, pp. 182–185, 2014.

[142] W. X. Wei, X. R. Li, K. W. Wang, Z. W. Zheng, and M. Zhou, "Lignans with anti-hepatitis B virus activities from *Phyllanthus niruri* L.," *Phytotherapy Research*, vol. 26, no. 7, pp. 964–968, 2012.

[143] R.-L. Huang, Y.-L. Huang, J.-C. Ou, C.-C. Chen, F.-L. Hsu, and C. Chang, "Screening of 25 compounds isolated from *Phyllanthus* species for anti-human hepatitis B virus in vitro," *Phytotherapy Research*, vol. 17, no. 5, pp. 449–453, 2003.

[144] D. F. P. Leite, C. A. L. Kassuya, T. L. Mazzuco et al., "The cytotoxic effect and the multidrug resistance reversing action of lignans from *Phyllanthus amarus*," *Planta Medica*, vol. 72, no. 15, pp. 1353–1358, 2006.

[145] C. A. L. Kassuya, D. F. P. Leite, L. V. de Melo, V. L. G. Rehder, and J. B. Calixto, "Anti-inflammatory properties of extracts, fractions and lignans isolated from *Phyllanthus amarus*," *Planta Medica*, vol. 71, no. 8, pp. 721–726, 2005.

[146] S. Liu, W. X. Wei, Y. B. Li et al., "In vitro and in vivo anti-hepatitis B virus activities of the lignan nirtetralin B isolated from *Phyllanthus niruri* L.," *Journal of Ethnopharmacology*, vol. 157, pp. 62–68, 2014.

[147] S.-S. Lee, M.-T. Lin, C.-L. Liu, Y.-Y. Lin, and K. C. S. C. Liu, "Six lignans from *Phyllanthus myrtifolius*," *Journal of Natural Products*, vol. 59, no. 11, pp. 1061–1065, 1996.

[148] G. R. Pettit and D. E. Schaufelberger, "Isolation and structure of the cytostatic lignan glycoside phyllanthostatin A," *Journal of Natural Products*, vol. 51, no. 6, pp. 1104–1112, 1988.

[149] J.-Q. Zhao, Y.-M. Wang, J.-J. Lv et al., "New phenolic glycosides from *Phyllanthus cochinchinensis*," *Journal of the Brazilian Chemical Society*, vol. 25, no. 8, pp. 1446–1454, 2014.

[150] S.-J. Wu and T.-S. Wu, "Cytotoxic arylnaphthalene lignans from *Phyllanthus oligospermus*," *Chemical & Pharmaceutical Bulletin*, vol. 54, no. 8, pp. 1223–1225, 2006.

[151] S.-H. Fang, Y. K. Rao, and Y.-M. Tzeng, "Anti-oxidant and inflammatory mediator's growth inhibitory effects of compounds isolated from *Phyllanthus urinaria*," *Journal of Ethnopharmacology*, vol. 116, no. 2, pp. 333–340, 2008.

[152] C.-Y. Wang, S.-W. Sun, and S.-S. Lee, "Pharmacokinetic and metabolic studies of retrojusticidin B, a potential anti-viral lignan, in rats," *Planta Medica*, vol. 70, no. 12, pp. 1161–1165, 2004.

[153] P. Satyanarayana, P. Subrahmanyam, K. N. Viswanatham, and R. S. Ward, "New seco- and hydroxy-lignans from *Phyllanthus niruri*," *Journal of Natural Products*, vol. 51, no. 1, pp. 44–49, 1988.

[154] E. Elfahmi, A. Koulman, R. Bos, and H. J. Woerdenbag, "Lignans from cell suspension cultures of *Phyllanthus niruri*, an Indonesian medicinal plant," *Journal of Natural Products*, vol. 69, no. 1, pp. 55–58, 2006.

[155] P. Satyanarayana and S. Venkateswarlu, "Isolation, structure and synthesis of new diarylbutane lignans from *Phyllanthus niruri*: synthesis of 5′-desmethoxy niranthin and an antitumour extractive," *Tetrahedron*, vol. 47, no. 42, pp. 8931–8940, 1991.

[156] P. Giridharan, S. T. Somasundaram, K. Perumal et al., "Novel substituted methylenedioxy lignan suppresses proliferation of cancer cells by inhibiting telomerase and activation of c-myc and caspases leading to apoptosis," *British Journal of Cancer*, vol. 87, no. 1, pp. 98–105, 2002.

[157] B. Singh, P. K. Agrawal, and R. S. Thakur, "Chemical-constituents of *Phyllanthus niruri* Linn," *Indian Journal of Chemistry, Section B—Organic Chemistry Including Medicinal Chemistry*, vol. 25, no. 6, pp. 600–602, 1986.

[158] C. A. L. Kassuya, A. Silvestre, O. Menezes-de-Lima Jr., D. M. Marotta, V. L. G. Rehder, and J. B. Calixto, "Antiinflammatory and antiallodynic actions of the lignan niranthin isolated from *Phyllanthus amarus*. Evidence for interaction with platelet activating factor receptor," *European Journal of Pharmacology*, vol. 546, no. 1–3, pp. 182–188, 2006.

[159] S. Chowdhury, T. Mukherjee, R. Mukhopadhyay et al., "The lignan niranthin poisons Leishmania donovani topoisomerase IB and favours a Th1 immune response in mice," *EMBO Molecular Medicine*, vol. 4, no. 10, pp. 1126–1143, 2012.

[160] B. Singh, P. K. Agrawal, and R. S. Thakur, "A new lignan and a new neolignan from *Phyllanthus niruri*," *Journal of Natural Products*, vol. 52, no. 1, pp. 48–51, 1989.

[161] K. L. Ooi, S. I. Loh, M. A. Sattar, T. S. T. Muhammad, and S. F. Sulaiman, "Cytotoxic, caspase-3 induction and in vivo hepatoprotective effects of phyllanthin, a major constituent of *Phyllanthus niruri*," *Journal of Functional Foods*, vol. 14, pp. 236–243, 2015.

[162] V. Murugaiyah and K.-L. Chan, "Antihyperuricemic lignans from the leaves of *Phyllanthus niruri*," *Planta Medica*, vol. 72, no. 14, pp. 1262–1267, 2006.

[163] I. Jantan, M. Ilangkovan, Yuandani, and H. F. Mohamad, "Correlation between the major components of *Phyllanthus amarus* and *Phyllanthus urinaria* and their inhibitory effects on phagocytic activity of human neutrophils," *BMC Complementary and Alternative Medicine*, vol. 14, article 429, 2014.

[164] G. Guha, T. Mandal, V. Rajkumar, and R. Ashok Kumar, "Antimycin A-induced mitochondrial apoptotic cascade is mitigated by phenolic constituents of *Phyllanthus amarus* aqueous extract in Hep3B cells," *Food and Chemical Toxicology*, vol. 48, no. 12, pp. 3449–3457, 2010.

[165] H. Chirdchupunseree and P. Pramyothin, "Protective activity of phyllanthin in ethanol-treated primary culture of rat hepatocytes," *Journal of Ethnopharmacology*, vol. 128, no. 1, pp. 172–176, 2010.

[166] C.-H. Kuo, S.-S. Lee, H.-Y. Chang, and S.-W. Sun, "Analysis of lignans using micellar electrokinetic chromatography," *Electrophoresis*, vol. 24, no. 6, pp. 1047–1053, 2003.

[167] Y. W. Chen, L. J. Ren, K. M. Li, and Y. W. Zhang, "Isolation and identification of novel polyphenolic compound from *Phyllanthus urinaria*," *Acta Pharmaceutica Sinica*, vol. 34, no. 7, pp. 526–529, 1999.

[168] O. Hnatyszyn, G. Ferraro, and J. D. Coussio, "Constituents of *Phyllanthus sellowianus*," *Fitoterapia*, vol. 66, no. 6, p. 543, 1995.

[169] C. Agyare, M. Lechtenberg, A. Deters, F. Petereit, and A. Hensel, "Ellagitannins from *Phyllanthus muellerianus* (Kuntze) Exell.: Geraniin and furosin stimulate cellular activity, differentiation and collagen synthesis of human skin keratinocytes and dermal fibroblasts," *Phytomedicine*, vol. 18, no. 7, pp. 617–624, 2011.

[170] X. Niu, L. Qi, W. Li, and X. Liu, "Simultaneous analysis of eight phenolic compounds in *Phyllanthus simplex* Retz by HPLC-DAD-ESI/MS," *Journal of Medicinal Plants Research*, vol. 6, no. 9, pp. 1512–1518, 2012.

[171] W. Luo, M. Zhao, B. Yang, G. Shen, and G. Rao, "Identification of bioactive compounds in *Phyllenthus emblica* L. fruit and their free radical scavenging activities," *Food Chemistry*, vol. 114, no. 2, pp. 499–504, 2009.

[172] Z. X. Wan, G. P. Zhou, and Y. H. Yi, "Chemical constituents of common leafflower (*Phyllanthus urinaria*)," *Zhongcaoyao*, vol. 25, no. 9, pp. 455–456, 1994.

[173] B. Ahmed, S. Khan, and A. Verma, "Antihepatotoxic activity of debelalactone, a new oxirano-furanocoumarin from *Phyllanthus debilis*," *Journal of Asian Natural Products Research*, vol. 11, no. 8, pp. 687–692, 2009.

[174] O. Hnatyszyn, G. Ferraro, and J. D. Coussio, "Coumarins of *Phyllanthus sellowianus*," *Fitoterapia*, vol. 64, no. 6, pp. 556–556, 1993.

[175] Y.-F. Xiang, H.-Q. Ju, S. Li, Y.-J. Zhang, C.-R. Yang, and Y.-F. Wang, "Effects of 1,2,4,6-tetra-O-galloyl-β-D-glucose from *P. emblica* on HBsAg and HBeAg secretion in HepG2.2.15 cell culture," *Virologica Sinica*, vol. 25, no. 5, pp. 375–380, 2010.

[176] K. Ishimaru, K. Yoshimatsu, T. Yamakawa, H. Kamada, and K. Shimomura, "Phenolic constituents in tissue cultures of *Phyllanthus niruri*," *Phytochemistry*, vol. 31, no. 6, pp. 2015–2018, 1992.

[177] C.-M. Yang, H.-Y. Cheng, T.-C. Lin, L.-C. Chiang, and C.-C. Lin, "The in vitro activity of geraniin and 1,3,4,6-tetra-O-galloyl-β-d-glucose isolated from *Phyllanthus urinaria* against herpes simplex virus type 1 and type 2 infection," *Journal of Ethnopharmacology*, vol. 110, no. 3, pp. 555–558, 2007.

[178] J. S. Londhe, T. P. A. Devasagayam, L. Y. Foo, and S. S. Ghaskadbi, "Antioxidant activity of some polyphenol constituents of the medicinal plant *Phyllanthus amarus* Linn," *Redox Report*, vol. 13, no. 5, pp. 199–207, 2008.

[179] L. Y. Foo, "Amariin, a di-dehydrohexahydroxydiphenoyl hydrolysable tannin from *Phyllanthus amarus*," *Phytochemistry*, vol. 33, no. 2, pp. 487–491, 1993.

[180] J. S. Londhe, T. P. A. Devasagayam, L. Y. Foo, P. Shastry, and S. S. Ghaskadbi, "Geraniin and amariin, ellagitannins from *Phyllanthus amarus*, protect liver cells against ethanol induced cytotoxicity," *Fitoterapia*, vol. 83, no. 8, pp. 1562–1568, 2012.

[181] J. S. Londhe, T. P. A. Devasagayam, L. Y. Foo, and S. S. Ghaskadbi, "Radioprotective properties of polyphenols from *Phyllanthus amarus* Linn," *Journal of Radiation Research*, vol. 50, no. 4, pp. 303–309, 2009.

[182] L. Yeap Foo, "Amariinic acid and related ellagitannins from *Phyllanthus amarus*," *Phytochemistry*, vol. 39, no. 1, pp. 217–224, 1995.

[183] L. Y. Foo, "Amarulone, a novel cyclic hydrolysable tannin from *Phyllanthus amarus*," *Natural Product Letters*, vol. 3, no. 1, pp. 45–52, 1993.

[184] Y.-J. Zhang, T. Abe, T. Tanaka, C.-R. Yang, and I. Kouno, "Phyllanemblinins A-F, new ellagitannins from *Phyllanthus emblica*," *Journal of Natural Products*, vol. 64, no. 12, pp. 1527–1532, 2001.

[185] W. Luo, L. Wen, M. Zhao et al., "Structural identification of isomallotusinin and other phenolics in *Phyllanthus emblica* L. fruit hull," *Food Chemistry*, vol. 132, no. 3, pp. 1527–1533, 2012.

[186] M.-T. Lin, S.-S. Lee, and K. C. S. C. Chen Liu, "Polar constituents from *Phyllanthus myrtifolius*," *Chinese Pharmaceutical Journal*, vol. 50, no. 6, pp. 327–336, 1998.

[187] A. Kumaran and R. J. Karunakaran, "Nitric oxide radical scavenging active components from *Phyllanthus emblica* L.," *Plant Foods for Human Nutrition*, vol. 61, no. 1, pp. 1–5, 2006.

[188] R. Gambari, M. Borgatti, I. Lampronti et al., "Corilagin is a potent inhibitor of NF-κB activity and downregulates TNF-α induced expression of IL-8 gene in cystic fibrosis IB3-1 cells," *International Immunopharmacology*, vol. 13, no. 3, pp. 308–315, 2012.

[189] D. X. Sha, Y. H. Liu, L. S. Wang et al., "Study on chemical constituents of *Phyllanthus urinaria*," *Shenyang Yaoke Daxue Xuebao*, vol. 17, no. 3, pp. 176–178, 2000.

[190] S.-G. Yeo, J. H. Song, E.-H. Hong et al., "Antiviral effects of *Phyllanthus urinaria* containing corilagin against human enterovirus 71 and Coxsackievirus A16 in vitro," *Archives of Pharmacal Research*, vol. 38, no. 2, pp. 193–202, 2015.

[191] Z.-Q. Shen, Z.-J. Dong, H. Peng, and J.-K. Liu, "Modulation of PAI-1 and tPA activity and thrombolytic effects of corilagin," *Planta Medica*, vol. 69, no. 12, pp. 1109–1112, 2003.

[192] S.-H. Lam, C.-Y. Wang, C.-K. Chen, and S.-S. Lee, "Chemical investigation of *Phyllanthus reticulatus* by HPLC-SPE-NMR and conventional methods," *Phytochemical Analysis*, vol. 18, no. 3, pp. 251–255, 2007.

[193] C. S. Joshi and E. Sanmuga Priya, "β-Glucuronidase inhibitory effect of phenolic constituents from *Phyllanthus amarus*," *Pharmaceutical Biology*, vol. 45, no. 5, pp. 363–365, 2007.

[194] F. Notka, G. R. Meier, and R. Wagner, "Inhibition of wild-type human immunodeficiency virus and reverse transcriptase inhibitor-resistant variants by *Phyllanthus amarus*," *Antiviral Research*, vol. 58, no. 2, pp. 175–186, 2003.

[195] A. Kumaran and R. J. Karunakaran, "Anti-oxidant activity of polyphenols from *Phyllanthus debilis* Klein ex Willd," *Journal of Natural Remedies*, vol. 6, no. 2, pp. 141–146, 2006.

[196] Y. W. Chen and L. J. Ren, "Studies on the anti-cancer active constituents of Matsumura leafflower (*Phyllanthus matsumurae*). II. Isolation and identification of polyphenolic compounds," *Chinese Traditional & Herbal Drugs*, vol. 28, no. 4, pp. 198–202, 1997.

[197] I. Ham, T. Wang, E. S. Cho, H. K. Cho, and W. K. Whang, "Phenolic compounds from *Phyllanthus ussuriensis*," *Yakhak Hoechi*, vol. 45, no. 3, pp. 237–244, 2001.

[198] S.-K. Chung, J.-A. Nam, S.-Y. Jeon et al., "A prolyl endopeptidase-inhibiting antioxidant from *Phyllanthus ussurensis*," *Archives of Pharmacal Research*, vol. 26, no. 12, pp. 1024–1028, 2003.

[199] H. Y. Cheng, C. M. Yang, T. C. Lin, L. T. Lin, L. C. Chiang, and C. C. Lin, "Excoecarianin, isolated from *Phyllanthus urinaria* Linnea, inhibits herpes simplex virus type 2 infection through inactivation of viral particles," *Evidence-Based Complementary and Alternative Medicine*, vol. 2011, Article ID 259103, 10 pages, 2011.

[200] O. G. Miguel, J. B. Calixto, A. R. S. Santos et al., "Chemical and preliminary analgesic evaluation of geraniin and furosin isolated from *Phyllanthus sellowianus*," *Planta Medica*, vol. 62, no. 2, pp. 146–149, 1996.

[201] X. L. Liu, C. Cui, M. M. Zhao et al., "Identification of phenolics in the fruit of emblica (*Phyllanthus emblica* L.) and their antioxidant activities," *Food Chemistry*, vol. 109, no. 4, pp. 909–915, 2008.

[202] D. Ndjonka, B. Bergmann, C. Agyare et al., "In vitro activity of extracts and isolated polyphenols from West African medicinal plants against *Plasmodium falciparum*," *Parasitology Research*, vol. 111, no. 2, pp. 827–834, 2012.

[203] V. Cechinel Filho, A. R. S. Santos, R. O. P. De Campos et al., "Chemical and pharmacological studies of *Phyllanthus caroliniensis* in mice," *Journal of Pharmacy and Pharmacology*, vol. 48, no. 12, pp. 1231–1236, 1996.

[204] C.-M. Yang, H.-Y. Cheng, T.-C. Lin, L.-C. Chiang, and C.-C. Lin, "Hippomanin A from acetone extract of *Phyllanthus urinaria* inhibited HSV-2 but not HSV-1 infection in vitro," *Phytotherapy Research*, vol. 21, no. 12, pp. 1182–1186, 2007.

[205] X. Liu, M. Zhao, K. Wu et al., "Immunomodulatory and anti-cancer activities of phenolics from emblica fruit (*Phyllanthus emblica* L.)," *Food Chemistry*, vol. 131, no. 2, pp. 685–690, 2012.

[206] N. N. Than, S. Fotso, B. Poeggeler, R. Hardeland, and H. Laatsch, "Niruriflavone, a new antioxidant flavone sulfonic acid from *Phyllanthus niruri*," *Zeitschrift fur Naturforschung-Section B: Journal of Chemical Sciences*, vol. 61, no. 1, pp. 57–60, 2006.

[207] M. A. Hossain and S. M. Mizanur Rahman, "Structure characterization and quantification of a new isoflavone from the arial parts of *Phyllanthus niruri*," *Arabian Journal of Chemistry*, 2015.

[208] L.-Z. Zhang, W.-H. Zhao, Y.-J. Guo, G.-Z. Tu, S. Lin, and L.-G. Xin, "Studies on chemical constituents in fruits of Tibetan medicine *Phyllanthus emblica*," *Zhongguo Zhongyao Zazhi*, vol. 28, no. 10, pp. 942–943, 2003.

[209] L.-Z. Zhang, Y.-J. Guo, G.-Z. Tu, W.-B. Guo, and F. Miao, "Studies on chemical constituents of *Phyllanthus urinaria* L.," *Zhongguo Zhongyao Zazhi*, vol. 25, no. 10, pp. 616–617, 2000.

[210] W. Luo, M. Zhao, B. Yang, J. Ren, G. Shen, and G. Rao, "Antioxidant and antiproliferative capacities of phenolics purified from *Phyllanthus emblica* L. fruit," *Food Chemistry*, vol. 126, no. 1, pp. 277–282, 2011.

[211] T. Yoshida, H. Itoh, S. Matsunaga, R. Tanaka, and T. Okuda, "Tannins and related polyphenols of Euphorbiaceous plants. IX. Hydrolyzable tannins with $^{1}C_{4}$ glucose core form *Phyllanthus flexuosus* MUELL. ARG," *Chemical & Pharmaceutical Bulletin*, vol. 40, no. 1, pp. 53–60, 1992.

[212] C.-B. Yang, F. Zhang, M.-C. Deng, G.-Y. He, J.-M. Yue, and R.-H. Lu, "A new ellagitannin from the fruit of *Phyllanthus emblica* L.," *Journal of the Chinese Chemical Society*, vol. 54, no. 6, pp. 1615–1618, 2007.

[213] L.-Z. Zhang, Y.-J. Guo, G.-Z. Tu, W.-B. Guo, and F. Miao, "Isolation and identification of a novel ellagitannin from *Phyllanthus urinaria* L.," *Yaoxue Xuebao*, vol. 39, no. 2, pp. 119–122, 2004.

[214] Y.-L. Huang, C.-C. Chen, F.-L. Hsu, and C.-F. Chen, "Two tannins from *Phyllanthus tenellus*," *Journal of Natural Products*, vol. 61, no. 4, pp. 523–524, 1998.

[215] T. K. Nara, J. Gleye, E. Lavergne de Cerval, and E. Stanislas, "Flavonoids of *Phyllanthus niruri* L., *Phyllanthus urinaria* L., and *Phyllanthus orbiculatus* L. C. Rich," *Plantes Medicinales et Phytotherapie*, vol. 11, no. 2, pp. 82–86, 1977.

[216] O. G. Miguel, V. C. Filho, M. G. Pizzolatti et al., "A triterpene and phenolic compounds from leaves and stems of *Phyllanthus sellowianus*," *Planta Medica*, vol. 61, no. 4, article 391, 1995.

[217] D. M. Wu, "Determination of quercetin content in the herba of *Phyllanthus matsumurae* Hayata by HPLC," *Zhongcaoyao*, vol. 38, no. 8, pp. 1259–1261, 2007.

[218] Y. W. Chen and L. J. Ren, "Studies on the anticancer constituents of matsumura leafflower (*Phyllanthus matsumurae*). I. Isolation and identification of flavonoid compounds," *Chinese Traditional & Herbal Drugs*, vol. 28, no. 1, pp. 5–7, 1997.

[219] C. Y. Liang, H. S. Zhen, X. L. Tong et al., "Studies on the chemical constituents from leaves of *Phyllanthus emblica*," *Zhongchengyao*, vol. 31, no. 5, pp. 761–763, 2009.

[220] Q. Q. Yao and C. X. Zuo, "Chemical studies on the constituents of *Phyllanthus urinaria* L.," *Acta Pharmaceutica Sinica*, vol. 28, no. 11, pp. 829–835, 1993.

[221] Habib-Ur-Rehman, K. A. Yasin, M. A. Choudhary et al., "Studies on the chemical constituents of *Phyllanthus emblica*," *Natural Product Research*, vol. 21, no. 9, pp. 775–781, 2007.

[222] C. Wu, C.-S. Wei, S.-F. Yu et al., "Two new acetylated flavonoid glycosides from *Phyllanthus urinaria*," *Journal of Asian Natural Products Research*, vol. 15, no. 7, pp. 703–707, 2013.

[223] Subeki, H. Matsuura, K. Takahashi et al., "Anti-babesial and anti-plasmodial compounds from *Phyllanthus niruri*," *Journal of Natural Products*, vol. 68, no. 4, pp. 537–539, 2005.

[224] V. T. Boeira, C. E. Leite, A. A. Santos Jr. et al., "Effects of the hydroalcoholic extract of *Phyllanthus niruri* and its isolated compounds on cyclophosphamide-induced hemorrhagic cystitis in mouse," *Naunyn-Schmiedeberg's Archives of Pharmacology*, vol. 384, no. 3, pp. 265–275, 2011.

[225] W. K. Whang, I. S. Oh, I. H. Ham, and D. R. Hahn, "The phenolic constituents of *Phyllanthus ussuriensis* leaves," *Saengyak Hakhoechi*, vol. 25, no. 2, pp. 113–116, 1994.

[226] D. T. Tran, Q. C. Bui, V. L. Hoang, and X. D. Nguyen, "Isolation and structural elucidation of some phenolic compounds from *Phyllanthus urinaria* L. in Vietnam," *Tap Chi Duoc Hoc*, vol. 47, no. 3, pp. 14–17, 2007.

[227] S. K. El-Desouky, R. S. Young, and K. Young-Kyoon, "A new cytotoxic acylated apigenin glucoside from *Phyllanthus emblica* L.," *Natural Product Research*, vol. 22, no. 1, pp. 91–95, 2008.

[228] T. Sarg, A. Abdel-Ghani, R. Zayed, and M. El-Sayed, "Bioactive compounds from *Phyllanthus atropurpureus*," *Journal of Natural Products*, vol. 5, pp. 10–20, 2012.

[229] D. R. Gupta and B. Ahmed, "Nirurin: a new prenylated flavanone glycoside from *Phyllanthus nirurii*," *Journal of Natural Products*, vol. 47, no. 6, pp. 958–963, 1984.

[230] Y.-J. Zhang, T. Abe, T. Tanaka, C.-R. Yang, and I. Kouno, "Two new acylated flavanone glycosides from the leaves and branches of *Phyllanthus emblica*," *Chemical & Pharmaceutical Bulletin*, vol. 50, no. 6, pp. 841–843, 2002.

[231] M. A. Hossain, "A new prenylated flavanol from the arial part of *Phyllanthus niruri* and confirmed by GC-MS/MS," *Nigerian Journal of Natural Products and Medicine*, vol. 11, pp. 85–86, 2007.

[232] W.-Y. Qi, Y. Li, L. Hua, K. Wang, and K. Gao, "Cytotoxicity and structure activity relationships of phytosterol from *Phyllanthus emblica*," *Fitoterapia*, vol. 84, no. 1, pp. 252–256, 2013.

[233] B. Ahmad and T. Alam, "Components from whole plant of *Phyllanthus amarus* Linn.," *Indian Journal of Chemistry*, vol. 42, no. 7, pp. 1786–1790, 2003.

[234] J. Gupta and M. Ali, "Four new seco-sterols of *Phyllanthus fraternus* roots," *Indian Journal of Pharmaceutical Sciences*, vol. 61, no. 1–6, pp. 90–96, 1999.

[235] S. A. Hassarajani and N. B. Mulchandani, "Securinine type of alkaloids from *Phyllanthus niruri*," *Indian Journal of Chemistry Section B: Organic Chemistry Including Medicinal Chemistry*, vol. 29, no. 9, pp. 801–803, 1990.

[236] N. Mulchandani and S. Hassarajani, "4-Methoxy-nor-securinine, a new alkaloid from *Phyllanthus niruri*," *Planta Medica*, vol. 50, no. 1, pp. 104–105, 1984.

[237] B. Sparzak, F. Dybowski, and M. Krauze-Baranowska, "Analysis of Securinega-type alkaloids from *Phyllanthus glaucus* biomass," *Phytochemistry Letters*, vol. 11, pp. 353–357, 2015.

[238] B. S. Joshi, D. H. Gawad, S. W. Pelletier, G. Kartha, and K. Bhandary, "Isolation and structure (X-ray analysis) of ent-norsecurinine, an alkaloid from *Phyllanthus niruri*," *Journal of Natural Products*, vol. 49, no. 4, pp. 614–620, 1986.

[239] M. Zhou, H. L. Zhu, K. W. Wang, W. X. Wei, and Y. Zhang, "Isolation and X-ray crystal structure of a securinega-type alkaloid from *Phyllanthus niruri* Linn," *Natural Product Research*, vol. 26, no. 8, pp. 762–764, 2012.

[240] P. J. Houghton, T. Z. Woldemariam, S. O'Shea, and S. P. Thyagarajan, "Two securinega-type alkaloids from *Phyllanthus amarus*," *Phytochemistry*, vol. 43, no. 3, pp. 715–717, 1996.

[241] P. Petchnaree, N. Bunyapraphatsara, G. A. Cordell et al., "X-ray crystal and molecular structure of nirurine, a novel alkaloid related to the securinega alkaloid skeleton, from *Phyllanthus niruri* (Euphorbiaceae)," *Journal of the Chemical Society, Perkin Transactions*, vol. 1, no. 9, pp. 1551–1556, 1986.

[242] Babady-Bila, T. E. Gedris, and W. Herz, "Niruroidine, a nor-securinine-type alkaloid from *Phyllanthus niruroides*," *Phytochemistry*, vol. 41, no. 5, pp. 1441–1443, 1996.

[243] I. Cesari, P. Grisoli, M. Paolillo, C. Milanese, G. Massolini, and G. Brusotti, "Isolation and characterization of the alkaloid Nitidine responsible for the traditional use of *Phyllanthus muellerianus* (Kuntze) Excell stem bark against bacterial infections," *Journal of Pharmaceutical and Biomedical Analysis*, vol. 105, pp. 115–120, 2015.

[244] S. Sahni, S. Maurya, U. P. Singh, A. K. Singh, V. P. Singh, and V. B. Pandey, "Antifungal activity of nor-securinine against some Phytopathogenic fungi," *Mycobiology*, vol. 33, no. 2, pp. 97–103, 2005.

[245] R. S. Negi and T. M. Fakhir, "Simplexine (14-hydroxy-4-methoxy-13,14-dihydronorsecurinine): an alkaloid from *Phyllanthus simplex*," *Phytochemistry*, vol. 27, no. 9, pp. 3027–3028, 1988.

[246] Z. Horii, T. Imanishi, M. Yamauchi, M. Hanaoka, J. Parello, and S. Munavalli, "Structure of phyllantidine," *Tetrahedron Letters*, vol. 13, no. 19, pp. 1877–1880, 1972.

[247] J. Parello, A. Melera, and R. Goutarel, "Phyllochrysine and securinine, alkaloids of *Phyllanthus discoides*," *Bulletin de la Societe Chimique de France*, no. 4, pp. 898–910, 1963.

[248] W.-X. Wei and Y.-J. Pan, "The crystal structure of one natural compound cyclo-(1,10-docandiamino-11,20-docanedioic) amide (1,12-diazacyclodocosane-2,11-dione)," *Bulletin of the Korean Chemical Society*, vol. 23, no. 11, pp. 1527–1530, 2002.

[249] E. Nicolis, I. Lampronti, M. C. Dechecchi et al., "Pyrogallol, an active compound from the medicinal plant *Emblica officinalis*, regulates expression of pro-inflammatory genes in bronchial epithelial cells," *International Immunopharmacology*, vol. 8, no. 12, pp. 1672–1680, 2008.

[250] A. A. Sittie, E. Lemmich, C. E. Olsen, L. Hviid, and S. B. Christensen, "Alkamides from *Phyllanthus fraternus*," *Planta Medica*, vol. 64, no. 2, pp. 192–193, 1998.

[251] M. S. Tempesta, D. G. Corley, J. A. Beutler et al., "Phyllanthimide, a new alkaloid from *Phyllanthus sellowianus*," *Journal of Natural Products*, vol. 51, no. 3, pp. 617–618, 1988.

[252] E. Miyoshi, Y. Shizuri, and S. Yamamura, "Isolation of potassium chelidonate as a bioactive substance concerning with circadian rhythm in nyctinastic plants," *Chemistry Letters*, vol. 16, no. 3, pp. 511–514, 1987.

[253] Y.-J. Zhang, T. Tanaka, C.-R. Yang, and I. Kouno, "New phenolic constituents from the fruit juice of *Phyllanthus emblica*," *Chemical and Pharmaceutical Bulletin*, vol. 49, no. 5, pp. 537–540, 2001.

[254] M. Puppala, J. Ponder, P. Suryanarayana, G. B. Reddy, M. Petrash, and D. V. LaBarbera, "The isolation and characterization of β-glucogallin as a novel aldose reductase inhibitor from *Emblica officinalis*," *PLoS ONE*, vol. 7, no. 4, Article ID e31399, 2012.

[255] W. X. Wei, Y. J. Pan, Y. Z. Chen, C. W. Lin, T. Y. Wei, and S. K. Zhao, "Carboxylic acids from *Phyllanthus urinaria*," *Chemistry of Natural Compounds*, vol. 41, no. 1, pp. 17–21, 2005.

[256] W.-X. Wei, Y.-J. Pan, H. Zhang, C.-W. Lin, and T.-Y. Wei, "Two new compounds from *Phyllanthus niruri*," *Chemistry of Natural Compounds*, vol. 40, no. 5, pp. 460–464, 2004.

[257] Z. A. Amin, M. A. Alshawsh, M. Kassim, H. M. Ali, and M. A. Abdulla, "Gene expression profiling reveals underlying molecular mechanism of hepatoprotective effect of *Phyllanthus niruri* on thioacetamide-induced hepatotoxicity in Sprague Dawley rats," *BMC Complementary and Alternative Medicine*, vol. 13, no. 1, article 160, 2013.

[258] X. Niu, W. Li, and L. He, "Pharmacokinetics and tissue distribution of 8,9-epoxy brevifolin in rats, a hepatoprotective constituent isolated from *Phyllanthus simplex* Retz by liquid chromatography coupled with mass spectrometry method," *Biopharmaceutics & Drug Disposition*, vol. 29, no. 5, pp. 251–258, 2008.

[259] H. P. Luo, L. R. Chen, Z. Q. Li, Z. S. Ding, and X. J. Xu, "Frontal immunoaffinity chromatography with mass spectrometric detection: a method for finding active compounds from traditional Chinese herbs," *Analytical Chemistry*, vol. 75, no. 16, pp. 3994–3998, 2003.

[260] X.-F. Niu, L.-C. He, T. Fan, and Y. Li, "Protecting effect of brevifolin and 8,9-single-epoxy brevifolin of *Phyllanthus simplex* on rat liver injury," *Zhongguo Zhongyao Zazhi*, vol. 31, no. 18, pp. 1529–1532, 2006.

[261] M. Shimizu, S. Horie, S. Terashima et al., "Studies on aldose reductase inhibitors from natural products. II. Active components of a Paraguayan crude drug "Para-parai mí," *Phyllanthus niruri*," *Chemical & Pharmaceutical Bulletin*, vol. 37, no. 9, pp. 2531–2532, 1989.

[262] J.-H. S. Pang, S.-T. Huang, C.-Y. Wang et al., "Ellagic acid, the active compound of *Phyllanthus urinaria*, exerts in vivo anti-angiogenic effect and inhibits MMP-2 activity," *Evidence-Based Complementary and Alternative Medicine*, vol. 2011, Article ID 215035, 10 pages, 2011.

[263] N. Paulino, M. G. Pizollatti, R. A. Yunes, T. B. Creczynski-Pasa, and J. B. Calixto, "The mechanisms underlying the relaxant effect of methyl and ethyl gallates in the guinea pig trachea in vitro: contribution of potassium channels," *Naunyn-Schmiedeberg's Archives of Pharmacology*, vol. 360, no. 3, pp. 331–336, 1999.

[264] S. Bhattacharya, S. Chatterjee, A. Bauri et al., "Immunopharmacological basis of the healing of indomethacin-induced gastric mucosal damage in rats by the constituents of *Phyllanthus emblica*," *Phytochemistry*, vol. 93, no. 1, pp. 47–53, 2007.

[265] S. Maity, N. Nag, S. Chatterjee, S. Adhikari, and S. Mazumder, "Bilirubin clearance and antioxidant activities of ethanol extract of *Phyllanthus amarus* root in phenylhydrazine-induced neonatal jaundice in mice," *Journal of Physiology and Biochemistry*, vol. 69, no. 3, pp. 467–476, 2013.

[266] A. R. Santos, R. O. De Campos, O. G. Miguel, V. Cechinel-Filho, R. A. Yunes, and J. B. Calixto, "The involvement of K^+ channels and Gi/o protein in the antinociceptive action of the gallic acid ethyl ester," *European Journal of Pharmacology*, vol. 379, no. 1, pp. 7–17, 1999.

[267] T. Iizuka, H. Moriyama, and M. Nagai, "Vasorelaxant effects of methyl brevifolincarboxylate from the leaves of *Phyllanthus niruri*," *Biological and Pharmaceutical Bulletin*, vol. 29, no. 1, pp. 177–179, 2006.

[268] T. Iizuka, M. Nagai, A. Taniguchi, H. Moriyama, and K. Hoshi, "Inhibitory effects of methyl brevifolincarboxylate isolated from *Phyllanthus niruri* L. on platelet aggregation," *Biological and Pharmaceutical Bulletin*, vol. 30, no. 2, pp. 382–384, 2007.

[269] Y. Zhorig, C. X. Zuo, F. Li et al., "Studies on chemical constituents of *Phyllanthus urinaria* L. and its antiviral activity against hepatitis B virus," *Zhongguo Zhongyao Zazhi*, vol. 23, no. 6, pp. 363–364, 1998.

[270] G. She, R. Cheng, L. Sha et al., "A novel phenolic compound from *Phyllanthus emblica*," *Natural Product Communications*, vol. 8, no. 4, pp. 461–462, 2013.

[271] L.-Z. Zhang, Y.-J. Guo, G.-Z. Tu, F. Miao, and W.-B. Guo, "Isolation and identification of a noval polyphenolic compound from *Phyllanthus urinaria* L," *Zhongguo Zhongyao Zazhi*, vol. 25, no. 12, pp. 725–725, 2000.

[272] M. T. H. Khan, I. Lampronti, D. Martello et al., "Identification of pyrogallol as an antiproliferative compound present in extracts from the medicinal plant *Emblica officinalis*: effects on in vitro cell growth of human tumor cell lines," *International journal of oncology*, vol. 21, no. 1, pp. 187–192, 2002.

[273] E. Ajaiyeoba and D. Kingston, "Cytotoxicity evaluation and isolation of a chroman derivative from *Phyllanthus amarus* aerial part extract," *Pharmaceutical Biology*, vol. 44, no. 9, pp. 668–671, 2006.

[274] M. A. Quader, M. Khatun, and M. Mosihuzzaman, "Isolation of 4-hydroxysesamin and ent-norsecurinine from *Phyllanthus niruri* and their chemotaxonomic significance," *Journal of Bangladesh Academy of Sciences*, vol. 18, no. 2, pp. 229–234, 1994.

[275] R. M. Kuster, W. B. Mors, and H. Wagner, "Cyclohexenyl butenolides from *Phyllanthus klotzschianus*," *Biochemical Systematics and Ecology*, vol. 25, no. 7, p. 675, 1997.

[276] Y. L. Huang, *Phytochemical pharmacological studies on* Phyllanthus multiflorus, Phyllanthus tenellus, *and* Phyllanthus virgatus *[Ph.D. thesis]*, Taipei Medical College, Taipei, Taiwan, 1999.

[277] R. Soman and P. P. Pillay, "Isolation of mucic acid from the fruits of *Emblica officinalis* [*Phyllanthus emblica*]," *Current Science*, vol. 31, pp. 13–14, 1962.

[278] J.-Q. Zhao, Y.-M. Wang, H.-P. He et al., "Two new highly oxygenated and rearranged limonoids from *Phyllanthus cochinchinensis*," *Organic Letters*, vol. 15, no. 10, pp. 2414–2417, 2013.

[279] M. Ueda, T. Shigemori-Suzuki, and S. Yamamura, "Phyllanthurinolactone, a leaf-closing factor of nyctinastic plant, *Phyllanthus urinaria* L.," *Tetrahedron Letters*, vol. 36, no. 35, pp. 6267–6270, 1995.

[280] H. L. Zhu, W. X. Wei, M. Zhou, D. Yang, X. W. Fan, and J. X. Liu, "Chemical constituents of *Phyllanthus niruri* L.," *Tianran Chanwu Yanjiu Yu Kaifa*, vol. 23, no. 2, pp. 401–403, 2011.

[281] E. O. Lima, V. M. F. Morais, S. T. A. Gomes, V. C. Filho, O. G. Miguel, and R. A. Yunes, "Preliminary evaluation of antifungal activity of xanthoxyline," *Acta Farmaceutica Bonaerense*, vol. 14, no. 3, pp. 213–216, 1995.

[282] C. Bothiraja, M. B. Shinde, S. Rajalakshmi, and A. P. Pawar, "In vitro anti-HIV-type 1 and antioxidant activity of *Emblica officinalis*," *Research Journal of Pharmacy and Technology*, vol. 2, no. 3, pp. 556–558, 2011.

[283] O. Hnatyszyn, A. Broussalis, G. Herrera et al., "Argentine plant extracts active against polymerase and ribonuclease H activities of HIV-1 reverse transcriptase," *Phytotherapy Research*, vol. 13, no. 3, pp. 206–209, 1999.

[284] B. H. Tai, N. D. Nhut, N. X. Nhiem et al., "An evaluation of the RNase H inhibitory effects of Vietnamese medicinal plant extracts and natural compounds," *Pharmaceutical Biology*, vol. 49, no. 10, pp. 1046–1051, 2011.

[285] Y. S. Ravikumar, U. Ray, M. Nandhitha et al., "Inhibition of hepatitis C virus replication by herbal extract: *Phyllanthus amarus* as potent natural source," *Virus Research*, vol. 158, no. 1-2, pp. 89–97, 2011.

[286] Á. L. Álvarez, G. del Barrio, V. Kourí, P. A. Martínez, B. Suárez, and F. Parra, "In vitro anti-herpetic activity of an aqueous extract from the plant *Phyllanthus orbicularis*," *Phytomedicine*, vol. 16, no. 10, pp. 960–966, 2009.

[287] G. Del Barrio and F. Parra, "Evaluation of the antiviral activity of an aqueous extract from *Phyllanthus orbicularis*," *Journal of Ethnopharmacology*, vol. 72, no. 1-2, pp. 317–322, 2000.

[288] K. B. Harikumar, G. Kuttan, and R. Kuttan, "Inhibition of viral carcinogenesis by *Phyllanthus amarus*," *Integrative Cancer Therapies*, vol. 8, no. 3, pp. 254–260, 2009.

[289] N. K. Jain, S. Lodhi, A. Jain, A. Nahata, and A. K. Singhai, "Effects of *Phyllanthus acidus* (L.) Skeels fruit on carbon tetrachloride-induced acute oxidative damage in livers of rats and mice," *Journal of Chinese Integrative Medicine*, vol. 9, no. 1, pp. 49–56, 2011.

[290] B. Rajkapoor, Y. Venugopal, J. Anbu, N. Harikrishnan, M. Gobinath, and V. Ravichandran, "Protective effect of *Phyllanthus polyphyllus* on acetaminophen induced hepatotoxicity in rats," *Pakistan Journal of Pharmaceutical Sciences*, vol. 21, no. 1, pp. 57–62, 2008.

[291] S. Gopi and O. H. Setty, "Protective effect of *Phyllanthus fraternus* against bromobenzene induced mitochondrial dysfunction in rat liver mitochondria," *Food and Chemical Toxicology*, vol. 48, no. 8-9, pp. 2170–2175, 2010.

[292] M. Ferrer, C. Cristófol, A. Sánchez-Lamar, J. L. Fuentes, J. Barbé, and M. Llagostera, "Modulation of rat and human cytochromes P450 involved in PhIP and 4-ABP activation by an aqueous extract of *Phyllanthus orbicularis*," *Journal of Ethnopharmacology*, vol. 90, no. 2-3, pp. 273–277, 2004.

[293] J. L. Fuentes, A. E. Alonso, E. Cuétara et al., "Usefulness of the SOS Chromotest in the study of medicinal plants as radioprotectors," *International Journal of Radiation Biology*, vol. 82, no. 5, pp. 323–329, 2006.

[294] M. Vernhes, M. González-Pumariega, L. Andrade et al., "Protective effect of a *Phyllanthus orbicularis* aqueous extract against UVB light in human cells," *Pharmaceutical Biology*, vol. 51, no. 1, pp. 1–7, 2013.

[295] N. Giribabu, P. V. Rao, K. P. Kumar, S. Muniandy, S. Swapna Rekha, and N. Salleh, "Aqueous extract of Phyllanthus niruri leaves displays in vitro antioxidant activity and prevents the elevation of oxidative stress in the kidney of streptozotocin-induced diabetic male rats," *Evidence-Based Complementary and Alternative Medicine*, vol. 2014, Article ID 834815, 10 pages, 2014.

[296] S. Kumar, D. Kumar, R. R. Deshmukh, P. D. Lokhande, S. N. More, and V. D. Rangari, "Antidiabetic potential of *Phyllanthus reticulatus* in alloxan-induced diabetic mice," *Fitoterapia*, vol. 79, no. 1, pp. 21–23, 2008.

[297] O. Hnatyszyn, J. Miño, G. Ferraro, and C. Acevedo, "The hypoglycemic effect of *Phyllanthus sellowianus* fractions in streptozotocin-induced diabetic mice," *Phytomedicine*, vol. 9, no. 6, pp. 556–559, 2002.

[298] A. Hashim, M. Salman Khan, and S. Ahmad, "Alleviation of hyperglycemia and hyperlipidemia by *Phyllanthus virgatus* forst extract and its partially purified fraction in streptozotocin induced diabetic rats," *EXCLI Journal*, vol. 13, pp. 809–824, 2014.

[299] J. Shabeer, R. S. Srivastava, and S. K. Singh, "Antidiabetic and antioxidant effect of various fractions of *Phyllanthus simplex* in alloxan diabetic rats," *Journal of Ethnopharmacology*, vol. 124, no. 1, pp. 34–38, 2009.

[300] A. Hashim, M. S. Khan, M. S. Khan, M. H. Baig, and S. Ahmad, "Antioxidant and α-amylase inhibitory property of *Phyllanthus virgatus* L.: an in vitro and molecular interaction study," *BioMed Research International*, vol. 2013, Article ID 729393, 12 pages, 2013.

[301] P. Buszniez, O. Di Sapio, and B. Riquelme, "Effects of phyllanthus sellowianus Müll Arg. extracts on the rheological properties of human erythrocytes," *Cell Biochemistry and Biophysics*, vol. 70, no. 2, pp. 1407–1416, 2014.

[302] C. Ngamkitidechakul, K. Jaijoy, P. Hansakul, N. Soonthornchareonnon, and S. Sireeratawong, "Antitumour effects of *Phyllanthus emblica* L.: induction of cancer cell apoptosis and inhibition of in vivo tumour promotion and in vitro invasion of human cancer cells," *Phytotherapy Research*, vol. 24, no. 9, pp. 1405–1413, 2010.

[303] H.-J. Zhao, T. Liu, X. Mao et al., "Fructus phyllanthi tannin fraction induces apoptosis and inhibits migration and invasion of human lung squamous carcinoma cells in vitro via MAPK/MMP pathways," *Acta Pharmacologica Sinica*, vol. 36, no. 6, pp. 758–768, 2015.

[304] S.-T. Huang, K.-W. Bi, H.-M. Kuo et al., "*Phyllanthus urinaria* induces mitochondrial dysfunction in human osteosarcoma 143B cells associated with modulation of mitochondrial fission/fusion proteins," *Mitochondrion*, vol. 17, pp. 22–33, 2014.

[305] S. H. Lee, I. B. Jaganath, S. M. Wang, and S. D. Sekaran, "Antimetastatic effects of *Phyllanthus* on human lung (A549) and breast (MCF-7) cancer cell lines," *PLoS ONE*, vol. 6, no. 6, Article ID e20994, 2011.

[306] Y.-Q. Tang, I. B. Jaganath, and S. D. Sekaran, "*Phyllanthus* spp. induces selective growth inhibition of PC-3 and mewo human cancer cells through modulation of cell cycle and induction of apoptosis," *PLoS ONE*, vol. 5, no. 9, Article ID e12644, 2010.

[307] Y.-Q. Tang, I. Jaganath, R. Manikam, and S. D. Sekaran, "*Phyllanthus* suppresses prostate cancer cell, PC-3, proliferation and induces apoptosis through multiple signalling pathways (MAPKs, PI3K/Akt, NF B, and Hypoxia)," *Evidence-Based Complementary and Alternative Medicine*, vol. 2013, Article ID 609581, 13 pages, 2013.

[308] S. Ramasamy, N. Wahab, N. Zainal Abidin, S. Manickam, and Z. Zakaria, "Growth inhibition of human gynecologic and colon cancer cells by *Phyllanthus watsonii* through apoptosis induction," *PLoS ONE*, vol. 7, no. 4, Article ID e34793, 2012.

[309] M. Ismail, G. Bagalkotkar, S. Iqbal, and H. A. Adamu, "Anticancer properties and phenolic contents of sequentially prepared extracts from different parts of selected medicinal plants indigenous to malaysia," *Molecules*, vol. 17, no. 5, pp. 5745–5756, 2012.

[310] S. Kumar, S. Sharma, D. Kumar, K. Kumar, and R. Arya, "Immunostimulant activity of *Phyllanthus reticulatus* Poir: a useful plant for infectious tropical diseases," *Asian Pacific Journal of Tropical Disease*, vol. 4, supplement 1, pp. S491–S495, 2014.

[311] A. R. S. Santos, V. C. Filho, R. Niero et al., "Analgesic effects of callus culture extracts from selected species of *Phyllanthus* in mice," *Journal of Pharmacy & Pharmacology*, vol. 46, no. 9, pp. 755–759, 1994.

[312] A. R. S. Santos, R. O. P. De Campos, O. G. Miguel et al., "Antinociceptive properties of extracts of new species of plants of the genus *Phyllanthus* (Euphorbiaceae)," *Journal of Ethnopharmacology*, vol. 72, no. 1-2, pp. 229–238, 2000.

[313] J. B. Perianayagam, S. K. Sharma, A. Joseph, and A. J. M. Christina, "Evaluation of anti-pyretic and analgesic activity of *Emblica officinalis* Gaertn," *Journal of Ethnopharmacology*, vol. 95, no. 1, pp. 83–85, 2004.

[314] S. M. Mali, A. Sinnathambi, C. U. Kapase, S. L. Bodhankar, and K. R. Mahadik, "Anti-arthritic activity of standardised extract of *Phyllanthus amarus* in Freund's complete adjuvant induced arthritis," *Biomedicine & Aging Pathology*, vol. 1, no. 3, pp. 185–190, 2011.

[315] H. S. Chouhan and S. K. Singh, "Phytochemical analysis, antioxidant and anti-inflammatory activities of *Phyllanthus simplex*," *Journal of Ethnopharmacology*, vol. 137, no. 3, pp. 1337–1344, 2011.

[316] M. H. Mehmood, H. S. Siddiqi, and A. H. Gilani, "The anti-diarrheal and spasmolytic activities of *Phyllanthus emblica* are mediated through dual blockade of muscarinic receptors and Ca^{2+} channels," *Journal of Ethnopharmacology*, vol. 133, no. 2, pp. 856–865, 2011.

[317] F. C. Amaechina and E. K. Omogbai, "Hypotensive effect of aqueous extract of the leaves of *Phyllanthus amarus* Schum and Thonn (Euphorbiaceae)," *Acta Poloniae Pharmaceutica*, vol. 64, no. 6, pp. 547–552, 2007.

[318] M. Sumitra, P. Manikandan, V. S. Gayathri, P. Mahendran, and L. Suguna, "Emblica officinalis exerts wound healing action through up-regulation of collagen and extracellular signal-regulated kinases (ERK1/2)," *Wound Repair and Regeneration*, vol. 17, no. 1, pp. 99–107, 2009.

[319] S. K. Bandyopadhyay, A. Chatterjee, and S. Chattopadhyay, "Biphasic effect of *Phyllanthus emblica* L. extract on NSAID-induced ulcer: An antioxidative trail weaved with immunomodulatory effect," *Evidence-Based Complementary and Alternative Medicine*, vol. 2011, Article ID 146808, 13 pages, 2011.

[320] G. Venkateshwarlu, S. K. Veliyath, K. Vijayabhaskar, K. Harishbabu, R. Malothu, and S. Sahoo, "Wound healing activity of *Phyllanthus niruri* in albino wistar rats," *Asian Journal of Chemistry*, vol. 24, no. 9, pp. 3929–3930, 2012.

[321] A. Bagavan, A. A. Rahuman, C. Kamaraj, N. K. Kaushik, D. Mohanakrishnan, and D. Sahal, "Antiplasmodial activity of botanical extracts against *Plasmodium falciparum*," *Parasitology Research*, vol. 108, no. 5, pp. 1099–1109, 2011.

[322] R. Appiah-Opong, A. K. Nyarko, D. Dodoo, F. N. Gyang, K. A. Koram, and N. K. Ayisi, "Antiplasmodial activity of extracts of Tridax procumbens and *Phyllanthus amarus* in in vitro *Plasmodium falciparum* culture systems," *Ghana Medical Journal*, vol. 45, no. 4, pp. 143–150, 2011.

[323] D. Dhingra, P. Joshi, A. Gupta, and R. Chhillar, "Possible involvement of monoaminergic neurotransmission in antidepressant-like activity of *Emblica officinalis* fruits in mice," *CNS Neuroscience and Therapeutics*, vol. 18, no. 5, pp. 419–425, 2012.

[324] M. Vasudevan and M. Parle, "Effect of Anwala churna (*Emblica offcinalis* GAERTN.): an ayurvedic preparation on memory deficit rats," *Journal of the Pharmaceutical Society of Japan*, vol. 127, no. 10, pp. 1701–1707, 2007.

[325] M. Vasudevan and M. Parle, "Memory enhancing activity of Anwala churna (*Emblica officinalis* Gaertn.): an Ayurvedic preparation," *Physiology and Behavior*, vol. 91, no. 1, pp. 46–54, 2007.

[326] G. Brusotti, I. Cesari, G. Gilardoni et al., "Chemical composition and antimicrobial activity of *Phyllanthus muellerianus* (Kuntze) Excel essential oil," *Journal of Ethnopharmacology*, vol. 142, no. 3, pp. 657–662, 2012.

[327] E. Goun, G. Cunningham, D. Chu, C. Nguyen, and D. Miles, "Antibacterial and antifungal activity of Indonesian ethnomedical plants," *Fitoterapia*, vol. 74, no. 6, pp. 592–596, 2003.

[328] M. Sousa, J. Ousingsawat, R. Seitz et al., "An extract from the medicinal plant *Phyllanthus acidus* and its isolated compounds induce airway chloride secretion: a potential treatment for cystic fibrosis," *Molecular Pharmacology*, vol. 71, no. 1, pp. 366–376, 2007.

[329] O. Hnatyszyn, J. Miño, S. Gorzalczany et al., "Diuretic activity of an aqueous extract of *Phyllanthus sellowianus*," *Phytomedicine*, vol. 6, no. 3, pp. 177–179, 1999.

[330] R. Kuttan and K. B. Harikumar, *Phyllanthus Species: Scientific Evaluation and Medicinal Applications*, CRC Press, 2011.

[331] M. A. Boim, I. P. Heilberg, and N. Schor, "*Phyllanthus niruri* as a promising alternative treatment for nephrolithiasis," *International Brazilian Journal of Urology*, vol. 36, no. 6, pp. 657–664, 2010.

[332] Y. A. Cheng, S. D. Wang, and S. S. Dang, "Clinical study of *Phyllanthus* pill on treating chronic hepatitis B," *Zhongxiyi Jiehe Ganbing Zazhi*, vol. 19, no. 17, pp. 195–197, 2009.

[333] G. A. Asare, P. Addo, K. Bugyei et al., "Acute toxicity studies of aqueous leaf extract of *Phyllanthus niruri*," *Interdisciplinary Toxicology*, vol. 4, no. 4, pp. 206–210, 2011.

[334] G. A. Asare, K. Bugyei, A. Sittie et al., "Genotoxicity, cytotoxicity and toxicological evaluation of whole plant extracts of the medicinal plant *Phyllanthus niruri* (Phyllanthaceae)," *Genetics & Molecular Research*, vol. 11, no. 1, pp. 100–111, 2012.

[335] G. A. Asare, K. Bugyei, I. Fiawoyi et al., "Male rat hormone imbalance, testicular changes and toxicity associated with aqueous leaf extract of an antimalarial plant: *Phyllanthus niruri*," *Pharmaceutical Biology*, vol. 51, no. 6, pp. 691–699, 2013.

[336] A. Josiah Obaghwarhieywo and N. Ezekiel Uba, "Histological effects of chronic administration of *Phyllanthus amarus* on the kidney of adult Wistar rat," *North American Journal of Medical Sciences*, vol. 2, no. 4, pp. 193–195, 2010.

[337] A. A. Bakare, G. O. Oguntolu, L. A. Adedokun et al., "*In vivo* evaluation of genetic and systemic toxicity of aqueous extracts of *Phyllanthus amarus* in mice and rats," *International Journal of Toxicological & Pharmacological Research*, vol. 7, no. 4, pp. 1–9, 2015.

[338] A. R. Chopade and F. Sayyad, "Toxicity studies and evaluation of *Phyllanthus amarus* and *Phyllanthus fraternus* extracts on the central nervous system and musculoskeletal function," *International Journal of Chemical and Pharmaceutical Sciences*, vol. 2, no. 3, pp. 1333–1338, 2013.

[339] S. K. Singh and V. Prakash, "Toxicity assessment of *Oxalis corniculata* and phyllanthus fraternus plants," *International Journal of Pharmacy & Pharmaceutical Sciences*, vol. 6, no. 4, pp. 388–392, 2014.

[340] L. R. Fukumoto and G. Mazza, "Assessing antioxidant and prooxidant activities of phenolic compounds," *Journal of Agricultural & Food Chemistry*, vol. 48, no. 8, pp. 3597–3604, 2000.

6

Involvement of 5-HT$_{1A}$ Receptors in the Anxiolytic-Like Effects of Quercitrin and Evidence of the Involvement of the Monoaminergic System

Jian Li,[1] Qian-tong Liu,[1] Yi Chen,[1] Jie Liu,[1] Jin-li Shi,[1] Yong Liu,[1] and Jian-you Guo[2]

[1]*School of Chinese Materia Medica, Beijing University of Chinese Medicine, Beijing 100102, China*
[2]*Key Laboratory of Mental Health, Institute of Psychology, Chinese Academy of Sciences, Beijing 100101, China*

Correspondence should be addressed to Jin-li Shi; shijl@vip.sina.com and Jian-you Guo; guojy@psych.ac.cn

Academic Editor: Victor Kuete

Quercitrin is a well-known flavonoid that is contained in Flos Albiziae, which has been used for the treatment of anxiety. The present study investigated the anxiolytic-like effects of quercitrin in experimental models of anxiety. Compared with the control group, repeated treatment with quercitrin (5.0 and 10.0 mg/kg/day, p.o.) for seven days significantly increased the percentage of entries into and time spent on the open arms of the elevated plus maze. In the light/dark box test, quercitrin exerted an anxiolytic-like effect at 5 and 10 mg/kg. In the marble-burying test, quercitrin (5.0 and 10.0 mg/kg) also exerted an anxiolytic-like effect. Furthermore, quercitrin did not affect spontaneous locomotor activity. The anxiolytic-like effects of quercitrin in the elevated plus maze and light/dark box test were blocked by the serotonin-1A (5-hydroxytryptamine-1A (5-HT$_{1A}$)) receptor antagonist WAY-100635 (3.0 mg/kg, i.p.) but not by the γ-aminobutyric acid-A (GABA$_A$) receptor antagonist flumazenil (0.5 mg/kg, i.p.). The levels of brain monoamines (5-HT and dopamine) and their metabolites (5-hydroxy-3-indoleacetic acid, 3,4-dihydroxyphenylacetic acid, and homovanillic acid) were decreased after quercitrin treatment. These data suggest that the anxiolytic-like effects of quercitrin might be mediated by 5-HT$_{1A}$ receptors but not by benzodiazepine site of GABA$_A$ receptors. The results of the neurochemical studies suggest that these effects are mediated by modulation of the levels of monoamine neurotransmitters.

1. Introduction

Anxiety is a state of excessive fear and characterized by psychomotor tension, sympathetic hyperactivity, and vigilance [1]. More than one of every four adults experience at least one anxiety disorder in his or her lifetime [2]. Benzodiazepines are the most common drugs that have been used for the treatment of anxiety, but these compounds have obvious side effects, such as sedation, muscle relaxation, amnesia, and dependence potential [3–5]. Therefore, more efficacious and better-tolerated anxiolytic agents need to be developed.

Albizia julibrissin Durazz., commonly called mimosa or silk trees, is widely distributed across China, Africa, Mid-Asia, East Asia, and North America [6]. Flos Albiziae is the dry flowers or flower buds of *Albizia julibrissin* Durazz., which have been used for the treatment of insomnia, amnesia,

sore throat, and contusion in traditional oriental medicine [7]. Our previous study showed that the total flavones contained in *Albizia julibrissin* exerted anxiolytic effects [8]. Quercitrin is the major component of flavonoids contained in Flos Albiziae [9]. Quercitrin has been reported to have many biological properties, including sedative [10], neuroprotective [11], anti-inflammatory [12, 13], antinociceptive [14], and antileishmanial [15] effects. However, the anxiolytic potential of quercitrin has not yet been reported.

Many currently available anxiolytic drugs are known to act through GABA-ergic or serotonergic systems [16, 17]. GABA plays an important role in anxiety disorders. Studies that use knockout and knock-in mice have been conducted to clarify the role of the GABA$_A$ receptor complex in the pathophysiology and management of anxiety [18]. Serotonin (5-hydroxytryptamine (5-HT)) is a key modulatory neurotransmitter that has been implicated in the pathophysiology and treatment of anxiety and mood disorders [19]. The proposed role of 5-HT$_{1A}$ receptors in modulating anxiety-related behavior is supported by recent studies that employed 5-HT$_{1A}$ receptor knockout mice [20, 21]. In addition, clinical and animal studies have provided evidence to support the involvement of central neurochemical systems, including neurotransmitter, neuromodulator, and neuroendocrine systems, in anxiety disorders [22]. Modulation of the monoaminergic system forms the basis for the actions of anxiolytic drugs [22], providing a framework for studying the pathophysiology of anxiety disorders and pharmacotherapies that target monoaminergic systems.

Animal models are indispensable tools for unraveling the neurobiological mechanisms that underlie anxiety and assessing the behavioral impact of new drug candidates that affect different aspects of anxiety [23–25]. In the present study, we explored the anxiolytic-like effects of quercitrin using the elevated plus maze (EPM), light/dark box (LDB) test, and marble-burying test. The open-field test (OFT) was used to evaluate spontaneous locomotor activity. We investigated the involvement of GABA$_A$ and 5-HT$_{1A}$ receptors in the anxiolytic-like properties of quercitrin. To explore the neuropharmacological mechanism, we assessed the influence of quercitrin on the levels of 5-HT and dopamine and their metabolites. Our results showed that quercitrin exerted an anxiolytic-like effect.

2. Materials and Methods

2.1. Animals. All of the experiments were performed using male ICR mice (19–21 g), which were obtained from the Vital River Company, Beijing, China. The mice were housed five per cage (25 cm × 15 cm × 14 cm) in a temperature- (23 ± 1˚C) and humidity- (55% ± 5%) controlled room under a 12 h/12 h light/dark cycle (lights on 7:00 AM–7:00 PM) with *ad libitum* access to food and water. All of the experiments were performed between 8 AM and 2 PM. The mice were introduced to the quiet experimental room under dim red light at least 1 h before testing. The experimental procedures were approved by the Animal Care and Use Committee of the Institute of Psychology, Chinese Academy of Sciences, and were in accordance with the National Institutes of Health Guide for Care and Use of Laboratory Animals.

2.2. Materials. Quercitrin was purchased from the China Food and Drug Inspection Institute. Diazepam was obtained from Yimin Pharmaceutical Factory (Beijing, China). 5-HT, 5-hydroxy-3-indoleacetic acid (5-HIAA), dopamine, 3,4-dihydroxyphenylacetic acid (DOPAC), and homovanillic acid (HVA) were purchased from Sigma (St. Louis, MO, USA). All of the other reagents were of analytical grade.

2.3. Treatments and Groups. The mice (n = 15 per group) were randomly assigned to eight experimental groups: vehicle control group, diazepam group, quercitrin groups (2.5, 5.0, and 10.0 mg/kg), diazepam + flumazenil group, quercitrin + flumazenil group, and quercitrin + WAY-100635 group. To evaluate the anxiolytic effects of quercitrin, quercitrin

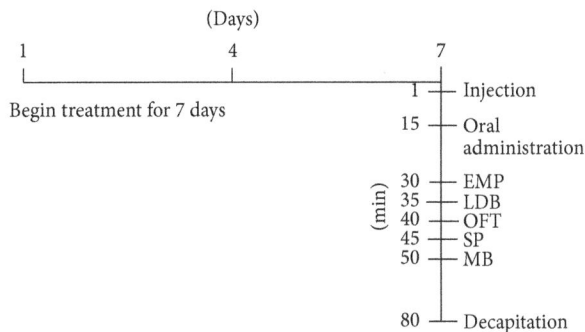

FIGURE 1: Schematic illustration of the experimental design. The vehicle (control), quercitrin (2.5, 5.0, and 10.0 mg/kg), and diazepam (DZP, 2 mg/kg) were orally administered daily for 7 days. On the last day, the antagonists flumazenil (F; 3 mg/kg, i.p.) and WAY-100635 (W; 0.5 mg/kg, i.p.) were injected 15 min before the oral treatments. The behavioral tests (EPM, LDB, OFT, SP, and MB tests) were performed, and tissue samples were collected on the same day.

(2.5, 5.0, and 10.0 mg/kg) and diazepam (2.0 mg/kg) were orally administered to the mice for 7 days. To explore the involvement of GABA$_A$ and 5-HT$_{1A}$ receptors in the effects of quercitrin, quercitrin (5.0 mg/kg) or diazepam (2.0 mg/kg) was administered to the mice for 7 days. On the last day, the GABA$_A$ receptor antagonist flumazenil (Sigma, St. Louis, MO, USA; 0.5 mg/kg, i.p.) or 5-HT$_{1A}$ receptor antagonist WAY-100635 (Sigma, St. Louis, MO, USA; 3 mg/kg, i.p.) was coadministered with quercitrin, and flumazenil was coadministered with diazepam 15 min before oral administration. The behavioral testing was conducted 30 min after oral administration. Diazepam at a dose of 2 mg/kg was chosen as a positive control drug. The dose and route of administration for diazepam and quercitrin were based on previous studies [8, 9, 26–28]. Quercitrin and diazepam were suspended in 0.9% physiological saline solution that contained 1% Tween 80, and flumazenil and WAY-100635 were dissolved in physiological saline. Control animals received vehicle orally and by injection. All of the drugs were prepared immediately before use and administered orally in a volume of 0.5 mL/25 g body weight for 7 days. All of the behavioral tests were performed on the 7th day of treatment. All groups of animals underwent all behavior tests. The study design is shown in Figure 1.

2.4. Experiments

2.4.1. Elevated Plus Maze. This validated test has been widely used to measure anxiety in rodents [24]. The EPM consisted of two open arms (30 cm × 5 cm × 15 cm) and two closed arms (30 cm × 5 cm) that were connected by a central platform (5 cm × 5 cm). It was elevated 45 cm above the floor. The open arms had a low edge (0.25 cm) that provided additional grip for the animals. The test was performed 30 min after oral administration. The mice were individually placed in the center of the maze, facing an open arm. The number of entries into the open and closed arms and time spent on the open and closed arms were recorded by AVTAS 3.0 software (Anilab, Ningbo, China) during a 5 min observation period. The percentage of entries into the open arms (% OE = entries into open arms/entries into open and closed arms) and percentage of time spent on the open arms (% OT = time spent on the open arms/time spent on the open and closed arms) were treated as an index of anxiety. Animals were excluded if they fell from the maze. The maze was cleaned thoroughly between trials using 10% ethanol.

2.4.2. Light/Dark Box Test. The LDB test was performed immediately after the EPM test. When the EPM test was completed, the mouse was immediately placed in the LDB. The apparatus consisted of two compartments, with one-third painted white and two-thirds painted black, which were divided by a plate with a small hole opening at floor level that allowed the mice to pass from one compartment to the other. A 60 W white light was placed 40 cm above the light chamber. The mouse was placed in the light compartment and allowed to freely explore the apparatus for 5 min. The number of transfers from the dark compartment to the light compartment and the time spent in the light compartment were recorded over 5 min by an observer using a chronometer. The observer remained quiet during the entire experiment. The apparatus was thoroughly cleaned between each test.

2.4.3. Open-Field Test. When the LDB test was completed, the mouse was immediately placed in the open field. The open field consisted of a square arena (60 cm × 60 cm). The entire apparatus was enclosed by 25 cm high walls made of black Plexiglas. The arena was illuminated by two 60 W red lamps that were placed over the center of the apparatus. The lamps were close to each other, 120 cm above the floor, and provided 100 lux illumination in the testing room. The test began by placing a single mouse in the middle of the arena and allowing it to move freely for 5 min. The total distance travelled was recorded by an automatic video tracking system and AVTAS 3.0 software (Anilab, Ningbo, China). After each trial, the apparatus was wiped clean with a 10% ethanol solution.

2.4.4. Spontaneous Activity. The spontaneous activity test was performed immediately after the open-field test. The locomotor test apparatus consisted of four clear acrylate test boxes (40 cm width × 40 cm length × 35 cm height) and four standard sound-attenuating cubicles with a camera and infrared lights. The mice were tested in a dim room that was illuminated with a 60 W red light (20 lux). To rule out any possible nonspecific locomotor effects of quercitrin on our measures of anxiety, spontaneous locomotor activity was recorded using a computer-based system (Anilab, Ningbo, China). During the observation period, the software detected infrared light beam breaks. The apparatus was thoroughly cleaned between each test.

2.4.5. Marble-Burying Test. The marble-burying test was performed immediately after the spontaneous activity test. Marble-burying behavior was assessed based on previously published methods [29]. The test was performed using transparent cages (37 cm length × 21 cm width × 15 cm height) that had 5 cm of bedding material and 20 glass marbles (1.5 cm diameter) that were equidistantly distributed throughout the cage. The marbles were placed in a 4 × 5 grid, with no marble closer than 1 cm from the wall of the cage. Testing was performed under normal ambient room lighting (>350 lux). The mice were individually placed in the cage, and transparent plastic was placed on top of the cage to prevent escape. At the end of the 30 min test, the mice were carefully removed from the chamber, and the number of marbles that were buried (i.e., more than two-thirds of the marble was covered by bedding) was determined.

2.4.6. Determination of Monoamines and Metabolites. The mice were decapitated by cervical dislocation immediately after the marble-burying test. The brains were dissected and immediately placed on ice. The tissue samples were weighed and stored at −80°C until homogenization. The brain tissue was manually homogenized with three volumes (w/v) of ice-cold 0.1 M perchloric acid (100 μL/mg wet weight) that contained 0.1 mM ethylenediaminetetraacetic acid (EDTA). After homogenization and centrifugation at 12,000 ×g at 4°C for 10 min, 20 μL of the tissue homogenate supernatant was injected directly into a high-performance liquid chromatography (HPLC) system that was equipped with an electrochemical detector (Waters ECD 2465, Milford, Massachusetts, USA). The mixed standard was used as a reference. The levels of monoamines (5-HT, dopamine, 5-HIAA, DOPAC, and HVA) in the samples were expressed as nanograms per gram fresh weight of tissue [30]. The HPLC system included a reversed-phase C18 column (2.1 mm × 150 mm, 3 μm, Waters Atlantis). The mobile phase consisted of 50 mM citric acid-sodium citrate (pH 3.5), 0.3 mM Na$_2$-EDTA, 1.8 mM dibutylamine, and 4% methanol. The flow rate was 0.35 mL/min, and the detector potential was +0.75 V.

2.5. Statistical Analysis. The data are expressed as mean ± SEM. The statistical analysis was performed using one- or two-way analysis of variance (ANOVA) followed by the Student-Newman-Keuls post hoc test and GraphPad Prism 5.0 software. In cases of significant variation, the individual values were compared using Dunnett's test. Values of $p < 0.05$ were considered statistically significant.

3. Results

3.1. Effect of Quercitrin in the Elevated Plus Maze. The one-way ANOVA revealed significant differences between groups in the time spent on the open arms ($F_{7,127} = 4.330$, $p < 0.01$, Figure 2(a)), percentage of open arm entries ($F_{7,127} = 3.123$, $p < 0.05$, Figure 2(b)), percentage of the time spent in the closed arms ($F_{7,127} = 4.140$, $p < 0.01$, Figure 2(c)), percentage of closed arm entries ($F_{7,127} = 3.342$, $p < 0.01$, Figure 2(d)), and percentage of the time spent in the central areas ($F_{7,127} = 1.692$, $p > 0.05$, Figure 2(e)). As shown in Figure 2(a), treatment with 5.0 and 10.0 mg/kg quercitrin significantly increased the percentage of time spent on the open arms (both $p < 0.01$). Diazepam (2 mg/kg) significantly increased the percentage of time spent on the open arms compared with the control group ($p < 0.01$). As shown in Figure 2(b), diazepam (both $p < 0.01$) and 5.0 and 10.0 mg/kg quercitrin ($p < 0.01$ and $p < 0.05$, resp.) significantly

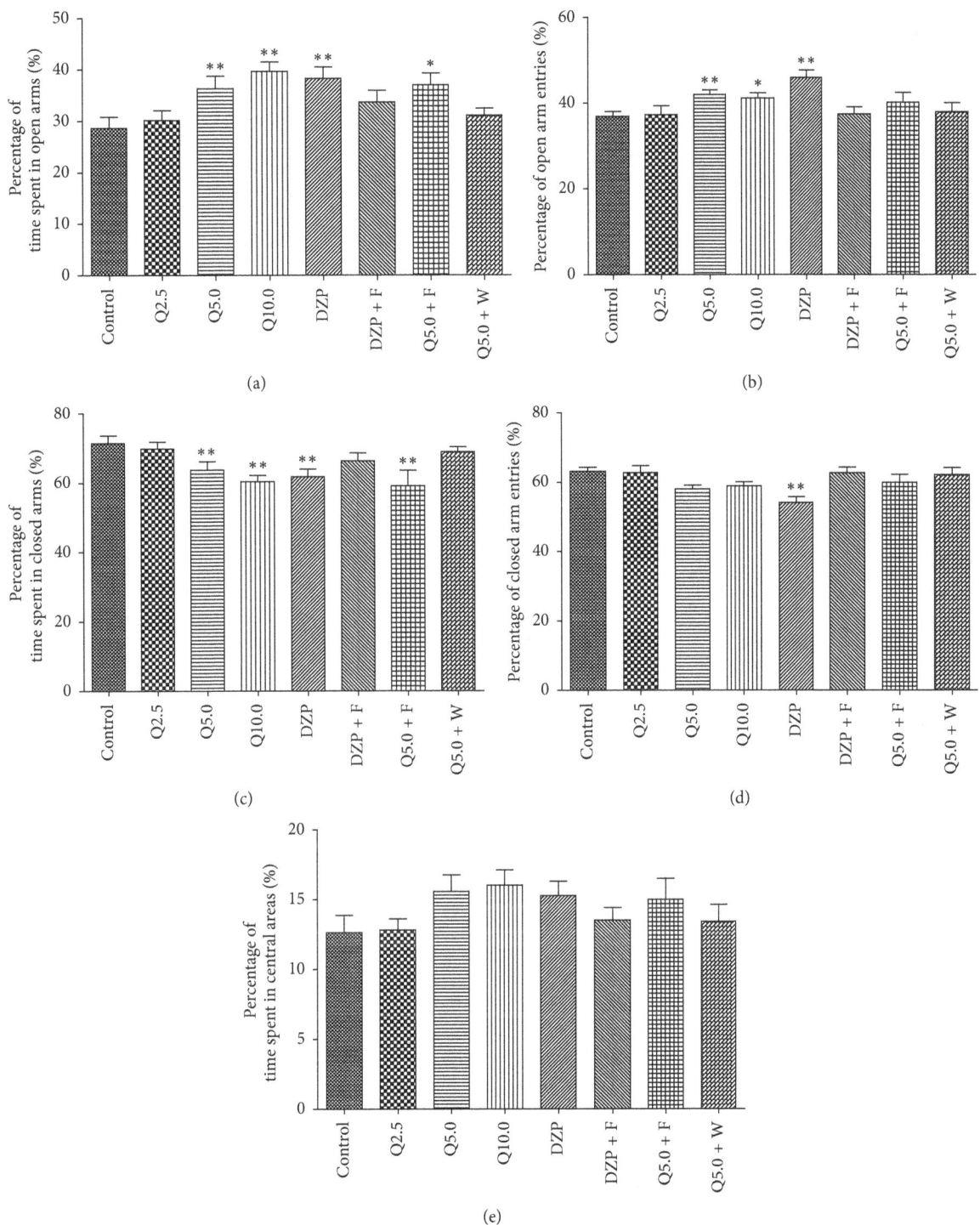

FIGURE 2: Behavioral performance of mice in a 5 min session in the elevated plus maze performed 0.5 h after the injection of vehicle (control, p.o.), quercitrin (2.5, 5.0, and 10.0 mg/kg, p.o.), diazepam (DZP, 2 mg/kg, p.o.), flumazenil (F; 3 mg/kg, i.p., 15 min after p.o. administration of positive control or quercitrin, Q), and WAY-100635 (W; 0.5 mg/kg, i.p., 15 min before p.o. administration of quercitrin, Q). (a) Percentage of time spent in the open arms, (b) percentage of open arm entries, (c) percentage of time spent in the closed arms, (d) percentage of closed arm entries, and (e) percentage of time spent in central areas. Columns represent the means ± SEM; $n = 15$ mice. $^{*}p < 0.05$ and $^{**}p < 0.01$ compared to the control group.

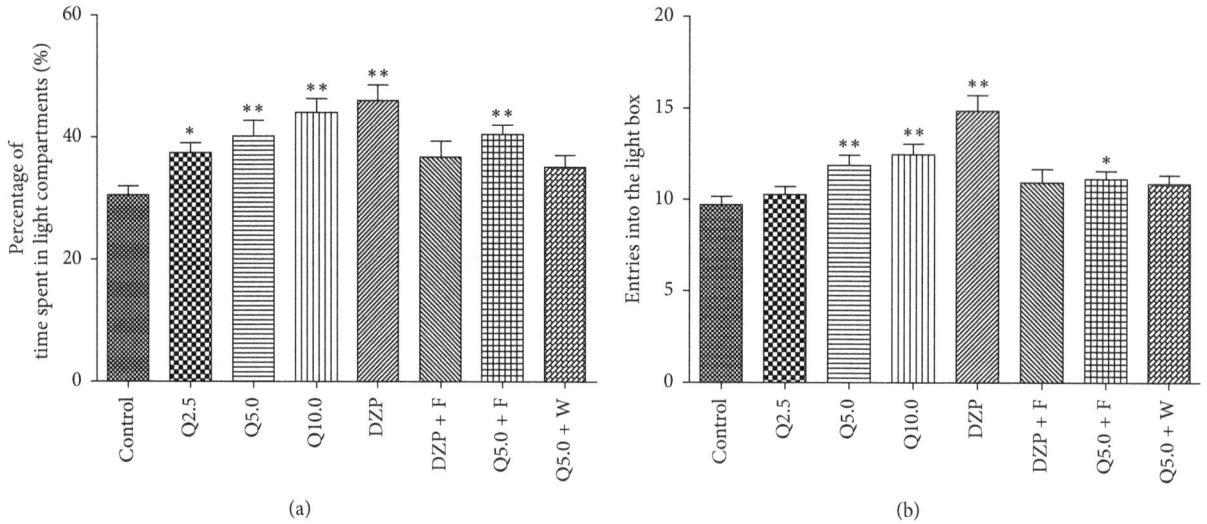

(a)

(b)

FIGURE 3: Behavioral performance of mice in a 5 min session in the light and dark box performed 0.5 h after the injection of vehicle (control, p.o.), quercitrin (2.5, 5.0, and 10.0 mg/kg, p.o.), diazepam (DZP, 2 mg/kg, p.o.), flumazenil (F; 3 mg/kg, i.p., 15 min after p.o. administration of positive control or quercitrin, Q), and WAY-100635 (W; 0.5 mg/kg, i.p., 15 min before p.o. administration of quercitrin, Q). (a) Percentage of time spent in light compartment and (b) entries into the light box. Columns represent the means ± SEM; $n = 15$ mice. $^{*}p < 0.05$ and $^{**}p < 0.01$ compared to the control group.

increased the number of entries into the open arms compared with the control group. As shown in Figure 2(c), treatment with 5.0 and 10.0 mg/kg quercitrin significantly decreased the percentage of time spent on the closed arms (both $p < 0.01$) as well as diazepam ($p < 0.01$). As shown in Figure 2(d), diazepam (both $p < 0.01$) significantly decreased the number of entries into the open arms compared with the control group whereas the entries into the closed arms in the quercitrin-treated group did not produce significant differences compared to the control group. No significant differences were found in the percentage of time spent in central areas ($p > 0.05$, Figure 2(e)).

3.2. Effect of Quercitrin in the Light/Dark Box Test. The one-way ANOVA revealed significant differences between groups in the time spent in the light compartment ($F_{7,127} = 5.174$, $p < 0.01$, Figure 3(a)) and number of entries into the light compartment ($F_{7,127} = 7.217$, $p < 0.01$, Figure 3(b)). As shown in Figure 3(a), 2.5, 5.0, and 10.0 mg/kg quercitrin significantly increased the time spent in the light compartment (all $p < 0.01$). Diazepam (2 mg/kg) significantly increased the percentage of time spent in the light compartment compared with the control group ($p < 0.01$). Additionally, 5.0 and 10.0 mg/kg quercitrin (both $p < 0.01$) and diazepam (both $p < 0.01$) significantly increased the number of entries into the light compartment compared with the control group.

3.3. Effect of Quercitrin in the Marble-Burying Test. The one-way ANOVA revealed significant differences between groups in the number of marbles buried ($F_{4,79} = 8.476$, $p < 0.01$, Figure 4). Diazepam (2.0 mg/kg) and quercitrin (5.0 and 10.0 mg/kg) significantly decreased the number of marbles

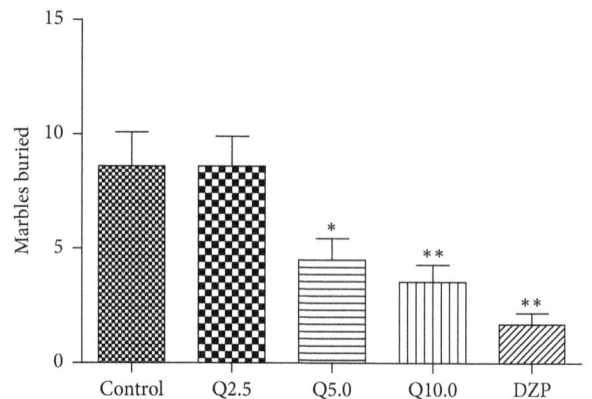

FIGURE 4: Marbles buried number of mice in a 30 min session in the marble-burying test performed 1.0 h after the injection of vehicle (control, p.o.), quercitrin (2.5, 5.0, and 10.0 mg/kg, p.o.), and diazepam (DZP, 2 mg/kg, p.o.). Columns represent the means ± SEM; $n = 15$ mice. $^{*}p < 0.05$ and $^{**}p < 0.01$ compared to the control group.

buried compared with the control group ($p < 0.01$), whereas 2.5 mg/kg quercitrin had no effect.

3.4. Effect of Quercitrin in the Open-Field Test. The one-way ANOVA revealed significant differences between groups in the total distance travelled ($F_{4,79} = 5.813$, $p < 0.01$, Figure 5). As shown in Figure 5, diazepam (2.0 mg/kg) significantly increased the total distance travelled compared with the control group ($p < 0.01$), whereas no differences were found between the quercitrin-treated groups and control group.

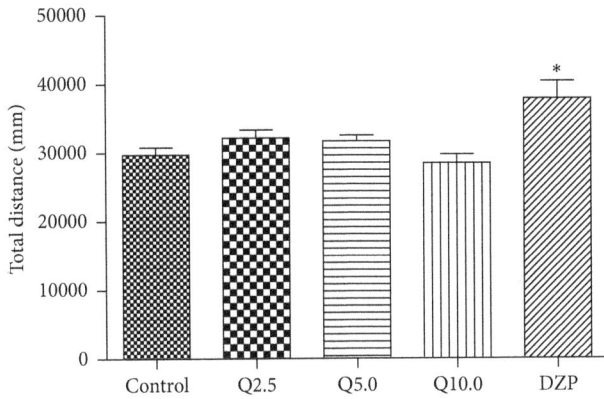

FIGURE 5: Total moving distance of mice in a 5 min session in the open-field test performed 0.5 h after the injection of vehicle (control, p.o.), quercitrin (2.5, 5.0, and 10.0 mg/kg, p.o.), and diazepam (DZP, 2 mg/kg, p.o.). Columns represent the means ± SEM; $n = 15$ mice. $^*p < 0.05$ and $^{**}p < 0.01$ compared to the control group.

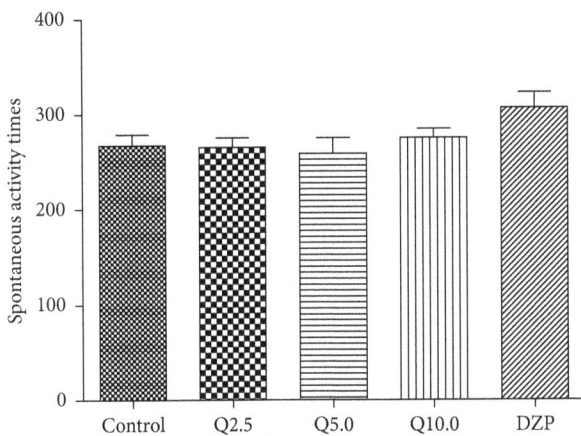

FIGURE 6: Number of activity times of mice in a 5 min session in the spontaneous activity test performed 0.5 h after the injection of vehicle (control, p.o.), quercitrin (2.5, 5.0, and 10.0 mg/kg, p.o.), and diazepam (DZP, 2 mg/kg, p.o.). Columns represent the means ± SEM; $n = 15$ mice. $^*p < 0.05$ and $^{**}p < 0.01$ compared to the control group.

3.5. Effect of Quercitrin in the Spontaneous Locomotor Activity Test. The one-way ANOVA revealed significant differences between groups in spontaneous locomotor activity ($F_{4,79} = 2.075$, $p < 0.05$, Figure 6). Diazepam (2 mg/kg) significantly increased spontaneous locomotor activity compared with the control group ($p < 0.01$). No differences in spontaneous locomotor activity were found between the quercitrin-treated groups and control group (Figure 6).

3.6. Influence of WAY-100635 on the Anxiolytic-Like Effects of Quercitrin. To determine whether the anxiolytic-like effects of quercitrin involve the serotonergic system, especially 5-HT$_{1A}$ receptors, diazepam- (2.0 mg/kg) and quercitrin- (5.0 mg/kg) treated mice were pretreated with the 5-HT$_{1A}$

receptor antagonist WAY-100635. The two-way ANOVA revealed significant differences between different treatments in the percentage of the time spent in the open arm ($F_{4,89} = 3.914$, $p < 0.05$, Figure 2(a)) and in the open arms entries ($F_{4,89} = 5.564$, $p < 0.01$, Figure 2(b)) and percentage of the time spent in the closed arm ($F_{4,89} = 3.914$, $p < 0.05$, Figure 2(c)) and in the closed arms entries ($F_{4,89} = 5.565$, $p < 0.01$, Figure 2(d)). The two-way ANOVA revealed significant differences between different pretreatments in the open arms entries ($F_{4,89} = 5.520$, $p < 0.01$, Figure 2(b)) and in the closed arms entries ($F_{4,89} = 5.510$, $p < 0.01$, Figure 2(d)), while there were no significant differences between different pretreatments in the percentage of the time spent in the open arm ($F_{4,89} = 2.916$, $p > 0.05$, Figure 2(a)) and in the percentage of the time spent in the closed arm ($F_{4,89} = 2.916$, $p > 0.05$, Figure 2(c)). As shown in Figure 2, 5.0 mg/kg quercitrin and diazepam significantly increased the percentage of time spent on the open arms and percentage of entries into the open arms compared with the vehicle-treated control group. 5.0 mg/kg quercitrin and diazepam significantly decreased the percentage of time spent on the closed arms compared to the vehicle-treated control group, but no significant difference was found in the percentage of closed arm entries. Pretreatment with WAY-100635 15 min before drug administration significantly blocked the effects of quercitrin, which significantly decreased the number of entries into the open arms and time spent on the open arms and increased the time spent in the closed arm. In the LDB test, the two-way ANOVA revealed significant differences between different treatments in the percentage of the time spent in the light compartment ($F_{4,89} = 9.905$, $p < 0.01$, Figure 3(a)) and in the light compartment entries ($F_{4,89} = 12.933$, $p < 0.01$, Figure 3(b)), and there were significant differences between different pretreatments in the percentage of the time spent in the light compartment ($F_{4,89} = 3.605$, $p < 0.05$, Figure 3(a)) and in the light compartment entries ($F_{4,89} = 7.089$, $p < 0.01$, Figure 3(b)). 5.0 mg/kg quercitrin and 2.0 mg/kg diazepam significantly increased the time spent in the light compartment and entries into the light compartment (Figure 3). Pretreatment with WAY-100635 15 min before administration significantly blocked the effects of quercitrin, which decreased the time spent in the light compartment and entries into the light compartment. These results indicate that the anxiolytic-like effects of quercitrin were blocked by WAY-100635.

3.7. Influence of Flumazenil on the Anxiolytic-Like Effects of Quercitrin. To determine whether the anxiolytic-like effects of quercitrin involve the GABA-ergic system, particularly the benzodiazepine site of GABA$_A$ receptors, diazepam- (2.0 mg/kg) and quercitrin- (5.0 mg/kg) treated mice were pretreated with the GABA$_A$ receptor antagonist flumazenil. As shown in Figure 2, in the EPM, diazepam and quercitrin (5 mg/kg) significantly increased the percentage of time spent on the open arms and percentage of open arm entries compared with the vehicle-treated control group. Diazepam and quercitrin (5 mg/kg) significantly decreased the percentage of time spent on the closed arms compared to the vehicle-treated control group, but no significant differences were

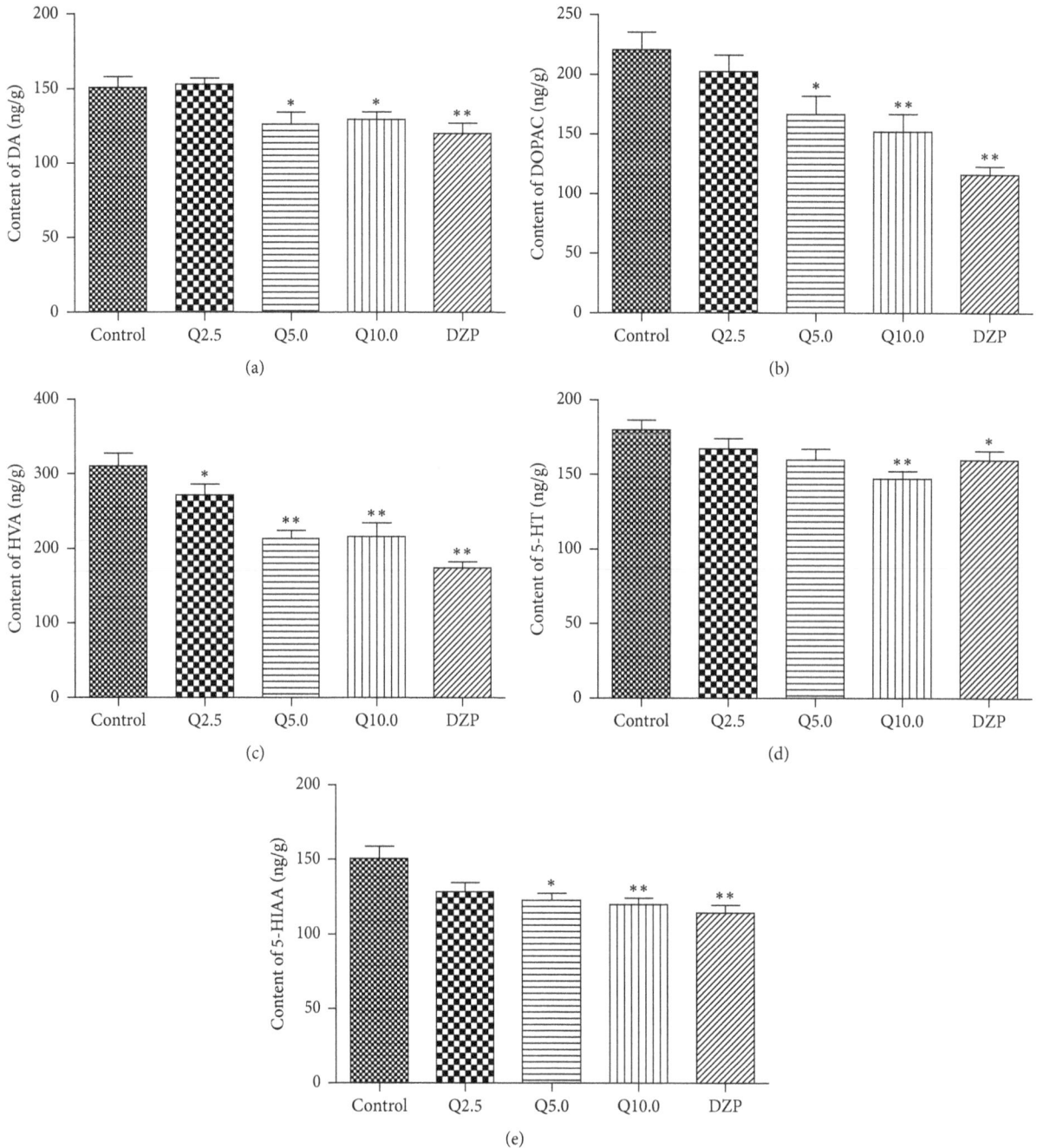

FIGURE 7: Effects of quercitrin on the monoamines neurotransmitters and their metabolites in the brains of mice. (a) The content of DA, (b) the content of DOPAC, (c) the content of HVA, (d) the content of 5-HT, and (e) the content of 5-HIAA. Results are expressed as mean ± SEM; $n = 8$ mice. $^{*}p < 0.05$ and $^{**}p < 0.01$ compared to the control group.

found in the percentage of closed arm entries. Pretreatment with flumazenil before drug administration blocked the effects of diazepam. Pretreatment with flumazenil did not block the effects of quercitrin. In the LDB test (Figure 3), 5.0 mg/kg quercitrin and 2.0 mg/kg diazepam significantly increased the time spent in the light compartment and entries into the light compartment. Pretreatment with flumazenil 15 min before drug administration significantly blocked the effects of diazepam but not quercitrin.

3.8. Effects of Quercitrin on Monoamine Neurotransmitters and Their Metabolites. The one-way ANOVA revealed significant differences in the levels of monoamine neurotransmitters and their metabolites ($F_{4,79} = 5.362$, $p < 0.01$, Figure 7(a); $F_{4,79} = 9.237$, $p < 0.01$, Figure 7(b); $F_{4,79} = 14.13$, $p < 0.01$, Figure 7(c); $F_{4,79} = 3.507$, $p < 0.01$, Figure 7(d); $F_{4,79} = 5.718$, $p < 0.01$, Figure 7(e)). Quercitrin (5.0 mg/kg) significantly decreased dopamine, DOPAC, HVA, and 5-HIAA levels (Figures 7(a)–7(c) and 7(e)); diazepam and quercitrin (10.0 mg/kg) significantly decreased the levels of both monoamines and their metabolites ($p < 0.01$, Figure 7).

4. Discussion

Flavonoids are secondary plant metabolites [31] that have a wide range of biological activities, such as antioxidant and anti-inflammatory effects, and readily cross the blood-brain barrier [32]. The anxiolytic effects of many flavone compounds that are derived from plants and synthetic sources, such as luteolin and apigenin, have been reported [33]. Our previous study showed that total flavones contained in *Albizia julibrissin* exerted anxiolytic-like effects [8]. Quercitrin is the main compound of total flavones [10]. The present results suggest that quercitrin exerts anxiolytic-like effects in animal models of anxiety and on the levels of monoamine neurotransmitters and their metabolites. In addition, the effects appeared to be mediated by 5-HT$_{1A}$ receptors.

Anxiety and fear can be induced by the novelty of a situation. They can be evaluated in mice by determining the intensity of behavior in an unfamiliar area, the quantity of unfamiliar food consumption [34], and social interactions with unfamiliar animals. The EPM is based on rodents' natural aversion to height and open spaces [24, 25]. The EPM is considered an ethologically valid animal model of anxiety because it uses natural stimuli (e.g., fear of novel open spaces and fear of balancing on a relatively narrow, raised platform) that can induce anxiety in humans [35]. In the present study, oral quercitrin administration induced an anxiolytic-like effect in mice. Quercitrin increased the percentage of entries into and time spent on the open arms of the EPM, while it decreased the percentage of time spent on the closed arms. These effects were blocked by the 5-HT$_{1A}$ receptor antagonist WAY-100635 and were unaffected by the GABA$_A$ receptor antagonist flumazenil. Our results suggest that quercitrin has anxiolytic properties in the EPM, and the 5-HT system may be involved in its effects.

The LDB test is based on rodents' innate aversion to brightly illuminated areas and spontaneous exploratory behavior in response to mild stressors (i.e., a novel environment and light). The effects of classic anxiolytics (e.g., benzodiazepines) and newer anxiolytic-like agents (e.g., serotonergic drugs or drugs that act on neuropeptide receptors) can be detected with this paradigm. In the present study, quercitrin significantly increased the number of transitions between the light and dark compartments and time spent in the light compartment in the LDB test. These results indicate that quercitrin has anxiolytic-like activity. Moreover, the anxiolytic effects were blocked by the 5-HT$_{1A}$ receptor antagonist WAY-100635.

The marble-burying test has been used to screen anxiolytics, including those for obsessive-compulsive disorder. Diazepam has been shown to decrease the number of marbles buried [36]. We found that 5 mg/kg quercitrin significantly decreased the number of marbles buried, indicating that quercitrin has anxiolytic-like activity in the marble-burying test.

To explore the possible mechanism of action of quercitrin, we performed antagonistic experiments. Many anxiolytic drugs exert their behavioral effects by binding to the benzodiazepine site on GABA receptors. In the EPM, we found that the anxiolytic effects of diazepam were completely blocked by flumazenil, whereas flumazenil pretreatment did not influence the effects of 5.0 mg/kg quercitrin. The quercitrin-treated group exhibited anxiolytic-like behavior in the LDB, and these anxiolytic-like effects were not blocked by flumazenil, in which the number of entries into and time spent in the light compartment increased compared with the control group. These results suggest that the anxiolytic-like effects of quercitrin might not be related to GABA$_A$ receptors.

5-HT$_{1A}$ receptor agonists, such as buspirone and gepirone, were developed for the treatment of anxiety and depression [37, 38]. To date, the only selective high-affinity antagonist of this receptor is WAY-100635 [39, 40]. In the present study, we confirmed the anxiolytic-like activity of diazepam as previously reported [41] in the EPM. Quercitrin (5.0 mg/kg) produced potent anxiolytic-like effects, and these effects of quercitrin were completely blocked by WAY-100635. Pretreatment with WAY-100635 resulted in percentages of open arm time, percentages of open arm entries, and percentages of closed arm time in the EPM that were not different from the control group. In the LDB test, quercitrin exerted an anxiolytic-like effect. Similarly, the anxiolytic-like effects were blocked by WAY-100635, in which the number of entries into and time spent in the light compartment were not different from the control group. These results suggest that the anxiolytic-like effects of quercitrin might be mediated by 5-HT$_{1A}$ receptors.

The central dopaminergic system is considered the crucial factor in anxiety disorders. Foot-shock and anxiogenic drugs markedly increase cortical dopamine output in normal rats, and chronic treatment with imipramine completely inhibits these changes [42]. The present results are consistent with these reports. Quercitrin significantly reduced the tissue concentration of dopamine in brain homogenates. The levels of DOPAC and HVA, the major metabolites of dopamine, significantly decreased. Therefore, we can speculate that the mechanism of action of quercitrin involves suppression of the synthesis and release of dopamine.

Changes in the serotonergic system were also observed in the present study. According to the classic serotonin hypothesis, anxiety is usually associated with increases in endogenous 5-HT, and anxiolytics tend to decrease endogenous 5-HT [43]. The selective 5-HT$_{1A}$ receptor agonist buspirone exerts anxiolytic effects by decreasing the concentration of 5-HT [44]. The present study is consistent with these reports. Quercitrin significantly decreased 5-HT levels in brain homogenates. The reduction of 5-HT levels might be attributable to the suppression of synthesis or release or an increase in metabolism [45]. Quercitrin also decreased the levels of the primary metabolite of 5-HT, 5-HIAA. These results suggest the quercitrin does not affect the metabolic pathway of 5-HT but decreases its synthesis or release. This mechanism will need to be explored further.

We chose only diazepam as a positive control to evaluate the effects of quercitrin. The 5-HT partial agonist buspirone was not used because it requires 1–4 weeks to show efficacy [46, 47]. Future studies should include buspirone as a positive control and compare its effects with a 5-HT$_{1A}$ receptor agonist. The present results cannot exclude the possibility that other binding sites of GABA and other neurotransmitter systems may play a role in the anxiolytic-like effects of quercitrin.

To reduce the number of animals used, we did not include groups in which WAY-100635 and flumazenil were administered alone. Antagonists usually do not induce any significant changes in behaviors in control animals [48]. In the present study, these drugs were administered by the same routes as quercitrin. We did not assess the effects of other routes of administration on anxiety-related behavior, nor did we assess bioavailability. These remain to be studied in the future.

5. Conclusions

In summary, the present results indicate that quercitrin exerts anxiolytic-like effects without affecting locomotor activity in mice. The anxiolytic effects of quercitrin appear to be mediated by 5-HT$_{1A}$ receptors and not involve the benzodiazepine binding site of GABA receptors. Our neurochemical studies suggest that these effects are mediated through the modulation of monoamine neurotransmitter levels. The present results suggest the potential usefulness of quercitrin for the treatment of anxiety disorders.

Competing Interests

The authors declare that they have no competing interests.

Acknowledgments

This work was supported by the Key New Drugs Innovation project from the Ministry of Science and Technology (2012ZX09102201-018).

References

[1] B. J. Sadock and V. A. Sadock, *Kplan and Sadock's Synopsis of Psychiatry-Behavioral Sciences/Clinical Psychiatry*, Lippincott Willams & Wilkins, Philadelphia, Pa, USA, 9th edition, 2003.

[2] R. C. Kessler, M. Angermeyer, J. C. Anthony et al., "Lifetime prevalence and age-of-onset distributions of mental disorders in the World Health Organization's World Mental Health Survey Initiative," *World Psychiatry*, vol. 6, no. 3, pp. 168–176, 2007.

[3] C. R. Gardner, W. R. Tully, and C. J. R. Hedgecock, "The rapidly expanding range of neuronal benzodiazepine receptor ligands," *Progress in Neurobiology*, vol. 40, no. 1, pp. 1–61, 1993.

[4] K. Rickels, F. Garcia-Espana, L. A. Mandos, and G. W. Case, "Physician withdrawal checklist (PWC-20)," *Journal of Clinical Psychopharmacology*, vol. 28, no. 4, pp. 447–451, 2008.

[5] N. A. Youssef and C. L. Rich, "Does acute treatment with sedatives/hypnotics for anxiety in depressed patients affect suicide risk? A literature review," *Annals of Clinical Psychiatry*, vol. 20, no. 3, pp. 157–169, 2008.

[6] J.-H. Kim, S. Y. Kim, S.-Y. Lee, and C.-G. Jang, "Antidepressant-like effects of Albizzia julibrissin in mice: involvement of

the 5-HT1A receptor system," *Pharmacology Biochemistry and Behavior*, vol. 87, no. 1, pp. 41–47, 2007.

[7] Editing Committee of Chinese Drugs Encyolpedia, *Chinese Drugs Encyclopedia*, Sangmu, Hong Kong, 1978.

[8] Q. T. Liu, J. Liu, J.-Y. Guo et al., "Anti-anxiety effect of total flavonoids of the flowers of Albizia julibrissin Durazz," *Research and Practice on Chinese Medicines*, vol. 29, no. 2, pp. 33–35, 2015.

[9] Y. L. Song and Z. P. Li, "Determination of quercitrin in Albizzia julibrissin durazz by RP-HPLC," *Lishizhen Medicine and Materia Medica Research*, vol. 17, no. 7, pp. 1139–1140, 2006.

[10] T. H. Kang, S. J. Jeong, N. Y. Kim, R. Higuchi, and Y. C. Kim, "Sedative activity of two flavonol glycosides isolated from the flowers of Albizzia julibrissin Durazz," *Journal of Ethnopharmacology*, vol. 71, no. 1-2, pp. 321–323, 2000.

[11] P. C. H. Hollman, J. H. M. De Vries, S. D. Van Leeuwen, M. J. B. Mengelers, and M. B. Katan, "Absorption of dietary quercetin glycosides and quercetin in healthy ileostomy volunteers," *The American Journal of Clinical Nutrition*, vol. 62, no. 6, pp. 1276–1282, 1995.

[12] D. Camuesco, M. Comalada, A. Concha et al., "Intestinal anti-inflammatory activity of combined quercitrin and dietary olive oil supplemented with fish oil, rich in EPA and DHA (n-3) polyunsaturated fatty acids, in rats with DSS-induced colitis," *Clinical Nutrition*, vol. 25, no. 3, pp. 466–476, 2006.

[13] H. J. Choi, J. H. Song, K. S. Park, and D. H. Kwon, "Inhibitory effects of quercetin 3-rhamnoside on influenza A virus replication," *European Journal of Pharmaceutical Sciences*, vol. 37, no. 3-4, pp. 329–333, 2009.

[14] M. S. Hasan, M. I. Ahmed, S. Mondal, S. J. Uddin, M. M. Masud, and S. K. Sadhu, "Antioxidant, antinociceptive activity and general toxicity study of Dendrophthoe falcata and isolation of quercitrin as the major component," *Oriental Pharmacy and Experimental Medicine*, vol. 6, no. 4, pp. 355–360, 2006.

[15] M. F. Muzitano, E. A. Cruz, A. P. De Almeida et al., "Quercitrin: an antileishmanial flavonoid glycoside from Kalanchoe pinnata," *Planta Medica*, vol. 72, no. 1, pp. 81–83, 2006.

[16] P. J. Whiting, "GABA-A receptors: a viable target for novel anxiolytics?" *Current Opinion in Pharmacology*, vol. 6, no. 1, pp. 24–29, 2006.

[17] V. Nunes-de-Souza, R. L. Nunes-de-Souza, R. J. Rodgers, and A. Canto-de-Souza, "5-HT$_2$ receptor activation in the midbrain periaqueductal grey (PAG) reduces anxiety-like behaviour in mice," *Behavioural Brain Research*, vol. 187, no. 1, pp. 72–79, 2008.

[18] U. Rudolph, F. Crestani, D. Benke et al., "Benzodiazepine actions mediated by specific γ-aminobutyric acid(A) receptor subtypes," *Nature*, vol. 401, no. 6755, pp. 796–800, 1999.

[19] A. Neumeister, A. Konstantinidis, J. Stastny et al., "Association between serotonin transporter gene promoter polymorphism (5HTTLPR) and behavioral responses to tryptophan depletion in healthy women with and without family history of depression," *Archives of General Psychiatry*, vol. 59, no. 7, pp. 613–620, 2002.

[20] L. K. Heisler, H.-M. Chu, T. J. Brennan et al., "Elevated anxiety and antidepressant-like responses in serotonin 5-HT$_{1A}$ receptor mutant mice," *Proceedings of the National Academy of Sciences of the United States of America*, vol. 95, no. 25, pp. 15049–15054, 1998.

[21] C. L. Parks, P. S. Robinson, E. Sibille, T. Shenk, and M. Toth, "Increased anxiety of mice lacking the serotonin$_{1A}$ receptor," *Proceedings of the National Academy of Sciences of the United States of America*, vol. 95, no. 18, pp. 10734–10739, 1998.

[22] Y. Zhang, W. Wang, and J. Zhang, "Effects of novel anxiolytic 4-butyl-alpha-agarofuran on levels of monoamine neurotransmitters in rats," *European Journal of Pharmacology*, vol. 504, no. 1-2, pp. 39–44, 2004.

[23] A. Shekhar, U. D. McCann, M. J. Meaney et al., "Summary of a national institute of mental health workshop: developing animal models of anxiety disorders," *Psychopharmacology*, vol. 157, no. 4, pp. 327–339, 2001.

[24] S. Pellow, P. Chopin, S. E. File, and M. Briley, "Validation of open: closed arm entries in an elevated plus-maze as a measure of anxiety in the rat," *Journal of Neuroscience Methods*, vol. 14, no. 3, pp. 149–167, 1985.

[25] R. G. Lister, "The use of a plus-maze to measure anxiety in the mouse," *Psychopharmacology*, vol. 92, no. 2, pp. 180–185, 1987.

[26] H. Han, Y. Ma, J. S. Eun et al., "Anxiolytic-like effects of sanjoinine A isolated from *Zizyphi Spinosi Semen*: possible involvement of GABAergic transmission," *Pharmacology Biochemistry and Behavior*, vol. 92, no. 2, pp. 206–213, 2009.

[27] J. B. Zou, Q. L. Kong, and L. L. Jiang, "Study on the effect of antianxiety of Passifloraeduli," *Chin Arch Tradit Chin Med*, vol. 31, pp. 1332–1333, 2013.

[28] X. J. Mi, S. W. Chen, W. J. Wang et al., "Anxiolytic-like effect of paeonol in mice," *Pharmacology Biochemistry and Behavior*, vol. 81, no. 3, pp. 683–687, 2005.

[29] R. M. J. Deacon, "Digging and marble burying in mice: simple methods for in vivo identification of biological impacts," *Nature Protocols*, vol. 1, no. 1, pp. 122–124, 2006.

[30] L. L. Hu, X. G. Zhao, J. Yang et al., "Chronic scream sound exposure alters memory and monoamine levels in female rat brain," *Physiology and Behavior*, vol. 137, pp. 53–59, 2014.

[31] J. B. Harborne and C. A. Williams, "Advances in flavonoid research since 1992," *Phytochemistry*, vol. 55, no. 6, pp. 481–504, 2000.

[32] L. A. Hilakivi-Clarke, J. Turkka, R. G. Lister, and M. Linnoila, "Effects of early postnatal handling on brain β-adrenoceptors and behavior in tests related to stress," *Brain Research*, vol. 542, no. 2, pp. 286–292, 1991.

[33] A. L. Piccinelli, M. G. Mesa, D. M. Armenteros et al., "HPLC-PDA-MS and NMR characterization of *C*-glycosyl flavones in a hydroalcoholic extract of *Citrus aurantifolia* leaves with antiplatelet activity," *Journal of Agricultural and Food Chemistry*, vol. 56, no. 5, pp. 1574–1581, 2008.

[34] H. Cappell and A. E. Le Blanc, "Punishment of saccharin drinking by amphetamine in rats and its reversal by chlordiazepoxide," *Journal of Comparative and Physiological Psychology*, vol. 85, no. 1, pp. 97–104, 1973.

[35] G. R. Dawson and M. D. Tricklebank, "Use of the elevated plus maze in the search for novel anxiolytic agents," *Trends in Pharmacological Sciences*, vol. 16, no. 2, pp. 33–36, 1995.

[36] L. B. Nicolas, Y. Kolb, and E. P. M. Prinssen, "A combined marble burying-locomotor activity test in mice: a practical screening test with sensitivity to different classes of anxiolytics and antidepressants," *European Journal of Pharmacology*, vol. 547, no. 1-3, pp. 106–115, 2006.

[37] G. Tunnicliff, "Molecular basis of buspirone's anxiolytic action," *Pharmacology and Toxicology*, vol. 69, no. 3, pp. 149–156, 1991.

[38] J. A. Den Boer, F. J. Bosker, and B. R. Slaap, "Serotonergic drugs in the treatment of depressive and anxiety disorders," *Human Psychopharmacology*, vol. 15, no. 5, pp. 315–336, 2000.

[39] E. A. Forster, I. A. Cliffe, D. J. Bill et al., "A pharmacological profile of the selective silent 5-HT_{1A} receptor antagonist, WAY 100635," *European Journal of Pharmacology*, vol. 281, no. 1, pp. 81–88, 1995.

[40] A. Fletcher, E. A. Forster, D. J. Bill et al., "Electrophysiological, biochemical, neurohormonal and behavioural studies with WAY-100635, a potent, selective and silent 5-HT1A receptor antagonist," *Behavioural Brain Research*, vol. 73, no. 1-2, pp. 337–353, 1995.

[41] Y.-H. Jung, R.-R. Ha, S.-H. Kwon et al., "Anxiolytic effects of Julibroside C1 isolated from Albizzia julibrissin in mice," *Progress in Neuro-Psychopharmacology and Biological Psychiatry*, vol. 44, pp. 184–192, 2013.

[42] L. Dazzi, M. Serra, F. Spiga, M. G. Pisu, J. D. Jentsch, and G. Biggio, "Prevention of the stress-induced increase in frontal cortical dopamine efflux of freely moving rats by long-term treatment with antidepressant drugs," *European Neuropsychopharmacology*, vol. 11, no. 5, pp. 343–349, 2001.

[43] Y. Clement and G. Chapouthier, "Biological bases of anxiety," *Neuroscience and Biobehavioral Reviews*, vol. 22, no. 5, pp. 623–633, 1998.

[44] F. F. Matos, C. Urban, and F. D. Yocca, "Serotonin (5-HT) release in the dorsal raphé and ventral hippocampus: raphé control of somatodendritic and terminal 5-HT release," *Journal of Neural Transmission*, vol. 103, no. 1-2, pp. 173–190, 1996.

[45] Q. Wang, X. Yang, B. Zhang, X. Yang, and K. Wang, "The anxiolytic effect of cinnabar involves changes of serotonin levels," *European Journal of Pharmacology*, vol. 565, no. 1-3, pp. 132–137, 2007.

[46] Z. M. Chen, X. Z. Hu, Y. L. Zhang, and J. H. Zhang, "Buspirone vs diazepam in treating anxiety disorders in a double-blind study," *Chinese Journal of New Drugs and Clinical Remedies*, vol. 17, no. 2, pp. 99–100, 1998.

[47] C. Wang, "Clinical observation of buspirone on treatment of 96 cases of anxiety," *Journal of Liaoning Medical University*, vol. 32, no. 6, p. 516, 2011.

[48] A. G. Sartim, F. S. Guimarães, and S. R. Joca, "Antidepressant-like effect of cannabidiol injection into the ventral medial prefrontal cortex—possible involvement of 5-HT_{1A} and CB1 receptors," *Behavioural Brain Research*, vol. 303, pp. 218–227, 2016.

7

Asparagus cochinchinensis Extract Alleviates Metal Ion-Induced Gut Injury in *Drosophila*: An In Silico Analysis of Potential Active Constituents

Weiyu Zhang and Li Hua Jin

College of Life Science, Northeast Forestry University, Harbin 150040, China

Correspondence should be addressed to Weiyu Zhang; zhangweiyu04@nefu.edu.cn

Academic Editor: Ghee T. Tan

Metal ions and sulfate are components of atmospheric pollutants that have diverse ways of entering the human body. We used *Drosophila* as a model to investigate the effect of *Asparagus cochinchinensis* (*A. cochinchinensis*) extracts on the gut and characterized gut homeostasis following the ingestion of metal ions (copper, zinc, and aluminum). In this study, we found that the aqueous *A. cochinchinensis* extract increased the survival rate, decreased epithelial cell death, and attenuated metal ion-induced gut morphological changes in flies following chronic exposure to metal ions. In addition, we screened out, by network pharmacology, six natural products (NPs) that could serve as putative active components of *A. cochinchinensis* that prevented gut injury. Altogether, the results of our study provide evidence that *A. cochinchinensis* might be an effective phytomedicine for the treatment of metal ion-induced gut injury.

1. Introduction

In recent years, atmospheric pollution has become a rapidly growing international trend. Atmospheric pollution not only is harmful to the Earth's climate, agriculture, and industry but also does immeasurable damage to humans. Atmospheric pollution can cause respiratory system damage, physiological abnormalities, neurological abnormalities, and digestive disorders [1, 2]. Metal ions and sulfate are components of atmospheric pollution stemming primarily from fuel combustion and large-scale industrial and mining enterprises, as well as from other man-made pollutants such as exhaust gas. Metal ions enter the human body in diverse ways, including inhalation, swallowing, and skin contact. Due to their nondegradation characteristics, metal ions accumulate in the body where they are converted into more toxic metal compounds by combining with organic matter. This triggers a series of damaging effects that result in physiological dysfunctions [3]. Previous studies have demonstrated that a dose of cadmium induces intestinal epithelial cell injury in the *Drosophila* midgut [4]. The intestinal epithelial is an important protective barrier between the internal and external environment. Mechanisms of immunity and tissue regeneration must be tightly regulated in order to maintain intestinal homeostasis [5, 6]. Dysregulation of inflammatory responses and tissue regeneration can lead to inflammatory bowel diseases and colorectal cancer in mammals [7]. In recent years, increasingly more people are plagued by intestinal inflammation, and prolonged inflammation and tissue damage can lead to intestinal carcinogenesis and tumor formation.

Asparagus cochinchinensis (*A. cochinchinensis*), referred to as Tiandong in China, is the root of *A. cochinchinensis* (Lour.) Merr. (Liliaceae) that is distributed among many provinces of China. *A. cochinchinensis* (AC) has been used in traditional Chinese medicine (TCM) for over 2,000 years. Its flavor is sweet, bitter, and cold. The channel tropism is the lungs, kidney, stomach, and large intestine meridian. *A. cochinchinensis* has often been used for the treatment of fever, cough, throat pain, swelling, constipation, and diabetes. The dried root has antibacterial, antipyretic, diuretic, expectorant, stomachic, nervous stimulant, and tonic properties [8]. Modern research has also demonstrated that *A. cochinchinensis* has antitumor activity, especially in lung cancer [9, 10].

However, the protective effect on intestinal injury and the active components of *A. cochinchinensis* affecting gut immunity remain poorly understood.

Drosophila is a well studied and highly tractable genetic model organism. Many basic biological and physiological properties are conserved between *Drosophila* and mammals, and nearly 75% of human disease-related genes have a functional homolog in the fly [11]. Thus, the *Drosophila* is widely used in basic and applied researches on a broad spectrum of human diseases including infectious diseases [12], cancers [13], neurodegenerative diseases [14], and metabolic diseases [15]. *Drosophila* and human intestine have similar anatomy and physiological function [16, 17], and they have also similarities in cell and composition and underlying signaling pathways that maintain intestinal homeostasis [18].

Chinese medicinal herbs exert their therapeutic actions through the synergistic effects of multiple compounds, targets, and channels. However, it has been difficult to isolate the effective components of these products and to identify specific therapeutic targets for treating disease. Network pharmacology has been used as an integrated approach to systematically investigate and explain the underlying molecular mechanisms of Chinese medicinal herbs. Using the Computerized Virtual Screening Technique to explore potential targets may help facilitate these investigations, while reducing manpower and material resources.

Drosophila has emerged as a potential whole animal model for drug screening [19, 20]. Through a large number of survival rate assays, we identified *A. cochinchinensis* as having good bioactivity against chemical reagents-induced stress in *Drosophila* (data was not shown). In this study, we revealed that the aqueous extract of *A. cochinchinensis* exerts a protective effect on gut injury in *Drosophila* induced by the chronic exposure to metal ions. In addition, we computationally identified the putative active ingredients of *A. cochinchinensis* using network pharmacology. Network analysis revealed six constituents of *A. cochinchinensis* that could potentially mediate its protective effects on gut injury. These results provide new insight into the pharmacological basis of the antigut injury activity of *A. cochinchinensis* and will provide impetus for preclinical drug discovery based on this medicinal plant.

2. Materials and Methods

2.1. Drosophila Fly Stocks. w^1118 flies were obtained from the Bloomington *Drosophila* Stock Center. Fly stocks were maintained on a 12 h light/12 h dark cycle at 25°C and 60% humidity.

2.2. A. cochinchinensis Extraction. *A. cochinchinensis* was identified by Professor Xiuhua Wang at the Herbarium of the College of Life Sciences, Northeast Forestry University, and purchased from Shiyitang Pharmacy of Harbin, China. The method of aqueous extraction of *A. cochinchinensis* has been previously described [21]. Total aqueous-derived extract was consolidated and concentrated to a final concentration of 20% (w/v).

2.3. Drosophila Food. Standard cornmeal-yeast medium used for the control group consisted of 5.6 g/L agar, 16.8 g/L yeast, 71.6 g/L polenta, 9.8 g/L soybean flour, and 60 g/L sucrose. Standard medium with 10% (w/v) aqueous *A. cochinchinensis* extract was used for the experimental group.

2.4. Survival Experiments. Procedures for the survival and feeding experiments were performed as previously described [21] with the difference that adult flies which aged 3–5 days (15 males and 15 females) were starved for 2 h without food before being transferred to a vial containing chemical compounds in 5% (w/v) sucrose solution serving as the control group for all experiments. The chemical compounds included cupric sulfate (7 mM, Sigma), zinc sulfate (7 mM, Sigma), and aluminum potassium disulfate dodecahydrate (20 mM, Sigma). The experimental group consists of flies fed with sucrose solutions incorporating the chemical compound with added AC extract at 10% (w/w). Fresh filter papers and solutions were provided every day, and dead flies were enumerated and evaluated daily.

2.5. 7-Amino-actinomycin D Staining and Imaging. 7-Amino-actinomycin D (7-AAD) staining and imaging were performed as previously described [21, 22].

2.6. Intestinal Morphological Analysis. Female flies were used for intestinal morphological studies due to their larger size.

Due to the bigger size of female flies, we used them for intestinal morphological analysis experiment. The guts of 3–5-day-old female flies that had orally ingested metal ions in 5% (w/v) sucrose with or without AC extract for 96 h were dissected at room temperature in phosphate buffered saline (PBS) and immediately observed under an Axioskop 2 plus microscope (Zeiss).

2.7. Targets Predictions of Natural Products (NPs) and Network Construction. The information pertaining to natural products (NPs) was obtained from the Universal Natural Products Database (UNPD) according to the scientific names of the herbs [23]. The information for approved drugs and drug targets was obtained from DrugBank [24]. We used the PharmMapper server to predict potential drug targets [25]. The network was constructed by Cytoscape 3.2.1 [26].

2.8. Statistics. For all experiments, data are representative of three independent experiments. Statistical analyses, including Student's t-test, the one-way ANOVA, and log-rank (Mantel-Cox) test, were performed using GraphPad Prism 5.0 software ($^*P < 0.05$; $^{**}P < 0.01$; $^{***}P < 0.001$; ns: no significant difference).

3. Results

3.1. A. cochinchinensis Increased Survival following the Ingestion of Metal Ions. As water decoction is the traditional formulation used in Chinese clinical medicine, we used aqueous extraction in this study. To assess the effect of *A. cochinchinensis* (AC) extract on the development of *Drosophila* larvae,

(a)

(b)

(c)

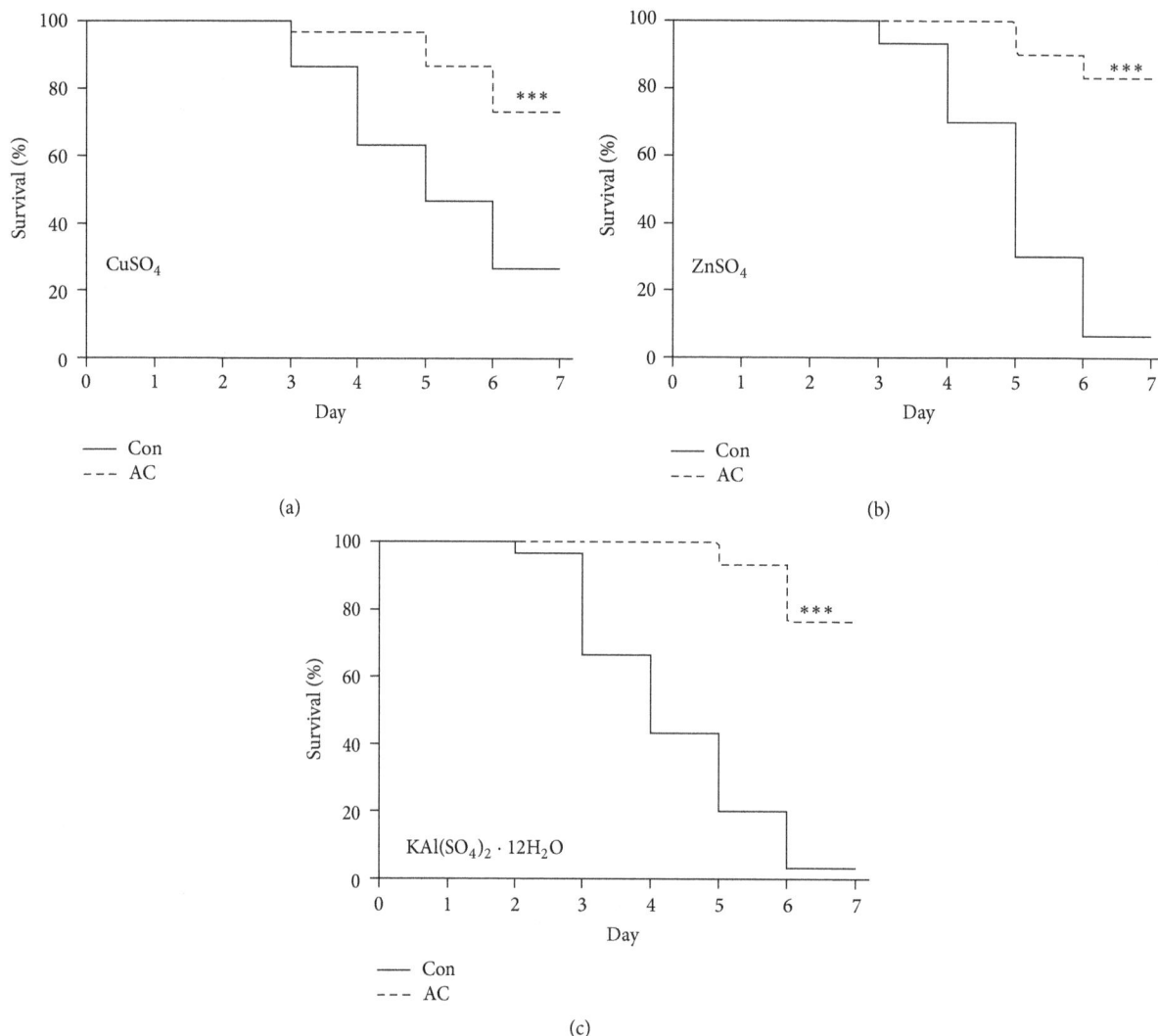

FIGURE 1: *A. cochinchinensis* improves the survival rate of flies that have ingested metal ions. (a) The survival rates of AC extract and control flies fed with 7 mM $CuSO_4$. (b) The survival rates of AC extract and control flies fed with 7 mM $ZnSO_4$. (c) The survival rates of AC extract and control flies fed with 20 mM $KAl(SO_4)_2 \cdot 12H_2O$. Three replicates were used for the determination of survival rates. *P* value was calculated by the log-rank test. ***$P < 0.001$ was considered statistically significant.

we orally administered different concentrations of AC extract to flies from egg until the adult stage. We found that AC extract demonstrated no cytotoxicity at doses of 10% (w/v) (data not shown); therefore, we used this concentration for the experiments described in this paper.

In order to investigate the effect of AC extract on the *Drosophila* gut following metal ion ingestion, we first examined whether AC extract affected survival. We observed that the survival rate of flies fed with AC extract was significantly greater compared with the control group following six days of metal ion ingestion. The survival rates associated with Cu ingestion were 74.4% for the AC extract group and 25% for the control group (Figure 1(a)). Six days following ingestion of Zn and Al, the survival rates were 83.3% and 77.8% in the AC extract group and 5.2% and 2.4% in the control group, respectively (Figures 1(b) and 1(c)). These results indicate that AC extract can increase survival in flies that have ingested

metal ions. Based on this observation, we hypothesized that AC extract might have a protective effect on metal ion-induced gut injury in *Drosophila*.

3.2. A. cochinchinensis Protects the Gut from Metal Ion-Induced Epithelial Cell Death in Drosophila. We further examined our hypothesis that AC has protective effects on metal ion-induced gut epithelial cell injury by evaluating gut epithelial cell death. After 4 days of ingesting various metal ions with or without AC extract, we found that Cu and Al feeding was associated with significantly more cell death compared with Zn feeding (Figure 2). Furthermore, only very few dead cells were detected in the AC extract group compared with the control group (Figure 2, red signal). These results demonstrate that AC extract can maintain host homeostasis by protecting gut epithelial cells from metal ion-induced damage.

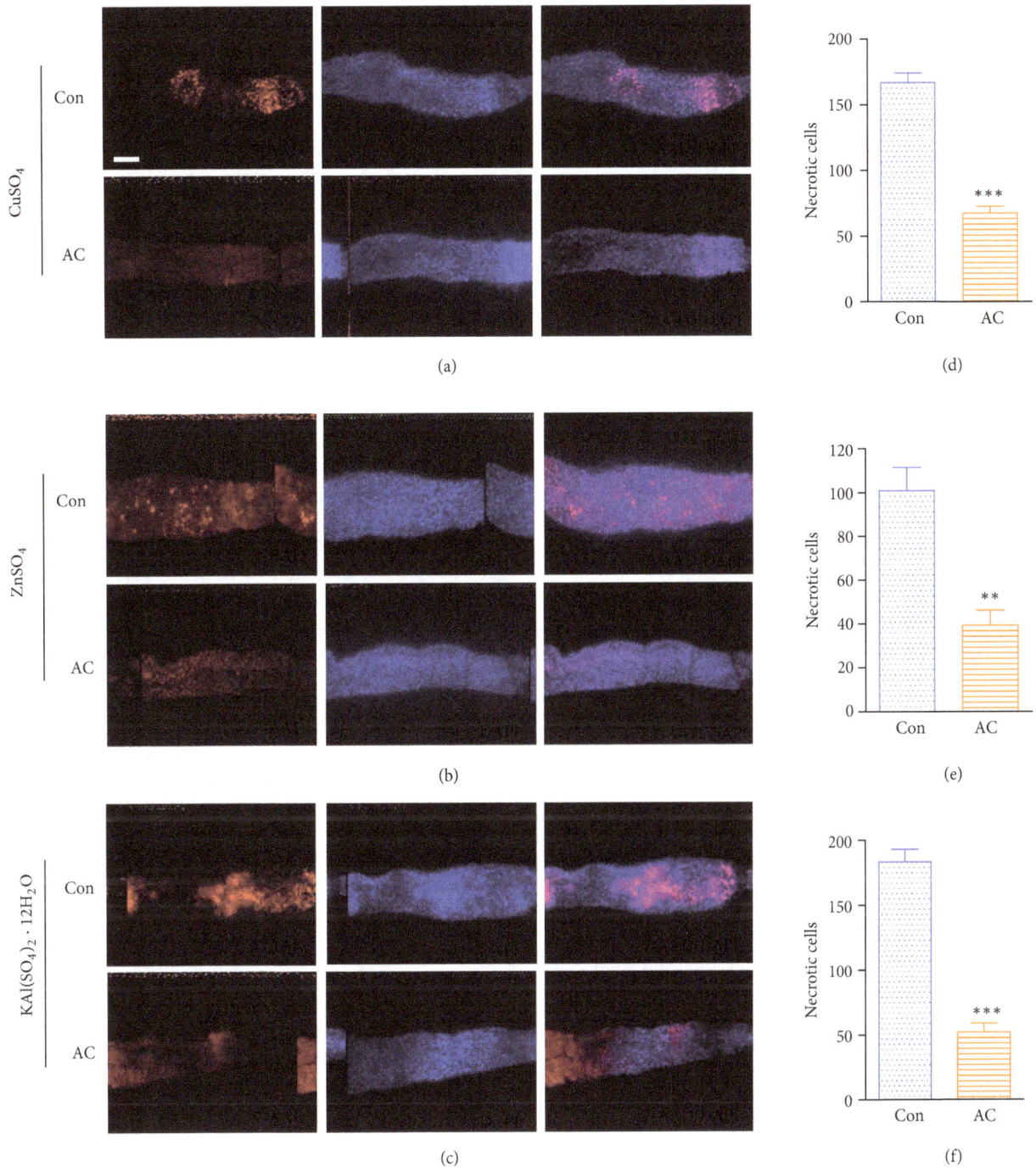

FIGURE 2: *A. cochinchinensis* protects gut epithelial cells from metal ion-induced cell death. (a) The effect of AC extract on Cu-induced epithelial cell death. (b) The effect of AC extract on Zn-induced epithelial cell death. (c) The effect of AC extract on Al-induced epithelial cell death. ((d)–(f)) The comparison of gut necrotic cell quantity between control and AC group. The number of necrotic cells was quantified using ImageJ software (10–15 guts were examined to quantify necrotic cells for each group). *P* value was calculated by Student's *t*-test. $^{***}P < 0.001$; $^{**}P < 0.01$. Con: control, flies fed with metal ions without AC for 96 h; AC: flies fed with metal ions with *A. cochinchinensis* (AC) for 96 h. 7-AAD: 7-amino-actinomycin D, dead cells (red signal); DAPI: 4′,6-diamidino-2-phenylindole, nucleus (blue signal); 7-AAD/DAPI (red and blue signal). Scale bar: 100 μm.

TABLE 1: The putative components of AC that mediate intestinal injury protection.

UNPD ID	Chemical name	CAS number	CID
UNPD133185	Coniferyl alcohol	32811-40-8|458-35-5	1549095
UNPD43533	Nyasol	230292-85-0	6438674
UNPD77220	Asparenydiol	166762-98-7	10084256
UNPD135865	$3'$-Hydroxy-$4'$-methoxy-$4'$-dehydroxynyasol	N/A	21575014
UNPD68648	$3''$-Methoxyasparenydiol	N/A	N/A
UNPD96599	$3''$-Methoxynyasol	N/A	25218067

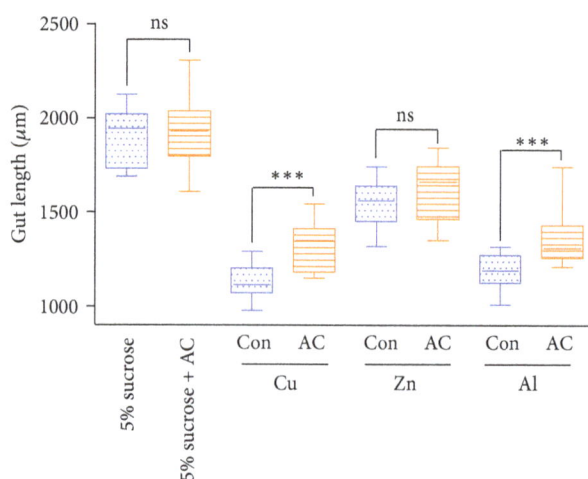

FIGURE 3: *A. cochinchinensis* prevents metal ion-induced gut atrophy. Con: control, flies fed with metal ion without AC for 96 h; AC: *A. cochinchinensis*, flies fed with metal ion with AC for 96 h. All experiments were independently performed three times. ***$P <$ 0.001; ns: no significant difference.

3.3. A. cochinchinensis Protects the Gut from Metal Ions-Induced Morphological Changes in Drosophila.

A large number of reactive oxygen species (ROS) were rapidly produced after feeding some toxic compounds [21, 22]. However, excessive ROS can damage the host intestinal epithelial cells. Study has shown that cadmium could change membrane permeability through inhibition of superoxide dismutase activity and result in necrotic organelles [27]. A previous study has shown that an increase in gut epithelial cell death associated with morphological changes in *Drosophila* [28]; therefore, we examined the gut morphology of flies that had been fed with metal ions. Four days after induction, we observed that the length of the adult gut from the control groups was significantly shorter than that of the group fed with 5% (w/v) sucrose (Figure 3). In contrast, the length of AC groups was alleviated compared with control groups which were fed with Cu and Al. However, there was no significant difference between the control group and the AC group following Zn feeding (Figure 3). These observations suggest that AC extract prevents metal ion-induced morphological changes in the adult fly gut, and, altogether, the results from our study demonstrate that AC extract has a protective effect on metal ion-induced gut injury in *Drosophila*.

3.4. The Prediction of Potential Targets of A. cochinchinensis Natural Products.

Based on our observations, we hypothesized that AC has potential implications for the discovery of new intestinal anti-inflammatory drugs. To test this hypothesis, we obtained 29 natural products (NPs) derived from AC from the UNPD. Next, we screened out 19 therapeutic proteins targeted by FDA-approved intestinal anti-inflammatory agents from DrugBank. Finally, using PharmMapper server, we found that 19 of the 29 NPs were predicted to bind to 3 of the 19 proteins targeted by FDA-approved intestinal anti-inflammatory agents (Supplementary Table S1 in Supplementary Material available online at http://dx.doi.org/10.1155/2016/7603746). These three targets were corticosteroid 11-beta-dehydrogenase isozyme 1 (11-DH), glucocorticoid receptor (GR), and peroxisome proliferator-activated receptor gamma (PPARγ). PharmMapper server is a web server for potential drug target identification using pharmacophore mapping approach [25, 29, 30].

Cytoscape software is a popular bioinformatics package for biological network visualization and data integration [26, 31]. According to the docking results, we constructed a NP and target network using the Cytoscape 3.2.1 network analysis software. The target protein was expressed by a node, and the edges represented the relationship between NPs and targets (Figure 4). Using this network, we found that 18 NPs targeted 11-DH, 16 NPs targeted GR, and 7 NPs targeted PPARγ. This result indicates that AC might serve as a useful new medicine for treating intestinal injury.

3.5. The Putative Components of A. cochinchinensis That Mediate Protection from Intestinal Injury.

Oral administration, a simple, low-cost option that does not directly damage mucous membranes, has become the most commonly used mode of drug administration. Our results demonstrated that 7 *A. cochinchinensis* NPs are predicted to bind three proteins targeted by FDA-approved intestinal anti-inflammatory agents simultaneously (Figure 4). We narrowed down the list of 7 candidates to 6 NPs by applying Lipinski's rule of five (Table 1) and considered these to be the putative components that mediate the protective effect of AC on intestinal injury.

3.6. The Drug-Likeness of the 6 NPs.

Molecular descriptors have been extensively used in cheminformatics research and the pharmaceutical industry for molecular clustering [32]. In order to explore the drug-likeness of the 6 NPs screened out from *A. cochinchinensis* (AC-NPs), we gathered information on 11 FDA-approved intestinal anti-inflammatory agents

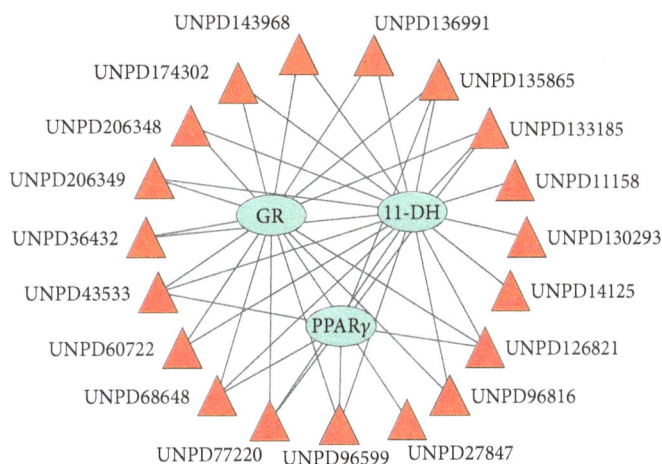

FIGURE 4: The NP-target network. The target protein was expressed by a node, and edges represented the relationship between NPs and the target protein. 11-DH: corticosteroid 11-beta-dehydrogenase isozyme 1; GR: glucocorticoid receptor; PPAR-gamma: peroxisome proliferator-activated receptor gamma. UNPD ID: Universal Natural Products Database identification.

from DrugBank (Supplementary Table S2) and calculated the following six descriptors: molecular weight, ALog$P$, number of hydrogen bond receptors (H Acceptors), number of hydrogen bond donors (H Donors), number of rotatable bonds (Rotatable Bonds), and number of rings (Rings) (Supplementary Tables S2 and S3). Using this information, we drew scatter plots to facilitate analysis of drug-likeness. As shown in Figure 5, the mean values of the descriptors of AC-NPs tended to be smaller than those of FDA-approved drugs. Nevertheless, ALog$P$ of AC-NPs was larger than that of approved drugs. The mean value of ALog$P$ was 3.6 ± 1.1 for AC-NPs and 2.3 ± 0.8 for the FDA-approved drugs. The numbers of H Acceptors and H Donors of approved drugs were primarily 5 and 3, but they were 3 and 2 for AC-NPs. The mean number of rotatable bonds for AC-NPs was slightly larger than those of the approved drugs, and this amounted to a significant difference. Most of the approved drugs had approximately 2 rotatable bonds, while the AC-NPs had approximately 5. These results indicate that the 6 AC-NPs have good drug-likeness and could potentially be used as intestinal anti-inflammatory drugs.

4. Discussion

A. cochinchinensis is primarily used in obstetrics and gynecology, otolaryngology, and ophthalmology. Its use in the clinical setting has revealed its remarkable antiaging, antitumor, and antiproliferative effects [33–35]. Previous studies have shown that AC ethanol extract might have therapeutic potential in immune-related cutaneous diseases [36]. However, the effect of AC aqueous extract on gut injury has not been previously characterized. In this study, AC significantly ameliorated epithelial cell damage in adult flies following chronic metal ion feeding (Figure 1). Due to the high level of conservation between *Drosophila* and mammalian intestinal properties [18], our results provide a theoretical basis for exploring the potential use of AC for the clinical treatment of inflammatory bowel disease.

Reverse docking of a small molecule compound (natural products, lead compounds, and chemicals) to a probe is an approach used to predict potential drug targets. It is an important tool for drug research and is indispensable for driving the modernization of new drug discovery. In this study, using the PharmMapper server, we observed AC-NP docking with targets that participate in several signaling pathways, including those associated with cancer, lipid metabolism, neurodegenerative diseases, the primary immunodeficiency pathway, and nitrogen metabolism. Moreover, some NPs demonstrated docking with intestinal anti-inflammatory targets. These observations support the hypothesis that AC exerts protective effects on metal ion-induced gut injury in *Drosophila*.

PPARγ belongs to a subfamily of the nuclear hormone receptor superfamily of ligand-inducible transcription factors [37]. PPARγ regulates genes related to lipid metabolism, as well as genes associated with immunity and inflammation [38–41]. In our study, we observed UNPD126821, UNPD133185, UNPD135865, UNPD43533, UNPD68648, UNPD77220, and UNPD96599 docking with PPARγ (Figure 4). This result further supported the hypothesis that AC has a protective effect on metal ion-induced gut injury in *Drosophila*. Moreover, this result provided a potential mechanism by which AC mediates its protective effects on gut injury. Altogether, our results suggest that AC extracts may employ similar pharmacological mechanisms as western medicines to prevent gut injury.

Nyasol was isolated from *A. cochinchinensis* many years ago, but there are few reports on its pharmacological properties [42]. Nyasol has demonstrated anti-inflammatory effects in LPS-activated BV-2 microglial cells [43]. In our study, we found that UNPD43533 (Nyasol) targeted 11-DH, GR, and PPARγ (Figure 4). This result demonstrates that AC has the potential to be used as an intestinal anti-inflammatory drug. The molecular descriptors of Nyasol were consistent with Lipinski's rules of five (Supplementary Table S3), indicating that Nyasol has good drug-likeness and is not likely to be

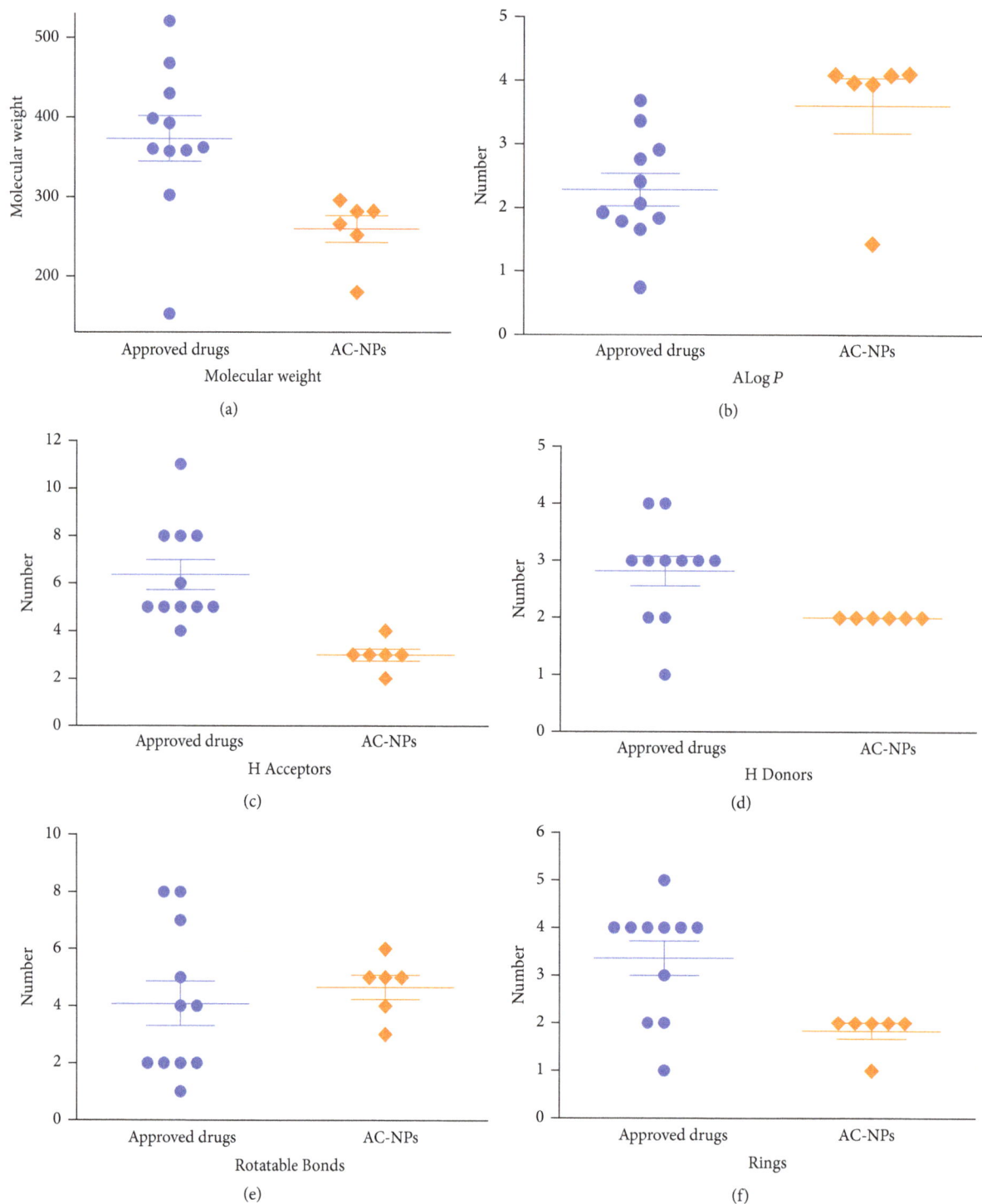

FIGURE 5: Distribution of the six molecular descriptors of AC-NPs and FDA-approved drugs. H Acceptors: number of hydrogen bond receptors; H Donors: number of hydrogen bond donors; Rotatable Bonds: number of rotatable bonds; Rings: number of rings. Approved drugs: FDA-approved drugs; AC-NPs: *A. cochinchinensis* natural products.

associated with absorption problems. Therefore, Nyasol has potential implications in intestinal anti-inflammatory drug discovery. In addition, we found that Nyasol docked with estradiol 17-beta-dehydrogenase 1 (HSD17B1), the insulin receptor, and other molecules. HSD17B1 is known to be involved in lipid transport and metabolism, and the insulin receptor is a key regulator of the insulin signaling pathway. Therefore, we predict that Nyasol may also have potential as an antidiabetic agent; however, this hypothesis requires further experimental verification.

5. Conclusion

Our results demonstrate that *A. cochinchinensis* aqueous extract exerts a protective effect on metal ion-induced gut injury in *Drosophila*. In addition, we screened out six constituents of *A. cochinchinensis* that could potentially mediate this effect. In addition, these NPs are associated with good drug-likeness. Further studies will be required to delineate the pharmacological properties associated with each of the putative active components of *A. cochinchinensis* and to determine the mechanism by which *A. cochinchinensis* mediates its protective effects in metal ion-induced gut injury. Taken together, our findings provide a basis to support the potential use of *A. cochinchinensis* for intestinal inflammation. Moreover, our studies provide helpful information and new insights into support of the application of TCM-derived natural products to drug discovery and development.

Competing Interests

The authors declare that they have no competing interests.

Acknowledgments

This work was supported by the Fundamental Research Funds for the Central Universities (DL13EA08-01).

References

[1] S. Genc, Z. Zadeoglulari, S. H. Fuss, and K. Genc, "The adverse effects of air pollution on the nervous system," *Journal of Toxicology*, vol. 2012, Article ID 782462, 23 pages, 2012.

[2] K. Matus, K.-M. Nam, N. E. Selin, L. N. Lamsal, J. M. Reilly, and S. Paltsev, "Health damages from air pollution in China," *Global Environmental Change*, vol. 22, no. 1, pp. 55–66, 2012.

[3] K. T. Palmer, R. McNeill-Love, J. R. Poole et al., "Inflammatory responses to the occupational inhalation of metal fume," *European Respiratory Journal*, vol. 27, no. 2, pp. 366–373, 2006.

[4] L. Zhefeng, C. Qiongjie, F. Yuqi et al., "Research on effects of cadmium induced intestinal epithelial cell injury and regulation on intestinal stem cells regeneration and differentiation in *Drosophila* mid-gut," *Chinese Journal of Cell Biology*, vol. 35, no. 5, pp. 602–608, 2013.

[5] N. Buchon, N. A. Broderick, S. Chakrabarti, and B. Lemaitre, "Invasive and indigenous microbiota impact intestinal stem cell activity through multiple pathways in *Drosophila*," *Genes and Development*, vol. 23, no. 19, pp. 2333–2344, 2009.

[6] J. Royet, "Epithelial homeostasis and the underlying molecular mechanisms in the gut of the insect model *Drosophila melanogaster*," *Cellular and Molecular Life Sciences*, vol. 68, no. 22, pp. 3651–3660, 2011.

[7] W. S. Garrett, J. I. Gordon, and L. H. Glimcher, "Homeostasis and inflammation in the intestine," *Cell*, vol. 140, no. 6, pp. 859–870, 2010.

[8] N. B. Samad, T. Debnath, A. Hasnat et al., "Phenolic contents, antioxidant and anti-inflammatory activities of *Asparagus cochinchinensis* (Loureiro) Merrill," *Journal of Food Biochemistry*, vol. 38, no. 1, pp. 83–91, 2014.

[9] M. Park, M. S. Cheon, S. H. Kim et al., "Anticancer activity of *Asparagus cochinchinensis* extract and fractions in HepG2 cells,"

[10] J. M. Chun, M. S. Cheon, B. C. Moon, A. Y. Lee, B. K. Choo, and H. K. Kim, "Anti-tumor activity of the ethyl acetate fraction from *Asparagus cochinchinensis* in HepG2-xenografted nude mice," *Journal of the Korean Society for Applied Biological Chemistry*, vol. 54, no. 4, pp. 538–543, 2011.

[11] T. E. Lloyd and J. P. Taylor, "Flightless flies: *Drosophila* models of neuromuscular disease," *Annals of the New York Academy of Sciences*, vol. 1184, pp. E1–E20, 2010.

[12] M. S. Dionne and D. S. Schneider, "Models of infectious diseases in the fruit fly *Drosophila melanogaster*," *Disease Models and Mechanisms*, vol. 1, no. 1, pp. 43–49, 2008.

[13] M. Vidal and R. L. Cagan, "*Drosophila* models for cancer research," *Current Opinion in Genetics and Development*, vol. 16, no. 1, pp. 10–16, 2006.

[14] M. E. Fortini and N. M. Bonini, "Modeling human neurodegenerative diseases in Drosophila: on a wing and a prayer," *Trends in Genetics*, vol. 16, no. 4, pp. 161–167, 2000.

[15] P. Leopold and N. Perrimon, "*Drosophila* and the genetics of the internal milieu," *Nature*, vol. 450, no. 7167, pp. 186–188, 2007.

[16] C. Pitsouli, Y. Apidianakis, and N. Perrimon, "Homeostasis in infected epithelia: stem cells take the lead," *Cell Host & Microbe*, vol. 6, no. 4, pp. 301–307, 2009.

[17] D. C. Rubin, "Intestinal morphogenesis," *Current Opinion in Gastroenterology*, vol. 23, no. 2, pp. 111–114, 2007.

[18] Y. Apidianakis and L. G. Rahme, "*Drosophila melanogaster* as a model for human intestinal infection and pathology," *Disease Models and Mechanisms*, vol. 4, no. 1, pp. 21–30, 2011.

[19] M. Gladstone and T. T. Su, "Chemical genetics and drug screening in *Drosophila* cancer models," *Journal of Genetics and Genomics*, vol. 38, no. 10, pp. 497–504, 2011.

[20] C. Gonzalez, "*Drosophila melanogaster*: a model and a tool to investigate malignancy and identify new therapeutics," *Nature Reviews Cancer*, vol. 13, no. 3, pp. 172–183, 2013.

[21] W. Li, Q. Luo, and L. H. Jin, "*Acanthopanax senticosus* extracts have a protective effect on *Drosophila* gut immunity," *Journal of Ethnopharmacology*, vol. 146, no. 1, pp. 257–263, 2013.

[22] C. Zhu, F. Guan, C. Wang, and L. H. Jin, "The protective effects of *Rhodiola crenulata* extracts on *Drosophila melanogaster* gut immunity induced by bacteria and SDS toxicity," *Phytotherapy Research*, vol. 28, no. 12, pp. 1861–1866, 2014.

[23] J. Gu, Y. Gui, L. Chen, G. Yuan, H.-Z. Lu, and X. Xu, "Use of natural products as chemical library for drug discovery and network pharmacology," *PLoS ONE*, vol. 8, no. 4, Article ID e62839, 2013.

[24] C. Knox, V. Law, T. Jewison et al., "DrugBank 3.0: a comprehensive resource for "Omics" research on drugs," *Nucleic Acids Research*, vol. 39, no. 1, pp. D1035–D1041, 2011.

[25] X. Liu, S. Ouyang, B. Yu et al., "PharmMapper server: a web server for potential drug target identification using pharmacophore mapping approach," *Nucleic Acids Research*, vol. 38, no. 2, pp. W609–W614, 2010.

[26] P. Shannon, A. Markiel, O. Ozier et al., "Cytoscape: a software Environment for integrated models of biomolecular interaction networks," *Genome Research*, vol. 13, no. 11, pp. 2498–2504, 2003.

[27] N. Buchon, N. A. Broderick, M. Poidevin, S. Pradervand, and B. Lemaitre, "*Drosophila* intestinal response to bacterial infection: activation of host defense and stem cell proliferation," *Cell Host & Microbe*, vol. 5, no. 2, pp. 200–211, 2009.

[28] S. Gupta, M. Athar, J. R. Behari, and R. C. Srivastava, "Cadmium-mediated induction of cellular defence mechanism: a novel example for the development of adaptive response against a toxicant," *Industrial Health*, vol. 29, no. 1, pp. 1–9, 1991.

[29] X. Li, X. Xu, J. Wang et al., "A system-level investigation into the mechanisms of chinese traditional medicine: compound danshen formula for cardiovascular disease treatment," *PLoS ONE*, vol. 7, no. 9, Article ID e43918, 2012.

[30] T. Liu, D. Lu, H. Zhang et al., "Applying high-performance computing in drug discovery and molecular simulation," *National Science Review*, vol. 3, no. 1, pp. 49–63, 2016.

[31] X. Liu, Z. Hu, B. Zhou, X. Li, and R. Tao, "Chinese herbal preparation xuebijing potently inhibits inflammasome activation in hepatocytes and ameliorates mouse liver ischemia-reperfusion injury," *PLoS ONE*, vol. 10, no. 7, Article ID e0131436, 2015.

[32] R. Todeschini and V. Consonni, *Handbook of Molecular Descriptors*, John Wiley & Sons, New York, NY, USA, 2008.

[33] J. Li, X. Liu, M. Guo, Y. Liu, S. Liu, and S. Yao, "Electrochemical study of breast cancer cells MCF-7 and its application in evaluating the effect of diosgenin," *Analytical Sciences*, vol. 21, no. 5, pp. 561–564, 2005.

[34] C. Corbiere, B. Liagre, A. Bianchi et al., "Different contribution of apoptosis to the antiproliferative effects of diosgenin and other plant steroids, hecogenin and tigogenin, on human 1547 osteosarcoma cells," *International Journal of Oncology*, vol. 22, no. 4, pp. 899–905, 2003.

[35] B. Liagre, J. Bertrand, D. Y. Leger, and J.-L. Beneytout, "Diosgenin, a plant steroid, induces apoptosis in COX-2 deficient K562 cells with activation of the p38 MAP kinase signalling and inhibition of NF-κB binding," *International Journal of Molecular Medicine*, vol. 16, no. 6, pp. 1095–1101, 2005.

[36] D. Y. Lee, B. K. Choo, T. Yoon et al., "Anti-inflammatory effects of *Asparagus cochinchinensis* extract in acute and chronic cutaneous inflammation," *Journal of Ethnopharmacology*, vol. 121, no. 1, pp. 28–34, 2009.

[37] L. Wang, B. Waltenberger, E.-M. Pferschy-Wenzig et al., "Natural product agonists of peroxisome proliferator-activated receptor gamma (PPARγ): a review," *Biochemical Pharmacology*, vol. 92, no. 1, pp. 73–89, 2014.

[38] I. Szatmari, E. Rajnavolgyi, and L. Nagy, "PPARγ, a lipid-activated transcription factor as a regulator of dendritic cell function," *Annals of the New York Academy of Sciences*, vol. 1088, pp. 207–218, 2006.

[39] L. Széles, D. Töröcsik, and L. Nagy, "PPARγ in immunity and inflammation: cell types and diseases," *Biochimica et Biophysica Acta-Molecular and Cell Biology of Lipids*, vol. 1771, no. 8, pp. 1014–1030, 2007.

[40] W. Huang and C. K. Glass, "Nuclear receptors and inflammation control: molecular mechanisms and pathophysiological relevance," *Arteriosclerosis, Thrombosis, and Vascular Biology*, vol. 30, no. 8, pp. 1542–1549, 2010.

[41] C. K. Glass and K. Saijo, "Nuclear receptor transrepression pathways that regulate inflammation in macrophages and T cells," *Nature Reviews Immunology*, vol. 10, no. 5, pp. 365–376, 2010.

[42] W.-Y. Tsui and G. D. Brown, "(+)-Nyasol from *Asparagus cochinchinensis*," *Phytochemistry*, vol. 43, no. 6, pp. 1413–1415, 1996.

[43] H. J. Lee, H. Li, H. R. Chang, H. Jung, D. Y. Lee, and J.-H. Ryu, "(−)-Nyasol, isolated from *Anemarrhena asphodeloides* suppresses neuroinflammatory response through the inhibition of I-κBα degradation in LPS-stimulated BV-2 microglial cells," *Journal of Enzyme Inhibition and Medicinal Chemistry*, vol. 28, no. 5, pp. 954–959, 2013.

8

Ex Vivo Stromal Cell-Derived Factor 1-Mediated Differentiation of Mouse Bone Marrow Mesenchymal Stem Cells into Hepatocytes Is Enhanced by Chinese Medicine Yiguanjian Drug-Containing Serum

Linlin Fu,[1] Bingyao Pang,[1] Ying Zhu,[1] Ling Wang,[2] Aijing Leng,[3] and Hailong Chen[4]

[1]*Department of Infectious Disease, The First Affiliated Hospital of Dalian Medical University, No. 222, Zhongshan Road, Xigang District, Dalian 116011, China*
[2]*Department of Digestive Disease, Gansu Provincial Hospital, Lanzhou 730000, China*
[3]*Department of Chinese Medicine, The First Affiliated Hospital of Dalian Medical University, Dalian 116011, China*
[4]*Department of General Surgery, The First Affiliated Hospital of Dalian Medical University, Dalian 116011, China*

Correspondence should be addressed to Ying Zhu; zhuyingsh52@126.com and Hailong Chen; hailongchen2007@hotmail.com

Academic Editor: Yuewen Gong

Yiguanjian is administered in traditional Chinese medicine for liver diseases and has been demonstrated to reduce liver fibrosis. This study investigated the effect of Yiguanjian drug-containing serum (YGJ) with Stromal Cell-Derived Factor 1 (SDF-1) and Hepatocyte Growth Factor (HGF) on the differentiation of murine bone-marrow-derived mesenchymal cells (BM-MSCs) into hepatocytes *in vitro*. Adherent MSCs were isolated from murine bone marrow. Differentiation was induced by 20 ng/mL HGF, 50 ng/mL SDF-1, and 20% Yiguanjian drug-containing serum for 7 to 28 days, and mature hepatocytes' marker albumin (ALB) and cholangiocytes' marker cytokeratin-18 (CK-18) were assessed by immunocytochemistry and western blot. BM-MSCs exhibited homogeneous spindle shape growth after subculture and stained positive for CD90 and negative for CD34. After induction with HGF + normal serum or YGJ for 14 days, HGF + SDF-1 + normal serum for 7 days, or HGF + SDF-1 + YGJ for 5 days, MSCs' morphology changed gradually and begun to resemble hepatocyte-like cells. Cultures supplemented with HGF + SDF-1 + YGJ contained significantly higher proportions of ALB and CK-18 positive cells than cultures supplemented with HGF + SDF-1 + normal serum at day 7. These observations corroborated the results of western blot. In conclusion, Yiguanjian drug-containing serum could facilitate the differentiation of murine BM-MSCs into hepatocytes *in vitro* and has a synergistic effect with SDF-1 and HGF.

1. Introduction

Liver transplantation is the most effective therapy for the patients with advanced liver diseases. However, the availability of donor livers limits application of this therapy [1, 2]. Recently, stem cell-based cytotherapy has been demonstrated to benefit some patients with liver disease [3–11].

BM-MSCs are relatively easy to separate and collect, exhibiting a relatively stable genetic background and extremely strong proliferative capacity and substantial plasticity and being capable of differentiation into liver parenchyma cells, liver sinus endothelial cells, Kupffer cells, stellate cells, and muscle fibroblasts [12–14]. Autologous BM-derived MSCs also induce only weakly immune rejection, and their use does not involve any complicated ethical or moral questions, recommending these cells for stem cell transplantation in the treatment of end-stage liver disease [12].

BM-MSCs can be readily isolated from bone marrow samples but represent a heterogeneous group, and responses in the clinic can vary accordingly [12]. Specific surface markers for MSCs are yet to be defined, limiting the capacity to isolate this population, and although effective transplantation likely requires large numbers of cells, *ex vivo* expansion methods which encourage differentiation into hepatocytes have not yet been perfected [3–11].

Stem cell microenvironment is a decisive factor to the differentiation specific of stem cells. Supplementing BM-derived MSC culture with HGF promoted mitosis by interaction with receptor c-met, enhancing migration capacity and promoting mesoderm and ectoderm-derived cell proliferation, thereby promoting cell mitosis and morphogenesis and directing differentiation into hepatocytes [15–18]. SDF-1, also known as pre-B cell stimulating factor (PBSF) or CXCL12, is a widely expressed chemokine differing by just one amino acid in human and murine forms. MSCs *in vitro* have been reported to express the SDF-1 receptor, CXCR4, and signaling induces MSC chemotaxis and homing to the liver [19–21]. We sought to further enhance this *ex vivo* culture environment to encourage proliferation of BM-derived MSC and direct differentiation towards hepatocytes.

The traditional Chinese medicine Yiguanjian (described in the "Liuzhou Medical Talks") is traditionally administered for liver diseases. It is comprised of radix glehniae, radix ophiopogonis, radix *Angelicae sinensis*, dried rehmannia root, *Lycium barbarum* L., and fructus meliae toosendan. This formula has a high concentration of polysaccharides, as each of *Lycium barbarum* L., radix *Angelicae sinensis*, radix ophiopogonis, and radix glehniae contains polysaccharides. There are 18 kinds of amino acids in this decoction, of which there are eight kinds of essential amino acids for humans. And it also contains many trace elements, microelements, saponins, phytosterols, triterpenoids, lactones, coumarins, and flavonoids. There are many researches indicating that, in both rat and mouse models of liver disease, Yiguanjian could reduce liver fibrosis [22–26], and oral administration of Yiguanjian decoction significantly reduced the serum aspartate aminotransferase (AST) and alanine transaminase (ALT) and inhibited accumulation of collagen I, tissue inhibitor of metalloproteinase-1, and α-smooth muscle actin (α-SMA) in hepatic tissues. Yiguanjian improves liver function in rats, reducing histological damage and increased expression of hepatic oval cells. Wang et al. [26] revealed that Yiguanjian inhibited liver fibrogenesis by inhibiting bone marrow cells differentiating into myofibroblasts in the liver. Hence, we sought to determine whether supplementing cultures with Yiguanjian drug-containing serum *ex vivo* could enhance BM-MSCs' differentiation towards hepatocytes and cholangiocytes in isolated mouse BM-MSCs.

2. Materials and Methods

2.1. Animals. Male Kunming mice ($n = 140$, body weight 18 ± 2 g) aged 4-5 weeks were obtained from the specific-pathogen-free (SPF) level animal experimental Center of Dalian Medical University (China) (license number: SCXK (Liao) 2008-0002). Animals were housed at 20–25°C and $50 \pm 5\%$ humidity with ad libitum access to food and water and a 12 : 12 h light/dark cycle. All procedures and animal experiments were approved by the Animal Care and Use Committee of Dalian Medical University (China). The mice were prepared for isolation of BM-MSCs and preparation of Yiguanjian drug-containing serum.

2.2. Preparation of Yiguanjian Decoction. A decocted concentrated liquid of Yiguanjian was produced using *radix glehniae* 9 g, *radix ophiopogonis* 9 g, *radix Angelicae sinensis* 9 g, *dried rehmannia root* 18 g, *Lycium barbarum* L. 9 g, and *fructus meliae toosendan* 5 g at the Chinese Medicine Center of the First Affiliated Hospital of Dalian Medical University. The decoction was prepared according to the original proportion and preparation method; then the filtrate was concentrated and dried into powder, and 1 g of the extract contained 2.3 g herbs.

2.3. Preparation of Yiguanjian Drug-Containing Serum. Mice were divided into two groups ($n = 50$ each group): normal control group and Yiguanjian decoction-treated group. 50 mice received Yiguanjian decoction in the dose of 0.016 mL/g body weight/day by gavage twice (with an interval of more than 6 hours) every day for 3 days. The daily dose is 10-fold as that of 60 kg adult, which is 10 mL/kg body weight. Animals in the normal control group received an equivalent volume of normal saline (NS). One hour after intragastric administration on the third day, blood was sampled from the eyeball, stored at 4°C for 4 hours, and then centrifuged at 1509 g for 20 min. The supernatant serum was mixed, sterilized and inactivated at 56°C for 30 min, and stored at −70°C.

2.4. Isolation and Culture of BM-MSCs. BM-MSCs were isolated from bone marrow, as previously described [27, 28]. Mice ($n = 40$) were sacrificed by cervical dislocation. The femur and tibia were removed and soaked in 75% alcohol for 3 min; then the bone marrow cavity was rinsed with DMEM/F 12 medium (HyClone). Bone marrow fluid was centrifuged at 377 g for 10 min, and the supernatant was discarded. Cells were resuspended at 1×10^9 cells/L in DMEM/F 12 medium containing 15% FBS (Gibco) and 100 U/mL penicillin-streptomycin and incubated at 37°C at an atmosphere of 5% CO_2. After 48 hours the culture medium was changed, and nonadherent hematopoietic cells were removed. The medium was then changed every 3-4 days, and cells were observed by Eclipse TS100 inverted microscopy (Nikon, Japan). When cells grew to 80–90% confluency (about 12–14 days), the monolayer was digested with 0.25% trypsin (Hyclone) containing 0.02% EDTA, and cells were passaged at the dilution of 1 : 2 for one to three rounds (P1 to P3).

2.5. Identification of BM-MSCs. CD90 expression in passage-two MSCs was determined by immunocytochemistry (rabbit anti-mouse CD90 and SP immunohistochemistry kit from Bioss Biotechnology Co., Ltd., Beijing, China), according to the manufacturer's instructions. Color was developed with 3,3'-diaminobenzidine (DAB) concentration reagent kit (Rope Lai Valuable Company, Beijing) by incubating at room temperature for 5 minutes in dark. Then coloration was finally finished by hematoxylin staining. The slides were observed under the Leica DMIL-LED inversion phase contrast microscope.

After two passages, 100 μL BM-MSCs (1×10^7 cells/mL) were stained with fluorescein isothiocyanate- (FITC-) labeled rabbit anti-mouse CD90 (eBioscience, San Diego, CA) or

PE-labeled rabbit anti-mouse CD34 (a BioLegend product, San Diego, CA) for 30 min at 4°C in the dark. Flow cytometry analysis was performed by FACS Vantage Flow Cytometer with CellQuest software (Becton Dickinson, USA).

2.6. Measurement of BM-MSCs' Growth. Second-passage BM-MSCs in the logarithmic growth phase were resuspended at 5×10^3/mL and 200 μL was plated in a 96-well plate. Blank wells were only medium without cells. The viability of cells was determined by the MTT method each day for 7 days. Briefly, 20 μL MTT solution (5 mg/mL, Ameresco, USA) was added to each well and incubated at 37°C with 5% CO_2 for 4 hours before the supernatant was replaced with 150 μL DMSO (Sigma, USA). After shaking for 10 min, the OD at 490 nm was measured on a microplate reader (Thermo, USA). This process was repeated for 3 times.

2.7. Induction of BM-MSCs' Differentiation In Vitro. Second-passage MSCs (4×10^5 cells/well) in the logarithmic phase of growth were cultured in 6-well plates. When having reached 70–90% confluency, cells were incubated with the following mediums for 7, 14, 21, and 28 days. Negative control cells were cultured in medium containing 15% normal serum, but cells at HGF + normal serum group (HGF group) received medium supplemented with a final concentration of 20 ng/mL HGF (Peprotech, USA) and 15% normal serum (as previously established [29, 30]). And cells at Yiguanjian drug-containing serum group (YGJ group) received medium supplemented with 20% Yiguanjian drug-containing serum. Cells at HGF + SDF-1 + normal serum group (HGF + SDF-1 group) received medium supplemented with a final concentration of 20 ng/mL HGF + 50 ng/mL SDF-1 (Peprotech, USA) and 15% normal serum (as previously established [31, 32]). Cells at HGF + SDF-1 + Yiguanjian drug-containing serum group (HGF + SDF + YGJ group) received medium supplemented with a final concentration of 20 ng/mL HGF + 50 ng/mL SDF-1 + 20% Yiguanjian drug-containing serum.

2.8. Characterization of Cells Differentiated from BM-Derived MSCs In Vitro

Morphological Observation. BM-derived MSC cultures were observed daily by inverted microscope. To assess differentiation, markers of hepatocyte-like differentiation, cellular ALB, and CK-18 expressions were assessed on 7, 14, 21, and 28 days after induction by immunocytochemistry and western blot.

For immunocytochemistry, cells were incubated with the following antibodies: rabbit anti-mouse ALB (1 : 200), rabbit anti-mouse CK-18 (1 : 200) (Bioss Biotechnology Co., Ltd., Beijing, China) overnight at 4°C followed by DAB staining. The numbers of total cells and ALB or CK-18 positive cells were counted in five randomly selected fields by three independent investigators blinded to grouping, and the percentage of ALB and CK-18 positive cells was calculated.

For western blot analysis, total protein was extracted in ice-cold lysis buffer (Beyotime, Haimen, China) containing proteinase inhibitor PMSF (KeyGEN BioTECH, Nanjing, China). The lysate were subjected to 10% SDS-PAGE and transferred to polyvinylidene fluoride membranes (Millipore,

Bedford, MA). The membranes were blocked and then incubated with anti-mouse ALB (1 : 2000) (Proteintech) and anti-mouse CK-18 (1 : 500) (Proteintech) overnight at 4°C. After washing, the membranes were incubated with horseradish peroxidase-conjugated IgG (diluted 1 : 10000, Bioss) at 37°C for 1 hour. The immunoreactive bands were detected by ECL system (Advansta, USA) and analyzed by AlphaView software (ProteinSimple, USA).

2.9. Statistical Analysis. SPSS13.0 software (SPSS Inc., Chicago, IL, USA) was used for statistical analysis, data are shown as mean ± standard deviation (SD), and comparisons among groups were performed using one-way analysis of variance (ANOVA) with q test for *post hoc* analysis. $P < 0.05$ was considered statistically significant.

3. Results

3.1. Characterization of Murine BM-MSCs. Adherent cells were isolated from murine bone marrow and passaged *in vitro*, termed BM-MSCs. Four hours after isolation, BM-MSCs began to adhere to the cell culture flask, and within 24 h the majority of cells were adhered (Figure 1(a)). During prolonged incubation, the cells aggregated into clusters, and with the exception that few cells were polygonal or round in shape, most cells were spindle-shaped (Figure 1(b)). MSCs tended gradually to confluency after growth of 12–14 days (Figure 1(c)). The MSCs were subcultured by trypsin digestion when the density reached 70% to 80%. After subculture, the MSCs refraction was better and spindle shape growth was more uniform (Figures 1(d), 1(e), and 1(f)).

The proliferation capacity of BM-MSCs (P3) was measured by MTT assay. While cells grew slowly within the first 2 days of culture, the number of cells increased between days 4 and 6 and then plateaued until day 7 (Figure 1(g)).

To determine the nature of the isolated cells (P2), they were stained for CD34 and CD90. Cells were positive for CD90 and negative for CD34 (Figure 2).

3.2. Morphology Change of BM-Derived MSCs during Differentiation. BM-MSCs (P2) cultured with 15% normal serum were spindle-shaped, spiral-shaped, or whirlpool-shaped (Figure 3(a)). After induction with 20 ng/mL HGF + 15% normal serum for 14 days or 20 ng/mL HGF + 50 ng/mL SDF-1 + 15% normal serum for 7 days, BM-MSCs proliferation gradually reduced, and cells clustered, projections retracted, and cell morphologically changed from irregular polygonal to large, round, less-adherent cells with clear nuclei and abundant cytoplasm, partially resembling hepatocyte-like cells (Figures 3(b) and 3(c)). Cells cultured with 20 ng/mL HGF, 50 ng/mL SDF-1, and 20% Yiguanjian drug-containing serum for 5 days were also circular, partially resembling hepatocyte-like cells (Figure 3(d)). After induction with 20% Yiguanjian drug-containing serum for 14 days, morphology of cells began to change (Figure 3(e)).

3.3. ALB Protein Level during Differentiation of BM-Derived MSCs. Immunocytochemical staining for ALB was observed

(a)

(b)

(c)

(d)

(e)

(f)

(g)

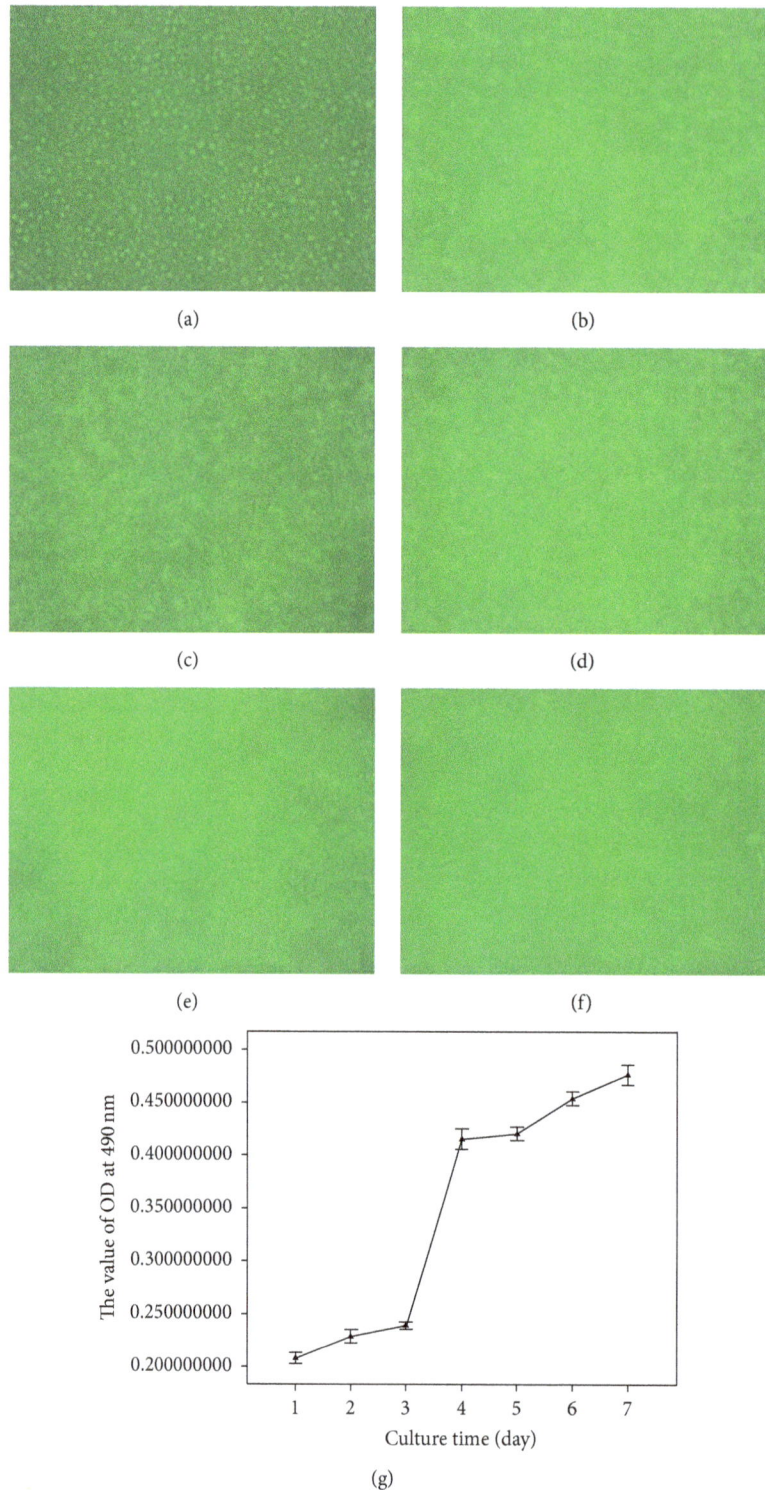

FIGURE 1: Morphology and growth of mouse bone-marrow- (BM-) derived Mesenchymal Stem Cells (MSCs). (a) BM-MSCs were isolated based on adherence and cultured for 24 hours. (b) Primary MSCs cultured for 7 days; the cells showed colony-like growth, shuttle shape with synapses, large and clear nuclei, and abundant cytoplasm. (c) Primary MSCs cultured for 15 days; cells gradually became fused. (d) MSCs at first passage (P1) cultured after 7 days; cells diffraction was better. (e) MSCs at second passage (P2) cultured after 7 days. (f) MSCs at third generation (P3) cultured after 7 days; P1, P2, and P3 MSCs were all in homogeneous spindle shape growth (magnification: ×10). (g) BM-derived MSCs at P3 grew slowly at 1-2 days; cells were in a logarithmic growth phase at 3-4 days; and cells entered a platform phase after 7 days.

(a)

Acquisition date: 8 April 2014

Marker	Left, right	Events	% gated	% total	Mean	Geo mean
All	1, 9647	5827	100.00	89.30	39.26	13.10
M1	21, 5623	2247	38.56	34.44	80.10	51.21

Acquisition date: 8 April 2014

Marker	Left, right	Events	% gated	% total	Mean	Geo mean
All	1, 9647	4079	100.00	88.87	8.33	3.88
M1	21, 5623	233	5.71	5.08	70.69	48.52

(b)

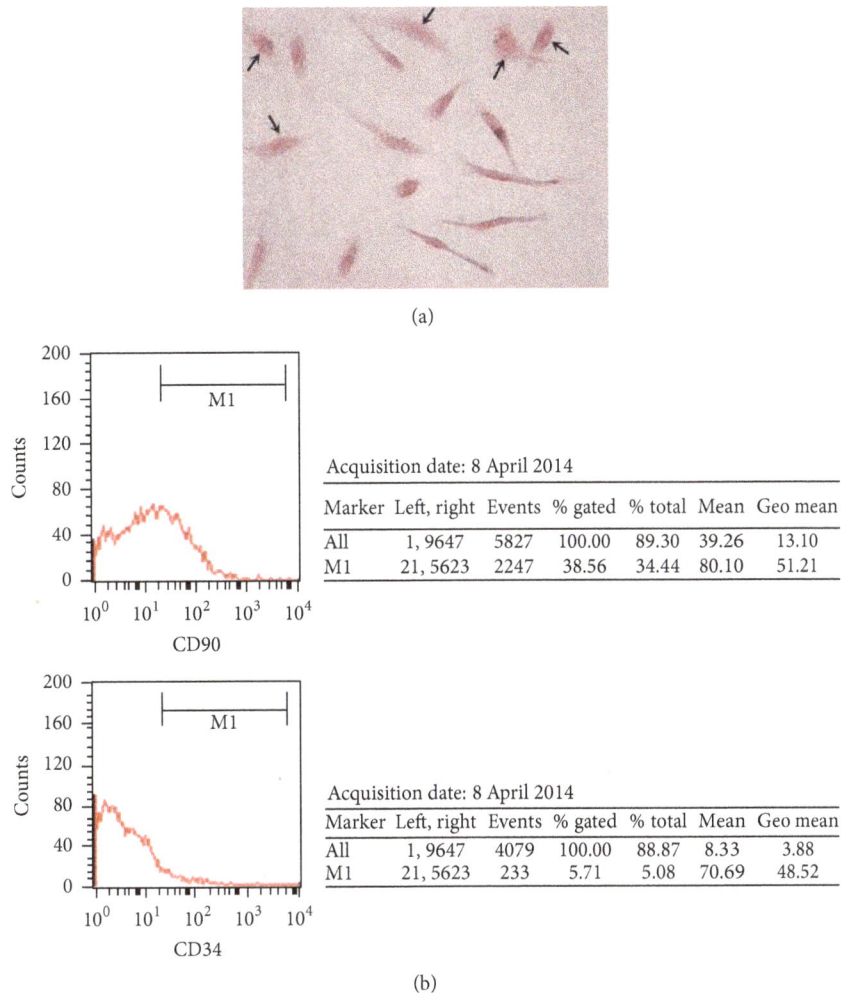

FIGURE 2: Characterization of BM-derived MSCs surface expression of CD90 and CD34. (a) CD90 expression at P3 MSCs determined by immunocytochemical staining (ICC) (magnification: ×40). Black arrows indicate MSCs positively stained for CD90 (brown staining, most obvious around the nuclei). (b) BM-MSCs' nature of these cells (P2) was confirmed based on positivity for CD90 (38.56%) and negativity for CD34 (5.71%).

at day 14 in cells cultured with 20 ng/mL HGF + 15% normal serum, and positive staining intensity increased until day 28 (Figure 4(a)). ALB positive staining was observed earlier in cells cultured with 20 ng/mL HGF + 50 ng/mL SDF-1 + 15% normal serum or those cultured with 20 ng/mL HGF + 50 ng/mL SDF-1 + 20% Yiguanjian drug-containing serum, and positive staining intensity increased from day 7 until day 28 (Figures 4(b) and 4(c)). And ALB positive staining cells in YGJ group could be observed at day 14 after induction and increased gradually to day 21, and there was a reduction at day 28 (Figure 4(d)). Cultures supplemented with HGF, SDF-1, and Yiguanjian drug-containing serum contained a significantly higher proportion of ALB positive cells than cultures supplemented with HGF, SDF-1, and normal serum at 7 ($51.96 \pm 3.17\%$ versus $19.27 \pm 1.91\%$), 14 ($65.53 \pm 2.02\%$ versus $47.22 \pm 1.62\%$), and 21 days ($72.95 \pm 0.95\%$ and $55.80 \pm 1.03\%$) (all $P < 0.05$), indicating that ALB expression appeared more rapidly in the former cultures (Table 1). However, by day 28, there was no significant difference in

the fraction of ALB positive cells in cultures supplemented with HGF, SDF-1, and normal serum or HGF, SDF-1, and Yiguanjian drug-containing serum (Table 1).

These observations corroborated the results of western blot quantification; ALB protein expression sharply increased at day 28 in cultures supplemented with HGF and normal serum (Table 2 and Figure 5(a)); however, ALB protein expression progressively increases from day 7 to day 28 in cultures supplemented with HGF, SDF-1, and normal serum, and protein expression at day 7 was significantly higher than that in cultures supplemented with HGF and normal serum (Table 2 and Figure 5(b)). ALB protein expression in cultures supplemented with HGF, SDF-1, and Yiguanjian drug-containing serum was higher than those in cultures supplemented with HGF, SDF-1, and normal serum at days 14 and 21 (Table 2 and Figure 5(c)). Expression of ALB increased from day 14 to 21 in culture supplemented with Yiguanjian drug-containing serum (Table 2 and Figure 5(d)).

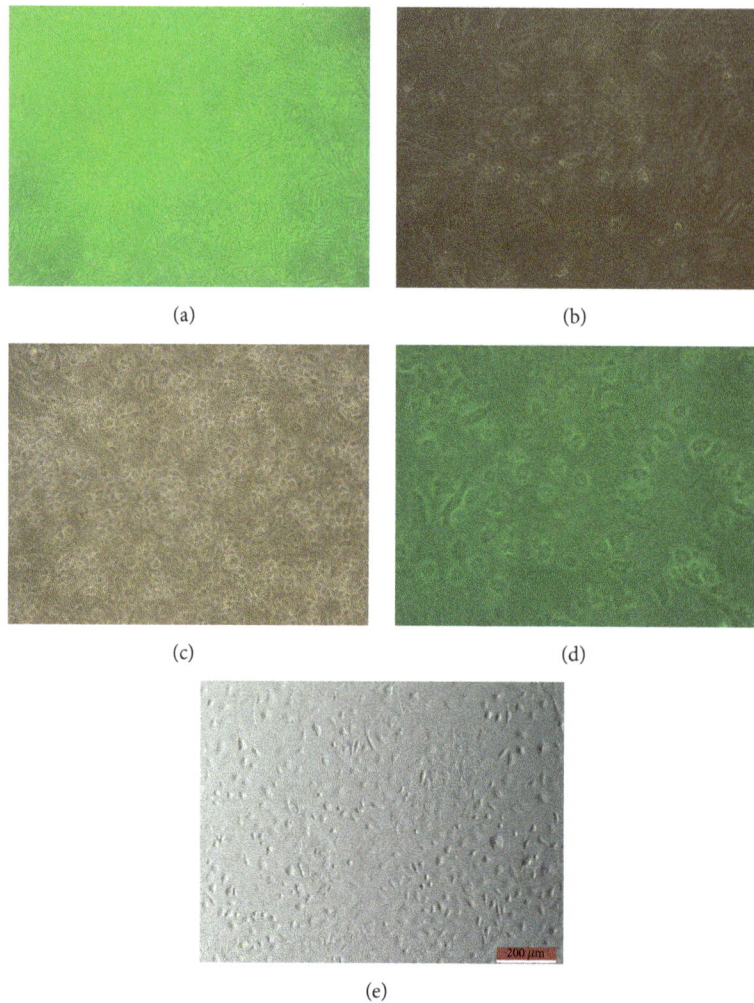

(a)

(b)

(c)

(d)

(e)

FIGURE 3: Differentiated cell morphology from P2 BM-derived MSCs. BM-derived MSCs (P2) were cultured with 15% normal serum (magnification: ×10) and were spindle-shaped, spiral-shaped, or whirlpool-shaped (a). MSCs cultured with 20 ng/mL HGF + 15% normal serum for 14 days (magnification: ×20) became polygonal and circular, partially resembling hepatocyte-like cells (b). MSCs cultured 20 ng/mL HGF + 50 ng/mL SDF-1 + 15% normal serum for 7 days (magnification: ×20) were polygonal and circular, partially resembling hepatocyte-like cells (c). MSCs cultured with 20 ng/mL HGF + 50 ng/mL SDF-1 + 20% Yiguanjian drug-containing serum for 5 days (magnification: ×20) were polygonal and circular, partially resembling hepatocyte-like cells (d). MSCs cultured with 20% Yiguanjian drug-containing serum for 14 days (magnification: ×10) (e).

TABLE 1: Albumin (ALB) in second-passage (P2) bone marrow- (BM-) derived Mesenchymal Stem Cells (MSCs) determined by immunocytochemical staining (ICC).

	ALB$^+$ BM-derived MSCs (%)			
	7 days	14 days	21 days	28 days
Negative controls	0	0	0	0
HGF + normal serum	0	24.96 ± 2.76	36.18 ± 1.45	$67.15 \pm 2.78^{\triangle}$
HGF + SDF-1 + normal serum	19.27 ± 1.91	47.22 ± 1.62	55.80 ± 1.03	$71.03 \pm 1.21^{\triangle}$
HGF + SDF-1 + YGJ	$51.96 \pm 3.17^{*}$	$65.53 \pm 2.02^{*}$	$72.95 \pm 0.95^{*}$	76.84 ± 1.70
YGJ	8.06 ± 0.59	$13.33 \pm 1.75^{\#}$	$21.43 \pm 1.08^{\#}$	16.36 ± 2.68

Note. Negative controls: MSCs were cultured in medium containing 15% normal serum; HGF + normal serum: MSCs were cultured in medium supplemented with a final concentration of 20 ng/mL HGF and 15% normal serum; HGF + SDF-1 + normal serum: MSCs were cultured in medium supplemented with a final concentration of 20 ng/mL HGF + 50 ng/mL SDF-1 and 15% normal serum; HGF + SDF-1 + Yiguanjian drug serum: MSCs were cultured in medium supplemented with a final concentration of 20 ng/mL HGF + 50 ng/mL SDF-1 and 20% Yiguanjian drug serum. YGJ: MSCs were cultured in medium supplemented with 20% Yiguanjian drug-containing serum. Data are shown as mean ± standard deviation (SD) from 5 independent experiments. $^{*}P < 0.05$ HGF + SDF-1 + Yinguanjian drug serum versus HGF + SDF-1 + normal serum at the same time. $^{\triangle}P < 0.05$: 28 days versus 7 days under the same induction condition. $^{\#}P < 0.05$: 14 days versus 7 days and 21 days versus 14 days under the same induction condition.

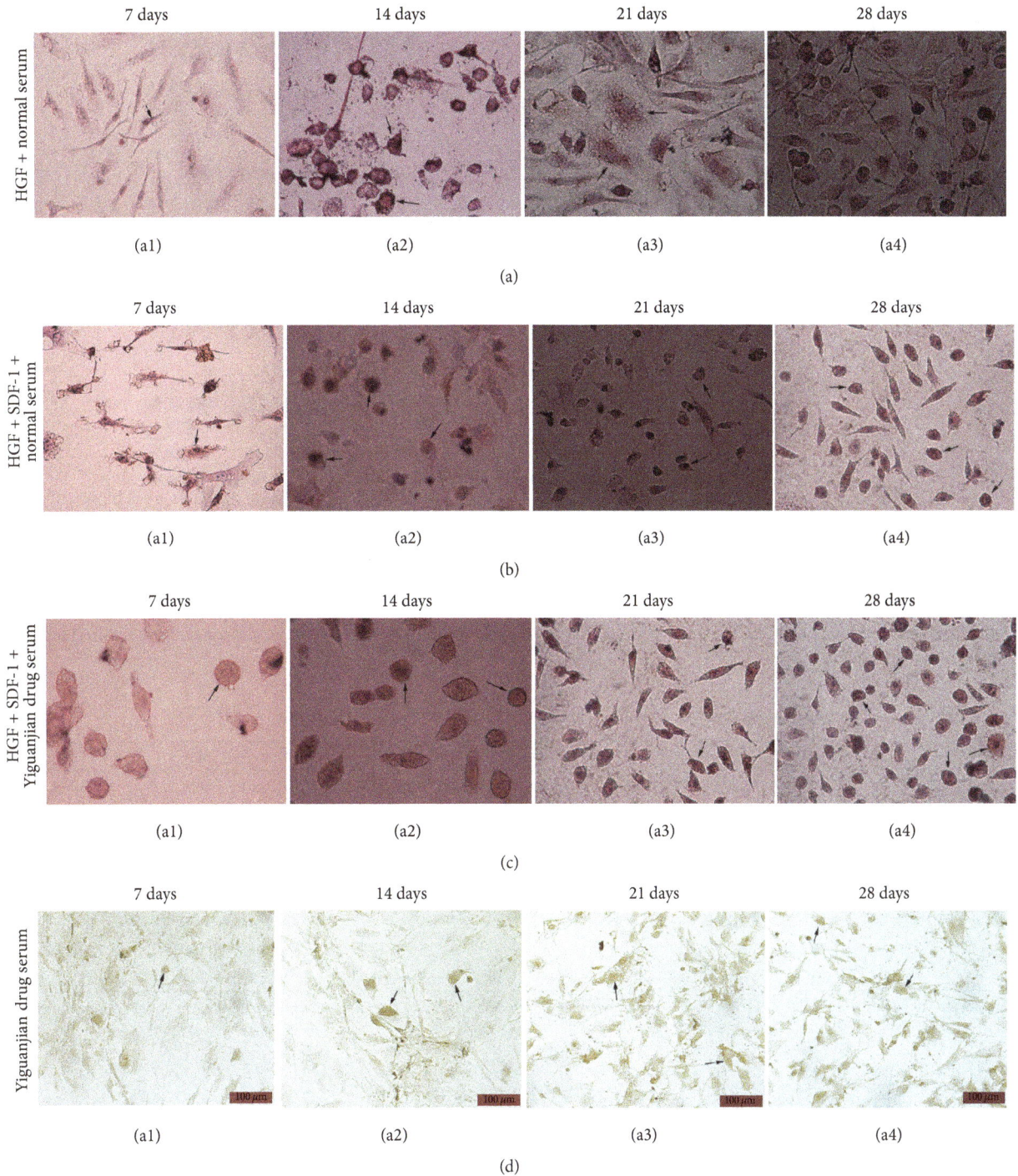

FIGURE 4: Albumin (ALB) expression in differentiated BM-derived MSCs (P2). MSCs were cultured in the presence of 20 ng/mL HGF + 15% normal serum (a), 20 ng/mL HGF + 50 ng/mL SDF-1 + 15% normal serum (b), 20 ng/mL HGF + 50 ng/mL SDF-1 + 20% Yiguanjian decoction (c), or 20% Yiguanjian drug-containing serum (d), and ALB was visualized by ICC at the indicated time points (magnification ×40: (a): (a3)-(a4) and (c): (a1)-(a2); magnification ×20: (a): (a1)-(a2), (b, c): (a3)-(a4), and (d)). ALB positive staining was observed at day 14 of culture in HGF + normal serum-treated BM-derived MSCs, and ALB staining density increased until day 28 (a). ALB staining was observed at day 7 of culture in HGF + SDF-1 + normal serum-treated BM-derived MSCs, and ALB staining density increased until day 28 (b). ALB staining was observed at day 7 of culture in HGF + SDF-1 + Yiguanjian decoction-treated BM-derived MSCs, and ALB staining density increased until day 28 (c). ALB positive staining cells in YGJ group could be observed at day 14 after induction, and increased gradually to day 21, and there was a reduction at day 28 (d).

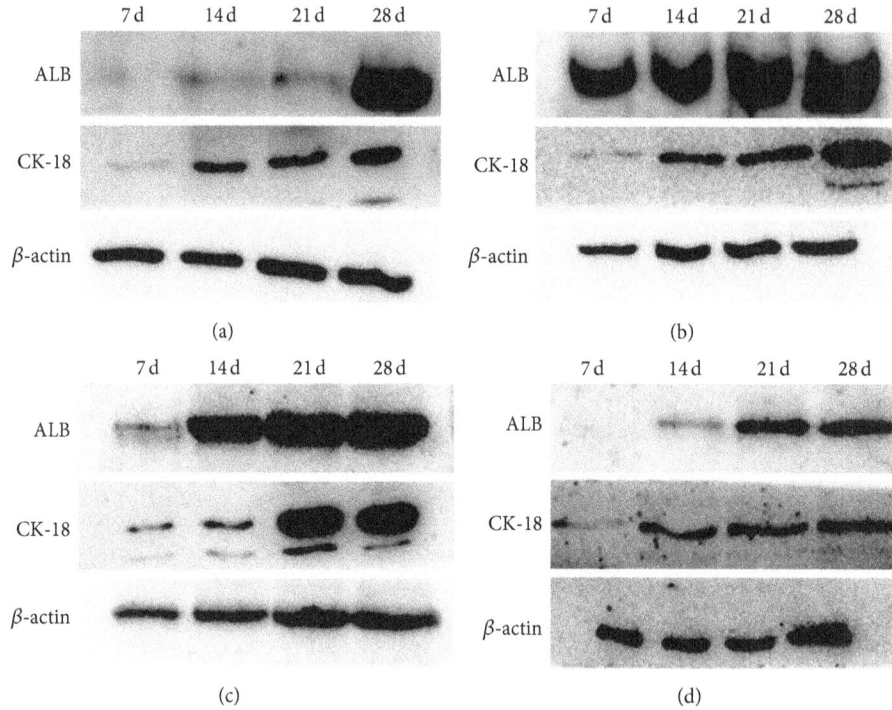

FIGURE 5: ALB and CK-18 protein expressions in differentiated BM-derived MSCs (P2). MSCs were cultured in the presence of 20 ng/mL HGF + 15% normal serum (a), 20 ng/mL HGF + 50 ng/mL SDF-1 + 15% normal serum (b), 20 ng/mL HGF + 50 ng/mL SDF-1 + 20% Yiguanjian drug-containing serum (c), or 20% Yiguanjian drug-containing serum (d), and protein expression was determined by western blot. β-actin was used as an inner control.

TABLE 2: Comparison of ALB and CK-18 expression of induced BM-MSCs by western blot.

Group		7 days	14 days	21 days	28 days
HGF + normal serum	ALB	0.33 ± 0.099	0.435 ± 0.064	0.51 ± 0.198	$2.515 \pm 0.375^{**}$
	CK-18	0.113 ± 0.064	0.443 ± 0.28	0.477 ± 0.294	$1.087 \pm 0.482^{**}$
HGF + SDF-1 + normal serum	ALB	$3.004 \pm 0.142^{**}$	$4.346 \pm 0.049^{**}$	$7.714 \pm 0.073^{**}$	$11.257 \pm 3.425^{**}$
	CK-18	0.099 ± 0.007	0.23 ± 0.013	0.238 ± 0.001	$0.562 \pm 0.21^{*}$
HGF + SDF-1 + YGJ	ALB	$0.769 \pm 0.04^{**}$	$2.286 \pm 0.038^{**}$	$2.411 \pm 0.002^{**}$	$2.826 \pm 0.014^{**}$
	CK-18	0.251 ± 0.167	0.387 ± 0.138	2.281 ± 0.741	2.712 ± 0.537
YGJ	ALB	0.452 ± 0.04	$1.145 \pm 0.09^{\#}$	2.143 ± 0.088	1.685 ± 0.357
	CK-18	0.312 ± 0.041	$0.963 \pm 0.145^{\#}$	$1.283 \pm 0.104^{\#}$	1.119 ± 0.198

The data are shown as mean ± SD. $^{*}P < 0.05$, $^{**}P < 0.01$ compared with other times in the same induction group. $^{\#}P < 0.05$: 14 days versus 7 days and 21 daysversus 14 days.

3.4. CK-18 Protein Level during Differentiation of BM-Derived MSCs.

Immunocytochemical staining for CK-18 was observed at day 14 in cells cultured with HGF and normal serum, and positive staining intensity increased until day 28 (Figure 6(a)). CK-18 positive staining was observed earlier in cells cultured with HGF, SDF-1, and normal serum or those cultured with HGF, SDF-1, and Yiguanjian drug-containing serum, and staining intensity increased from day 7 until day 28 (Figures 6(b) and 6(c)). Positive staining for CK-18 was observed at day 14 in cells cultured with YGJ, and staining intensity increased until day 28 (Figure 6(d)). Cultures supplemented with HGF, SDF-1, and YGJ contained significantly higher proportion of CK-18 positive cells than cultures supplemented with HGF, SDF-1, and normal serum

at day 7 (45.76 ± 2.20% versus 34.00 ± 1.85%) ($P < 0.05$), indicating that CK-18 expression appeared more rapidly in the former cultures (Table 3). However, by day 14 onward, there was no significant difference in the fraction of CK-18 positive cells in cultures supplemented with HGF, SDF-1, and normal serum or HGF, SDF-1, and YGJ (Table 3).

These observations corroborated the results of western blot quantification. CK-18 protein expression in cultures supplemented with HGF at the 28th day had a significant difference compared with the other time (all $P < 0.01$) (Table 2 and Figure 5(a)). CK-18 protein expression in HGF + SDF-1 + normal serum at the 28th day had a significant difference compared with the other time (all $P < 0.05$) (Table 2 and Figure 5(b)). CK-18 protein expression in

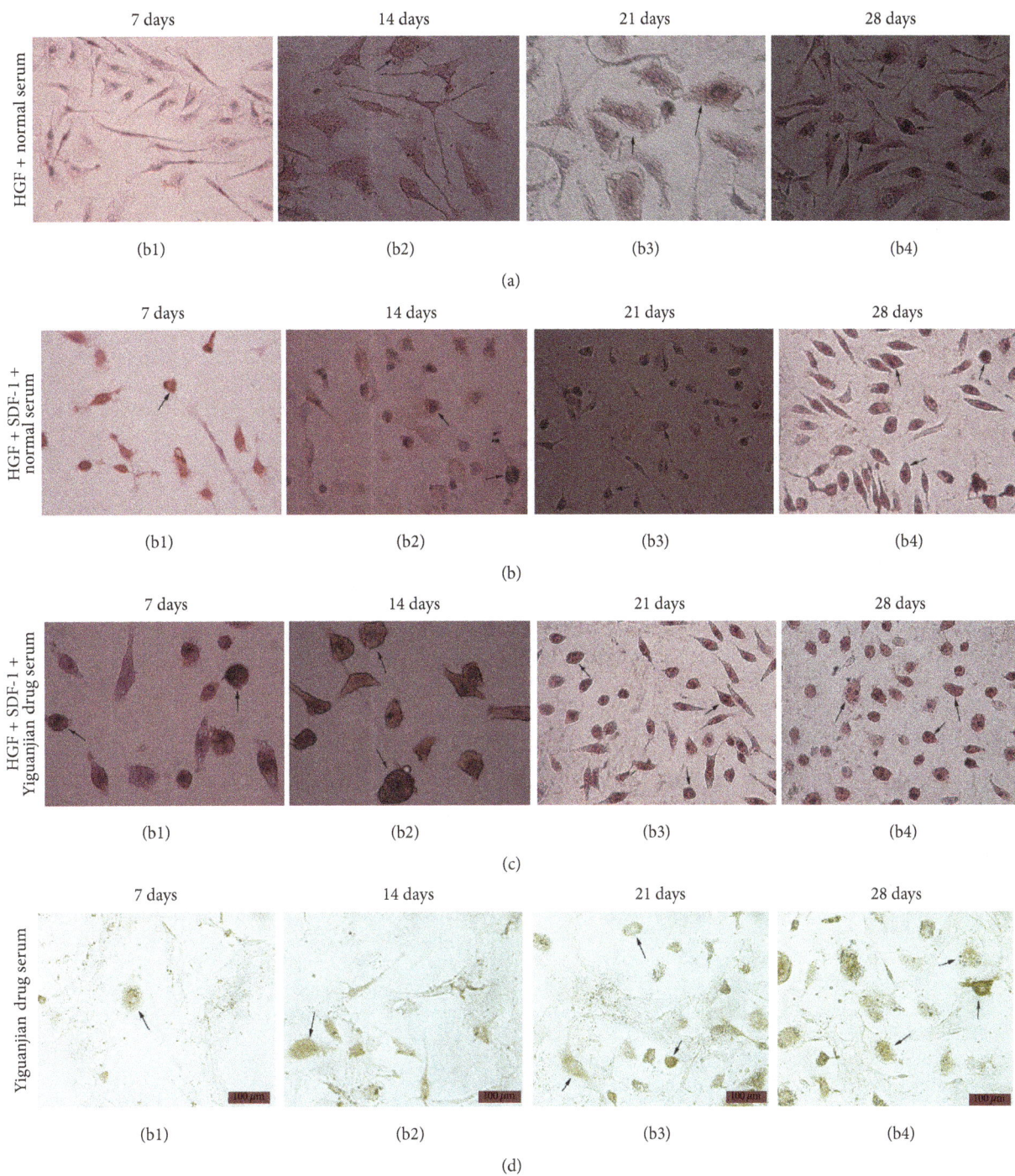

FIGURE 6: Cytokeratin-18 (CK-18) expression in differentiated BM-derived MSCs (P2). BM-MSCs were cultured in the presence of 20 ng/mL HGF + 15% normal serum (a), 20 ng/mL HGF + 50 ng/mL SDF-1 + 15% normal serum (b), 20 ng/mL HGF + 50 ng/mL SDF-1 + 20% YGJ (c), or 20% YGJ (d), and CK-18 was visualized by ICC at the indicated time points (magnification ×40: (a): (b2)-(b3) and (c): (b1)-(b2); magnification ×20: (a): (b1) and (b4), (b, c): (b3)-(b4), and (d)). CK-18 staining was observed at day 14 of culture in HGF + normal serum-treated BM-MSCs, and CK-18 staining density increased until day 28 (a). CK-18 staining was observed at day 7 of culture in HGF + SDF-1 + normal serum-treated BM-MSCs, and CK-18 staining density increased until day 28 (b). CK-18 staining was observed at day 7 of culture in HGF + SDF-1 + YGJ-treated BM-MSCs, and CK-18 staining density increased until day 28 (c). Positive staining for CK-18 was observed at day 14 in cells cultured with YGJ, and staining intensity increased until day 28 (d).

TABLE 3: Cytokeratin-18 (CK-18) in P2 BM-derived MSCs determined by ICC.

| | CK-18$^+$ BM-derived MSCs (%) | | | |
	7 days	14 days	21 days	28 days
Negative controls	0	0	0	0
HGF + normal serum	0	42.19 ± 3.78	47.46 ± 2.75	68.61 ± 1.23$^\triangle$
HGF + SDF-1 + normal serum	34.00 ± 1.85	47.68 ± 1.75	50.55 ± 1.01	72.45 ± 4.01$^\triangle$
HGF + SDF-1 + YGJ	45.76 ± 2.20*	56.24 ± 3.51	71.36 ± 1.02	76.72 ± 2.18$^\triangle$
YGJ	4.05 ± 1.28	11.25 ± 2.31$^\#$	18.92 ± 1.89$^\#$	21.21 ± 3.27

Note. Data are shown as mean ± SD from 5 independent experiments. $^*P < 0.05$ HGF + SDF-1 + Yiguanjian drug serum versus HGF + SDF-1 + normal serum at the same time point. $^\triangle P < 0.05$: 28 days versus 7 days under the same induction condition. $^\# P < 0.05$: 14 days versus 7 days and 21 days versus 14 days.

HGF + SDF-1 + YGJ-treated cells at the 21st day was significantly higher than those at 7th and 14th days (both $P < 0.01$); furthermore, CK-18 protein expression at the 28th day was higher than those at the 7th and 14th days (both $P < 0.001$) (Table 2 and Figure 5(c)). CK-18 protein expression in YGJ-treated cells increased from the 14th day to the 21st day ($P < 0.05$) (Table 2 and Figure 5(d)).

4. Discussion

We sought to determine whether supplementing cultures with Yiguanjian drug-containing serum could enhance isolated murine BM-MSCs' differentiation towards hepatocytes and cholangiocytes. We prepared the Yiguanjian drug-containing serum by giving mice Yiguanjian decoction by gavage for 3 days and obtained their blood to prepare the drug-containing serum. We isolated MSCs from murine bone marrow by adhesion. Differentiation towards hepatocytes and cholangiocytes was induced by supplementing culture medium with 20 ng/mL HGF, 50 ng/mL SDF-1, and/or 20% Yiguanjian drug-containing serum.

Albumin is expressed in the embryonic liver, increasing gradually with the liver maturation, and is one of the most commonly used reliable indicators of mature hepatocytes. It is mainly secreted and synthesized by hepatocytes [33]. As a specific marker of biliary epithelial cells, CK-18 is not expressed in infantile hepatic progenitor cells but is a relatively specific marker of mature hepatocytes [33]. So we detected a hepatocyte phenotype by staining for albumin and a cholangiocyte phenotype by staining for CK-18. We found that medium added to HGF + SDF-1 or Yiguanjian drug-containing serum alone could induce BM-MSCs' hepatic differentiation as we detected the expression of ALB and CK-18 in group HGF + SDF-1 and group YGJ in addition to cells' morphological changes during induction, and supplementation with YGJ induced differentiation more rapidly than using HGF and SDF-1 alone, although after 28 days in culture there was no significant difference in the fraction of cells positively expressing ALB or CK-18 between the cultures supplemented with HGF + SDF-1 and those supplemented with HGF + SDF-1 + YGJ.

These findings suggest that HGF + SDF-1 or Yiguanjian drug-containing serum alone could induce BM-MSCs' differentiation to hepatocytes and cholangiocytes, and Yiguanjian has a synergistic effect with SDF-1 and HGF as it could enhance the process of differentiation.

HGF binding its receptor HGFR would increase the interaction between the cytokine receptor and ligand and accelerate stem cell mitosis, strengthening differentiation of stem cells into hepatic cells. MSCs can express CXCR4 and c-met cytokine receptor; when exogenous SDF-1 and HGF are added to the cell culture, the MAPK pathway is stimulated [34–36]. Activation of protein kinase MSK1 enhances ALB and CK-18 gene promoter phosphorylation and epigenetic modification can induce multidirectional differentiation. Addition of Yiguanjian drug-containing serum enhanced this effect, and as CXCR4 is the specific receptor of SDF-1, we speculated that YGJ induces BM-MSCs' hepatic differentiation via SDF-1/CXCR4 pathway. However further work will be required to determine the mechanism of Yiguanjian action and explore the active substances of Yiguanjian through performing the chemical analysis in this formula.

5. Conclusions

In conclusion, we found that addition of Yiguanjian drug-containing serum can enhance the speed to induce differentiation of murine BM-derived MSCs into hepatocytes by supplementing HGF and SDF-1 *in vitro*. Yiguanjian might promote liver cell maturation, protect mature hepatocytes, or inhibit hepatic apoptosis. However, these findings in this study are preliminary, and the special mechanism of Yiguanjian and the properties of these *ex vivo* expanded differentiated cells in transplant experiments on animals will need to be further investigated as well.

Competing Interests

The authors declare that they have no competing interests.

Acknowledgments

This work was supported by the National Natural Science Foundation of China (nos. 81273925 and 81573751). The authors wish to sincerely thank Professor Zhu from the First Affiliated Hospital of Dalian Medical University for her thoughtful comments. They also sincerely thank all the staff in Center Laboratory and Pathology Department of the First Affiliated Hospital of Dalian Medical University for support.

References

[1] J. P. Iredale, "Cirrhosis, new research provides a basis for rational and targeted treatments," *The British Medical Journal*, vol. 327, no. 7407, pp. 143–147, 2003.

[2] D. S. Lee, W. H. Gil, H. H. Lee et al., "Factors affecting graft survival after living donor liver transplantation," *Transplantation Proceedings*, vol. 36, no. 8, pp. 2255–2256, 2004.

[3] M.-E. M. Amer, S. Z. El-Sayed, W. A. El-Kheir et al., "Clinical and laboratory evaluation of patients with end-stage liver cell failure injected with bone marrow-derived hepatocyte-like cells," *European Journal of Gastroenterology and Hepatology*, vol. 23, no. 10, pp. 936–941, 2011.

[4] M. El-Ansary, I. Abdel-Aziz, S. Mogawer et al., "Phase II trial: undifferentiated versus differentiated autologous mesenchymal stem cells transplantation in Egyptian patients with HCV induced liver cirrhosis," *Stem Cell Reviews and Reports*, vol. 8, no. 3, pp. 972–981, 2012.

[5] Y. O. Jang, Y. J. Kim, S. K. Baik et al., "Histological improvement following administration of autologous bone marrow-derived mesenchymal stem cells for alcoholic cirrhosis: a pilot study," *Liver International*, vol. 34, no. 1, pp. 33–41, 2014.

[6] P. Kharaziha, P. M. Hellström, B. Noorinayer et al., "Improvement of liver function in liver cirrhosis patients after autologous mesenchymal stem cell injection: a phase I-II clinical trial," *European Journal of Gastroenterology and Hepatology*, vol. 21, no. 10, pp. 1199–1205, 2009.

[7] M. Mohamadnejad, K. Alimoghaddam, M. Mohyeddin-Bonab et al., "Phase 1 trial of autologous bone marrow mesenchymal stem cell transplantation in patients with decompensated liver cirrhosis," *Archives of Iranian Medicine*, vol. 10, no. 4, pp. 459–466, 2007.

[8] M. Mohamadnejad, M. Namiri, M. Bagheri et al., "Phase 1 human trial of autologous bone marrow-hematopoietic stem cell transplantation in patients with decompensated cirrhosis," *World Journal of Gastroenterology*, vol. 13, no. 24, pp. 3359–3363, 2007.

[9] M. Mohamadnejad, K. Alimoghaddam, M. Bagheri et al., "Randomized placebo-controlled trial of mesenchymal stem cell transplantation in decompensated cirrhosis," *Liver International*, vol. 33, no. 10, pp. 1490–1496, 2013.

[10] C.-H. Park, S. H. Bae, H. Y. Kim et al., "A pilot study of autologous CD34-depleted bone marrow mononuclear cell transplantation via the hepatic artery in five patients with liver failure," *Cytotherapy*, vol. 15, no. 12, pp. 1571–1579, 2013.

[11] S. Terai, T. Ishikawa, K. Omori et al., "Improved liver function in patients with liver cirrhosis after autologous bone marrow cell infusion therapy," *Stem Cells*, vol. 24, no. 10, pp. 2292–2298, 2006.

[12] L.-J. Dai, H. Y. Li, L.-X. Guan, G. Ritchie, and J. X. Zhou, "The therapeutic potential of bone marrow-derived mesenchymal stem cells on hepatic cirrhosis," *Stem Cell Research*, vol. 2, no. 1, pp. 16–25, 2009.

[13] X.-Q. Kang, W.-J. Zang, T.-S. Song et al., "Rat bone marrow mesenchymal stem cells differentiate into hepatocytes in vitro," *World Journal of Gastroenterology*, vol. 11, no. 22, pp. 3479–3484, 2005.

[14] X.-L. Shi, Y.-D. Qiu, X.-Y. Wu et al., "In vitro differentiation of mouse bone marrow mononuclear cells into hepatocyte-like cells," *Hepatology Research*, vol. 31, no. 4, pp. 223–231, 2005.

[15] N. Lin, J. Lin, L. Bo, P. Weidong, S. Chen, and R. Xu, "Differentiation of bone marrow-derived mesenchymal stem cells into hepatocyte-like cells in an alginate scaffold," *Cell Proliferation*, vol. 43, no. 5, pp. 427–434, 2010.

[16] S. Oyagi, M. Hirose, M. Kojima et al., "Therapeutic effect of transplanting HGF-treated bone marrow mesenchymal cells into CCl4-injured rats," *Journal of Hepatology*, vol. 44, no. 4, pp. 742–748, 2006.

[17] S. Snykers, J. De Kock, V. Tamara, and V. Rogiers, "Hepatic differentiation of mesenchymal stem cells: in vitro strategies," *Methods in Molecular Biology*, vol. 698, pp. 305–314, 2011.

[18] P. P. Wang, J. H. Wang, Z. P. Yan et al., "Expression of hepatocyte-like phenotypes in bone marrow stromal cells after HGF induction," *Biochemical and Biophysical Research Communications*, vol. 320, no. 3, pp. 712–716, 2004.

[19] S. Bhakta, P. Hong, and O. Koc, "The surface adhesion molecule CXCR4 stimulates mesenchymal stem cell migration to stromal cell-derived factor-1 in vitro but does not decrease apoptosis under serum deprivation," *Cardiovascular Revascularization Medicine*, vol. 7, no. 1, pp. 19–24, 2006.

[20] Y. Matsuda-Hashii, K. Takai, H. Ohta et al., "Hepatocyte growth factor plays roles in the induction and autocrine maintenance of bone marrow stromal cell IL-11, SDF-1α, and stem cell factor," *Experimental Hematology*, vol. 32, no. 10, pp. 955–961, 2004.

[21] I. Petit, D. Jin, and S. Rafii, "The SDF-1-CXCR4 signaling pathway: a molecular hub modulating neo-angiogenesis," *Trends in Immunology*, vol. 28, no. 7, pp. 299–307, 2007.

[22] W. Chen, J.-Y. Chen, Y.-T. Tung et al., "High-frequency ultrasound imaging to evaluate liver fibrosis progression in rats and yi guan jian herbal therapeutic effects," *Evidence-Based Complementary and Alternative Medicine*, vol. 2013, Article ID 302325, 11 pages, 2013.

[23] X. Gou, Q. Tao, Q. Feng et al., "Urine metabolic profile changes of CCl4-liver fibrosis in rats and intervention effects of Yi Guan Jian Decoction using metabonomic approach," *BMC Complementary and Alternative Medicine*, vol. 13, article 123, 2013.

[24] H.-J. Lin, J.-Y. Chen, C.-F. Lin et al., "Hepatoprotective effects of Yi Guan Jian, an herbal medicine, in rats with dimethylnitrosamine-induced liver fibrosis," *Journal of Ethnopharmacology*, vol. 134, no. 3, pp. 953–960, 2011.

[25] H. J. Lin, C. P. Tseng, C. F. Lin et al., "A Chinese herbal decoction, modified Yi Guan Jian, induces apoptosis in hepatic stellate cells through an ROS-mediated mitochondrial/caspase pathway," *Evidence-Based Complementary and Alternative Medicine*, vol. 2011, Article ID 459531, 8 pages, 2011.

[26] X.-L. Wang, D.-W. Jia, H.-Y. Liu et al., "Effect of Yiguanjian decoction on cell differentiation and proliferation in CCl$_4$-treated mice," *World Journal of Gastroenterology*, vol. 18, no. 25, pp. 3235–3249, 2012.

[27] A. J. Friedenstein, R. K. Chailakhyan, and U. V. Gerasimov, "Bone marrow osteogenic stem cells: in vitro cultivation and transplantation in diffusion chambers," *Cell and Tissue Kinetics*, vol. 20, no. 3, pp. 263–272, 1987.

[28] H. Zhu, Z.-K. Guo, X.-X. Jiang et al., "A protocol for isolation and culture of mesenchymal stem cells from mouse compact bone," *Nature Protocols*, vol. 5, no. 3, pp. 550–560, 2010.

[29] Y. Kuang, "Regulation of different concentrations of hepatocyte growth factor and fibroblast growth factor on rat liver stem cell proliferation," *International Journal of Pathology and Clinical Medicine*, vol. 30, pp. 106–109, 2010.

[30] L. Zeng, L. Yang, and J. Yuan, "Experimental study of HGF, EGF effect on proliferation of cultured rat hepatocytes in vitro,"

Laboratory Animal and Comparative Medicine, vol. 29, pp. 361–364, 2009.

[31] P. Ding, Z. Feng, and Z. Yang, "In vitro study of the migration of marrow stromal cells induced by SDF-1," *Chinese Journal of Neuromedicine*, vol. 6, pp. 225–227, 2007.

[32] D. Kong, N. Gao, and Y. Zhang, "Migration experiment in vitro of bone marrow mesenchymal stem cells by CXCR4 gene modification," *Journal of Biomedical Engineering*, vol. 26, pp. 595–600, 2009.

[33] C. Lange, P. Bassler, M. V. Lioznov et al., "Liver-specific gene expression in mesenchymal stem cells is induced by liver cells," *World Journal of Gastroenterology*, vol. 11, no. 29, pp. 4497–4504, 2005.

[34] J. Li, Z. Zhao, J. Liu et al., "MEK/ERK and p38 MAPK regulate chondrogenesis of rat bone marrow mesenchymal stem cells through delicate interaction with TGF-β1/Smads pathway," *Cell Proliferation*, vol. 43, no. 4, pp. 333–343, 2010.

[35] S. Peng, G. Zhou, K. D. K. Luk et al., "Strontium promotes osteogenic differentiation of mesenchymal stem cells through the Ras/MAPK signaling pathway," *Cellular Physiology and Biochemistry*, vol. 23, no. 1–3, pp. 165–174, 2009.

[36] S. Zhou, S. Lechpammer, J. S. Greenberger, and J. Glowacki, "Hypoxia inhibition of adipocytogenesis in human bone marrow stromal cells requires transforming growth factor-β/Smad3 signaling," *Journal of Biological Chemistry*, vol. 280, no. 24, pp. 22688–22696, 2005.

9

Icariin Inhibits Pulmonary Hypertension Induced by Monocrotaline through Enhancement of NO/cGMP Signaling Pathway in Rats

Li-sheng Li,[1] Yun-mei Luo,[1] Juan Liu,[2] Yu Zhang,[1] Xiao-xia Fu,[1] and Dan-li Yang[1]

[1]*Department of Pharmacology, Key Lab of Basic Pharmacology of Education Ministry, Zunyi Medical College, No. 201 Dalian Road, Zunyi, Guizhou 563099, China*
[2]*Institute of Clinical Medicine, Affiliated Hospital of Zunyi Medical College, No. 149 Dalian Road, Zunyi, Guizhou 563099, China*

Correspondence should be addressed to Li-sheng Li; medlls@sina.com

Academic Editor: Shun-Wan Chan

It has been reported that icariin (ICA) increased contents of nitric oxide (NO) and cyclic guanosine monophosphate (cGMP) by improving expression of endothelial nitric oxide synthase (eNOS) and inhibition of phosphodiesterase type 5 (PDE5). In addition, dysfunction of the NO/cGMP pathway may play a crucial role in the pathogenesis of pulmonary hypertension (PH). In this study, the potential protective effects of ICA on PH induced by monocrotaline (MCT, 50 mg/kg) singly subcutaneous injection were investigated and the possible mechanisms involved in NO/cGMP pathway were explored in male Sprague Dawley rats. The results showed that ICA (20, 40, and 80 mg/kg/d) treatment by intragastric administration could significantly ameliorate PH and upregulate the expression of eNOS gene and downregulate the expression of PDE5 gene in MCT-treated rats. Both ICA (40 mg/kg/d) and L-arginine (200 mg/kg/d), a precursor of NO as positive control, notably increased the contents of NO and cGMP in lung tissue homogenate, which were inversed by treatment with ^{N}G-nitro-L-arginine-methyl ester (L-NAME), a NOS inhibitor, and L-NAME-treatment could also inhibit the protective effects of ICA (40 mg/kg/d) on mean pulmonary artery pressure and artery remodeling and tends to inhibit right ventricle hypertrophy index. In summary, ICA is effective in protecting against MCT-induced PH in rats through enhancement of NO/cGMP signaling pathway in rats.

1. Introduction

Pulmonary hypertension (PH) is a chronic progressive and devastating disease in which mean pulmonary arterial pressure (mPAP) increases by more than 25 mmHg in the resting state and finally leads to right ventricular failure [1]. The disease is characterized by the difficulty in determining its origination and diagnosis, poor prognosis, and a high mortality rate (about 15% annually) [2]. Although the exact pathogenesis of PH is not fully understood, the considerable evidence from PH animal experiments and patients suggest nitric oxide/cyclic guanosine monophosphate (NO/cGMP) signaling pathway dysfunction is a key event in the PH pathophysiology process [3, 4], which leads to vasoconstriction and arterial remodeling of small pulmonary arteries. The vicious cycle being formed between arterial remodeling

and elevation of pulmonary arterial obstruction promotes gradually development of the disease. So it is helpful towards the treatment of PH to investigate any reagents that ameliorate vascular remodeling and/or decrease pulmonary arterial obstruction [5]. On the other hand, recent studies in animal model of PH induced by monocrotaline (MCT) show unchanged NO content and endothelial nitric oxide synthase (eNOS) expression in the early MCT treatment [6]; Sawamura et al. found also there was no significant change in pulmonary cGMP levels 3 weeks after MCT (60 mg/kg) injection [7], but it is worth to be sure that to enhance function of NO/cGMP signaling pathway can improve PH. The function of NO/cGMP signaling pathway is modulated by three key enzymes in the cardiovascular system, namely, eNOS, soluble guanylate cyclase (sGC), and phosphodiesterase type 5 (PDE5) [8–10]. NO in blood serum is mainly produced by eNOS through the conversion of L-arginine (L-arg) into L-citrulline in vascular endothelial cells, and NO in turn activates sGC; the latter promotes conversion of guanosine triphosphate (GTP) to cGMP [11]. cGMP further activates protein kinase G and subsequently develops the wide range of bioactivities, including vascular relaxation and inhibition of vascular smooth cell proliferation in the cardiovascular system [12–14]. PDE5 can terminate the action of cGMP by improving hydrolysis of cGMP, which is expressed at a higher level in the pulmonary circulation than in systemic vessels [15]. The presented facts clearly demonstrated that NO/cGMP signaling pathway dysfunction is involved in the pathogenesis of PH and also is an important target for the development of new drugs such as PDE5 inhibitor sildenafil or soluble guanylate cyclase (sGC) stimulator BAY 63-252.

Icariin (ICA, PubCHem CID: 5318997), a major compound of *herb epimedium*, is a well-known and popular traditional Chinese medicine to treat erectile dysfunction. At present, abundant pharmacological functions of ICA have been identified including anti-inflammation, antioxidative stress reduction, anticancer, cardiovascular protection, stimulation of osteoblast proliferation, and enhanced immune function [16, 17]. Recently, ICA has been demonstrated to act as a PDE5 inhibitor with IC_{50} values of 1.0, 0.75, and 1.1 μM, respectively, an inhibitor of PDE5A1, A2, and A3, and to increase cGMP concentration in cavernous smooth muscle cells *in vitro* [18, 19], and it can also notably upregulate eNOS expression in porcine aorta endothelial cells [20]. On the basis of these facts, we hypothesize that ICA may function as anti-PH. The present study was designed to investigate (1) the potential effect of ICA on PH induced by subcutaneous injection MCT in rats and (2) the relationship between the possible anti-PH effect and NO/cGMP signaling pathway.

2. Materials and Methods

2.1. Animals and Reagents. Adult male Sprague-Dawley rats ($n = 108$, weight 200 to 250 g, SPF) were purchased from the Experiment Animal Center of Institute of Surgery Research of the Third Military Medical University (Chongqing, China) and were housed in SPF-grade animal facilities (Certificate Number: SYXK 2011-004) of Zunyi Medical College (Guizhou, China). Animals were allowed free access to a standard laboratory rat diet and water ad libitum. ICA (purity: 98%) was obtained from Nanjing Zelang Medical Technology Co., Ltd. (Nanjing, China). Sildenafil (SIL) was product of Pfizer Inc. (New York, USA). Monocrotaline (MCT), L-arg, and NG-nitro-L-arginine-methyl ester (L-NAME) were bought from Sigma-Aldrich Co. (St. Louis, MO, USA). The study protocol was approved by the ethics committee of Zunyi Medical College.

2.2. PH Model and Experimental Protocol. The rats were given single subcutaneous injection with either MCT (50 mg/kg) or equal vehicle as a control after they were acclimatized for 1 week [21]. Then, all rats were randomly divided into 8 groups with 12 rats allocated to each group as follows: control, model, ICA (20, 40, and 80 mg/kg/d, intragastric administration), and SIL (25 mg/kg/d, intragastric administration). For

analyzing whether the effects of ICA on PH model were related to NO/cGMP signaling pathway, two groups were given L-NAME (20 mg/kg/d, intragastric administration) combined with ICA (40 mg/kg/d, intragastric administration) or L-arg (200 mg/kg/d, intraperitoneal injection), respectively. All animals received equal volume of vehicle for different reagents. On the 8th day after MCT injection, the animals were treated according to the above protocol for 3 consecutive weeks. All rats were weighed every 2 days to enable dose adjustment during this period.

2.3. mPAP Measurement. All surviving rats were anesthetized with pentobarbital sodium (50 mg/kg, intraperitoneal injection). For assessment of mPAP, a central venous catheter (Secalon, 16 G/1.6 × 400 mm, Viggo pruducts, Swindon, UK) was bent about 90 degrees with the help of a thin metallic wire and took shape in 60°C water for 10 min at tip of catheter in advance. The catheter connected to a pressure transducer was inserted firstly into the right subclavian vein at 0.5 cm overhead clavicle and advanced into the RA, RV, and PA. Whether the catheter had reached the pulmonary artery was judged on the basis of changes of the pressure curve shown on a monitor connected to a Powerlab system (ADInstruments, Sydney, Australia).

2.4. Surgical Operation and Tissue Harvest. After the final hemodynamic assessment, arterial blood (0.5 mL) was collected from another catheter placed in right carotid artery and isolated completely from air for measurement of partial pressure of oxygen and carbon dioxide by Cobas b123 type Blood Gas Analyzer (Roche, Basel, Switzerland). Then, all animals were euthanized by exsanguination. The heart was removed quickly, and RV and the left ventricle with septum were separated and weighed separately, and the right ventricle hypertrophy index (RVHI) for each rat was calculated using the following formula: RV weight/(LV + septum) weight × 100%. The right lung tissue and pulmonary artery were together separated, the lung tissue was subsequently perfused with 30 mmHg perfusion pressure by pulmonary artery with 10% buffered formalin until without blood in lavage fluid, and then the right lower pulmonary lobe was fixed in 10% buffered formalin for histological analysis. The left lungs were separated, washed with cold physiological salt solution, and kept in liquid nitrogen for biochemical analysis.

2.5. Measurement of cGMP and NO Level in Lung Tissue. Lung tissues separated for cGMP and NO level assay were put into 1 mL PBS buffer solution (137 mM NaCl, 2.7 mM KCl, 4.3 mM NaH_2PO_4, and 1.4 mM K_2HPO_4, pH 7.4) and homogenized using a manual tissue homogenizer and then centrifuged (3000 rpm, 4°C, 10 min). The supernatant was collected, and the protein concentrations in supernatant were detected using the BCA protein assay Kit (Beyotime, Shanghai, China). The contents of the target substance per milligram of protein were standardized in accordance with the protein concentration of corresponding samples. The levels of cGMP were detected using Enzyme-linked Immunosorbent Assay Kits (R&D System, Minneapolis, USA). NO is rapidly oxidized to nitrite and nitrate which are used to quantitate

NO production, and nitrite and nitrate levels were assayed by a Nitric Oxide Colorimetric Assay Kit (Biovision, Milpitas, USA) according to the manufacturer's instruction. In the text nitrite and nitrate levels were still expressed in NO.

2.6. Western Blot Assay. The frozen lung tissue samples conserved in liquid nitrogen were cut into pieces and put into 1 mL RIPA lysing buffer supplement with 1 nM PMSF (Beyotime, Shanghai, China). The samples were homogenized using a manual tissue homogenizer and then centrifuged (12000 ×g, 4°C, 10 min) and the supernatants were collected. Total protein in supernatants was quantified by BCA protein assay Kit (Beyotime, Shanghai, China) and subjected to Western blot analysis. Each sample (containing protein 100 µg) was hyperthermally denatured at 95°C for 5 min and electrophoretically separated on 5 to 10% gradient SDS-PAGE gels and transferred to a PVDF (0.45 µm) membrane. The membranes were blocked with 5% defatted milk in PBS buffer for 2 h at room temperature and then incubated, respectively, with anti-PDE5 polyclonal antibody (1 : 500, Abcam, Cambridge, USA), anti-eNOS polyclonal antibody (1 : 1000, Abcam, Cambridge, USA), and anti-β-actin monoclonal antibody (1 : 2000, Abcam, Cambridge, USA) at 4°C overnight, followed by incubation with an appropriate horseradish peroxidase conjugated secondary antibody at room temperature for 2 h with gentle rotation. The membranes were visualized using chemiluminescence reagent BeyoECL Plus (Beyotime, Shanghai, China). The image was scanned and band densities were quantified using Quantity One 1D analysis software v4.52 (BioRad, Hercules, USA). β-actin was used to normalize protein loading.

2.7. RNA Isolation and Real-Time RT-PCR. Total RNA was isolated from lung tissue using Trizol™ (Beyotime, Shanghai, China) and purified by RNeasy mini kit (Qiagen Co., Valencia, USA). Reverse transcription of total RNA was performed with MuLV reverse transcriptase and OligodT primer. iCycler iQ Real-Time PCR Detection System (BIO-RAD Co., CA, USA) was employed to execute Real-Time Polymerase Chain Reaction (PCR) with SYBR® Green PCR Master Mix (ABI Co., Foster, USA). The primers were designed and synthesized by TaKaRa Biological Engineering Com (TaKaRa, Dalian, China). The following primers were used: eNOS (GenBank Acc. NM_021838.2) forward, 5-CAA GAC CGA TTA CAC GAC ATT GAGA-3, reverse, 5-TGA GGA CTT GTC CAA ACA CTC CAC-3 (148 bp product); PDE5 (GenBank Acc. NM_133584.1) forward, 5-AAT TGG AGG CAC GCC TTT AACA-3; reverse, 5-TCA TGG CTT AAA GCG GCA ATC-3 (122 bp product); β-actin (GenBank Acc. NM_031144.2) forward, 5-GGA GAT TAC TGC CCT GGC TCC TA-3; reverse, 5-GAC TCA TCG TAC TCC TGC TTG CTG-3 (150 bp product). The reactions conditions were as follows: (1) 95°C 8 min 1 cycle; (2) 95°C 15 s 60°C 1 min 40 cycles. The results (Ct values) of target gene were normalized with β-actin of the same sample and expressed relative to controls.

2.8. Histomorphology Assay. Lung tissues from the same location (marginal right lower pulmonary lobes) were harvested from the surviving rats and immersed fully and fixed with 4% paraformaldehyde solution for 8 h and then embedded in paraffin wax. Tissue blocks were sectioned to 5 µm in thickness and stained with hematoxylin & eosin (H&E) according to common histopathological procedures. Pulmonary artery remodeling was assessed by measuring the area of vessels wall (diameter 50 to 100 µm) [17]. Arterial wall and section areas were measured by an observer, who was blinded to the treatments of the rats; the measurements were conducted under 200x magnification with a microscope (Leica, Wetzlar, Germany) and computerized morphometric system with the software LAS 3.8 (Leica microsystem, Heerbrugg, Switzerland). The percentage of arterial wall area was calculated according to the following formula: arterial wall area/arterial section area × 100% [18].

2.9. Statistical Analysis. All data were presented as mean ± SD and analyzed statistically using the SPSS 19.0 software (SPSS Inc., Chicago, USA). Survival curves were derived by the Kaplan-Meier method and compared by Log-Rank tests. The normality of other data was analyzed statistically by the K-S test. The normal-distributed data firstly were analyzed statistically via one-way analysis of variance (ANOVA), and the statistical significance of difference between two groups was determined using LSD method if equal variance or Dunnett's T3 method if missing variance. Statistical significance was accepted at $p < 0.05$.

3. Results

3.1. ICA Administration Enhances Survival Rates of MCT-PH Model Rats. Just 10 days after MCT injection, rats started to die in model group and ICA20 group; subsequently rats in all groups intermittently died except control group. The survival rate of model group was 42% at the 28th day after MCT treatment, which was notably lower than control group (100%) ($p < 0.05$); the survival rates in ICA and L-arg treatment groups increase (they were 58.3%, 75%, 75%, and 66.7% in ICA20, ICA40, ICA80, and L-arg groups, resp.). The survival rate of L-arg (200 mg/kg/d) with L-NAME (20 mg/kg/d) group and ICA (40 mg/kg/d) with L-NAME (20 mg/kg/d) group was, respectively, 66.7% and 58.3%, but there was no statistical difference in comparison with that in the ICA40 group and the L-arg group ($p > 0.05$).

3.2. ICA Treatment Decreases mPAP and Ameliorates Right Ventricle Hypertrophy in MCT-PH Model Rats. The effects of ICA on mPAP and RVHI are shown in Figures 2 and 3. The mPAP value in model group was 53.5 ± 6.7 mmHg, showing a significant elevation compared with the control group (16.2 ± 3.2 mmH) ($p < 0.05$), and RVHI also increased from 16.2 ± 3.1% in the control group to 32.8 ± 3.8% in the model group ($p < 0.05$). Sildenafil (25 mg/kg/d), a PDE-5 inhibitor, conspicuously decreased the mPAP (26.2 ± 8.5 mmHg) and ameliorated right ventricle hypertrophy (RVHI 25.9%) ($p < 0.05$). The data have shown that PH model was successfully

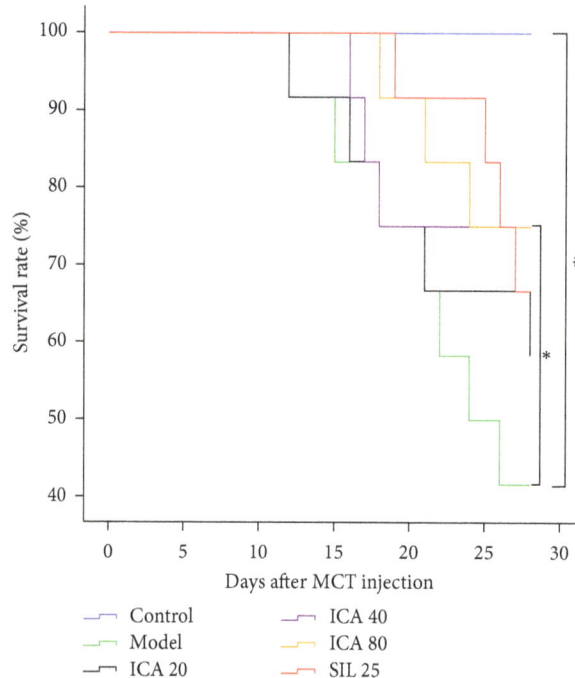

FIGURE 1: Effect of ICA on survival rates. Dose: mg/kg/d. Mortality was observed daily and the figure shows the survival rate at each time point, setting the survival rate at the start of model established as 100%. In order to easily read, the survival rates data of L-arg treatment groups, L-arg (200 mg/kg/d) with L-NAME (20 mg/kg/d) group, and ICA (40 mg/kg/d) with L-NAME (20 mg/kg/d) group are not presented in Figure 1. Compared with control group $^{#}p < 0.05$, compared with model group $^{*}p < 0.05$, Log-Rank test.

established and the test system was reliable. Administration of ICA (20, 40, and 80 mg/kg/d) suppressed the mPAP in a dose-dependent manner. L-arg (200 mg/kg/d) treatment had a similar effect on mPAP. It was notable that L-NAME (20 mg/kg/d), a NOS inhibitor, could significantly inhibit the effect of ICA (40 mg/kg/d) and L-arg on mPAP ($p < 0.05$). The inhibitory effects of ICA and L-arg on RVHI were similar to that of mPAP in a consistent manner, and L-NAME had a tendency to inhibit both ICA (40 mg/kg/d) and L-arg effects on RVHI, but there was no statistical difference ($p > 0.05$).

3.3. ICA Treatment Suppresses Lung Vascular Remodeling Induced by MCT in Rats. The normal histomorphology of pulmonary artery was shown in Figure 4(a). It was shown that MCT injection led to a conspicuous artery remodeling, which was characterized by intimal hyperplasia and medial hypertrophy and vascular lumen stenosis in the distal arterioles (Figure 4(b)). ICA-treatment could alleviate the artery remodeling (Figures 4(c), 4(d), and 4(e)) as well as sildenafil and L-arg (Figures 4(f) and 4(g)); the intimal hyperplasia was improved more significantly than medial hypertrophy. When the protective effect of ICA on MCT-induced pulmonary vascular remodeling was analyzed quantitatively by calculating the percentage of the artery wall area and its cross-sectional area, it was found that MCT treatment evoked an increase in percentage to approximately 4 times, administration of ICA significantly decreased the elevated percentage ($p < 0.05$), and it was the same in sildenafil and L-arg groups ($p < 0.05$). L-NAME markedly inhibited protective function of

ICA (40 mg/kg/d) and L-arg ($p < 0.05$) on MCT-induced pulmonary vascular remodeling (Figure 4(j)), similar to its influence on the effects of ICA on mPAP and RVHI.

3.4. ICA Administration Ameliorates Lung Function in MCT-PH Model Rats. In the present study, the partial pressures of arterial blood oxygen and carbon dioxide, a pair of very important indices reflecting the pulmonary function, were checked. It was found that, compared with the control, the arterial blood partial pressure of oxygen significantly decreased (98.7 ± 2.4 mmHg to 62.9 ± 8.5 mmHg) with the retention of carbon dioxide in model group. Administration of ICA could reverse the deterioration of pulmonary function resulting from MCT injection ($p < 0.05$) (Figure 5).

3.5. ICA Enhances Function of NO/cGMP Signaling Pathway in MCT-PH Model Rats. For investigating whether protective effects of ICA on PH induced by MCT were associated with NO/cGMP signaling pathway, mRNA and protein expression of eNOS and PDE5 were investigated, although protein expression of both eNOS and PDE5 had no notable difference between control group and model group ($p > 0.05$), ICA (20, 40, and 80 mg/kg/d) administrations caused a significant difference in protein expression of eNOS ($p < 0.05$), and ICA (40, 80 mg/kg/d) and sildenafil (25 mg/kg/d) treatment decrease the protein expression of PDE5 (Figures 6(a), 6(b), and 6(c)) ($p < 0.05$). The result of Real-Time RT-PCR indicates that ICA upregulates expression of eNOS mRNA and downregulates expression of PDE5 mRNA compared

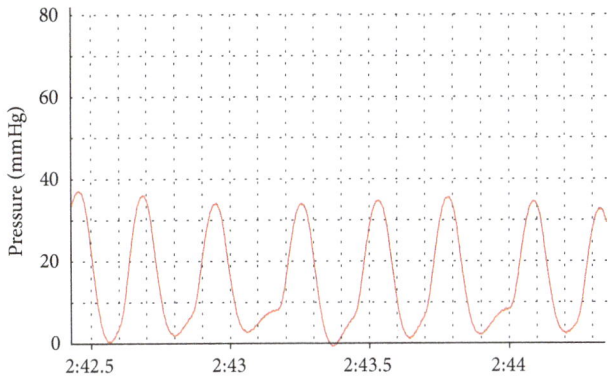

(a)

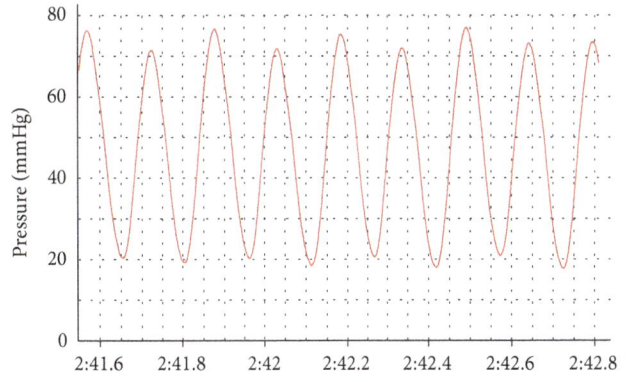

(b)

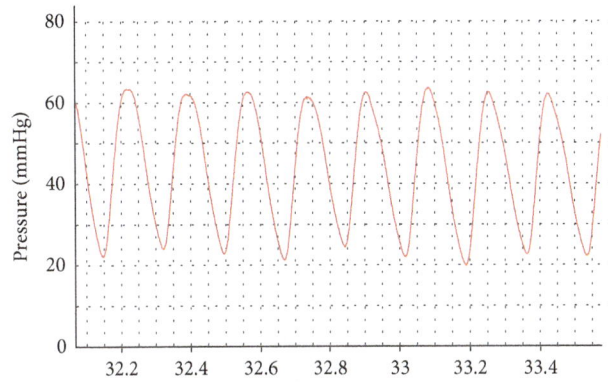

(c)

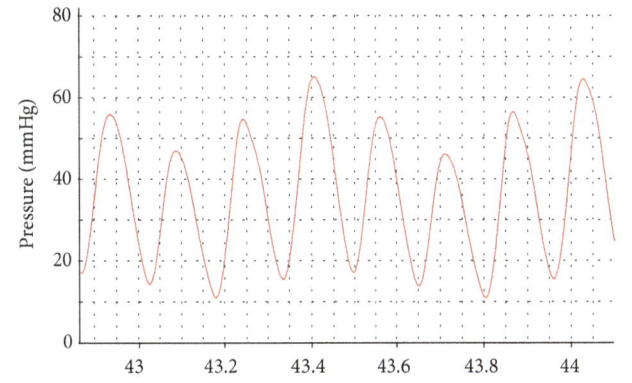

(d)

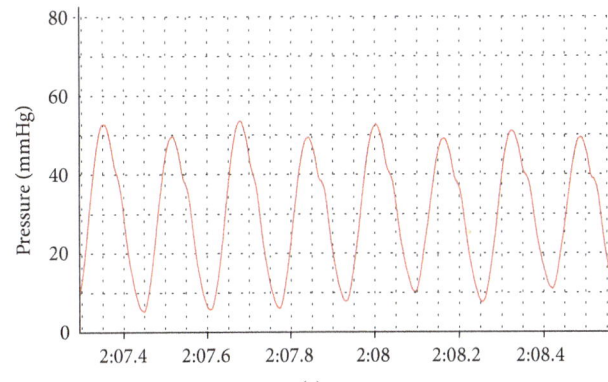

(e)

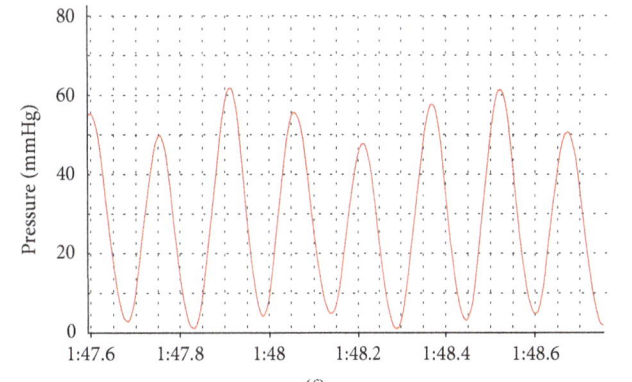

(f)

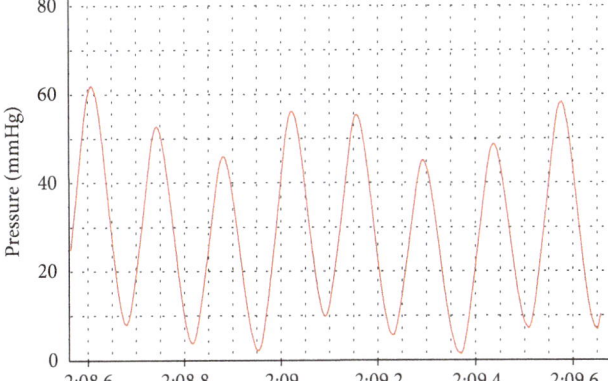

(g)

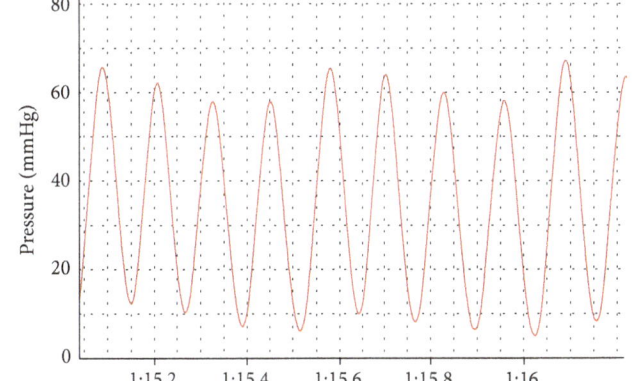

(h)

FIGURE 2: Continued.

(i)

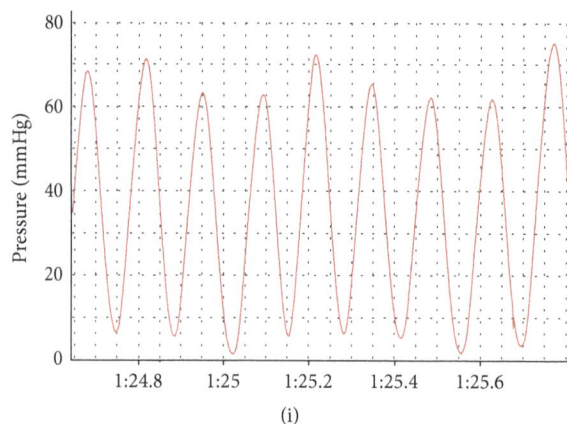

FIGURE 2: Representative pulmonary arterial pressure curve. Groups: (a) control; (b) model; (c) ICA (20 mg/kg/d); (d) ICA (40 mg/kg/d); (e) ICA (80 mg/kg/d); (f) SIL (25 mg/kg/d); (g) L-arg (200 mg/kg/d); (h) ICA (40 mg/kg/d) combining with L-arg (200 mg/kg/d); (i) L-NAME combining with L-arg (200 mg/kg/d).

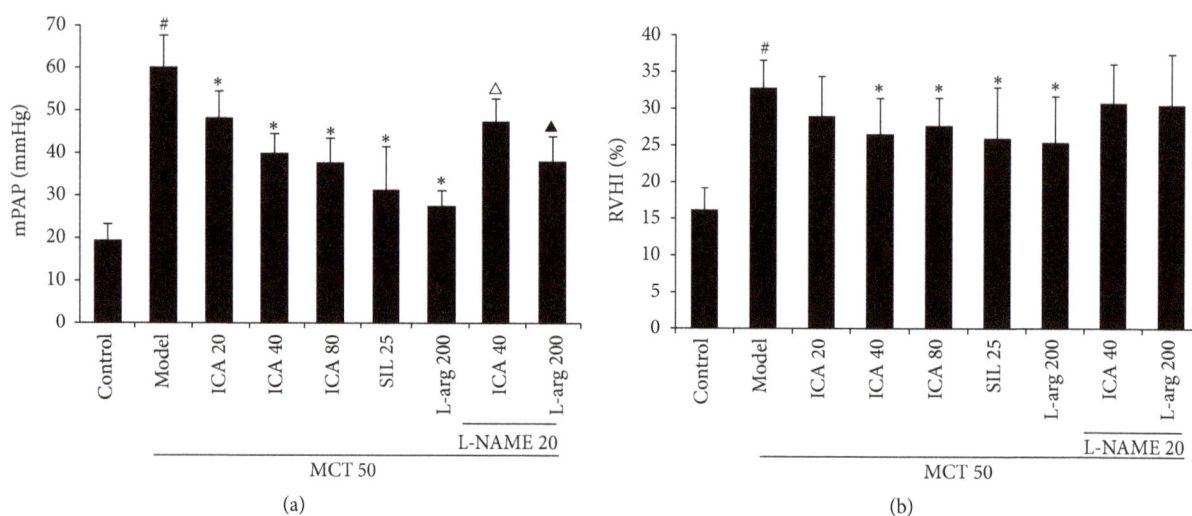

(a)

(b)

FIGURE 3: Effects of ICA treatment on mPAP (a) and RVHI (b) (mean ± SD, n = 5–12). Dose: mg/kg/d. mPAP: mean pulmonary artery pressure; RVHI: right ventricular hypertrophy index. Compared with control group $^{#}p < 0.01$; compared with model group $^{*}p < 0.05$; compared with ICA (40 mg/kg/d) group $^{△}p < 0.05$; compared with L-arg (200 mg/kg/d) group $^{▲}p < 0.05$.

with model group (Figure 6(d)). For further confirming effect of ICA on NO/cGMP signaling pathway, the content of NO and cGMP in lung tissue was measured. Figures 6(e) and 6(f) showed that administration of ICA (40 mg/kg/d) or L-arg (200 mg/kg/d) could significantly increase the contents of NO and cGMP in lung tissue versus model group ($p <$ 0.05). Treatment of L-NAME (20 mg/kg/d), a NOS inhibitor, could abolish the effects of ICA and L-arg on NO and cGMP contents ($p < 0.05$).

4. Discussion

Although the causes and pathogenesis of PH have still not been fully elucidated, the understanding of PH in the recent three decades has made the rapid progress in pathobiological processes and therapeutic targets, which partly benefited from development of PH animal models [22]. The classical rat MCT-PH model was introduced more than 50 years ago [23]. MCT is metabolized by hepatic cytochrome P450 3A and changed to monocrotaline pyrrole, an active form, which injures pulmonary vascular endothelium and causes PH [24], which is characterized by gradually increasing pulmonary arterial pressures and secondary vascular remodeling in 1~2 weeks after MCT single subcutaneous injection [25]. The typical histological changes present in MCT model include intimal hyperplasia, medial hypertrophy, adventitial proliferation/fibrosis, and occlusion of small arteries [26]. With development of the disease, the impairment of heart and lung structures occurs and finally leads to heart failure and respiratory failure [22]. Our study found that, at the end

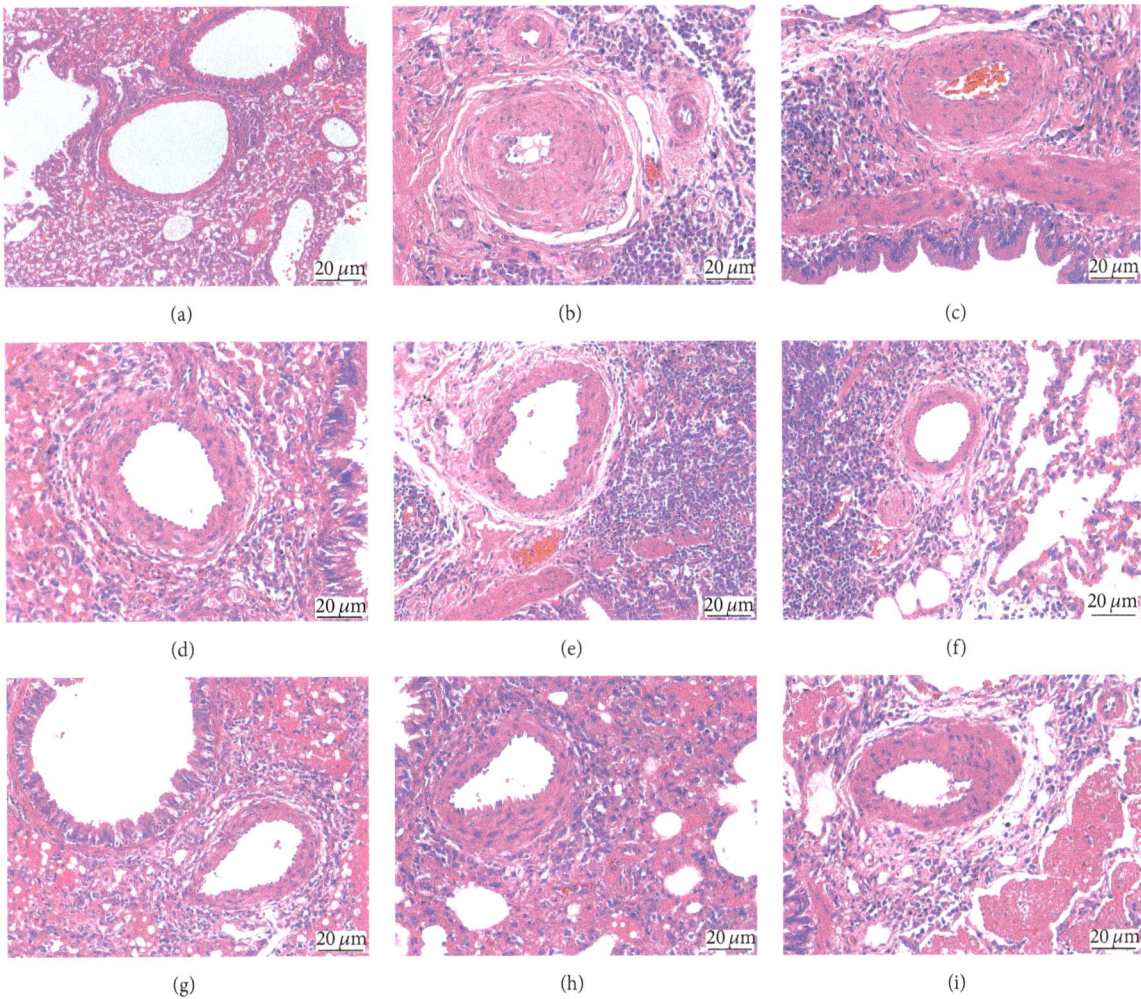

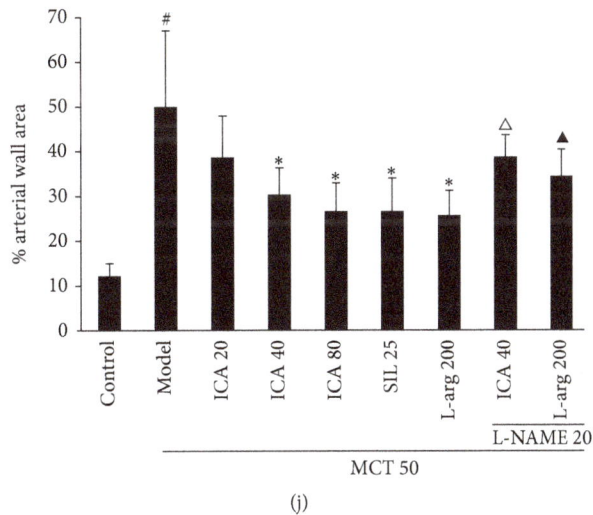

FIGURE 4: Effect of ICA on lung vascular remodeling induced by MCT in rats (mean ± SD, n = 5–12). Dose: mg/kg/d. (a)~(i) Representative images of H&E staining lung sections from every group rats. (j) Bar graph of % pulmonary artery wall area (diameter: 50 to 100 μm). Groups: (a) control; (b) model; (c) ICA (20 mg/kg/d); (d) ICA (40 mg/kg/d); (e) ICA (80 mg/kg/d); (f) SIL (25 mg/kg/d); (g) L-arg (200 mg/kg/d); (h) ICA (40 mg/kg/d) combining with L-arg (200 mg/kg/d); (i) L-NAME combining with L-arg (200 mg/kg/d). Compared with control group [#] $p < 0.05$; compared with model group [*] $p < 0.05$; compared with ICA (40 mg/kg/d) group [△] $p < 0.05$; compared with L-arg (200 mg/kg/d) group [▲] $p < 0.05$.

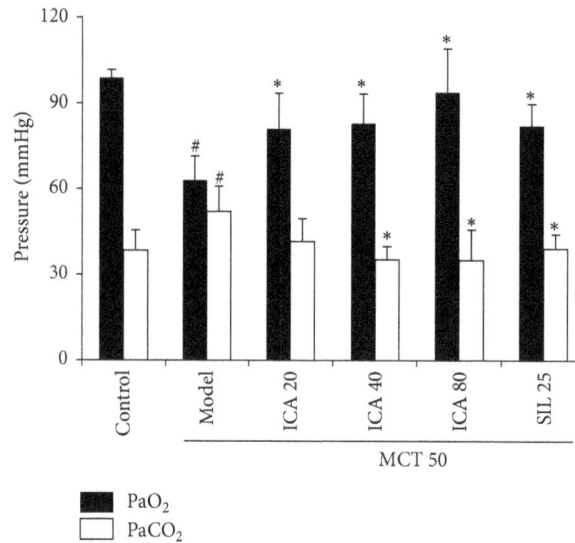

FIGURE 5: Effect of ICA on arterial blood partial pressure of oxygen and carbon dioxide (mean ± SD, $n = 5$–12). Dose: mg/kg/d. PaO_2: arterial blood partial pressure of oxygen; $PaCO_2$: arterial blood partial pressure of carbon dioxide. Compared with control group $^{\#}p < 0.05$; compared with model group $^{*}p < 0.05$.

of the 4th week after MCT injection, a series of pathological changes in rats could be detected, including elevated mPAP, pulmonary artery remodeling, right ventricle hypertrophy, and deteriorated respiratory exchange function, with a lower survival rate. These findings suggested that the model was successfully established.

In the present study, the effects of ICA on PH progression and survival benefit were investigated in MCT-induced PH rats, employing the sildenafil as a positive control. ICA was given by intragastric administration for a period from the 8th day to 28th day after MCT injection, which is the aggressive phase of progression of MCT-PH model and is usually chosen as the therapeutic time window by some investigators. To our attention, ICA 20 mg/kg/d significantly suppressed the increases in mPAP, whereas suppressing effects of ICA 20 mg/kg/d on RVHI and % arterial wall area were not complete in our experiment, suggesting that ICA 20 mg/kg/d dosage was close to minimum effective dose of attenuating MCT-induced PH in rats. Enhancement of reactivity of pulmonary artery to vasoconstrictive substances and pulmonary artery remodeling caused by monocrotaline pyrrole toxicity result in increase of mPAP and compensatory hypertrophy of the right ventricle due to overload in MCT-PH rat model [7], ICA treatment could decrease mPAP in a dose-dependent fashion at doses of 20, 40, and 80 mg/kg/d, and however ameliorated effect of ICA on pulmonary artery remodeling was not significant compared with model group at doses of 20 mg/kg/d level, suggesting that decrease in mPAP in ICA-treated group did not fully result from attenuation of vascular remodeling. On the other hand, degree of right ventricle hypertrophy was notably ameliorated in ICA-treated group due to shrinking of afterload. ICA treatment also significantly extended survival time in dose-dependent fashion with statistical difference at the highest dose. These

results strongly suggested that ICA is an effective reagent of anti-PH induced by MCT.

With the increased understanding of the pathogenesis of PH, many investigators have focused on NO/cGMP signaling pathway as the target of new drug development. In this study, in spite of NO and cGMP content, protein expression of eNOS and PDE5 in lung tissue had no notable statistical difference except expression of eNOS mRNA downregulation and expression of PDE5 mRNA upregulation in the MCT-treated group in comparison to that in the control group. We found that ICA administration could upregulate the expression of eNOS gene at 20, 40, and 80 mg/kg/d dose levels and downregulated the expression of PDE5 gene at 40 and 80 mg/kg/d dose levels in lung tissue of the MCT-injection rats. Further research found that the contents of NO of lung tissue homogenate were significantly increased by ICA with the dose level of 40 mg/kg/d, which coincided with expression changes in the eNOS, and the contents of cGMP were also elevated by ICA with the same dose level that resulted from increasing of NO contents and downregulated the expression of PDE5 protein. For further confirmation of whether or not the anti-PH effect of ICA related to its enhancement of NO/cGMP pathway, we used L-NAME, a NOS inhibitor, to interfere with the effects of ICA on the NO/cGMP pathway, and L-arg was taken in this experiment protocol as a positive control. The results showed that L-NAME could inhibit anti-PH effect of ICA: abolishing the decreasing effect of ICA and L-arg on mPAP, attenuating amelioration of ICA and L-arg on artery remodeling, and abolishing the enhancing effects of ICA and L-arg on NO and cGMP contents. It is similar to the influence of L-NAME on L-arg anti-PH effect. L-NAME-treatment could have tendencies to inhibit the decreasing effect of ICA and L-arg on right ventricle hypertrophy, although there was no

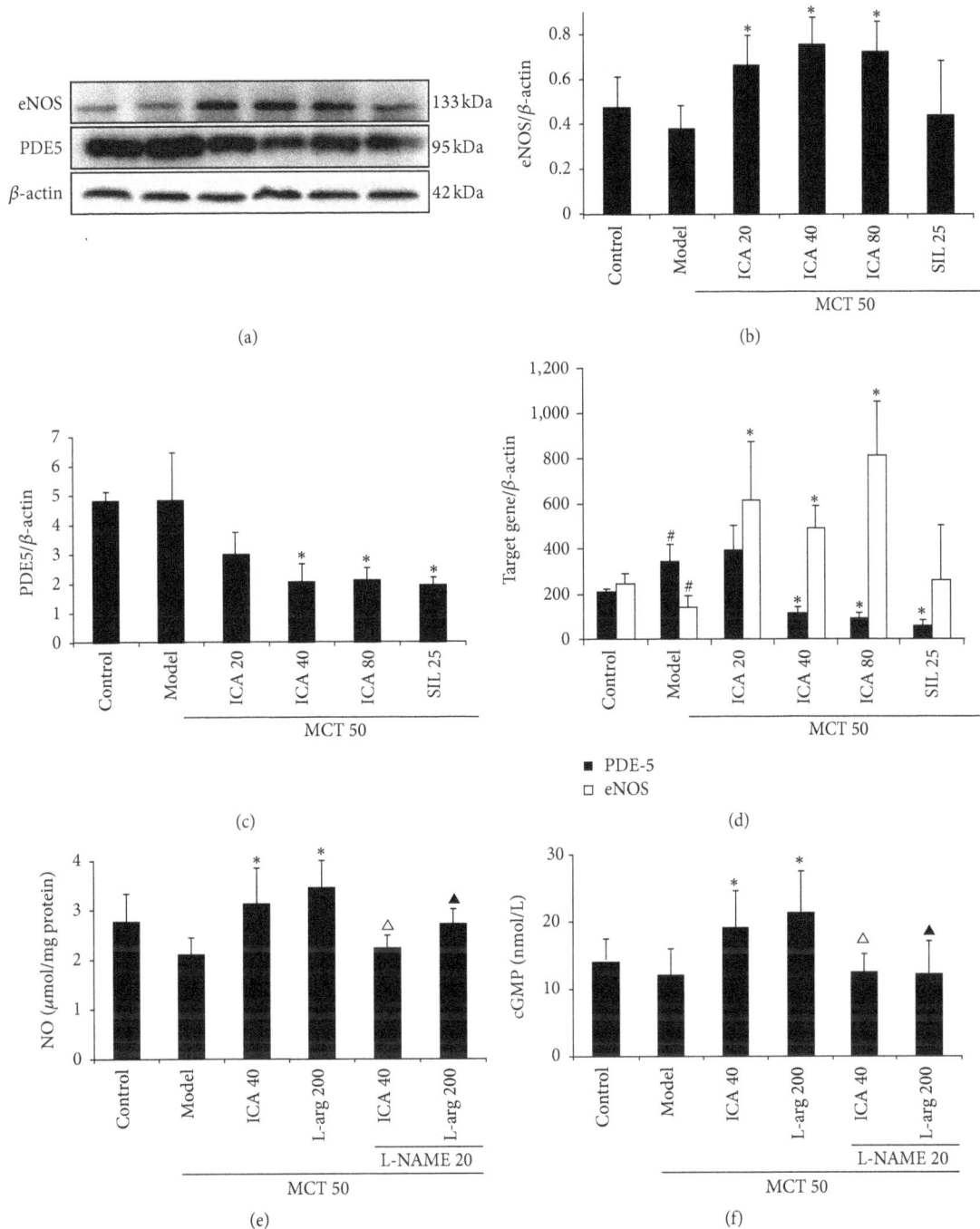

FIGURE 6: ICA enhances function of NO/cGMP signaling pathway in MCT-PH model rats (mean ± SD, n = 5–12). Dose: mg/kg/d. (a) Representative Western blots from lung homogenate; (b) quantitative bar graph of eNOS expression of lung tissue; (c) quantitative bar graph of PDE5 expression of lung tissue. (d) Bar graph of eNOS and PDE5 mRNA expression; (e) bar graph of NO content of lung tissue; (f) bar graph of cGMP content of lung tissue; compared with control group $^{#}p < 0.05$; compared with model group $^{*}p < 0.05$; compared with ICA (40 mg/kg/d) group $^{\triangle}p < 0.05$; compared with L-arg (200 mg/kg/d) group $^{\blacktriangle}p < 0.05$.

statistical difference. From the results, it was very clearly suggested that ICA enhanced the NO/cGMP signal pathway in the lung tissue. Therefore, we believe that the anti-PH effect of ICA is involved in the enhancement of the NO/cGMP pathway.

5. Conclusions

In conclusion, ICA is effective in protecting against MCT-induced PH in rats; the mechanism for its anti-PH may be involved in the enhancement of the NO/cGMP signaling pathway.

Competing Interests

The authors declare that they have no competing interests.

Acknowledgments

This work was supported by National Natural Science Foundation of China (no. 81260654), Guizhou Provincial Department of Education Natural Science Research Projects (Qian Jiao Ke, no. 2011019), and Guizhou Provincial Science and Technology Plan (Subjects SY, Qian Zi (2011) no. 3019).

References

[1] T. Satoh, "Current practice for pulmonary hypertension," *Chinese Medical Journal*, vol. 127, no. 19, pp. 3491–3495, 2014.

[2] S. L. Archer, E. K. Weir, and M. R. Wilkins, "Basic science of pulmonary arterial hypertension for clinicians: new concepts and experimental therapies," *Circulation*, vol. 121, no. 18, pp. 2045–2066, 2010.

[3] C. Guignabert, L. Tu, B. Girerd et al., "New molecular targets of pulmonary vascular remodeling in pulmonary arterial hypertension: importance of endothelial communication," *Chest*, vol. 147, no. 2, pp. 529–537, 2015.

[4] C.-N. Chen, G. Watson, and L. Zhao, "Cyclic guanosine monophosphate signalling pathway in pulmonary arterial hypertension," *Vascular Pharmacology*, vol. 58, no. 3, pp. 211–218, 2013.

[5] J. R. Klinger, S. H. Abman, and M. T. Gladwin, "Nitric oxide deficiency and endothelial dysfunction in pulmonary arterial hypertension," *American Journal of Respiratory and Critical Care Medicine*, vol. 188, no. 6, pp. 639–646, 2013.

[6] Y.-Y. Zhao, Y. D. Zhao, M. K. Mirza et al., "Persistent eNOS activation secondary to caveolin-1 deficiency induces pulmonary hypertension in mice and humans through PKG nitration," *The Journal of Clinical Investigation*, vol. 119, no. 7, pp. 2009–2018, 2009.

[7] F. Sawamura, M. Kato, K. Fujita, T. Nakazawa, and A. Beardsworth, "Tadalafil, a long-acting inhibitor of PDE5, improves pulmonary hemodynamics and survival rate of monocrotaline-induced pulmonary artery hypertension in rats," *Journal of Pharmacological Sciences*, vol. 111, no. 3, pp. 235–243, 2009.

[8] F. Jin, Q.-H. Gong, Y.-S. Xu et al., "Icariin, a phoshphodiesterase-5 inhibitor, improves learning and memory in APP/PS1 transgenic mice by stimulation of NO/cGMP signalling," *International Journal of Neuropsychopharmacology*, vol. 17, no. 6, pp. 871–881, 2014.

[9] K. B. Neves, N. S. Lobato, R. A. M. Lopes et al., "Chemerin reduces vascular nitric oxide/cGMP signalling in rat aorta: a link to vascular dysfunction in obesity?" *Clinical Science*, vol. 127, no. 2, pp. 111–122, 2014.

[10] S. H. Francis, J. L. Busch, J. D. Corbin, and D. Sibley, "cGMP-dependent protein kinases and cGMP phosphodiesterases in nitric oxide and cGMP action," *Pharmacological Reviews*, vol. 62, no. 3, pp. 525–563, 2010.

[11] U. Förstermann and T. Münzel, "Endothelial nitric oxide synthase in vascular disease: from marvel to menace," *Circulation*, vol. 113, no. 13, pp. 1708–1714, 2006.

[12] L. L. Dupont, C. Glynos, K. R. Bracke, P. Brouckaert, and G. G. Brusselle, "Role of the nitric oxide-soluble guanylyl cyclase pathway in obstructive airway diseases," *Pulmonary Pharmacology and Therapeutics*, vol. 29, no. 1, pp. 1–6, 2014.

[13] P. Crosswhite and Z. Sun, "Nitric oxide, oxidative stress and inflammation in pulmonary arterial hypertension," *Journal of Hypertension*, vol. 28, no. 2, pp. 201–212, 2010.

[14] C. Napoli, G. Paolisso, A. Casamassimi et al., "Effects of nitric oxide on cell proliferation: novel insights," *Journal of the American College of Cardiology*, vol. 62, no. 2, pp. 89–95, 2013.

[15] K. Omori and J. Kotera, "Overview of PDEs and their regulation," *Circulation Research*, vol. 100, no. 3, pp. 309–327, 2007.

[16] H. Koizumi, J. Yu, R. Hashimoto, Y. Ouchi, and T. Okabe, "Involvement of androgen receptor in nitric oxide production induced by icariin in human umbilical vein endothelial cells," *FEBS Letters*, vol. 584, no. 11, pp. 2440–2444, 2010.

[17] L. Li, J. Sun, C. Xu et al., "Icariin ameliorates cigarette smoke induced inflammatory responses via suppression of NF-κB and modulation of GR in vivo and in vitro," *PLoS ONE*, vol. 9, no. 8, Article ID e102345, 2014.

[18] M. Dell'Agli, G. V. Galli, E. Dal Cero et al., "Potent inhibition of human phosphodiesterase-5 by icariin derivatives," *Journal of Natural Products*, vol. 71, no. 9, pp. 1513–1517, 2008.

[19] H. Ning, Z.-C. Xin, G. Lin, L. Banie, T. F. Lue, and C.-S. Lin, "Effects of icariin on phosphodiesterase-5 activity in vitro and cyclic guanosine monophosphate level in cavernous smooth muscle cells," *Urology*, vol. 68, no. 6, pp. 1350–1354, 2006.

[20] T. Liu, X.-C. Qin, W.-R. Li et al., "Effects of icariin and icariside II on eNOS expression and NOS activity in porcine aorta endothelial cells," *Beijing Da Xue Xue Bao*, vol. 43, no. 4, pp. 500–504, 2011.

[21] J. Li, C. Long, W. Cui, and H. Wang, "Iptakalim ameliorates monocrotaline-induced pulmonary arterial hypertension in rats," *Journal of Cardiovascular Pharmacology and Therapeutics*, vol. 18, no. 1, pp. 60–69, 2013.

[22] M. G. Dickinson, B. Bartelds, M. A. J. Borgdorff, and R. M. F. Berger, "The role of disturbed blood flow in the development of pulmonary arterial hypertension: lessons from preclinical animal models," *American Journal of Physiology—Lung Cellular and Molecular Physiology*, vol. 305, no. 1, pp. L1–L14, 2013.

[23] J. J. Lalich and L. A. Ehrhart, "Monocrotaline-induced pulmonary arteritis in rats," *Journal of Atherosclerosis Research*, vol. 2, pp. 482–492, 1962.

[24] M. J. Reid, M. W. Lamé, D. Morin, D. W. Wilson, and H. J. Segall, "Involvement of cytochrome P450 3A in the metabolism and covalent binding of 14C-monocrotaline in rat liver microsomes," *Journal of Biochemical and Molecular Toxicology*, vol. 12, no. 3, pp. 157–166, 1998.

[25] B. Meyrick, W. Gamble, and L. Reid, "Development of Crotalaria pulmonary hypertension: hemodynamic and structural study," *The American Journal of Physiology*, vol. 239, no. 5, pp. H692–H702, 1980.

[26] L. Li, C. Wei, I.-K. Kim, Y. Janssen-Heininger, and S. Gupta, "Inhibition of nuclear factor-κB in the lungs prevents monocrotaline-induced pulmonary hypertension in mice," *Hypertension*, vol. 63, no. 6, pp. 1260–1269, 2014.

10

Effects of Zusanli and Ashi Acupoint Electroacupuncture on Repair of Skeletal Muscle and Neuromuscular Junction in a Rabbit Gastrocnemius Contusion Model

Zhan-ge Yu,[1] Rong-guo Wang,[2] Cheng Xiao,[3] Jun-yun Zhao,[4] Qian Shen,[5] Shou-yao Liu,[6] Qian-wei Xu,[7] Qing-xi Zhang,[8] and Yun-ting Wang[9]

[1]*Department of Graduate School, Beijing University of Chinese Medicine, Beijing 100029, China*
[2]*College of Acupuncture-Moxibustion and Tuina, Beijing University of Chinese Medicine, Beijing 100029, China*
[3]*Institute of Clinical Medicine, China-Japan Friendship Hospital, Beijing 100029, China*
[4]*School of Basic Medical Science, Beijing University of Chinese Medicine, Beijing 100029, China*
[5]*Department of Tuina, Dongfang Hospital, Beijing University of Chinese Medicine, Beijing 100078, China*
[6]*Department of Traditional Chinese Medicine Surgery, China-Japan Friendship Hospital, Beijing 100029, China*
[7]*Department of Traditional Chinese Medicine, Northern Hospital, Beijing 100029, China*
[8]*Department of Graduate School, Peking University of Health Science Center, Beijing 100029, China*
[9]*Department of Orthopedics, China-Japan Friendship Hospital, Beijing 100029, China*

Correspondence should be addressed to Yun-ting Wang; yunting1118@sina.com

Academic Editor: Manel Santafe

Objective. To explore the effects of electroacupuncture (EA) at ST36 (EA-ST36) and at Ashi acupoints (EA-Ashi) on skeletal muscle repair. *Methods.* Seventy-five rabbits were randomly divided into five groups: normal, contusion, EA-Ashi, EA-ST36, and EA at Ashi acupoints and ST36 (EA-AS). EA (0.4 mA, 2 Hz, 15 min) was applied after an acute gastrocnemius contusion. The morphology of myofibers and neuromuscular junctions (NMJs) and expressions of growth differentiation factor-8 (GDF-8), acetylcholinesterase (AChE), Neuregulin 1 (NGR1), and muscle-specific kinase (MuSK) were assessed 7, 14, and 28 days after contusion. *Results.* Compared with that in contusion group, there was an increase in the following respective parameters in treatment groups: the number and diameter of myofibers, the mean staining area, and continuities of NMJs. A comparison of EA-Ashi and EA-ST36 groups indicated that average myofiber diameter, mean staining area of NMJs, and expressions of AChE and NRG1 were higher in EA-Ashi group, whereas expression of GDF-8 decreased on day 7. However, increases in myofiber numbers, expressions of MuSK and AChE, as well as decreases in GDF-8 expression, and the discontinuities were observed in EA-ST36 group on the 28th day. *Conclusion.* Both EA-ST36 and EA-Ashi promoted myofiber regeneration and restoration of NMJs. EA-Ashi was more effective at earlier stages, whereas EA-ST36 played a more important role at later stages.

1. Introduction

A contusion is a common sports injury and involves approximately 12.1% of all skeletal muscles disorders [1]. Contusions considerably impact people's lives and productivity [2]. The current treatment for acute skeletal muscle injury typically leads to secondary injury due to scar tissue formation [3].

In recent years, researches have focused on treating skeletal muscle injuries with growth factors, genetic engineering, and stem cell therapy. However, they have side effects and their clinical application is controversial [4]. Based on the meridian theory of traditional Chinese medicine (TCM), electroacupuncture (EA) plays a therapeutic role in conjunction with trace current wave stimulation to acupoints. Due to the curative effects of EA for skeletal muscle injuries [5], there is an increasing amount of research on skeletal muscle regeneration via EA [6].

Our preliminary study confirmed that EA at both Ashi acupoints and Zusanli (ST36) acupoint (EA-AS) could promote the regeneration of muscle [7] and improve the electrophysiological properties of the rabbit gastrocnemius (GM) after contusion [8]. However, the respective roles and mechanisms of EA at Ashi acupoint (EA-Ashi) and ST36 (EA-ST36) in skeletal muscle repair remain unclear.

In order to understand more details of the treatment and provide a laboratory basis for making better clinical decisions, we designed the present study to (1) determine whether EA-ST36 or EA-Ashi could improve skeletal muscle and neuromuscular junctions (NMJs) repair and (2) investigate the individual characteristics of EA-ST36 treatment and EA-Ashi treatment in the repair in a rabbit model with a GM contusion. To attain these goals, we evaluated the morphology of myofibers and NMJs. Furthermore, the mechanisms of the treatments were assessed by the following parameters: the expression of growth differentiation factor-8 (GDF-8) for muscle fiber regeneration, acetylcholinesterase (AChE) content, muscle-specific kinase (MuSK), and Neuregulin 1 (NGR1) for NMJ restoration.

2. Materials and Methods

2.1. Animal Models, Experimental Groups, and Treatment.
Seventy-five New Zealand white rabbits (male or female, 2.0 ± 0.5 kg) were randomly divided into five groups: the normal group ($n = 15$), contusion group ($n = 15$), EA-Ashi group ($n = 15$), EA-ST36 group ($n = 15$), and EA-AS group ($n = 15$). All animals had access to food and water ad libitum in temperature ($23 \pm 1^{\circ}$C) and humidity ($50 \pm 5\%$) controlled rooms with 12-hour light-dark cycles. The experimental procedures were approved by the Ethical Committee of the Academy of Medical Sciences and were conducted in accordance with internationally accepted principles for laboratory animal use and care.

The rabbits were positioned with their right sides fixed to the experimental table after anesthesia with 3% pentobarbital sodium (30 mg/kg of body weight) through the marginal vein of the ear. The hindlimb was set by extending the knee and dorsiflexing the ankle to 90° to fully display the GM. The crushing machine was used to create a contusion with the drop-mass technique using 9.555 J of energy. The injured area was approximately 1 cm^2 on the muscle bellies of the GM. The skin was confirmed to be intact, and there were no fractures.

To keep the injury site dry and avoid infection, 25 g/L anerdian was applied topically once per day. The animals were treated with EA 24 hours after contusion. In the EA-ST36 group, the main needle (anode (diameter: 0.25 mm, length: 25 mm), Zhongyan Taihe Medical Instruments Co. Ltd., Beijing, China) was inserted into ST36 (according to World Health Organization standards) [9] of the normal hindlimb with a depth of 15 mm. Then, the auxiliary needle (cathode) was placed 5 mm away from the main needle. On the injured hindlimb of rabbit in the EA-Ashi group, Ashi

acupoints were located 10 mm from the proximal end (as the anode) and distal end (as the cathode) of the contusion midpoint. The acupoints in EA-AS group selected ST36 in the normal hindlimb and Ashi acupoints of the injured hindlimb of rabbit. When the needles were placed, all of the electrodes were stimulated synchronously with identical parameters (0.4 mA, 2 Hz, 15 min) using Han's acupoint nerve stimulator (Han's 200E, Nanjing Jisheng Medical Co. Ltd., Jiangsu, China) (Figure 1(b)). The rabbits in the contusion group and normal group received mock EA treatments, with the fixed position and time in the treatment groups but without EA treatments [10] (Figure 1(a)).

2.2. Material Collection.
Five rabbits from each group were sacrificed by the air embolism method randomly on the 7th, 14th, and 28th day after contusion. The injured area of the GM was cut vertically into four equal parts after being washed by prechilled PBS. The first tissue (approximately $1.5 \times 1.0 \times 0.5$ cm) was fixed in 4% paraformaldehyde for 24 hours. Then, the specimen was placed in 15% or 30% sucrose solution (mass fraction) until it sank down to the bottom of the container. After being embedded by optimum cutting temperature compound (4583, SAKURA, CA, USA), the samples were cut into 30 μm sections parallel to the direction of the myofibers. The sections were stored at 4°C after drying at room temperature for immunofluorescence staining. Another set of samples was fixed in 4% formalin for 3 days and then processed via gradient alcohol dehydration and paraffin embedding. Then cut into 5 μm sections, alcohol dewaxing and hydration were performed for hematoxylin-eosin (HE) and immunohistochemical staining. The remaining tissue portions were wrapped in foil, frozen in liquid nitrogen, and stored at −80°C for enzyme-linked immunosorbent assay (ELISA) and quantitative real-time polymerase chain reaction (QRT-PCR).

2.3. HE Staining of the Myofiber Morphology.
After hydrating the tissue, the slides were dipped into a Coplin jar containing Mayer's hematoxylin and agitate for 30 sec. The slides were stained with 1% eosin Y solution for 10–30 sec via agitation and then rinsed in H$_2$O for 1 min. The sections were then dehydrated with two applications of 95% alcohol and two applications of 100% alcohol for 30 sec each. The alcohol was then extracted with two applications of xylene. One drop of mounting medium was added, and the samples were covered with a coverslip. The slides were recorded and analyzed by microscopy (Zeiss Scope. AI, Carl Zeiss, Germany) with a 20x objective lens. Five random fields of each section were chosen for the analysis of morphological changes of injured skeletal muscles. The number of muscle fibers was recorded while the average diameter was measured in the obtained pictures using Image-Pro Plus Image (IPP, Version 6.0, Media Cybernetics, USA).

2.4. Immunohistochemical Staining of GDF-8.
Tissue sections were placed in 3% H$_2$O$_2$ at room temperature for 10 min, rinsed with distilled water, and immersed in confining liquid for sealing. For the first antibody incubation, GDF-8 (1 : 50)

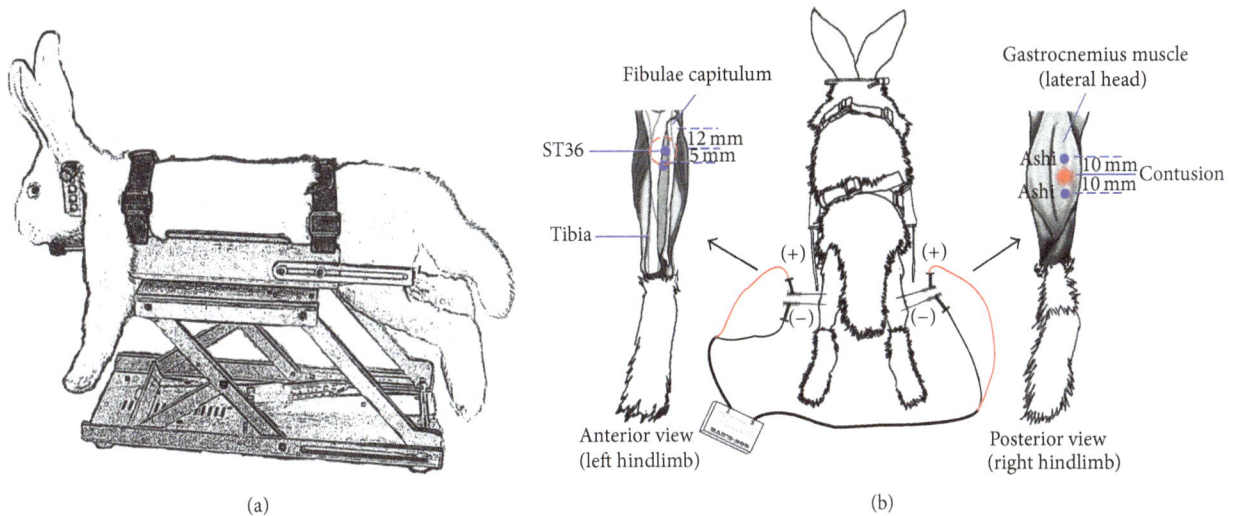

(a) (b)

FIGURE 1: Outline of rabbit restraint and electroacupuncture (EA) stimulation. A specially designed fixator was applied to restrain the rabbits undergoing EA (a). A schematic diagram showing EA stimulation at ST36 and Ashi acupoints (b). ST 36 is located between the tibia and fibula, approximately 12 mm beneath the fibulae capitulum. Acupuncture needles were inserted perpendicularly as deep as 15 mm at left ST36 (anode) and 5 mm away from that (cathode) and kept in place. Another pair of acupuncture needles were inserted into the Ashi acupoints of right hindlimb at a depth of 15 mm, which were located 10 mm from the proximal (anode) and distal (cathode) end of the contusion midpoint. Each of the paired needles was then subjected to a current (0.4 mA, 2 Hz, 15 min) by Han's acupoint nerve stimulator.

rabbit polyclonal antibody (Santa Cruz, CA, USA) was incubated overnight at 4°C. After rinsing with distilled water, the second antibody, horseradish peroxidase- (HRP-) conjugated anti-rabbit IgG (Wuhan Boster Biological Engineering Co. Ltd., China), was incubated at 37°C for 30 min. After rinsing, histochemical stain 3,3′-diaminobenzidine (DAB, Wuhan Boster Biological Engineering Co. Ltd., China) was applied for visualization at room temperature for 10 min. After recording, five fields of each section were chosen, and the mean optical density (MOD) was computed using IPP.

2.5. Assessment of NMJ Morphology. A typical NMJ results from several twisting branches of the motor neurons. Each branch is enlarged to form the terminal synaptic boutons, which contain synaptic vesicles full of the acetylcholine (ACh). Boutons are located over stabilizing invaginations called junctional folds, where high-density clusters of acetylcholine receptors (AChRs) reside [11]. α-bungarotoxin (α-BTX) can bind to AChR. With help of fluorescent dye labeling, the morphological characteristics of NMJs can be observed and measured visually through fluorescent microscopy. The sections were washed with PBS fluid, and, then, marker profiles were obtained using Pap Pen, stained with α-BTX conjugated to rhodamine (T0195, Sigma, USA) (1 : 100, diluted by PBS) and protected from light for 1 hour. The sections were mounted with fluorescence-free glycerol after being washed with PBS fluid. Digital images of the NMJs were obtained with an OLYMPUS FV1000 confocal laser-scanning microscope with an excitation of 480 nm (40x objective for viewing and 60x objective for representative images). Five random NMJs were captured for each section; the maximum intensity flat plane projection was made from Z-stacked images in Image J software (NIH). Only NMJs in

a complete *en face* view were selected for analysis. A Gaussian Blur filter with $\sigma = 2.00$ was applied after background was subtracted and noise despeckled. Mean stained area was quantified from binary images (Figure 2, processed). The connectivity of NMJs was described from skeletonized images (Figure 2, skeletonized) for each pixel via the number of neighbouring pixels. One neighbour implied a terminal pixel, two neighbours implied a pixel along a single branch, and three or more neighbours indicated that a pixel exists at a branch node. The terminal pixels were counted within the NMJ to describe discontinuities [12].

2.6. ELISA of AChE. The protein levels of AChE in the samples were quantified using ELISA. Homogenized tissues blending with equivalent 0.05 mol/L PBS (PH = 8) were coated to microtiter ELISA plates and incubated at 4°C overnight. After washing, the plates were blocked by a 1 h room temperature with 3% BSA. The AChE antibody (ab2803, Abcam Co. Ltd., UK) (0.2 mg/mL) was added to the plates, which were then incubated for 1 h at 37°C. HRP-conjugated anti-rabbit IgG was added to quantify the binding of the secondary antibody. After chromogenic assay by 0.03% o-phenylenediamine and stopping the reaction by the addition of 2 mol/L sulphuric acid, the optical density (OD) was measured on a microplate reader (DNM-9602, Perlong, Beijing, China) at 492 nm. This experiment was carried out twice on different dates under uniform laboratory conditions to avoid internal variations and thus to determine the reproducibility of the assay.

2.7. QRT-PCR for MuSK and NRG1. We used QRT-PCR to evaluate the RNA according to the fluorescence value of

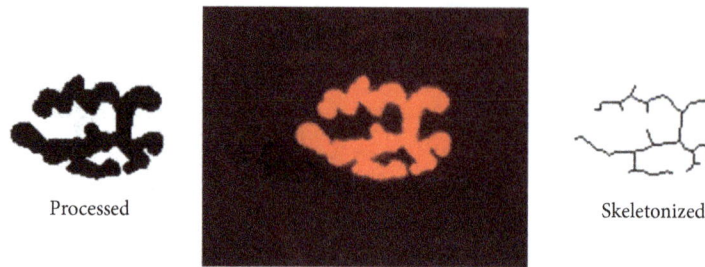

FIGURE 2: Processed and skeletonized images of neuromuscular junction (NMJ). Confocal photomicrograph of the NMJ (middle) was obtained with an OLYMPUS FV1000 confocal laser-scanning microscope. The staining area of NMJ was measured from processed binary images (left) and discontinuity was quantified using pixel positions of skeletonized images (right) generated in Image J (NIH) software.

the amplified exponential phase. Samples were homogenized in Trizol reagent (15596-018, Invitrogen, USA), and total RNA was extracted according to the manufacturer's instructions. Subsequently, RNA was reverse transcribed (Revertaid First Strand cDNa Synthesis Kit, Thermo Scientific K1622, USA), and qRT-PCR was carried out with an ABI 7900HT Sequence Detection System (Applied Biosystems, USA) using SYBR green (SYBR FAST qPCR Kit Master Mix (2x) Universal, KAPA Biosystems, USA). Relative expression was determined by simultaneous comparison to the "housekeeping" gene, actin, using the geNorm software (v3.5, Ghent, Belgium). Transcriptions for MuSK and NGR1 were assessed. The primer sets used for PCR amplification were as follows: Actin-F1, CACACTCCCGCTCAGCTCAC and Actin-R1 GCTTGCTCTGGGCCTCGT; NGR1-F, CTTCGCTGT-GAGACCAGTTCAG and NGR1-R CCAGTGATGCTT-TGTTGATGC; Musk-F TGTTCTCCTGCCTGAGCCTG and Musk-R TTGCGGGTAGGATTCCACTG.

2.8. Statistics. The results were presented as the mean ± standard deviation. The data from each time point were analyzed with the SPSS 20.0 statistical software (SPSS Inc., Chicago, IL, USA). The normal distribution was analyzed using single factor analysis of variance. The groups were compared using the LSD method. The outcomes were evaluated using double-sided inspection. $P < 0.05$ was considered to be statistically significant.

3. Result

3.1. Evaluation of Muscle Regeneration after Contusion. During muscle regeneration, new skeletal muscle fibers exhibited their central nuclei and then matured into periphery nucleated fibers. The regenerative myofiber cytoplasm and large hyperchromatic nuclei were identified in the center of cell using basophilic blue staining [13]. The HE staining results showed that the diameter and volume of the myofibers increased gradually and that the nucleus deviated toward the periphery during the repair process (Figure 3).

3.2. Expression of GDF-8 in Each Group. GDF-8 was a muscle-specific factor in the TGF-β super family and an important myostatin that not only inhibits the regeneration of myofibers but also stimulates the differentiation of

myofibroblasts [14]. Positive immunohistochemical staining of GDF-8 was observed in the cytoplasm of myofibers and fibrocytes (Figure 4).

3.3. Changes in NMJ Morphology in Each Group. Sections were stained with α-BTX for quantification and visualization. NMJs contained many wrinkles and appear to be plump and large "rosette-shaped" under normal conditions. In the samples, the NMJs degenerated and fragmented into oval-shaped patches one week after contusion, resulting in many dispersed synapses. With AChR aggregation, some of the synapses connected to one another, similar to short rods, and became larger in size a week later. NMJs in the contusion area exhibited a higher number of folds and were better stacked on the 28th day (Figure 5(a)). In addition, EA at different acupoints caused the mean stained area and discontinuities of the NMJs to change, as shown in Figures 5(b) and 5(c), respectively.

3.4. AChE Expression in the Muscles. AChE is a pivotal enzyme in cholinergic nerve conduction and an important marker for the function of cholinergic neurons [15]. The protein levels of AChE were assessed by ELISA. The results showed that AChE content was considerably reduced after 7 days in the contusion group compared with that of the normal group. The content increased gradually in the following 3 weeks and approached normal by the 28th day (Figure 6).

3.5. MuSK mRNA and NRG1 mRNA Expressions in the Muscles. NMJs occur in a specialized area of the sarcolemma called the motor end-plate (MEP). Reconstruction of NMJ function requires a large number of AChRs aggregated in the MEP. This process is mainly regulated by the Agrin/MuSK pathway [16]. MuSK is a transmembrane protein tyrosine kinase (PTK) that is expressed and aggregated in the post-synaptic membrane coupled with AChR, which is more important for AChR clusterization regulation than Agrin [17]. Moreover, transcriptional regulation has a pivotal role in AChR clusterization. Recent evidence has indicated that the NRG-1/ErbB pathway is the main signal responsible for the increased transcription of AChR [18]. The expressions of key genes in the aforementioned pathways were tested by QRT-PCR, as presented in Figure 7.

(a)

(b)

(c)

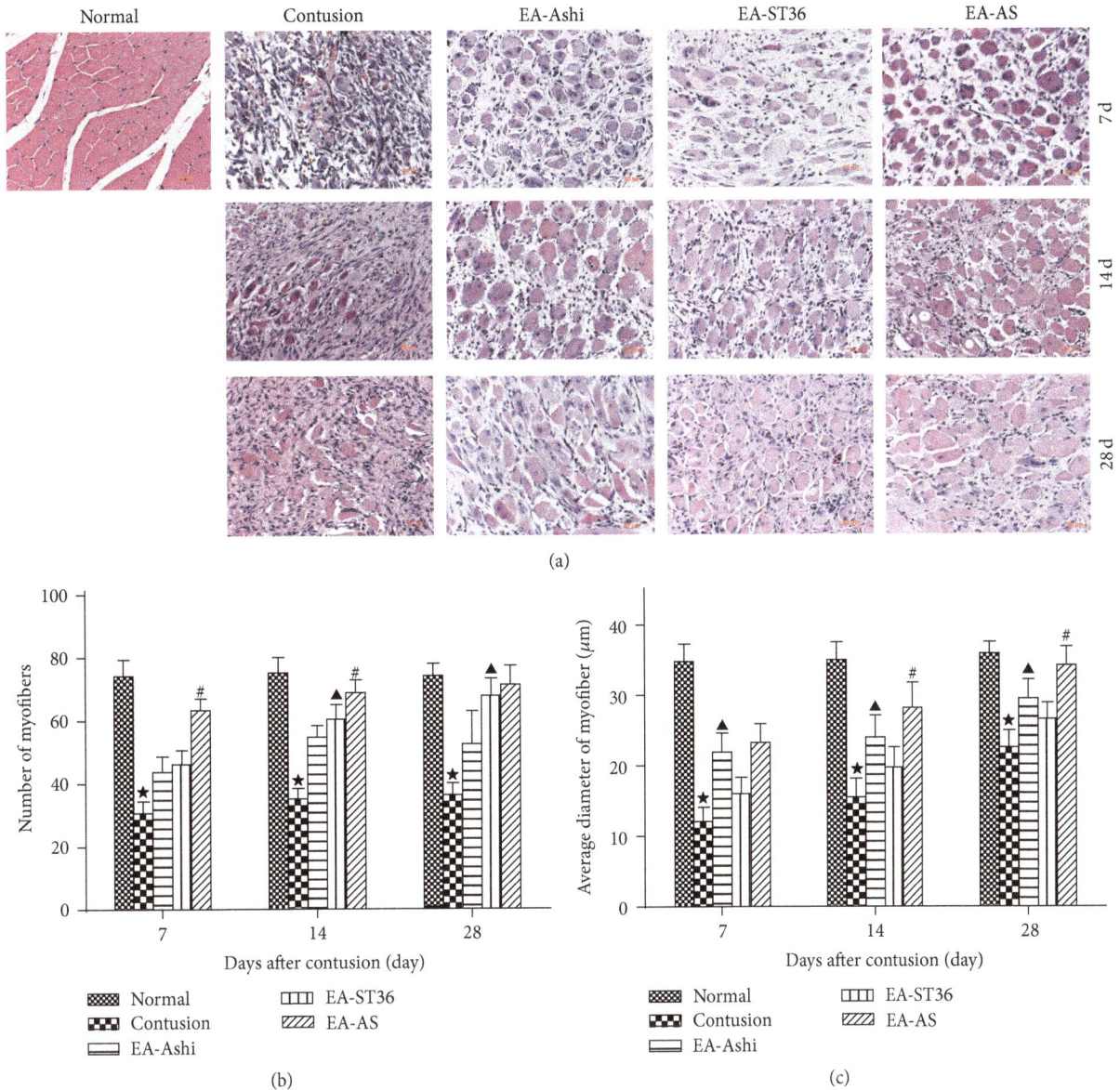

FIGURE 3: Tissue sections were stained with hematoxylin and eosin (HE) to evaluate the general morphology of muscle fibers. HE staining (×200) of normal skeletal muscle revealed fibers uniform in size containing peripherally located nuclei. After contusion, there was skeletal muscle degeneration and necrosis characterized by variation in the size and shape of skeletal muscle fibers, granular and/or hyalinized eosinophilic cytoplasm. Enhanced mononuclear cell infiltration was detected in the connective tissue between muscle fibers. Over time, regenerating myofibers that are centrally nucleated and heterogeneous in size could be detected. By day 28 after contusion, some regenerating fibers were mature, especially in the group receiving EA-AS, peripherally nucleated, and homogeneous in size (a). Quantitative analyses of the number (b) and average diameter (c) of skeletal muscle fibers were administrated on the 7th, 14th, and 28th day after contusion. Compared to the untreated group (contusion), the treatment groups (EA-Ashi, EA-ST36, and EA-AS) showed an increase in number and average diameter of myofibers ($P < 0.05$). EA-ST36 increased more myofiber number especially from two weeks ($P < 0.05$) and EA-Ashi was more effective on enhancing average diameter of myofibers ($P < 0.05$) by comparison between them (EA-Ashi versus EA-ST36, ▲$P < 0.05$; EA-AS versus EA-Ashi and EA-ST36, #$P < 0.05$; contusion group versus treatment groups, ★$P < 0.05$; EA-Ashi, electroacupuncture at Ashi acupoints; EA-ST36, electroacupuncture at ST36; EA-AS, electroacupuncture at Ashi acupoints and ST36; treatment groups (EA-Ashi, EA-ST36, and EA-AS)).

4. Discussion

Clinically, EA is widely applied in skeletal muscle injury treatment [5], and research on the mechanism of EA has attracted increasing attention. TCM held that the basic pathological change after contusion was "qi-stagnation and blood stasis." Therefore, "activating blood and regulating qi" were the key to treatment. According to the theory that "where there is pain, there is an acupoint" in "Miraculous Pivot," the Ashi acupoint near the injured area is typically chosen to treat traumatic injury [19–21]. ST36 is he-sea acupoint on the stomach meridian of foot-yangming, and the yangming

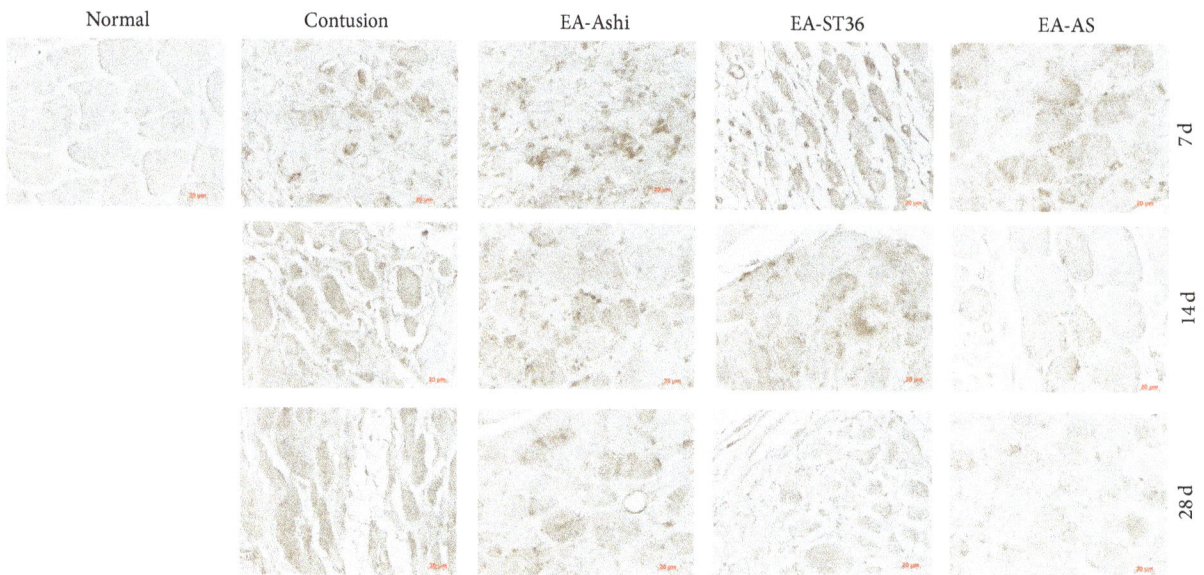

(a)

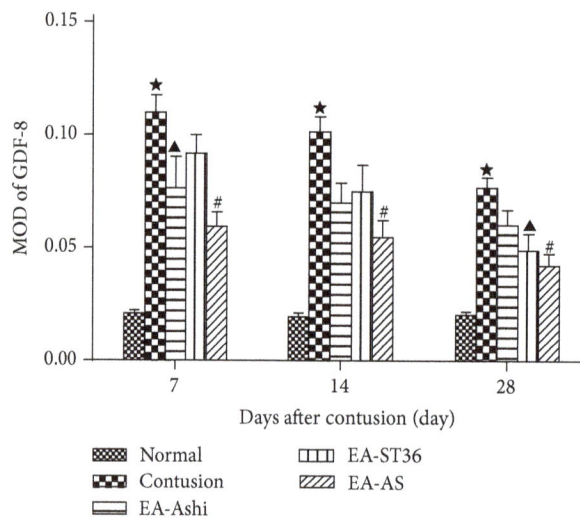

(b)

FIGURE 4: Immunohistochemical staining of growth differentiation factor-8 (GDF-8) in the skeletal muscle. Muscle cytoplasm reacting with GDF-8 was stained brown. The staining of GDF-8 was very weak in the normal muscle tissue. But, after contusion, muscle fibers showed strong immunoreaction for GDF-8 (a, ×400). The expression peaked on the 7th and 14th day and decreased significantly by the 28th day. The mean optical density (MOD) was assessed to quantify expression of GDF-8 in different groups. GDF-8 expression was higher in the contusion group compared to the treatment groups (EA-ST36, EA-Ashi, and EA-AS groups) ($P < 0.05$). Compared with the EA-ST36 group, GDF-8 expression in the EA-Ashi group was lower ($P < 0.05$) on day 7 but became higher on the 28th day ($P < 0.05$) (b) (EA-Ashi versus EA-ST36, ▲$P < 0.05$; EA-AS versus EA-Ashi and EA-ST36, #$P < 0.05$; contusion group versus treatment groups, ★$P < 0.05$; EA-Ashi, electroacupuncture at Ashi acupoints; EA-ST36, electroacupuncture at ST36; EA-AS, electroacupuncture at Ashi acupoints and ST36; treatment groups (EA-Ashi, EA-ST36, and EA-AS)).

meridian is full of blood and qi in meridian theory. Therefore, acupuncture at ST36 could regulate the overall qi and blood circulation and strengthen the healthy qi of the body. Modern research has also demonstrated that acupuncture at Ashi acupoint could activate blood and disperse blood stasis [22]. EA-ST36 could not only protect organisms from injury [23] but also promote general body recovery after injury [24, 25].

In injured skeletal muscle, it is generally accepted that the Ashi acupoint is the injured region. To avoid new injury generated from needles inserted into injured area, Ashi acupoints were not located in the exact contusion midpoint, but rather 10 mm [26] from the proximal and distal end of it in our treatment protocol. To regulate the overall qi (remote effect of ST36) and avoid interfering Ashi acupoints (near to one of the Ashi acupoints), ST36 of the normal hindlimb was selected. Because the distance between the two needles is 1 mm in rat, if there is only one acupoint located ipsilaterally, according to common use in previous

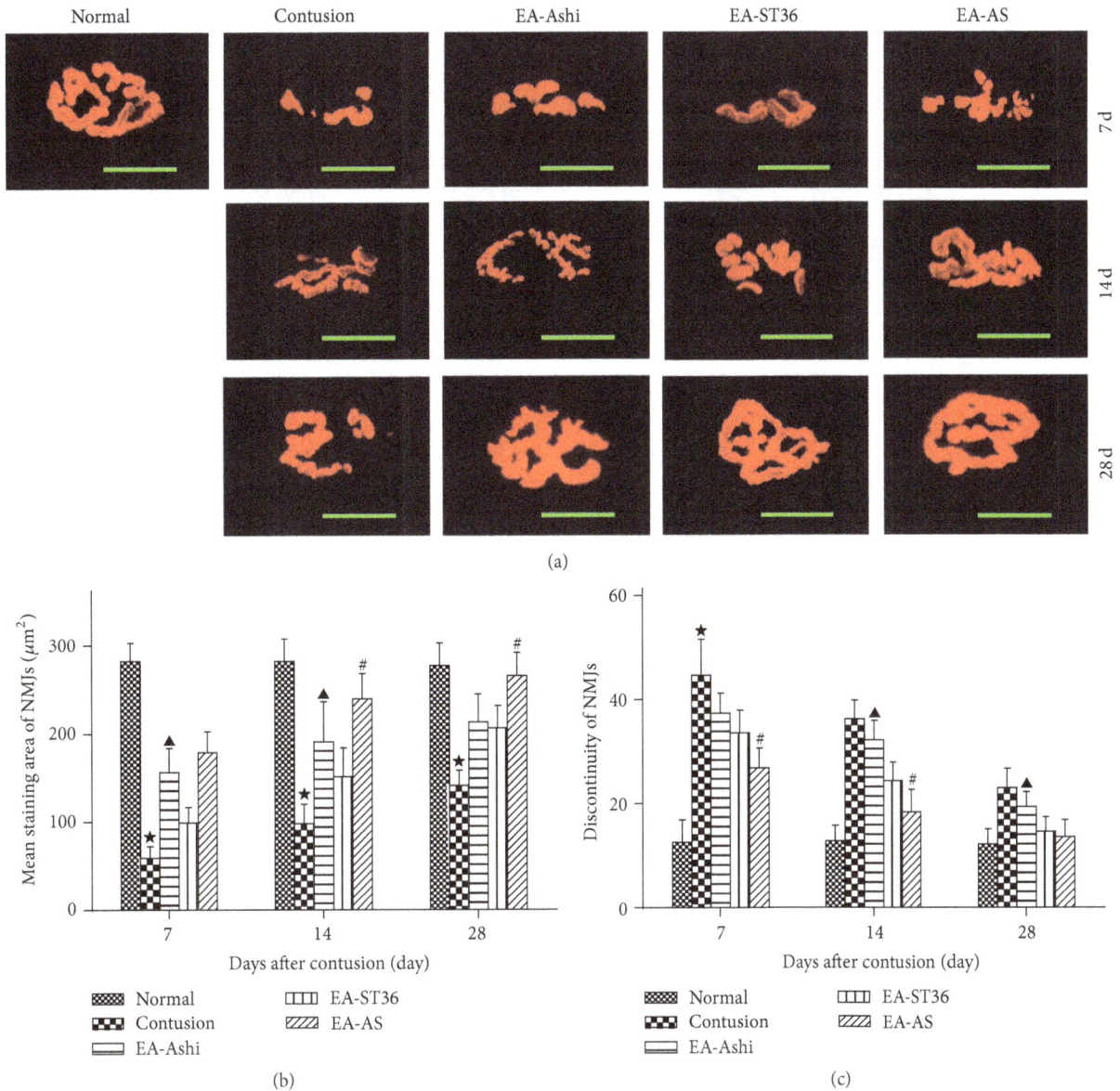

FIGURE 5: Morphology of neuromuscular junctions (NMJs) at different time points after contusion. Postsynaptic NMJ was identified by rhodamine α-bungarotoxin staining for acetylcholine receptors (AChRs) and observed by confocal microscopy. Representative confocal photomicrographs of NMJ (scale scar: 20 μm) displayed the differences among all groups following contusion (a). In normal muscle fibers, AChR clusters were organized in a classical pretzel-shaped structure. NMJs showed a frequent fragmented appearance on day 7 after contusion: AChR staining in muscles was generally dramatically disorganized, with its branches barely discernable. On the 14th and 28th day, NMJs appeared to have some branches and be less fragmented, and the size of the postsynaptic apparatus had increased. Quantitative analysis of NMJs revealed that the mean stained area (b) increased and discontinuities (c) of NMJs decreased gradually during repair. The treatment (EA-Ashi, EA-ST36, and EA-AS) increased mean stained area and reduced discontinuity of NMJs compared to contusion. EA-ST36 decreased more discontinuity ($P < 0.05$), especially at the second and third week, and EA-Ashi was more effective during the first two weeks on enhancing mean stained area of NMJs, by comparison ($P < 0.05$) (EA-Ashi versus EA-ST36, $\blacktriangle P < 0.05$; EA-AS versus EA-Ashi and EA-ST36, $^{\#}P < 0.05$; contusion group versus treatment groups, $\star P < 0.05$; EA-Ashi, electroacupuncture at Ashi acupoints; EA-ST36, electroacupuncture at ST36; EA-AS, electroacupuncture at Ashi acupoints and ST36; treatment groups (EA-Ashi, EA-ST36, and EA-AS)).

studies [27, 28], we made the distance 5 mm in rabbit by a combination of comparative anatomy, simulated bone length measurement, and experimental observation. Earlier experiments confirmed that EA following this treatment protocol could improve the regeneration [7] and electrophysiological properties [8] of myofibers. However, it was unclear whether EA-ST36 and EA-Ashi could individually play a role in promoting the repair. Furthermore, the respective characteristics and mechanism of the effects of the EA-ST36 and EA-Ashi were unclear. This experiment explored the above topics by observing the effects of EA-ST36 and EA-Ashi acupoints on the morphology of skeletal muscle fibers and NMJs as well

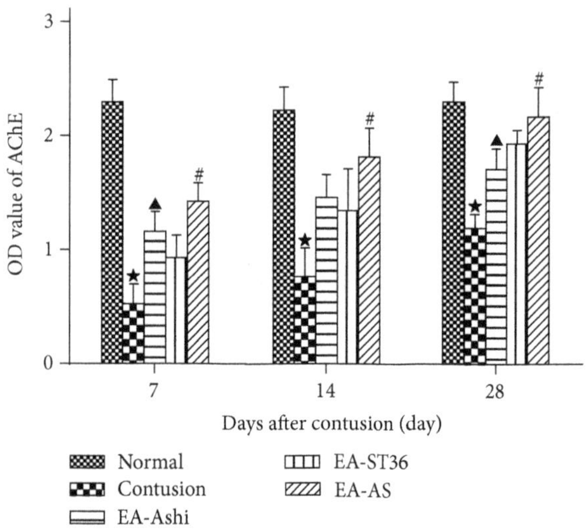

FIGURE 6: Content of acetylcholinesterase (AChE) in the recruited muscles. The optical density (OD) value at 492 nm obtained by ELISA was provided for skeletal muscle samples for the AChE protein. Increases in AChE content were observed in the treatment groups compared to that of contusion group at different time points during repair ($P < 0.05$). Compared with that of the EA-ST36 group, AChE content in the EA-Ashi group was higher on day 7 but became lower on the 28th day ($P < 0.05$) (EA-Ashi versus EA-ST36, ▲$P < 0.05$; EA-AS versus EA-Ashi and EA-ST36), #$P < 0.05$; contusion group versus treatment groups, ★$P < 0.05$; EA-Ashi, electroacupuncture at Ashi acupoints; EA-ST36, electroacupuncture at ST36; EA-AS, electroacupuncture at Ashi acupoints and ST36; treatment groups (EA-Ashi, EA-ST36, and EA-AS)).

as the expressions of GDF-8, AChE, NRG1, and MuSK at different times over the course of repair.

4.1. By Inhibiting the Expressions of GDF-8, EA-ST36 and EA-Ashi Acupoints Could Increase the Number and Diameter of Myofibers. The Effect of EA-ST36 Was Delayed with respect to That of EA-Ashi, but the Long-Term Effect Was Better. After contusion, the number and diameter of muscle fibers in the treatment groups were significantly increased compared to the contusion group, indicating that both EA-ST36 and EA-Ashi could promote skeletal muscle regeneration. The diameter increased more significantly in the EA-Ashi group. This greater increase in diameter might be related to the fact that the electrodes were placed on the distal and proximal ends of the contusions, as muscle fibers might adaptively thicken against the mechanical stretching generated by electrodes [29, 30]. In addition, regional electrical stimulation promoted the growth of denervated muscles [10, 31] or indirectly inhibited the metabolism of myofibers so that they were relatively enlarged [32]. EA-ST36 was more effective in increasing the number of muscle fibers than EA-Ashi, likely because EA-ST36 was more effective in promoting cell proliferation [33] and angiogenesis [24]. The precise mechanisms of action need to be investigated in future research. EA-Ashi was more effective in reducing the expression of GDF-8 on the 7th day, whereas EA-ST36 was more effective two weeks later.

The effect of EA-ST36 was delayed compared to that of EA-Ashi, but the long-term effect was better. A previous study found that regional EA at "Heyang and Feiyang" acupoints (amounting to Ashi acupoints in this study) could lower the expression of myostatin [24]. This research has found that EA-ST36 had a similar function and was more effective on inhibiting the expression of GDF-8 compared to EA-Ashi in the last two weeks.

4.2. Both EA-ST36 and EA-Ashi Promoted the Reconstruction of NMJ and EA-Ashi Could Increase the Expressions of AChR and AChE in the Earlier Stage, Whereas EA-ST36 Could Promote AChR Clusterization and the Expression of AChE at a Later Stage. The most important event in the restoration of a NMJ is the expression and aggregation of AChR on the MEP. In this study, stained α-BTX was used to measure the MEP of the rabbit GM at different time points after muscle damage by confocal laser-scanning microscopy. The mean staining area and discontinuities of the MEPs were calculated. The discontinuities reflected the clusterization of AChRs, whereas the mean staining area represents the volume of AChRs in each NMJ. The majority of NMJs in damage muscle had degraded, appearing as scattered oval-shaped plaques at 7 days after injury, indicating secondary damage to the NMJs after muscle contusion. As AChRs gradually gathered, the NMJ was partially reconstructed after 2 weeks and some cracks appeared. The scattered AChRs connected into sheets, and the NMJ became oval at 4 weeks after contusion, although many NMJs exhibited shrinking and dispersed shapes. Meanwhile, the mean stained area of the NMJs had become larger and the discontinuities had decreased. Aside from shape changes, we also observed that AChE increased gradually from days 7 to 28, indicating that the function of injured NMJs had been restored step by step. In contrast, the NMJs in the treatment groups exhibited fuller shapes with more folds, larger mean staining area, lower discontinuities, and a higher content of AChE, indicating that EA may promote the survival of NMJs and thus play a pertinent role in accelerating their recovery. Previous studies have shown that EA could promote the survival of injured neurons after transection of the neural stem [34] and that electrical stimulation accelerated NMJ formation [35]. These findings provide further support that EA improves the reconstruction of NMJ degeneration following skeletal muscle damage.

Furthermore, increases in the mean stained area of the NMJs and AChE expression were observed in the EA-Ashi and EA-AS groups on days 7 and 14, compared to that of the other groups. The treatments in these groups may potentially be better at increasing the proliferation of AChR in the early stage of repair. Although the mean stained area in EA-ST36 group was lower, the continuities and AChE content increased on 14 and 28 days after contusion, suggesting that the clusterization of AChR and NMJ's function had been enhanced.

We next explored the molecular mechanism of how this happens. As we know, AChR first proliferated after injury and then regressed following clusterization in the reconstruction

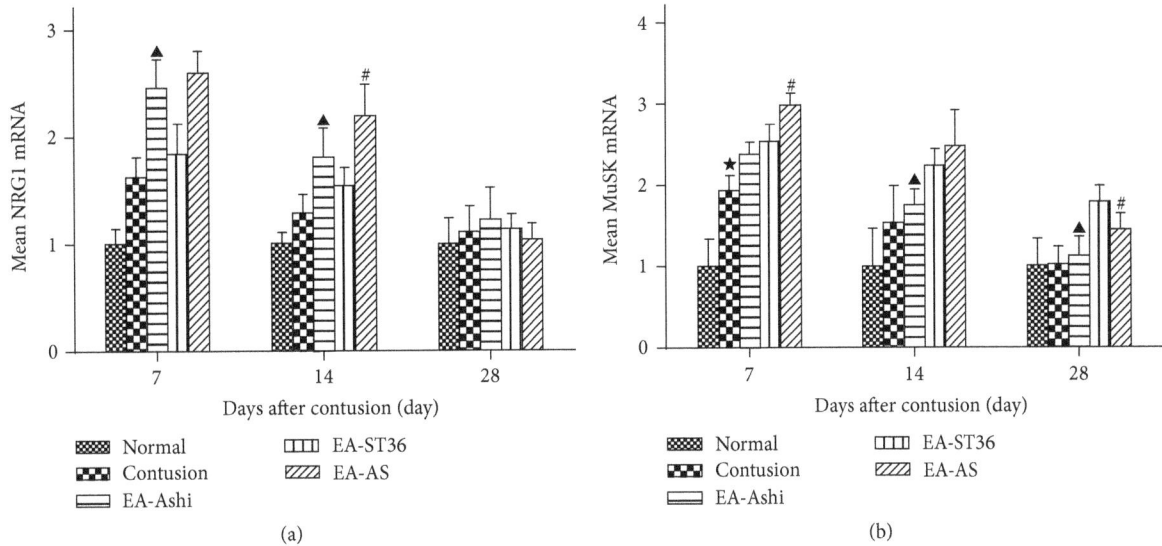

(a)

(b)

FIGURE 7: Comparison of the expression of Neuregulin 1 (NGR1) and muscle-specific kinase (MuSK) at different time points after contusion. QRT-PCR assays were conducted with samples from rabbits to demonstrate the gene expressions of NRG1 (a) and MuSK (b). Both MuSK and NRG1 expressions were increased on the 7th day after contusion and gradually decreased near to normal in the following 3 weeks. Comparison between EA-Ashi and EA-ST36 groups showed that mean NRG1 mRNA in EA-Ashi group was higher than that of EA-ST36 group on day 7 and day 14 after contusion ($P < 0.05$), while mean MuSK mRNA in the EA-ST36 group was lower on the 14th and 28th day ($P < 0.05$) (EA-Ashi versus EA-ST36, ▲$P < 0.05$; EA-AS versus EA-Ashi and EA-ST36, #$P < 0.05$; contusion group versus treatment groups, ★$P < 0.05$; EA-Ashi, electroacupuncture at Ashi acupoints; EA-ST36, electroacupuncture at ST36; EA-AS, electroacupuncture at Ashi acupoints and ST36; treatment groups (EA-Ashi, EA-ST36, and EA-AS)).

and development processes of the NMJ [36]. NRG1 is the key factor responsible for the increased transcription of AChRs and MuSK regulates AChRs clusterization [37]. In this study, expressions of NRG1 and MuSK gradually decreased and remained higher than the normal level on day 14 after contusion, possibly because the injured muscle stayed in a relaxed state after the loss of control from motor neurons, such that the muscle nuclei lost their inhibition by muscle activity [38]. On day 28, the expressions had decreased significantly, whereas the mean staining area of the NMJs and AChE expression had increased, possibly due to the synapse regression to improve the efficiency of synaptic transmission [36]. What is more, increases in the expression of NRG1 were observed in the EA-Ashi and EA-AS groups on days 7 and 14, while the MuSK increased significantly in EA-ST36 and EA-AS groups at the 14th and 28th day, compared to the other groups. These results may illustrate that EA-Ashi was more effective in improving the proliferation of AChR through regulating NRG1 mainly at earlier stages, whereas EA-ST36 was more effective in promoting the clusterization of AChR by regulating MuSK at later stages. By applying ST36 and Ashi acupoints simultaneously, EA could proliferate and cluster AChR more effectively within an appropriate timeframe.

5. Conclusion

In conclusion, in this study, we demonstrate via morphological and molecular biological approaches that both EA-Ashi and EA-ST36 have an effect on the regeneration of

myofibers and restoration of NMJ, leading to muscle repair, possibly through the regulation of GDF-8, AChE, NRG1, and MuSK. EA-Ashi was more effective at earlier stages, whereas EA-ST36 was more effective later on. The combination of these two acupoints achieved a better effect than either one. Therefore, EA-AS is a suggested method for skeletal muscle injury treatment, which combines regional and distal acupoints. Additional molecular investigations are needed to clarify whether it is more effective to increase the stimuli of EA-Ashi and decrease EA-ST36 stimuli at earlier stages and reverse later on than the same stimuli of EA-AS.

Competing Interests

The authors declare that there is no conflict of interests regarding the publication of this paper.

Authors' Contributions

Zhan-ge Yu and Rong-guo Wang contributed equally to this work.

Acknowledgments

This paper is supported by the National Science Foundation of China (no. 81173343) and the "Youth Talent Plan" of Beijing Municipal Colleges and Universities (no. YETP 0795).

References

[1] W. G. Fernandez, E. E. Yard, and R. D. Comstock, "Epidemiology of lower extremity injuries among U.S. high school athletes," *Academic Emergency Medicine*, vol. 14, no. 7, pp. 641–645, 2007.

[2] S.-J. Lee, S. Tak, T. Alterman, and G. M. Calvert, "Prevalence of musculoskeletal symptoms among agricultural workers in the United States: an analysis of the National Health Interview Survey, 2004–2008," *Journal of Agromedicine*, vol. 19, no. 3, pp. 268–280, 2014.

[3] T. M. Best, B. Gharaibeh, and J. Huard, "Stem cells, angiogenesis and muscle healing: a potential role in massage therapies?" *British Journal of Sports Medicine*, vol. 47, no. 9, pp. 556–560, 2013.

[4] L. Baoge, E. Van Den Steen, S. Rimbaut et al., "Treatment of skeletal muscle injury: a review," *ISRN Orthopedics*, vol. 2012, Article ID 689012, 7 pages, 2012.

[5] X.-S. Xu, W.-P. Lin, J.-Y. Chen, L.-C. Yu, and Z.-H. Huang, "Efficacy observation on rear thigh muscles strain of athletes treated with surrounding needling of electroacupuncture and hot compress of Chinese medicine," *Zhongguo Zhen Jiu*, vol. 32, no. 6, pp. 511–514, 2012.

[6] N. Guo, "Treatment of sprain by electro-acupuncture," *Journal of Traditional Chinese Medicine*, vol. 23, no. 2, pp. 119–120, 2003.

[7] R. Wang, D. Luo, C. Xiao et al., "The time course effects of electroacupuncture on promoting skeletal muscle regeneration and inhibiting excessive fibrosis after contusion in rabbits," *Evidence-Based Complementary and Alternative Medicine*, vol. 2013, Article ID 869398, 16 pages, 2013.

[8] S. Liu, R. Wang, D. Luo et al., "Effects of electroacupuncture on recovery of the electrophysiological properties of the rabbit gastrocnemius after contusion: an in vivo animal study," *BMC Complementary and Alternative Medicine*, vol. 15, no. 1, article 69, 2015.

[9] W. Lin and P. Wang, *Experiment Acupuncture Science*, Shanghai Science and Technology Press, Shanghai,China, 1st edition, 1999.

[10] H. Xing, M. Zhou, P. Assinck, and N. Liu, "Electrical stimulation influences satellite cell differentiation after sciatic nerve crush injury in rats," *Muscle and Nerve*, vol. 51, no. 3, pp. 400–411, 2015.

[11] A. G. Engel, "The neuromuscular junction," in *Handbook of Clinical Neurology*, vol. 91, chapter 3, pp. 103–148, 2008.

[12] S. J. P. Pratt, S. B. Shah, C. W. Ward, M. P. Inacio, J. P. Stains, and R. M. Lovering, "Effects of in vivo injury on the neuromuscular junction in healthy and dystrophic muscles," *Journal of Physiology*, vol. 591, no. 2, pp. 559–570, 2013.

[13] D. A. Fischman, "Chapter 7 the synthesis and assembly of myofibrils in embryonic muscle," *Current Topics in Developmental Biology*, vol. 5, pp. 235–280, 1970.

[14] J. Zhu, Y. Li, W. Shen et al., "Relationships between transforming growth factor-β1, myostatin, and decorin: implications for skeletal muscle fibrosis," *Journal of Biological Chemistry*, vol. 282, no. 35, pp. 25852–25863, 2007.

[15] R. L. Rotundo, C. A. Ruiz, E. Marrero et al., "Assembly and regulation of acetylcholinesterase at the vertebrate neuromuscular junction," *Chemico-Biological Interactions*, vol. 175, no. 1–3, pp. 26–29, 2008.

[16] E. Ferraro, F. Molinari, and L. Berghella, "Molecular control of neuromuscular junction development," *Journal of Cachexia, Sarcopenia and Muscle*, vol. 3, no. 1, pp. 13–23, 2012.

[17] S. R. Hubbard and K. Gnanasambandan, "Structure and activation of MuSK, a receptor tyrosine kinase central to neuromuscular junction formation," *Biochimica et Biophysica Acta*, vol. 1834, no. 10, pp. 2166–2169, 2013.

[18] X.-L. Yang, Y. Z. Huang, W. C. Xiong, and L. Mei, "Neuregulin-induced expression of the acetylcholine receptor requires endocytosis of ErbB receptors," *Molecular and Cellular Neuroscience*, vol. 28, no. 2, pp. 335–346, 2005.

[19] J. W. Zhou, F. Zhang, J. J. Zhao, Y. Zhang, and M. Wang, "Clinical observation on Ashi points Sihua needling method for treatment of acute soft tissue injury," *Zhongguo Zhen Jiu*, vol. 25, no. 11, pp. 753–756, 2005.

[20] J.-A. Lee, H. J. Jeong, H.-J. Park, S. Jeon, and S.-U. Hong, "Acupuncture accelerates wound healing in burn-injured mice," *Burns*, vol. 37, no. 1, pp. 117–125, 2011.

[21] F. Yuanzhi and W. Yaochi, "Effect of electroacupuncture on muscle state and infrared thermogram changes in patients with acute lumbar muscle sprain," *Journal of Traditional Chinese Medicine*, vol. 35, no. 5, pp. 499–506, 2015.

[22] M. Tsuchiya, E. F. Sato, M. Inoue, and A. Asada, "Acupuncture enhances generation of nitric oxide and increases local circulation," *Anesthesia and Analgesia*, vol. 104, no. 2, pp. 301–307, 2007.

[23] M.-H. Du, H.-M. Luo, Y.-J. Tian et al., "Electroacupuncture ST36 prevents postoperative intra-abdominal adhesions formation," *Journal of Surgical Research*, vol. 195, no. 1, pp. 89–98, 2015.

[24] J.-K. Luo, H.-J. Zhou, J. Wu, T. Tang, and Q.-H. Liang, "Electroacupuncture at Zusanli (ST36) accelerates intracerebral hemorrhage-induced angiogenesis in rats," *Chinese Journal of Integrative Medicine*, vol. 19, no. 5, pp. 367–373, 2013.

[25] M.-H. Nam, C. S. Yin, K.-S. Soh, and S.-H. Choi, "Adult neurogenesis and acupuncture stimulation at ST36," *Journal of Acupuncture and Meridian Studies*, vol. 4, no. 3, pp. 153–158, 2011.

[26] V. Parmen, C. Pestean, C. Ober, M. Mircean, L. Ognean, and L. Oana, "Influence of electroacupuncture on thermal changes in a soft tissue defect," *JAMS Journal of Acupuncture and Meridian Studies*, vol. 7, no. 5, pp. 238–242, 2014.

[27] S. T. Koo, K. S. Lim, K. Chung, H. Ju, and J. M. Chung, "Electroacupuncture-induced analgesia in a rat model of ankle sprain pain is mediated by spinal α-adrenoceptors," *Pain*, vol. 135, no. 1-2, pp. 11–19, 2008.

[28] G. Lv, R. Liang, J. Xie, Y. Wang, and G. He, "Role of peripheral afferent nerve fiber in acupuncture analgesia elicited by needling point zusanli," *Science in China, Series A*, vol. 22, no. 6, pp. 680–692, 1979.

[29] C. A. Powell, B. L. Smiley, J. Mills, and H. H. Vandenburgh, "Mechanical stimulation improves tissue-engineered human skeletal muscle," *American Journal of Physiology-Cell Physiology*, vol. 283, no. 5, pp. C1557–C1565, 2002.

[30] L. H. Batista, A. C. Vilar, J. J. de Almeida Ferreira, J. R. Rebelatto, and T. F. Salvini, "Active stretching improves flexibility, joint torque, and functional mobility in older women," *American Journal of Physical Medicine and Rehabilitation*, vol. 88, no. 10, pp. 815–822, 2009.

[31] H. Kern, S. Boncompagni, K. Rossini et al., "Long-term denervation in humans causes degeneration of both contractile and excitation-contraction coupling apparatus, which is reversible by functional electrical stimulation (FES): a role for myofiber regeneration?" *Journal of Neuropathology and Experimental Neurology*, vol. 63, no. 9, pp. 919–931, 2004.

[32] F. Kanaya and T. Tajima, "Effect of electrostimulation on denervated muscle," *Clinical Orthopaedics and Related Research*, no. 283, pp. 296–301, 1992.

[33] I. K. Hwang, J. Y. Chung, D. Y. Yoo et al., "Comparing the effects of acupuncture and electroacupuncture at zusanli and baihui on cell proliferation and neuroblast differentiation in the rat hippocampus," *Journal of Veterinary Medical Science*, vol. 72, no. 3, pp. 279–284, 2010.

[34] W.-J. Li, S.-M. Li, Y. Ding et al., "Electro-acupuncture upregulates CGRP expression after rat spinal cord transection," *Neurochemistry International*, vol. 61, no. 8, pp. 1397–1403, 2012.

[35] T. Fukazawa, M. Matsumoto, T. Imura et al., "Electrical stimulation accelerates neuromuscular junction formation through ADAM19/neuregulin/ErbB signaling in vitro," *Neuroscience Letters*, vol. 545, pp. 29–34, 2013.

[36] S. Koirala and C.-P. Ko, "Pruning an axon piece by piece: a new mode of synapse elimination," *Neuron*, vol. 44, no. 4, pp. 578–580, 2004.

[37] S. d'Houtaud, E. Sztermer, K. Buffenoir et al., "Synapse formation and regeneration," *Neurochirurgie*, vol. 55, supplement 1, pp. S49–S62, 2009.

[38] J. N. Sleigh, R. W. Burgess, T. H. Gillingwater, and M. Z. Cader, "Morphological analysis of neuromuscular junction development and degeneration in rodent lumbrical muscles," *Journal of Neuroscience Methods*, vol. 227, pp. 159–165, 2014.

11

Flavonoids Extraction from Propolis Attenuates Pathological Cardiac Hypertrophy through PI3K/AKT Signaling Pathway

Guang-wei Sun,[1,2] Zhi-dong Qiu,[3] Wei-nan Wang,[3] Xin Sui,[3] and Dian-jun Sui[1,3]

[1]*China-Japan Union Hospital of Jilin University, Changchun 130033, China*
[2]*Chinese Traditional Medicine Institute of Ji Lin Province, Changchun 130021, China*
[3]*Changchun University of Chinese Medicine, Changchun 130117, China*

Correspondence should be addressed to Dian-jun Sui; 834321375@qq.com

Academic Editor: Yoshiji Ohta

Propolis, a traditional medicine, has been widely used for a thousand years as an anti-inflammatory and antioxidant drug. The flavonoid fraction is the main active component of propolis, which possesses a wide range of biological activities, including activities related to heart disease. However, the role of the flavonoids extraction from propolis (FP) in heart disease remains unknown. This study shows that FP could attenuate ISO-induced pathological cardiac hypertrophy (PCH) and heart failure in mice. The effect of the two fetal cardiac genes, atrial natriuretic factor (ANF) and β-myosin heavy chain (β-MHC), on PCH was reversed by FP. Echocardiography analysis revealed cardiac ventricular dilation and contractile dysfunction in ISO-treated mice. This finding is consistent with the increased heart weight and cardiac ANF protein levels, massive replacement fibrosis, and myocardial apoptosis. However, pretreatment of mice with FP could attenuate cardiac dysfunction and hypertrophy *in vivo*. Furthermore, the cardiac protection of FP was suppressed by the pan-PI3K inhibitor wortmannin. FP is a novel cardioprotective agent that can attenuate adverse cardiac dysfunction, hypertrophy, and associated disorder, such as fibrosis. The effects may be closely correlated with PI3K/AKT signaling. FP may be clinically used to inhibit PCH progression and heart failure.

1. Introduction

Cardiac hypertrophy is frequently observed in various clinical conditions, including hypertension and aortic stenosis. It can progressively lead to heart failure (HF). HF is the most frequent cause of cardiovascular death worldwide. HF is caused by a pathological state that results in insufficient cardiac output [1–6]. Although there has been great progress in therapy, the mortality and morbidity of HF place it in the top 5 lethal diseases. Currently, the high mortality of HF imposes a significant economic burden in both China and Western countries [7]. Thus, identifying novel preventive and/or therapeutic strategies to counteract this deadly disease is of importance.

Cardiac hypertrophy, which is characterized by increased cell volume and metabolic and biochemical disorders, can also lead to reactivation of fetal cardiac genes such as atrial natriuretic factor (ANF) and β-myosin heavy chain (β-MHC) [8–10]. Currently, cardiac hypertrophy is attracting

attention because it can progressively lead to HF [11–15]. Some specific factors with cardioprotective properties have been identified through the preventative mechanisms of minimizing cardiac hypertrophy. Some cellular/molecular pathways, including the mitochondrial pathway, phosphoinositide 3-kinase (PI3K), AKT, and mammalian target of rapamycin (mTOR), are involved in the progression of cardiac hypertrophy [1, 4, 16].

Propolis, a complex mixture of naturally sticky, gummy, and resinous components, is produced by honeybees from plant materials [17]. Propolis contains various compounds, such as flavonoids, terpenes, β-steroids, aromatic aldehydes, and alcohols [18]. Propolis exhibits a wide range of biological activities, including antibacterial, antifungal, anti-inflammatory, immunostimulatory, antitumor, and antioxidant effects [18]. Therefore, propolis is extensively used in food and beverages to improve health and prevent diseases.

In recent years, considerable efforts have been focused on identifying naturally occurring herbal medicines [19–22].

The flavonoid fraction is the main component of propolis. Many flavonoids exhibit strong antioxidant activity [17]. Our research has focused on studying the cardioprotective properties of the flavonoids extraction from propolis (FP). Our preliminary results showed that FP exerts an effective role in cardiac protection. However, the protective effect of FP on pathological cardiac hypertrophy (PCH) and HF remains unknown. This study shows that FP is a novel cardioprotective agent. First, FP significantly attenuates adverse cardiac dysfunction, hypertrophy, and associated disorder, such as fibrosis. Secondly, FP significantly attenuates apoptotic damage and cardiac remodeling, which is correlated with the PI3K/AKT signaling. Thus, FP may be clinically used to inhibit PCH progression and prevent HF.

2. Materials and Methods

2.1. Preparation of FP.
Propolis was purchased from the An Guo herbal medicine market in Hebei province, China. The propolis was authenticated by Professor Dacheng Jiang from the Changchun University of Chinese Medicine and a voucher specimen (number 1019907) was deposited at the Jilin museum of Materia Medica, Jilin province, China. The sample was frozen at 4°C before being ground into a powder. Then, 10x of 75% ethanol/water was added to extract the active fractions. This process was conducted twice and the fractions were filtered through a 0.45 μm membrane after being combined. The filtrate was evaporated to dryness at 80°C under reduced pressure. One g of the powder was dissolved in 100 mL chloroform-ethanol (10 : 1) and was extracted twice by the same volume of 1% NaOH solution. The aqueous alkali was adjusted to pH 6 by 1% HCl and then left at room temperature for another 24 h for precipitation. The FP were then obtained through filtration, rinsed in water to neutral pH, and dried under reduced pressure.

2.2. High Performance Liquid Chromatography-High-Resolution Mass Spectrometry (HPLC-HRMS) Analysis of FP.
The FP was dissolved in pure methanol and filtered through a 0.22 μm membrane before HPLC-Q-TOF-MS analysis. The liquid chromatography separation was performed on an Agilent SB-Aq column (250 mm × 4.6 mm, 4.5 μm, 400 bar) at 30°C. For HPLC analysis, 0.1% formic acid/water (v/v) and 0.1% formic acid/methanol were used as the mobile phases A and B, respectively. The gradient elution was programmed as follows: 0–110 min (35–90% B) and 110–120 min (90% B). The flow rate was 1.0 mL/min and the injected sample volume was 10 μL. The Q-TOF-MS scan range was set at m/z 100–1200 in positive modes. The dry gas (N_2) flow rate was 9.0 L/min, the dry gas temperature was 350°C, the nebulizer gas was set at 30 psi, the capillary voltage was 3500 V, the fragmentor was 175 V, and the skimmer was 65 V.

Standard pinocembrin, kaempferol, isosakuranetin, pinobanksin-3-O-acetate, 12-acetoxyviscidone, galangin, and chrysin (purity > 98% by HPLC) were purchased from the National Institutes for Food and Drug Control of China. They were mixed and dissolved in pure methanol at the concentration of 2 μM per compound prior to use.

Data analysis was performed on an Agilent MassHunter Workstation Software-Qualitative Analysis (version B.04.00, Build 4.0.479.5, Service Pack 3, Agilent Technologies, Inc., 2011).

2.3. Animals and In Vivo Pharmacological Treatment.
The mice used in this study were handled in compliance with the guidelines for the care and use of laboratory animals established by the Chinese Council on Animal Care, and all animal protocols were approved by the Jilin University Animal Care and Use Committee. Eight-week-old male mice were anesthetized with 1.5% isoflurane. The adult mice were intragastrically given different doses of FP (1–50 mg·kg^{-1}·d^{-1}) for 7 d. Alzet osmotic minipumps containing PBS or isoproterenol (ISO) were surgically implanted subcutaneously in the interscapular region of the mouse. ISO was calibrated to release the drug at a rate of 25 mg·kg^{-1}·d^{-1} for 7 d to experimentally induce heart hypertrophy. The dose-dependent effect of FP on ISO-induced gene reactivation was determined. FP (50 mg·kg^{-1}·d^{-1}) did not exert an additional benefit to reduce heart hypertrophy; thus, we selected 25 mg·kg^{-1}·d^{-1} for the following experiments. In a separate experiment, mice were pretreated with the selective PI3K antagonist wortmannin (WM) (1 mg·kg^{-1}) at 1 h before ISO administration. The PI3K inhibitor doses were selected based on the results of previous studies.

2.4. Determination of Cardiac Dysfunction through Echocardiography.
The animals were euthanized and the hearts were removed for hypertrophic evaluation. The analysis showed no effect on cardiac function. Cardiac function was examined through echocardiography using a Vevo 770 microultrasound system (VisualSonics, Toronto, Ontario, Canada) as described previously [17]. Briefly, an in vivo transthoracic echocardiography of the left ventricle was performed using a 30 MHz scan head interfaced with a Vevo 770. An ultrasound beam was placed on the heart and near the papillary muscles. High-resolution two-dimensional electrocardiogram-based kilohertz visualization was achieved. The parameters of cardiac function were digitally measured on the M-mode tracings and then averaged from three to five cardiac cycles.

2.5. Histological Analyses.
The animals were euthanized and the hearts were removed for hypertrophic evaluation. Serial sections (4 mm) of heart tissues were stained with hematoxylin-eosin [20] or Masson's trichrome and then visualized using a light microscope as previously described.

2.6. Transmission Electron Microscopy.
The animals were euthanized and the hearts were removed for hypertrophic evaluation. Heart tissue sections were collected and observed by transmission electron microscopy.

2.7. Real-Time RT-PCR.
Total RNA was extracted using TRIzol (Invitrogen, Carlsbad, CA). Briefly, 2 mg of total RNA was reverse transcribed using the SuperScript first-strand synthesis system (Invitrogen, Carlsbad, CA, USA). cDNA was synthesized from the isolated RNA. Cycle time values were obtained using real-time RT-PCR with the Power SYBR

TABLE 1: Primers used for real-time RT-PCRs.

Target genes	Primer pairs (5′-3′)	
	Forward	Reverse
ANF	AGCATGGGCTCCTTCTCCAT	TGGCCTGGAAGCCAAAAG
β-MHC	CCTACAAGTGGCTGCCTGTGT	ATGGACTGATTCTCCCGATCTG
α-SKA	GGAGAAGATCTGGCACCATACATT	AGCAGGGTTGGGTGTTCCT
MMP-9	GGACGACGTGGGCTACGT	CACGGTTGAAGCAAAGAAGGA
p53	CAAAAGAAAAAACCACTTGATGGA	CGGAACATCTCGAAGCGTTTA
TNFR	CTCAGGTACTGCGGTGCTGTT	GCACATTAAACTGATGAAGATAAAGGA
Fas	GCTGCGCCTCGTGTGAA	GCGATTTCTGGGACTTTGTTTC
GAPDH	AACGACCCCTTCATTGAC	TCCACGACATACTCAGCAC

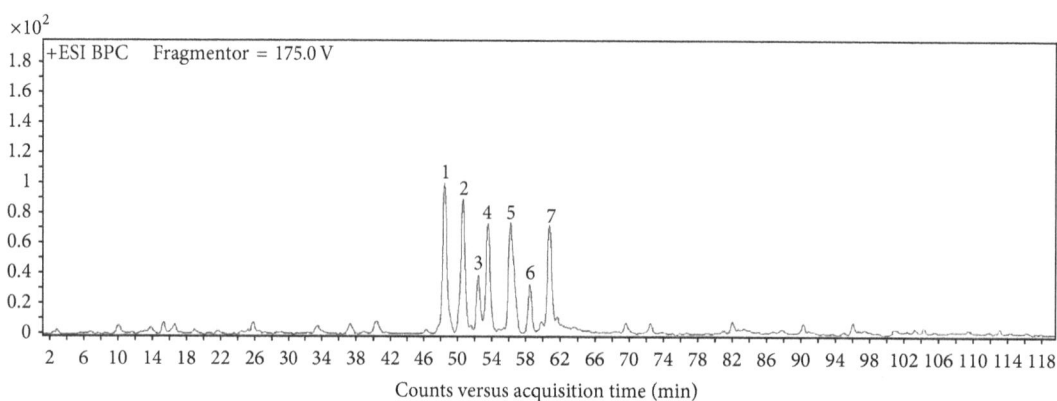

FIGURE 1: LC-MS base peak chromatograms of FP. The peak numbers refer to Table 1. FP (0–120 min).

green PCR master mix (Applied Biosystems, Foster City, CA, USA), the iQ5 real-time PCR detection system, and analysis software (Bio-Rad, Hercules, CA, USA) as previously described [23]. Primers were designed using the Applied Biosystems Primer Express Software (version 2.0) (Table 1).

2.8. Western Blot Analysis. Heart tissues were lysed on ice with T-PER tissue or cell protein extraction reagent (Pierce Chemical Co., Rockford, IL) containing 0.1 mM dithiothreitol and proteinase inhibitor cocktail. Lysate preparation and Western blot analysis were performed as previously described [21]. Protein concentration was determined using a Bio-Rad DC protein determination kit with BSA as the standard. Immunoblots were developed using an ECL kit.

2.9. Caspase-3, Caspase-8, and Caspase-9 Activity Assay. Caspase-3, caspase-8, and caspase-9 activities were measured using a fluorometric assay kit (BioVision, Mountain View, CA, USA) according to the manufacturer's instructions. The samples were subjected to a Fluoroskan Ascent FL fluorometer (Thermo Fisher Scientific, Waltham, MA, USA) with 400 nm excitation and 505 nm emission wavelengths. The results were expressed as fold change compared to the control.

2.10. Biochemical Measurements. The protein levels of ANF and β-MHC were quantified using ELISA according to

the manufacturer's instructions (R&D Systems, Wiesbaden, Germany).

2.11. Data Analysis. The data are expressed as the mean ± SE. The significance of the differences between the means was assessed using Student's t-test, and p values lower than 0.05 were considered significant. One-way ANOVA and Bonferroni corrections were used to determine the significance for multiple comparisons. Calculations were performed using SPSS (version 11.0) statistical software.

2.12. Materials. All chemicals were purchased from Sigma (St. Louis, MO) and all antibodies were purchased from Santa Cruz Biotechnology (Santa Cruz, CA).

3. Results

3.1. Chemical Profiling of FP. By HPLC-Q-TOF-MS analysis, 7 well-separated chromatographic peaks in propolis flavonoids were identified in the BPC of FP (Figure 1). Six of the peaks were characterized as pinocembrin, kaempferol, isosakuranetin, pinobanksin-3-O-acetate, 12-acetoxyviscidone, galangin, and chrysin by comparison to the external standards and the mass data relative abundance and fragmentation rules according to reported references [24–27] (Table 2). And the extraction efficiency of the flavonoids

TABLE 2: Characteristics of chemical components of TFP by HPLC-HRMS.

Peak number	Retention time (min)	m/z for $[M + H]^+$	MS^n $[M + H]^+$	Formula	Identification	Relative abundance (%)
1	48.499	257.0824	215, 153, 131	$C_{15}H_{12}O_4$	Pinocembrin	6.74
2	50.621	287.0950	165, 153, 121	$C_{15}H_{10}O_6$	Kaempferol	6.01
3	52.497	287.0931	245, 217	$C_{16}H_{14}O_5$	Isosakuranetin	1.71
4	53.480	315.0867	273, 255	$C_{17}H_{14}O_6$	Pinobanksin-3-O-acetate	4.1
5	56.231	277.0852	232, 216	$C_{15}H_{16}O_5$	12-Acetoxyviscidone	6.51
6	58.527	271.0615	165, 153, 105	$C_{15}H_{10}O_5$	Galangin	1.77
7	60.755	255.0676	209, 153, 129	$C_{15}H_{10}O_4$	Chrysin	4.47

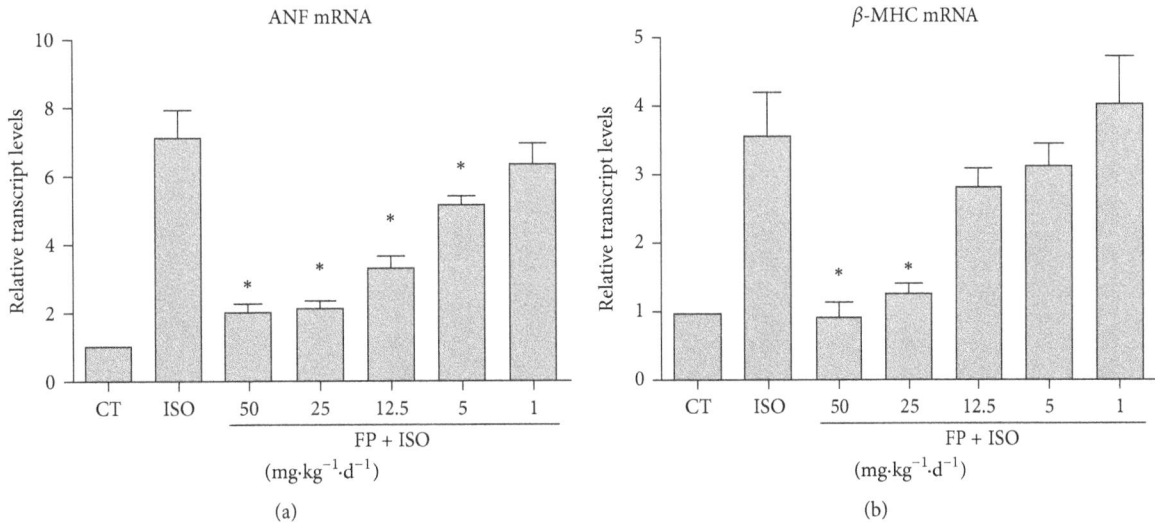

FIGURE 2: FP represses isoproterenol-induced fetal gene reactivation in a dose-dependent manner. Intragastric injection of various doses of FP (1–50 mg·kg^{-1}·d^{-1}) for 7 days was followed by continuous infusion with isoproterenol (ISO, 25 mg·kg^{-1}·d^{-1}) for 7 days to experimentally induce heart hypertrophy. Heart tissues were collected and assayed for ANF (a) and β-MHC expression (b). The results are expressed as the means ± SE; $n = 10$ mice per group ($^*p < 0.05$ compared with isoproterenol group).

extraction from propolis is 31.32% as determined by colorimetric methods. The purity of flavonoids is 56.13% in chloroform-ethanol solution and increased to 79.88% after extracted by NaOH solution.

3.2. FP Dose-Dependently Repressed ISO-Induced Fetal Gene Reactivation.
Figure 2(a) shows that intragastric injection of various doses of FP (1–50 mg·kg^{-1}·d^{-1}) for 7 days was followed by continuous infusion with isoproterenol (ISO, 25 mg·kg^{-1}·d^{-1}) for 7 days to experimentally induce heart hypertrophy. Heart tissues were collected and assayed to determine ANF and β-MHC expression. FP (50 mg·kg^{-1}·d^{-1}) exerted no additional benefit to reduce heart hypertrophy; thus, we selected 25 mg·kg^{-1}·d^{-1} for the following experiments.

3.3. FP Attenuated ISO-Induced Cardiac Dysfunction in Mice.
To determine whether FP could inhibit cardiac dysfunction *in vivo*, we performed echocardiography in the mice treated with various drugs. The representative echocardiographic parameters are depicted in Table 3. The mice infused with ISO showed an enlarged left ventricular chamber size, indicated by the significant increase in the left ventricular internal

dimension values at the end diastole (LVIDd) and end systole (LVIDs) compared to those treated with saline (Table 3). Consistently, these structural alterations were accompanied with marked impairment in cardiac contractile function, represented by the decrease in the left ventricular fractional shortening (FS) and ejection fraction (EF). The treatment with FP significantly reversed the changes stimulated by ISO in these parameters (Table 3).

3.4. Reduced Cardiac Hypertrophy in Mice Treated with FP.
To further verify the antihypertrophic effect of FP, we directly measured the heart weight (HW) and heart-to-body weight (HW/BW) ratio after the animals were euthanized. As shown in Figure 3(a), after 7 d of ISO infusion, HW significantly increased in ISO-treated mice compared to saline-treated mice. However, FP treatment attenuated the increased HW and HW/BW ratio.

Histological sections were also analyzed using hematoxylin-eosin staining (Figures 3(b)–3(d)), whereas ANF mRNA and protein levels were quantified through qPCR (Figure 3(e)) and ELISA assay (Figure 3(e)). As shown in Figure 3(d), the CM cross-sectional area was larger in ISO-treated mice than in saline-treated mice. FP treatment attenuated

(a)

(b)

(c)

(d)

(e)

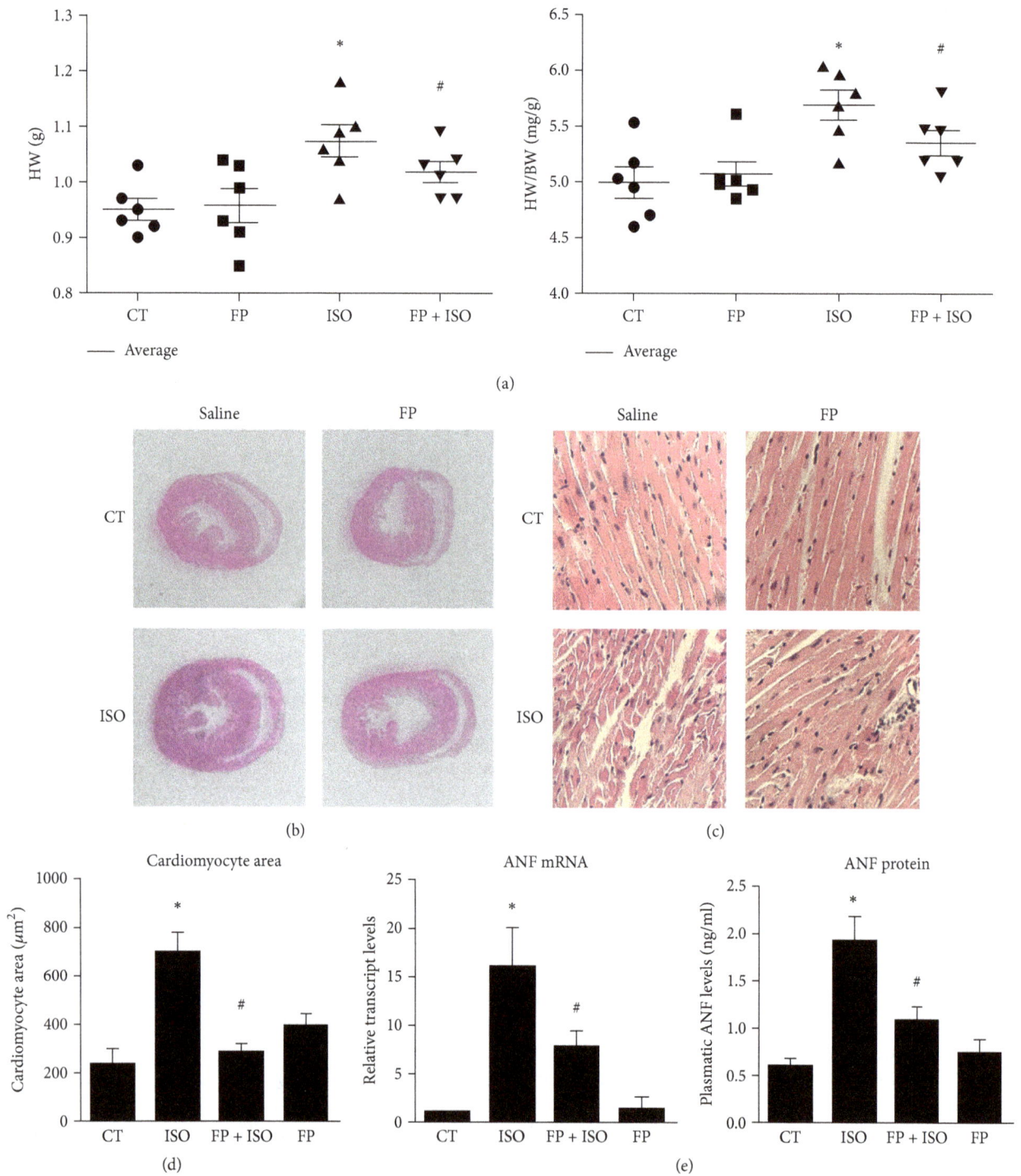

FIGURE 3: Cardiac hypertrophy is reduced in mice treated by FP. Intragastric injection of FP ($25\,\mathrm{mg\cdot kg^{-1}\cdot d^{-1}}$) for 7 days followed by continuous infusion with isoproterenol (ISO, $25\,\mathrm{mg\cdot kg^{-1}\cdot d^{-1}}$) for 7 days was sued to experimentally induce heart hypertrophy. (a) Animals were euthanized and the hearts were removed for hypertrophic evaluation. A comparison of HW (g) and HW/BW ratios (mg/g) for the animals is shown. (b) Representative histological sections of hearts stained with H&E. (c) Magnified images of histological sections in (b) used to determine CM cross-sectional area. (d) Quantification of CM cross-sectional area in the left ventricular wall. (e) mRNA expression and plasma protein levels of the hypertrophy marker ANF. The results are expressed as the means ± SE; $n = 10$ mice per group ($^{*}p < 0.05$ compared to the control group; $^{\#}p < 0.05$ compared to the isoproterenol group).

TABLE 3: Echocardiography data after ISO-induced hypertrophy.

	Saline		TFP	
	CT ($n = 5$)	ISO ($n = 5$)	CT ($n = 5$)	ISO ($n = 5$)
LVIDs (mm)	2.09 ± 0.31	$3.01 \pm 0.28^*$	2.11 ± 0.21	$2.25 \pm 0.35^{\#}$
LVIDd (mm)	3.60 ± 0.56	$4.34 \pm 0.34^*$	3.72 ± 0.42	$3.95 \pm 0.51^{\#}$
LVVs (μL)	14.29 ± 3.17	$35.3 \pm 8.04^*$	18.35 ± 4.20	$17.26 \pm 5.12^{\#}$
LVVd (μL)	54.28 ± 10.63	84.74 ± 19.28	63.89 ± 13.11	76.44 ± 14.51
EF (%)	75.23 ± 8.34	$58.34 \pm 5.91^*$	71.28 ± 11.55	$77.42 \pm 10.01^{\#}$
FS (%)	43.20 ± 6.03	$30.58 \pm 4.67^*$	39.94 ± 6.98	$45.76 \pm 9.20^{\#}$
SV (μL)	39.99 ± 11.56	49.44 ± 12.64	45.55 ± 13.11	59.18 ± 10.03

LVIDs, left ventricular internal diameter at systolic phase; LVIDd, left ventricular internal diameter at diastolic phase; LVVs, left ventricle end-systolic volume; LVVd, left ventricle end-diastolic volume; EF, ejection fraction; FS, fractional shortening; SV, stroke volume. All measurements are means $\pm$ SE. The data were analyzed by one-way ANOVA ($^*p < 0.05$ compared to saline controls; $^{\#}p < 0.05$ compared to ISO-induced saline-treated animals).

the increased cross-sectional area in ISO-treated mice. The expression of the hypertrophic marker ANF also increased in ISO-treated mice compared to saline-treated mice. Moreover, FP treatment reduced the increased mRNA and protein levels of ANF. However, FP alone had no significant effect on these processes.

3.5. FP Treatment Reduced Associated Disorder, Such as Fibrosis. To evaluate fibrosis, we evaluated the expression of α-skeletal actin (α-SKA) mRNA and matrix metalloproteinase-9 by using Masson's trichrome staining (Figure 4). Consistently, the ISO-treated hearts presented massive cell death with replacement fibrosis (Figure 4(b)). In contrast, FP treatment abbreviated ISO-elicited cardiac cell death/fibrosis. Using both measures, ISO substantially increased the mRNA levels of α-SKA (Figure 4(a)). Moreover, FP treatment attenuated the ISO-induced α-SKA levels. However, ISO and FP did not significantly affect the MMP-9 levels. Collectively, FP treatment attenuated cardiac hypertrophy and the associated disorder, such as fibrosis.

3.6. Effects of ISO and FP on Apoptotic Damage and Apoptosis-Related Gene Expression in Heart Tissues. Apoptotic damage has been implicated in cardiac hypertrophy. To determine the relationship between the cardioprotection of FP against ISO-induced cardiac hypertrophy and apoptosis, we assessed the morphology of mouse heart tissues using transmission electron microscopy (Figure 5(a)). The results showed evident heart tissue abnormalities, including cytoplasmic vacuolization, myofibrillar loss, mitochondrial edema, chromatin condensation, and cardiomyocyte necrosis, in the cardiac sections of ISO-induced mice. The structural abnormalities in the hearts were partially prevented by cotreatment with FP (Figure 5(a)). Moreover, the activation of caspase-3 resulted in the cleavage of PARP. Caspase-3 activation is one of the key processes involved in apoptosis and contributes to myocardial dysfunction and cardiac hypertrophy. Figure 5(b) shows that myocardial caspase-3 activation was reduced in the mice cotreated with FP and ISO compared to the mice treated with ISO alone, as indicated by the increased activity. Figure 5(c) shows that apoptotic damage was activated in the myocardium of ISO-infused mice. This finding was depicted by the elevated caspase-8, caspase-9, and caspase-3 activities

(Figure 5(b)) and the increased mRNA levels in p53, TNF-R1, and Fas, which were attenuated by FP treatment (Figure 5(c)).

3.7. FP Prevented ISO-Induced Cardiac Remodeling In Vivo, Which Is Correlated with the PI3K/AKT Signaling. As shown in Figure 6(a), Western blot analysis revealed significantly enhanced AKT phosphorylation in the FP-treated hearts even if the total AKT protein was similar in all animal groups. FP-ISO cotreated mice exhibited higher p-AKT in the hearts than those treated with FP alone; however, the difference was not significant. These results indicated that the cardioprotective effect of FP could be attributed to the antihypertrophic and antiapoptotic activities, which possibly involved the PI3K-AKT signaling pathway.

We also determined the functional consequences of disrupting the PI3K-AKT signaling pathway in pathological hypertrophy induction. WM, a selective PI3K inhibitor, was used to suppress PI3Ks. The results were consistent with the findings shown in Figure 2. ISO immediately upregulated the expression of ANF and β-MHC (Figure 6(b)), whereas FP treatment markedly antagonized ISO-induced fetal gene expression (Figure 6(b)). However, the ISO-induced increase in the ANF and β-MHC mRNAs was attenuated by FP in the mice pretreated with WM (Figure 6(b)), whereas FP and WM showed no significant effect compared to the control. Furthermore, as is shown in supplementary figure (see Supplementary Material available online at http://dx.doi.org/10.1155/2016/6281376), cardiac hypertrophy phenotype is not altered by WM. These results suggested that the inhibition of PI3Ks with WM could suppress the FP-induced antihypertrophic effect.

4. Discussion

Natural drugs that exert cardioprotective properties have gained worldwide attention [9, 13]. Propolis, a traditional medicine, has been widely used for a thousand years as an anti-inflammatory and antioxidant drug. However, the role of propolis in cardiovascular diseases remains unknown. Propolis possesses a wide range of biological activities. Total flavonoids are the main active component of propolis and exhibit strong antioxidant activities. Therefore, this study assessed the cardioprotective effects of FP in the ISO-induced

(a)

(b)

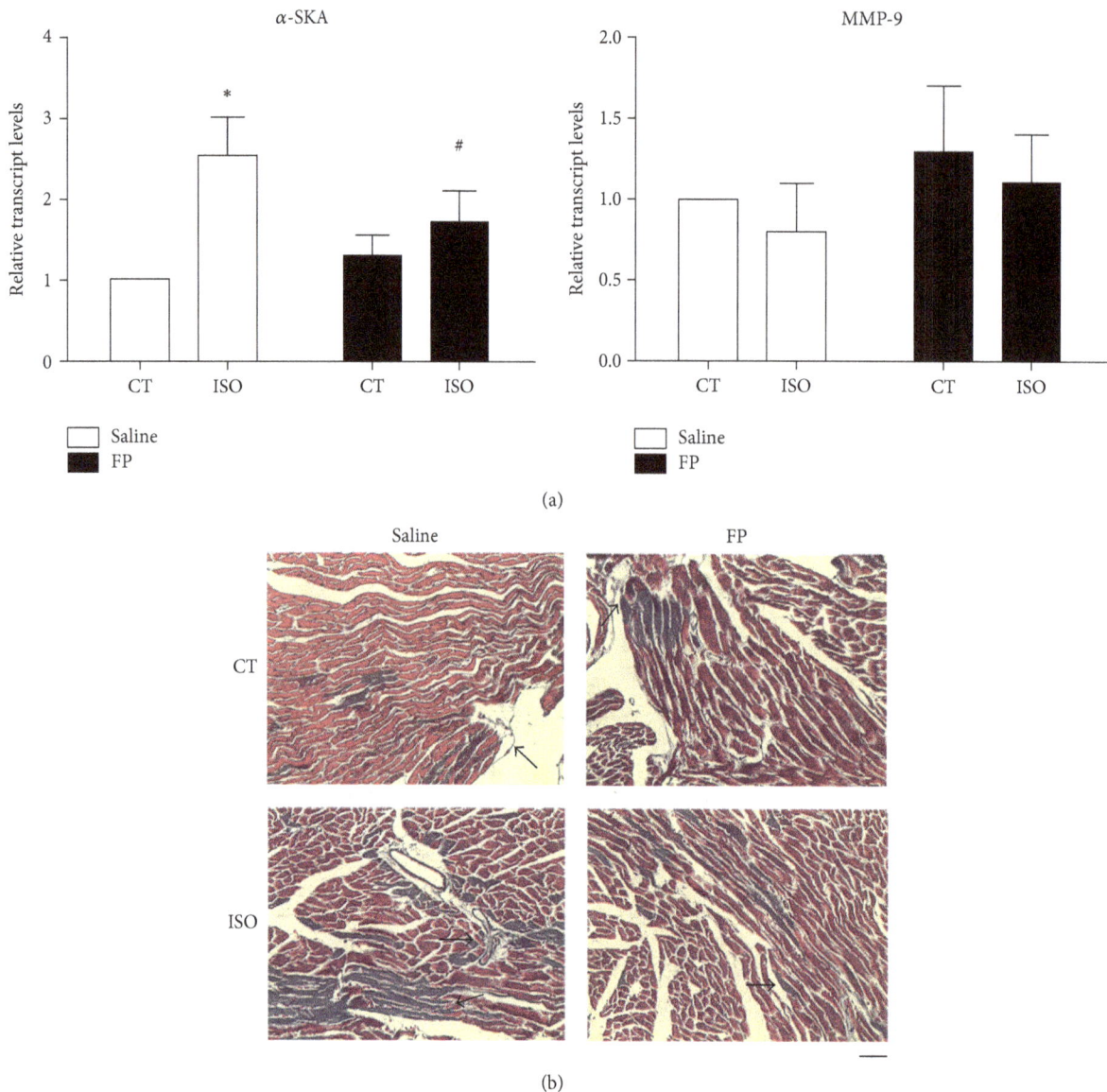

FIGURE 4: FP treatment reduced associated disorder, such as fibrosis. (a) mRNA expression levels of the hypertrophy marker a-SKA and the fibrosis marker matrix metalloproteinase-9 (MMP-9). (b) Determination of fibrosis in histological sections by Masson's trichrome staining. Scale bar, 50 μm. The arrows show fibrotic areas. The results are expressed as the means ± SE; $n = 10$ mice per group ($^*p < 0.05$ compared with control group; $^\#p < 0.05$ compared with isoproterenol group).

C57BL/6 mouse model, as well as the mechanisms that mediate the therapeutic activities of this drug. The significant findings of this study were as follows: (1) FP treatment significantly attenuated adverse cardiac dysfunction, hypertrophy, and associated disorder, such as fibrosis; (2) FP treatment significantly attenuated apoptotic damage and cardiac remodeling, which were correlated with the PI3K/AKT signaling.

Cardiac hypertrophy can be divided into two categories, physiological hypertrophy and pathological hypertrophy. It is generally recognized that ANP level is increased in hypertrophic hearts. However, some results also supported that factors can protect against pathological cardiac hypertrophy by activating PI3K/AKT signaling [28]. In accordance with our study, factors can also attenuate pathological cardiac

hypertrophy by increasing AKT, and effects can be blocked with PI3K inhibition [23, 29, 30]. Furthermore, some factors such as Cav-3 protect against cardiac hypertrophy and ischemia by increasing p-AKT signaling and ANP, partially due to mimicking ischemia-induced preconditioning [31, 32]. These seemingly opposite results may be partially ascribed to multiple functions of PI3K and complicated experimental conditions varied in the settings of cardiac hypertrophy. Although PI3K is a well-known survival factor which can inhibit cardiac apoptosis and cell death, in some conditions such as exercise it can activate PI3K/AKT signaling and leads to cardiac hypertrophy, with little effect on cell death. Previous experiments have shown that insulin or IGF-I may regulate heart development [33]. PI3K of the IA group could

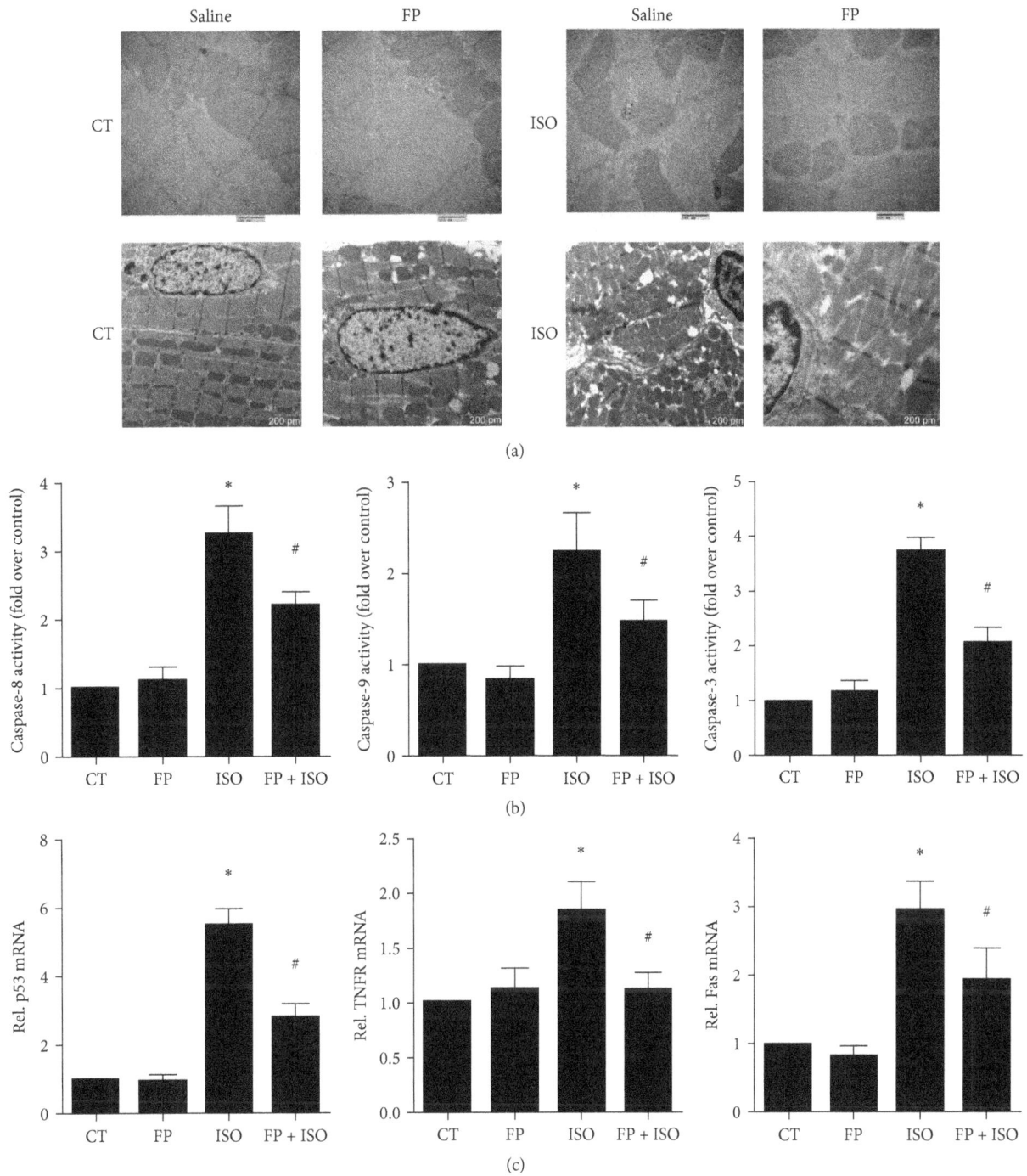

FIGURE 5: Effects of isoproterenol and FP on apoptotic damage and apoptosis-related gene expression in heart tissues. (a) Transmission electron microscopy of heart tissues. (b) The activities of caspase-8, caspase-9, and caspase-3 were measured using a fluorometric assay and expressed as the fold change over the control. (c) mRNA levels of p53, TNFR1, and Fas were determined by real-time RT-PCR. The levels of mRNA were normalized to GAPDH. Relative mRNA levels are shown using arbitrary units, and the value of the control group (CT) is defined as 1. The results are expressed as the means ± SE; $n = 10$ mice per group ($^*p < 0.05$ compared to the control group; $^\#p < 0.05$ compared to the isoproterenol group).

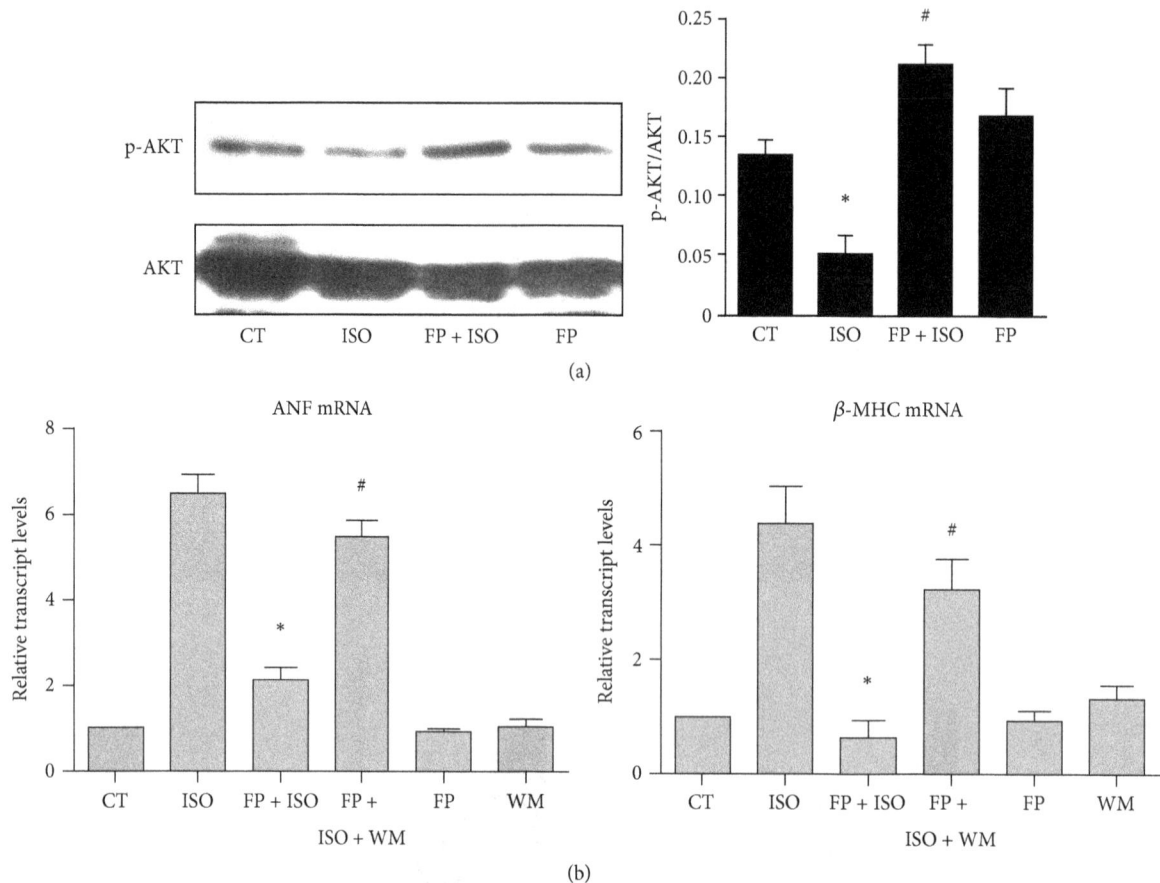

FIGURE 6: FP prevents isoproterenol-induced cardiac remodeling *in vivo*, which is correlated with PI3K/AKT signaling. (a-b) Intragastric injection of FP (25 mg·kg^{-1}·d^{-1}) or saline (CT) for 7 days was followed by continuous infusion with isoproterenol (ISO, 25 mg·kg^{-1}·d^{-1}) for 7 days to experimentally induce heart hypertrophy. The animals were euthanized and the hearts were removed for hypertrophic evaluation. (a) Representative Western blotting assays and quantitative analysis of phosphorylated AKT in the hearts by drug treatment ($^*p < 0.05$ compared to the control group; $^#p < 0.05$ compared to the isoproterenol group). (b) Effect of a selective PI3K antagonist, wortmannin (WM), on isoproterenol-induced gene reactivation. The heart tissues were collected and assayed for ANF and β-MHC expression. The results are expressed as the means ± SE; $n = 10$ mice per group ($^*p < 0.05$ compared to the isoproterenol group; $^#p < 0.05$ compared to the FP-isoproterenol cotreated group).

be activated by IGF-I through the binding of ligands to PI3Kα [34, 35]. After activation of PI3K, plasma membrane lipid phosphatidylinositol-4,5-bisphosphate is converted to phosphatidylinositol-3,4,5-triphosphate, which may lead to the activation of a series of signaling components. To the best of our knowledge, our present study indicates that FP preserves cardiac function with a decrease in levels of ANF and β-MHC, and effects can be inhibited by PI3K antagonist, wortmannin. And FP induces activation in PI3K/AKT signaling and induction in antiapoptotic and antioxidative properties may also have complex effects on cardiac hypertrophy signaling.

Pathological cardiac hypertrophy (PCH) is a vital and independent predictor of cardiovascular mortality and is also a key target in the treatment of HF [36–39]. Studies have shown that ISO-induced HF is associated with an array of metabolic and biomedical disorders in experimental animals [2, 23]. ISO infusion causes myocardial ischemia and cardiomyocyte necrosis and progressively leads to diastolic

and systolic dysfunction in the heart, which eventually results in PCH and HF [3]. In the present study, we also observed a significant cardiac dysfunction caused by ISO infusion, as indicated by the enlarged left ventricular chamber size and marked impairment in cardiac contractile function, which can be partially attenuated by FP. This finding was closely correlated with our data that FP can attenuate PCH and fibrosis marker expression. PCH is characterized by increased cell volume and metabolic and biochemical disorders, accompanied by reactivation of fetal cardiac genes such as ANF and β-MHC. In this study, we first investigated the effects of FP on the mRNA expression of these two fetal cardiac genes. PCH is a maladaptive response that could result in HF when unmatched cardiac cell death and fibrosis occur. Collectively, our study revealed that FP treatment attenuated cardiac hypertrophy and associated disorder, such as fibrosis.

Apoptotic damage has been implicated in cardiac hypertrophy [40, 41]. Apoptosis of cardiac cells is caused by biomedical stimuli that eventually lead to morphological changes in these cells. The signals involved in cardiac hypertrophy may finally result in cell death. Because cardiomyocytes are nondividing cells, the apoptotic cardiomyocyte may be largely replaced by fibrous tissues [42]. Hence, cardiac cell death has a close association with the transition of hypertrophy to irreversible HF [41, 42]. Our present study clearly showed that FP attenuated the apoptotic damage activated in the myocardium of ISO-induced mice, as evidenced by attenuating structural abnormities and decreasing the elevated caspase-8, caspase-9, and caspase-3 activities and the increased mRNA levels of p53, TNF-R1, and Fas. These results revealed that the recovery of PCH and cardiac dysfunction induced by ISO infusion may be closely associated with diminished cardiac cell apoptosis after FP pretreatment. To the best of our knowledge, this study is the first to demonstrate the beneficial effects of FP on ISO-induced PCH in mice.

5. Conclusions

In summary, this study demonstrates that FP has potent cardioprotective activities against ISO-induced HF in the C57BL/6 mouse, and these activities are correlated with PI3K/AKT signaling. Additional experiments should be performed to investigate the cardiac protection properties of FP. FP may be a novel therapeutic agent for inhibiting the progression of PCH and HF.

Competing Interests

The authors declare that there is no conflict of interests.

Acknowledgments

This research was supported by the National Natural Science Foundation of China (no. 81173543). The authors are grateful to Professor Dacheng Jiang from Changchun University of Chinese Medicine for kindly authenticating the propolis.

References

[1] E. D. Abel and T. Doenst, "Mitochondrial adaptations to physiological vs. pathological cardiac hypertrophy," *Cardiovascular Research*, vol. 90, no. 2, pp. 234–242, 2011.

[2] M. A. Allwood, R. T. Kinobe, L. Ballantyne et al., "Heme oxygenase-1 overexpression exacerbates heart failure with aging and pressure overload but is protective against isoproterenol-induced cardiomyopathy in mice," *Cardiovascular Pathology*, vol. 23, no. 4, pp. 231–237, 2014.

[3] M. Anderson, D. Moore, and D. F. Larson, "Comparison of isoproterenol and dobutamine in the induction of cardiac hypertrophy and fibrosis," *Perfusion*, vol. 23, no. 4, pp. 231–235, 2008.

[4] T. Aoyagi and T. Matsui, "Phosphoinositide-3 kinase signaling in cardiac hypertrophy and heart failure," *Current Pharmaceutical Design*, vol. 17, no. 18, pp. 1818–1824, 2011.

[5] M. M. Benjamin, R. L. Smith, and P. A. Grayburn, "Ischemic and functional mitral regurgitation in heart failure: natural history and treatment," *Current Cardiology Reports*, vol. 16, no. 8, p. 517, 2014.

[6] B. C. Bernardo, K. L. Weeks, L. Pretorius, and J. R. McMullen, "Molecular distinction between physiological and pathological cardiac hypertrophy: experimental findings and therapeutic strategies," *Pharmacology and Therapeutics*, vol. 128, no. 1, pp. 191–227, 2010.

[7] C. Cook, G. Cole, P. Asaria, R. Jabbour, and D. P. Francis, "The annual global economic burden of heart failure," *International Journal of Cardiology*, vol. 171, no. 3, pp. 368–376, 2014.

[8] M. G. Rosca, B. Tandler, and C. L. Hoppel, "Mitochondria in cardiac hypertrophy and heart failure," *Journal of Molecular and Cellular Cardiology*, vol. 55, no. 1, pp. 31–41, 2013.

[9] A. C. de Groot, "Propolis: a review of properties, applications, chemical composition, contact allergy, and other adverse effects," *Dermatitis*, vol. 24, no. 6, pp. 263–282, 2013.

[10] H. S. Lim and M. Theodosiou, "Exercise ventilatory parameters for the diagnosis of reactive pulmonary hypertension in patients with heart failure," *Journal of Cardiac Failure*, vol. 20, no. 9, pp. 650–657, 2014.

[11] T. A. McKinsey and D. A. Kass, "Small-molecule therapies for cardiac hypertrophy: moving beneath the cell surface," *Nature Reviews Drug Discovery*, vol. 6, no. 8, pp. 617–635, 2007.

[12] L. Bacharova, H. Chen, E. H. Estes et al., "Determinants of discrepancies in detection and comparison of the prognostic significance of left ventricular hypertrophy by electrocardiogram and cardiac magnetic resonance imaging," *American Journal of Cardiology*, vol. 115, no. 4, pp. 515–522, 2015.

[13] A. Prathapan, V. P. Vineetha, and K. G. Raghu, "Protective effect of *Boerhaavia diffusa* L. against mitochondrial dysfunction in angiotensin II induced hypertrophy in H9c2 cardiomyoblast cells," *PLoS ONE*, vol. 9, no. 4, Article ID e96220, 2014.

[14] P. S. Saba, M. Cameli, G. Casalnuovo et al., "Ventricular-vascular coupling in hypertension: methodological considerations and clinical implications," *Journal of Cardiovascular Medicine*, vol. 15, no. 11, pp. 773–787, 2014.

[15] B. Swynghedauw and B. Chevalier, "Biological characteristics of the myocardium during the regression of cardiac hypertrophy due to mechanical overload," *Journal of Heart Valve Disease*, vol. 4, supplement 2, pp. S154–S159, 1995.

[16] C. Tarin, B. Lavin, M. Gomez, M. Saura, A. Diez-Juan, and C. Zaragoza, "The extracellular matrix metalloproteinase inducer EMMPRIN is a target of nitric oxide in myocardial ischemia/reperfusion," *Free Radical Biology and Medicine*, vol. 51, no. 2, pp. 387–395, 2011.

[17] A. Mavri, H. Abramovič, T. Polak et al., "Chemical properties and antioxidant and antimicrobial activities of slovenian propolis," *Chemistry and Biodiversity*, vol. 9, no. 8, pp. 1545–1558, 2012.

[18] V. C. Toreti, H. H. Sato, G. M. Pastore, and Y. K. Park, "Recent progress of propolis for its biological and chemical compositions and its botanical origin," *Evidence-Based Complementary and Alternative Medicine*, vol. 2013, Article ID 697390, 13 pages, 2013.

[19] P. K. Gupta, D. J. DiPette, and S. C. Supowit, "Protective effect of resveratrol against pressure overload-induced heart failure," *Food Science & Nutrition*, vol. 2, no. 3, pp. 218–229, 2014.

[20] T. Wang, X. Yu, S. Qu, H. Xu, B. Han, and D. Sui, "Effect of ginsenoside Rb3 on myocardial injury and heart function impairment induced by isoproterenol in rats," *European Journal of Pharmacology*, vol. 636, no. 1–3, pp. 121–125, 2010.

[21] H. Xu, X. Yu, S. Qu, Y. Chen, Z. Wang, and D. Sui, "Protective effect of Panax quinquefolium 20(S)-protopanaxadiol saponins, isolated from Pana quinquefolium, on permanent focal cerebral ischemic injury in rats," *Experimental and Therapeutic Medicine*, vol. 7, no. 1, pp. 165–170, 2013.

[22] H. Yang, Y. Dong, H. Du, H. Shi, Y. Peng, and X. Li, "Antioxidant compounds from propolis collected in Anhui, China," *Molecules*, vol. 16, no. 4, pp. 3444–3455, 2011.

[23] L. Yang, X. Cai, J. Liu et al., "CpG-ODN attenuates pathological cardiac hypertrophy and heart failure by activation of PI3Kα-Akt signaling," *PLoS ONE*, vol. 8, no. 4, Article ID e62373, 2013.

[24] C. Sun, Z. Wu, Z. Wang, and H. Zhang, "Effect of ethanol/water solvents on phenolic profiles and antioxidant properties of Beijing propolis extracts," *Evidence-Based Complementary and Alternative Medicine*, vol. 2015, Article ID 595393, 9 pages, 2015.

[25] K. Midorikawa, A. H. Banskota, Y. Tezuka et al., "Liquid chromatography-mass spectrometry analysis of propolis," *Phytochemical Analysis*, vol. 12, no. 6, pp. 366–373, 2001.

[26] F. Pellati, G. Orlandini, D. Pinetti, and S. Benvenuti, "HPLC-DAD and HPLC-ESI-MS/MS methods for metabolite profiling of propolis extracts," *Journal of Pharmaceutical and Biomedical Analysis*, vol. 55, no. 5, pp. 934–948, 2011.

[27] N. Volpi and G. Bergonzini, "Analysis of flavonoids from propolis by on-line HPLC-electrospray mass spectrometry," *Journal of Pharmaceutical and Biomedical Analysis*, vol. 42, no. 3, pp. 354–361, 2006.

[28] G. Y. Oudit, M. A. Crackower, U. Eriksson et al., "Phosphoinositide 3-kinase γ-deficient mice are protected from isoproterenol-induced heart failure," *Circulation*, vol. 108, no. 17, pp. 2147–2152, 2003.

[29] Y. S. Weng, H. F. Wang, P. Y. Pai et al., "Tanshinone IIA prevents Leu27IGF-II-induced cardiomyocyte hypertrophy mediated by estrogen receptor and subsequent Akt activation," *The American Journal of Chinese Medicine*, vol. 43, no. 8, pp. 1567–1591, 2015.

[30] P. Chang, Q. Wang, H. Xu et al., "Tetrahydrobiopterin reverse left ventricular hypertrophy and diastolic dysfunction through the PI3K/p-Akt pathway in spontaneously hypertensive rats," *Biochemical and Biophysical Research Communications*, vol. 463, no. 4, pp. 1012–1020, 2015.

[31] Y. T. Horikawa, M. Panneerselvam, Y. Kawaraguchi et al., "Cardiac-specific overexpression of caveolin-3 attenuates cardiac hypertrophy and increases natriuretic peptide expression and signaling," *Journal of the American College of Cardiology*, vol. 57, no. 22, pp. 2273–2283, 2011.

[32] H. Okawa, H. Horimoto, S. Mieno, Y. Nomura, M. Yoshida, and S. Sasaki, "Preischemic infusion of alpha-human atrial natriuretic peptide elicits myoprotective effects against ischemia reperfusion in isolated rat hearts," *Molecular and Cellular Biochemistry*, vol. 248, no. 1-2, pp. 171–177, 2003.

[33] J. Heineke and J. D. Molkentin, "Regulation of cardiac hypertrophy by intracellular signalling pathways," *Nature Reviews Molecular Cell Biology*, vol. 7, no. 8, pp. 589–600, 2006.

[34] G. Y. Oudit, H. Sun, B.-G. Kerfant, M. A. Crackower, J. M. Penninger, and P. H. Backx, "The role of phosphoinositide-3 kinase and PTEN in cardiovascular physiology and disease," *Journal of Molecular and Cellular Cardiology*, vol. 37, no. 2, pp. 449–471, 2004.

[35] L. C. Cantley, "The phosphoinositide 3-kinase pathway," *Science*, vol. 296, no. 5573, pp. 1655–1657, 2002.

[36] S. Unzek and G. S. Francis, "Management of heart failure: a brief review and selected update," *Cardiology Clinics*, vol. 26, no. 4, pp. 561–571, 2008.

[37] E. Braunwald, "Heart failure," *JACC: Heart Failure*, vol. 1, no. 1, pp. 1–20, 2013.

[38] J. R. McMullen and G. L. Jennings, "Differences between pathological and physiological cardiac hypertrophy: novel therapeutic strategies to treat heart failure," *Clinical and Experimental Pharmacology & Physiology*, vol. 34, no. 4, pp. 255–262, 2007.

[39] D. L. Mann, R. Bogaev, and G. D. Buckberg, "Cardiac remodelling and myocardial recovery: lost in translation?" *European Journal of Heart Failure*, vol. 12, no. 8, pp. 789–796, 2010.

[40] A. Haunstetter and S. Izumo, "Apoptosis: basic mechanisms and implications for cardiovascular disease," *Circulation Research*, vol. 82, no. 11, pp. 1111–1129, 1998.

[41] T. Kubota, M. Miyagishima, C. S. Frye et al., "Overexpression of tumor necrosis factor-α activates both anti- and pro-apoptotic pathways in the myocardium," *Journal of Molecular and Cellular Cardiology*, vol. 33, no. 7, pp. 1331–1344, 2001.

[42] T. Hang, Z. Huang, S. Jiang et al., "Apoptosis in pressure overload-induced cardiac hypertrophy is mediated, in part, by adenine nucleotide translocator-1," *Annals of Clinical & Laboratory Science*, vol. 36, no. 1, pp. 88–95, 2006.

12

Anti-HMG-CoA Reductase, Antioxidant, and Anti-Inflammatory Activities of *Amaranthus viridis* Leaf Extract as a Potential Treatment for Hypercholesterolemia

Shamala Salvamani,[1] **Baskaran Gunasekaran,**[1] **Mohd Yunus Shukor,**[1]
Noor Azmi Shaharuddin,[1] **Mohd Khalizan Sabullah,**[2] **and Siti Aqlima Ahmad**[1]

[1]*Department of Biochemistry, Faculty of Biotechnology and Biomolecular Sciences, Universiti Putra Malaysia (UPM), 43400 Serdang, Selangor, Malaysia*
[2]*Faculty of Science and Natural Resources, Universiti Malaysia Sabah, Jalan UMS, 88400 Kota Kinabalu, Sabah, Malaysia*

Correspondence should be addressed to Siti Aqlima Ahmad; aqlima@upm.edu.my

Academic Editor: Ki-Wan Oh

Inflammation and oxidative stress are believed to contribute to the pathology of several chronic diseases including hypercholesterolemia (elevated levels of cholesterol in blood) and atherosclerosis. HMG-CoA reductase inhibitors of plant origin are needed as synthetic drugs, such as statins, which are known to cause adverse effects on the liver and muscles. *Amaranthus viridis* (*A. viridis*) has been used from ancient times for its supposedly medically beneficial properties. In the current study, different parts of *A. viridis* (leaf, stem, and seed) were evaluated for potential anti-HMG-CoA reductase, antioxidant, and anti-inflammatory activities. The putative HMG-CoA reductase inhibitory activity of *A. viridis* extracts at different concentrations was determined spectrophotometrically by NADPH oxidation, using HMG-CoA as substrate. *A. viridis* leaf extract revealed the highest HMG-CoA reductase inhibitory effect at about 71%, with noncompetitive inhibition in Lineweaver-Burk plot analysis. The leaf extract showed good inhibition of hydroperoxides, 2,2-diphenyl-1-picrylhydrazyl (DPPH), nitric oxide (NO), and ferric ion radicals in various concentrations. *A. viridis* leaf extract was proven to be an effective inhibitor of hyaluronidase, lipoxygenase, and xanthine oxidase enzymes. The experimental data suggest that *A. viridis* leaf extract is a source of potent antioxidant and anti-inflammatory agent and may modulate cholesterol metabolism by inhibition of HMG-CoA reductase.

1. Introduction

Various forms of free radicals, such as alkoxy (RO) and nitric oxide (NO) radicals, are believed to contribute to the pathogenesis of chronic diseases. Hypercholesterolemia, which is characterized by the presence of high levels of cholesterol in the blood, is also believed to arise from oxidative stress. The enzyme, 3-hydroxy-3-methylglutaryl-coenzyme A (HMG-CoA) reductase, is a rate-limiting enzyme that catalyzes the conversion of HMG-CoA to mevalonate in the cholesterol biosynthesis pathway [1]. Statins competitively inhibit HMG-CoA reductase and are efficient in reducing the serum levels of low density lipoprotein (LDL) cholesterol. However, long-term consumption of statins causes serious side effects such as liver and muscles damage [2].

Edible medicinal plants with antioxidant and anti-inflammatory abilities can play a crucial role in the management of hypercholesterolemia [3]. Essentially, practicing healthy diets, including the consumption of desirable quantities of edible antioxidants, enables the body to neutralize radicals and offset damage associated with oxidative stress [4]. Flavonoids and phenolic acids are classes of polyphenolic substances with known antioxidant properties, including inhibition of oxidative enzymes, scavenging of free radicals, and induction of anti-inflammatory actions [5]. The advantages of using plants for medicinal purposes relate to their safety, availability, and economical benefits [6].

Amaranthus viridis L. (*A. viridis*), locally known as "bayam pasir," belongs to the family of Amaranthaceae. It is a branched glabrous herb which is distributed in most of the tropical countries [7]. *A. viridis* has been traditionally used to reduce labour pain and as an antipyretic in India and Nepal [8]. Other traditional usages are as analgesic, antiulcer, antirheumatic, antileprotic, and antiemetic agent [9]. It is also believed to treat eye diseases, psoriasis, eczema, asthma, and respiratory problems [10].

In the present study, the HMG-CoA reductase inhibitory activity of different parts of *A. viridis* (leaf, stem, and seed) was tested. Ferric thiocyanate (FTC), thiobarbituric acid (TBA), 2,2-diphenyl-1-picrylhydrazyl (DPPH) and nitric oxide (NO) scavenging activity, and ferric-reducing antioxidant power (FRAP) assays were used to measure the antioxidant activity while hyaluronidase, xanthine oxidase, and lipoxygenase inhibition assays were performed to determine the anti-inflammatory potential of *A. viridis* extract. The objectives of this study are to investigate anti-HMG-CoA reductase, antioxidant, and anti-inflammatory effects of *A. viridis*, focusing on the therapeutic potential relating to hypercholesterolemia.

2. Materials and Methods

2.1. Chemicals. All the chemicals and reagents used in this study were of analytical reagent grade and were purchased from Sigma-Aldrich and Merck.

2.2. Extraction of A. viridis. *A. viridis* was collected from various regions of Selangor, Malaysia. The plant was botanically identified and the plant voucher specimen was deposited in the Institute of Bioscience, Universiti Putra Malaysia. The plant was washed and separated into leaf, stem, and seed. The parts of *A. viridis* were air-dried and ground using a blender (Panasonic MX 8967) and subjected to methanol 50% (v/v) distillation for 48 h. After filtration, the extracts were isolated using a separatory funnel. The crude methanol extracts were then concentrated using a rotary evaporator (Heidolph) under reduced pressure at 40°C and freeze-dried at −40°C [11].

2.3. Enzyme Assay. HMG-CoA reductase inhibitory activities of *A. viridis* (leaf, stem, and seed) were determined based on spectrophotometric measurements. Each crude extract (50 μg) was mixed with reaction mixture containing NADPH (400 μM), HMG-CoA substrate (400 μM), and potassium phosphate buffer (100 mM, pH 7.4) containing KCl (120 mM), EDTA (1 mM), and DTT (5 mM), followed by the addition of HMG-CoA reductase (2 μL). The reactants were incubated at 37°C and absorbance was measured at 340 nm after 10 min. Simvastatin (Sigma, Missouri, US) was used as positive control and distilled water as negative control. The HMG-CoA

reductase inhibition (%) was calculated using the following formula [12]:

$$\text{Inhibition \%} = \left(\frac{\Delta \text{ Absorbance control} - \Delta \text{ Absorbance test}}{\Delta \text{ Absorbance control}} \right) \quad (1)$$

$$\times 100.$$

2.4. Kinetic Study. The inhibition mode of *A. viridis* leaf extract was determined using various concentrations of HMG-CoA reductase (0.3, 0.6, 0.9, and 1.2 mmol/L) and three different concentrations of *A. viridis* (0.05, 0.15, and 0.25 mg/mL). The assay was analyzed using Lineweaver-Burk plot analysis according to the Michaelis-Menten kinetics [12].

2.5. Total Phenolic Content (TPC). The TPC of *A. viridis* extracts was determined according to Meda et al. [13] using Folin-Ciocalteu assay. Briefly, *A. viridis* extracts (100 mg) were dissolved in methanol (10 mL). The extracts (100 μL), sodium carbonate (7.5% (w/v), 2 mL), and Folin-Ciocalteu reagent (tenfold dilution, 2.5 mL) were mixed, vortexed, and incubated at 40°C for 30 min. The absorbance was measured at 760 nm using a UV-visible spectrophotometer (Pharmaspec UV-1650 PC, Shimadzu, Japan). TPC of *A. viridis* extracts were expressed as mg gallic acid equivalents/g dry weight.

2.6. Total Flavonoid Content (TFC). The TFC of *A. viridis* leaf extracts was determined according to Ismail et al. [14] using aluminium calorimetric method. *A. viridis* extracts (100 mg) were dissolved in methanol (10 mL). The extracts (100 μL) were mixed with sodium nitrite (5% (w/v), 300 μL) and incubated at room temperature for 5 min. Aluminium chloride (10% (w/v), 300 μL) and sodium hydroxide (1 N, 2 mL) were then added followed by the addition of distilled water up to a total volume of 5 mL. The absorbance was measured using a UV-visible spectrophotometer (Pharmaspec UV-1650 PC, Shimadzu, Japan) at 510 nm. TFC of *A. viridis* extracts were expressed as mg rutin equivalents/g dry weight.

2.7. Antioxidant Activity of A. viridis Extracts

2.7.1. Ferric Thiocyanate (FTC). FTC assay was performed according to the method described by Ismail et al. [14]. *A. viridis* extracts (4 mg) were dissolved in methanol (4 mL) and mixed with linoleic acid (2.5%, 4.1 mL), phosphate buffer (50 mM, pH 7, 8 mL), and distilled water (3.9 mL). The mixtures were kept in screw-cap vials which were placed in an oven maintained at 40°C in the dark. The mixtures (100 μL) were added to ethanol (75%, 9.7 mL) and ammonium thiocyanate (30%, 100 μL). Three minutes after the addition of ferrous chloride solution (2×10^2 M in 3.5% hydrochloric acid, 100 μL) to the reaction mixtures, the absorbance was measured at 500 nm using a UV-visible spectrophotometer (Pharmaspec UV-1650 PC, Shimadzu, Japan). The procedure was repeated (at 24 h interval) until the absorbance of the control sample reached its maximum value. Ascorbic acid and α-tocopherol were used as the standard antioxidants.

2.7.2. Thiobarbituric Acid (TBA).

TBA assay on *A. viridis* extracts was carried out according to the method described by Hendra et al. [15]. The test was performed instantly after the control sample (from FTC test) reached the maximum absorbance value. Aqueous trichloroacetic acid (20%, 1 mL) and aqueous thiobarbituric acid (0.67%, 2 mL) were added to the sample solution (2 mL) acquired from the FTC test. The mixtures were incubated in a boiling water bath for 10 min. After cooling, the mixtures were spun at 3000 rpm for 20 min. Absorbance of the supernatants was read at 532 nm using a UV-visible spectrophotometer (Pharmaspec UV-1650 PC, Shimadzu, Japan). For both FTC and TBA assays, the antioxidant activity was expressed as % inhibition as in the following formula:

$$\% \text{ inhibition} = \frac{(\text{Ab}_c - \text{Ab}_s)}{\text{Ab}_c} \times 100\%, \qquad (2)$$

where Ab_c is the absorbance of control and Ab_s is the absorbance of sample.

2.7.3. 2,2-Diphenyl-1-picrylhydrazyl (DPPH) Radical Scavenging Activity.

The free radical scavenging activity of *A. viridis* extracts was determined as described by Ismail et al. [14] using the DPPH assay. *A. viridis* extracts (100 μL) at various concentrations (50, 100, 150, 200, 250, and 300 μg/mL) were added to methanol (490 μL) and DPPH methanolic solution (4 mg/100 mL, 390 μL). The mixtures were then vortexed and allowed to stand at room temperature in the dark for 60 min. Absorbance of the mixtures was measured using a UV-visible spectrophotometer (Pharmaspec UV-1650 PC, Shimadzu, Japan) at 515 nm. Ascorbic acid and α-tocopherol were used as the standard antioxidants. Free radical scavenging activity of *A. viridis* extracts was expressed as % inhibition as in formula (2).

2.7.4. Nitric Oxide (NO) Scavenging Activity.

The NO scavenging activity of *A. viridis* extracts was determined according to the method of Tsai et al. [16]. *A. viridis* extracts (60 μL) at various concentrations (50, 100, 150, 200, 250, and 300 μg/mL) were mixed with sodium nitroprusside (10 mM in phosphate buffered saline, 60 μL) in a flat-bottomed microtiter plate and incubated in the light for 150 min at room temperature. An equal volume of the Griess reagent was added to the wells to measure the nitrite content. A_{546} was measured with a microtiter plate reader (Stat Fax 3200 Microplate Reader, Awareness Technology Inc., USA). Ascorbic acid and α-tocopherol were used as the standard antioxidants. The NO scavenging activity was expressed as % inhibition as in formula (2).

2.7.5. Ferric-Reducing Antioxidant Power (FRAP) Assay.

The ferric-reducing effect of *A. viridis* extracts was determined according to the method suggested by Yen and Chen [17]. *A. viridis* extracts (1 mL) at various concentrations (50, 100,

150, 200, 250, and 300 μg/mL) were mixed with potassium phosphate buffer (0.2 M, pH 6.6, 2.5 mL) and potassium ferricyanide (1 g/100 mL, 2.5 mL). The mixtures were then incubated at 50°C for 20 min. After incubation, trichloroacetic acid (10%) was added to stop the reaction. An equal volume of distilled water was added to the mixtures followed by the addition of ferum chlorate (0.1 g/100 mL, 500 μL). The mixtures were then allowed to stand at room temperature for 30 min. A_{700} was determined with a UV-visible spectrophotometer (Pharmaspec UV-1650PC, Shimadzu, Japan). The procedures were performed in triplicate and repeated with the standard antioxidants (ascorbic acid and α-tocopherol). The antioxidant activity (%) of the samples in FRAP assay was expressed as reducing power (%) according to the following formula:

$$\text{Reducing power } (\%) = \frac{(\text{Ab}_s \times \text{Ab}_c)}{\text{Ab}_s} \times 100\%, \qquad (3)$$

where Ab_c is the absorbance of control and Ab_s is the absorbance of sample.

2.8. In Vitro Anti-Inflammatory Assay

2.8.1. Hyaluronidase Inhibition Assay.

The assay was carried out according to the method described by Yahaya and Don [18] with slight modifications. All the solutions were freshly prepared before the assay. *A. viridis* samples (5 mg) were dissolved in dimethylsulphoxide (250 μL). The samples were prepared at various concentrations (100, 200, 300, 400, and 500 μg/mL) by dissolving in sodium phosphate buffer (200 mM, pH 7). Hyaluronidase (4 U/mL, 100 μL) was mixed with sample solution (25 μL) incubated at 37°C for 10 min. The reaction was initiated with the addition of substrate, hyaluronic acid solution (0.03% in 300 mM sodium phosphate, pH 5.4, 100 μL), and incubated at 37°C for 45 min. The undigested hyaluronic acid was then precipitated with acid albumin solution (bovine serum albumin (0.1%) in sodium acetate (24 mM), pH 3.8, 1 mL). After 10 min incubation at room temperature, A_{600} was measured using a spectrophotometer (XMA 1200V, Seoul, Korea). The absorbance measurement in the absence of enzyme was used as a control value. Quercetin was used as the positive control to verify the performance of the assay. The assay was performed in triplicate. The percentage of hyaluronidase inhibition was determined using the following formula:

$$\% \text{ Inhibition} = \frac{\text{Ab}_s}{\text{Ab}_c} \times 100\%, \qquad (4)$$

where Ab_c is the absorbance of control and Ab_s is the absorbance of sample.

2.8.2. Lipoxygenase Inhibition Assay.

Lipoxygenase inhibitory activity was performed according to the method suggested by Pin et al. [19] with slight modification. *A. viridis* samples (10 mg) were dissolved in dimethylsulphoxide (500 μL). The samples were prepared at various concentrations (100, 200, 300, 400, and 500 μg/mL) by dissolving in sodium phosphate buffer (100 mM, pH 8). Sodium phosphate buffer (100 mM, pH 8, 2.46 mL), *A. viridis* samples (10 μL), and soybean lipoxygenase solution (167 U/mL, 20 μL) were mixed and incubated at 25°C for 10 min. The reaction was initiated with the addition of substrate, sodium linoleic acid solution (10 μL). The enzymatic conversion of sodium linoleic acid to (9Z,11E)-(13S)-13-hydroperoxyoctadeca-9,11-dienoate was measured by observing the change of absorbance at 234 nm for 6 min using a UV-vis spectrophotometer (Evolution 201, Madison, USA). A control was prepared by replacing samples (10 μL) with mixture of sodium phosphate buffer (2.74 mL) and dimethylsulphoxide (25 μL) into the quartz. Quercetin was used as the positive control to verify the performance of the assay. The assay was performed in triplicate. The percentage of lipoxygenase inhibition was determined according to formula (2).

2.8.3. Xanthine Oxidase Inhibition Assay.
Xanthine oxidase inhibitory activity was determined according to the method of Yahaya and Don [18], with slight modifications. *A. viridis* samples (10 mg) were dissolved in dimethylsulphoxide (500 μL). The samples were prepared at various concentrations (100, 200, 300, 400, and 500 μg/mL) by dissolving in potassium phosphate buffer (50 mM, pH 7.5). Potassium phosphate buffer (50 mM, pH 7.5, 2.38 mL), *A. viridis* samples (10 μL), and xanthine oxidase solution (0.4 U/mL, 10 μL) were mixed and incubated at 25°C for 10 min. The reaction was initiated by the addition of the substrate, xanthine solution (100 μM, 100 μL). The enzymatic conversion of xanthine to uric acid and hydrogen peroxides was measured at A_{295} using UV-vis spectrophotometer (Evolution 201, Madison, USA). A control was prepared by replacing samples (10 μL) with a mixture of potassium phosphate buffer (2.39 mL) and dimethylsulphoxide (25 μL) into the quartz. Quercetin was used as a positive control to validate the performance of the assay. The assay was performed in triplicate. The percentage of xanthine oxidase inhibition was determined according to formula (2).

2.9. IC$_{50}$ Value Determination.
The sample concentration providing 50% of inhibition (IC$_{50}$) was determined through interpolation of linear regression analysis, with lower IC$_{50}$ values suggesting higher antioxidant and anti-inflammatory activities, and vice versa.

2.10. Statistical Analysis.
Data were expressed as mean ± SD from values determined in triplicate. One-way analysis of variance (ANOVA) and the accompanying Dunnett test (SPSS, version 19) were applied to compare values of *A. viridis* extracts with those of the positive controls, and IC$_{50}$ was analyzed by using nonlinear regression.

3. Results

3.1. HMG-CoA Reductase Inhibitory Effect.
A. viridis leaf, seed, and stem showed 72%, 35%, and 22% inhibitory effects, respectively, on HMG-CoA reductase activities (Figure 1). The leaf extract showed the highest inhibition and was further

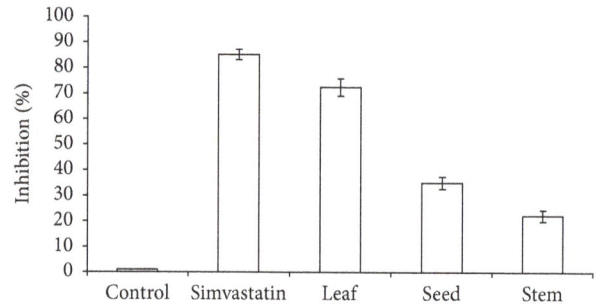

FIGURE 1: Inhibition of HMG-CoA reductase by *A. viridis* extracts. Distilled water was used as a negative control and simvastatin was used as a positive control. All data are presented as the mean ± SD of samples tested in triplicate.

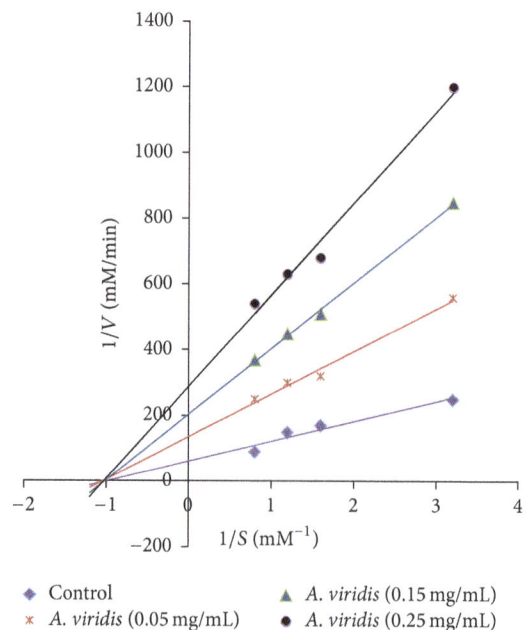

FIGURE 2: The Lineweaver-Burk plot analysis of HMG-CoA reductase in the presence of *A. viridis* leaf extract (0.05, 0.15, and 0.25 mg/mL) and HMG-CoA (0.3, 0.6, 0.9, and 1.2 mmol/L) at 340 nm.

analyzed using Lineweaver-Burk plot analysis. Enzyme kinetics revealed noncompetitive inhibition on HMG-CoA reductase activity (Figure 2). Km value of HMG-CoA for HMG-CoA reductase was 1.0 mM. V_{max} value of the control was 0.0164. V_{max} values for *A. viridis* leaf extract at concentrations of 0.05, 0.15, and 0.25 mg/mL were 0.0074, 0.0049, and 0.0035, respectively.

3.2. Total Phenolic and Total Flavonoid Content.
Total phenolic and total flavonoid content was determined using Folin-Ciocalteu and aluminium calorimetric assays, respectively. *A. viridis* leaf extract showed the highest phenolic and flavonoid content, which was approximately 85.83 mg GAE/g DW and 152.12 mg rutin equivalent/g DW, respectively. The results are summarized in Table 1.

TABLE 1: Total phenolic and flavonoid content of different parts of *A. viridis*.

Sample	Total phenolic content[a] (mg/g DW)	Total flavonoid content[b] (mg/g DW)
Leaf	85.83 ± 1.56	152.12 ± 1.41
Stem	26.38 ± 0.34	50.97 ± 0.75
Seed	38.12 ± 0.89	81.36 ± 0.36

a: gallic acid equivalent; b: rutin equivalent. The analyses were performed in three replications.

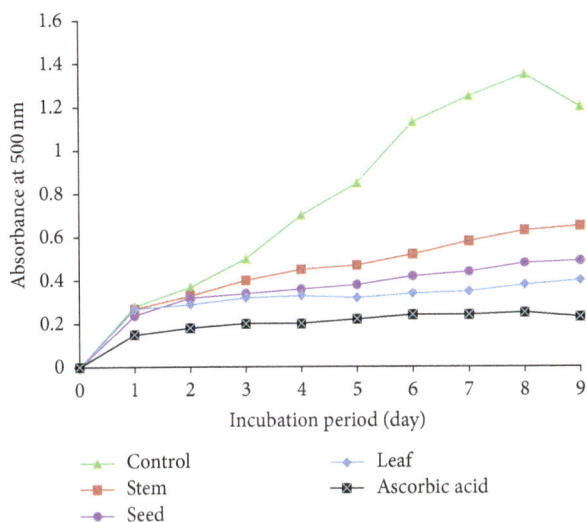

FIGURE 4: Total antioxidant activity assayed by ferric thiocyanate and thiobarbituric acid methods on day 9. The data represent the mean $\pm$ SD measurements of samples tested in triplicate.

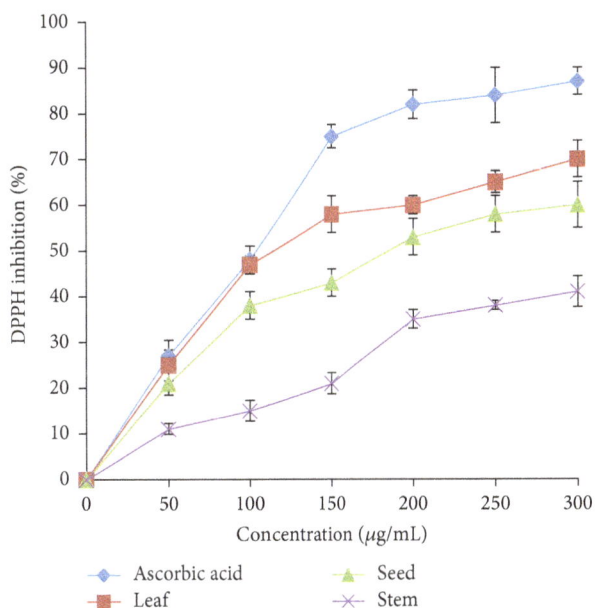

FIGURE 3: The inhibitory activity of *A. viridis* extracts on hydroperoxides in the ferric thiocyanate test.

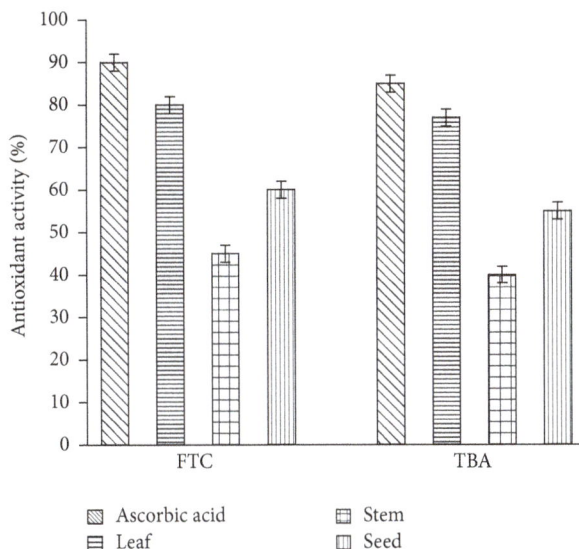

FIGURE 5: DPPH radical scavenging activity of *A. viridis* extracts at various concentrations. The data represent the mean $\pm$ SD measurements of sample tested in triplicate.

3.3. Antioxidant Activities.

The inhibitory activity of *A. viridis* extracts with respect to hydroperoxides was measured by the ferric thiocyanate assay (Figure 3). The leaf extract was found to have the best tendency to inhibit hydroperoxides compared to stem and seed. The results from FTC and TBA were almost similar in the sense that leaf extract was superior to stem and seed in terms of the potential to inhibit hydroperoxides (Figure 4).

A. viridis extracts exhibited DPPH radical scavenging activity at various concentrations (Figure 5). All samples exhibited DPPH scavenging activity in a dose-dependent manner. Leaf extract achieved its highest inhibition at about 70%, followed by seed (58%) and stem (39%) at a concentration of 300 μg/mL. IC_{50} values of leaf, seed, and stem were 115.74 μg/mL, 189.21 μg/mL, and >300 μg/mL, respectively.

All samples exhibited NO scavenging activity in a dose-dependent manner (Figure 6). The leaf extract exhibited the highest inhibition, about 60%, followed by seed (48%) and stem (22%) at a concentration of 300 μg/mL. IC_{50} values of leaf, seed, and stem were 244.36 μg/mL, 299.40 μg/mL, and >300 μg/mL, respectively.

A. viridis extracts also exhibited satisfactory potential to reduce ferric ions at different concentrations (Figure 7). A drastic increase in the reducing power was observed at a concentration of 100 μg/mL. The leaf extract exhibited the highest inhibition, about 85%, followed by seed (72%) and stem (48%) at a concentration of 300 μg/mL. IC_{50} values of leaf, seed, and stem were 77.32 μg/mL, 83.47 μg/mL, and >300 μg/mL, respectively. Table 2 summarizes IC_{50} values of *A. viridis* extracts and standards for DPPH and NO radical scavenging and ferric-reducing activities.

3.4. Anti-Inflammatory Activities.

The hyaluronidase inhibitory activity of the *A. viridis* extracts was investigated at different concentrations and was compared to quercetin

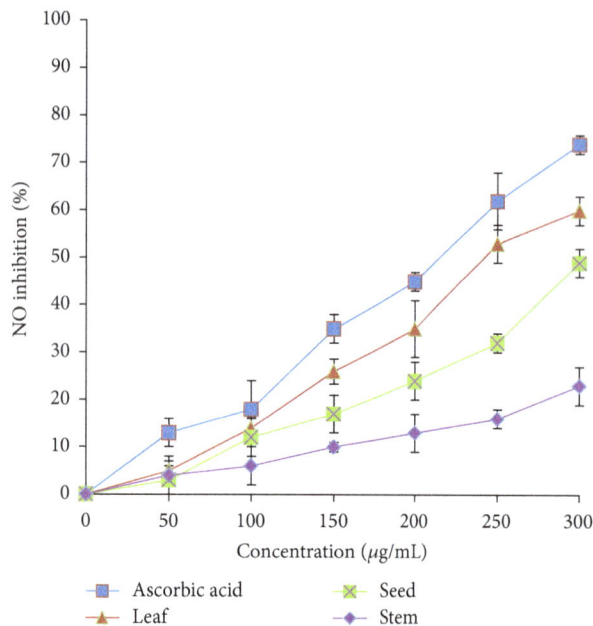

FIGURE 6: Nitric oxide scavenging activity of *A. viridis* extracts at various concentrations. The data represent the mean ± SD measurements of samples tested in triplicate.

TABLE 2: IC$_{50}$ values (μg/mL) of *A. viridis* extracts and standard on radical scavenging and reducing power activities.

Sample	DPPH	NO	FRAP
Ascorbic acid	105.03 ± 1.31	217.64 ± 0.79	63.49 ± 1.75
Leaf	115.74 ± 1.64	244.36 ± 2.15	77.32 ± 0.96
Stem	>300	>300	>300
Seed	189.21 ± 1.25	299.40 ± 1.26	83.47 ± 1.25

The analyses were performed in three replications.

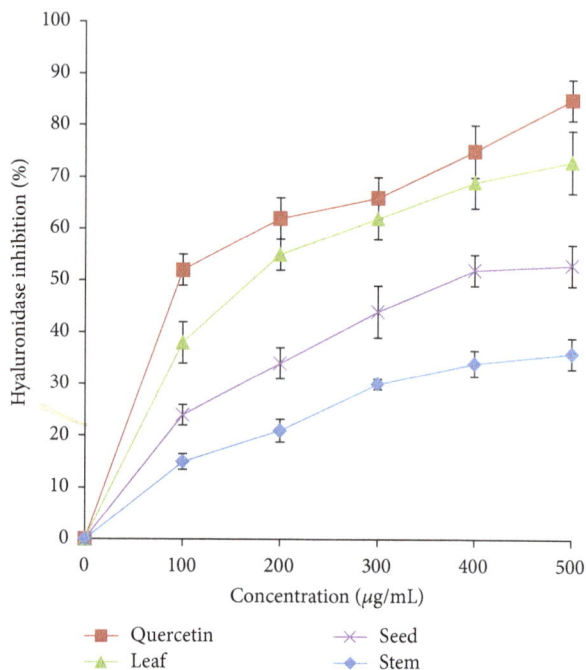

FIGURE 8: Hyaluronidase inhibitory activity of *A. viridis* extracts at various concentrations. The data represent the mean ± SD measurements of samples tested in triplicate.

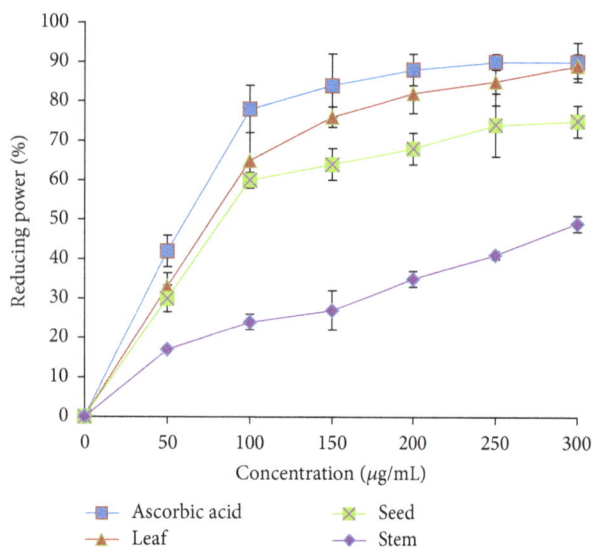

FIGURE 7: Ferric-reducing activity of *A. viridis* extracts at various concentrations. The data represent the mean ± SD measurements of samples tested in triplicate.

(Figure 8). The inhibitory activity of the *A. viridis* extracts showed a gradual increase as the concentration increased. The leaf extract achieved about 70% inhibition at a concentration of 500 μg/mL, followed by seed (50%) and stem (35%). IC$_{50}$ values of leaf extract and quercetin were 186.23 μg/mL and 101.64 μg/mL, respectively.

Similarly, the investigation on lipoxygenase inhibitory activity revealed that *A. viridis* extracts inhibited the lipoxygenase enzyme in a dose-dependent manner. The highest

inhibition, 82%, was exhibited by the leaf extract, followed by seed (60%) and stem (35%) at a concentration of 500 μg/mL (Figure 9). IC$_{50}$ values of leaf extract and quercetin were 151.59 μg/mL and 98.36 μg/mL, respectively.

A. viridis extracts exhibited anti-xanthine oxidase activity in a concentration-dependent manner (Figure 10). The highest inhibition, approximately 80%, was achieved by the leaf extract at a concentration of 500 μg/mL, followed by seed (58%) and stem (43%). IC$_{50}$ values of leaf extract and quercetin were approximately 101.62 μg/mL and 68.67 μg/mL, respectively. Table 3 summarizes IC$_{50}$ values of *A. viridis* extracts and standards for hyaluronidase, lipoxygenase, and xanthine oxidase inhibition assays.

4. Discussion

Among the *A. viridis* extracts, the leaf extract showed the highest inhibition of 71% on HMG-CoA reductase activity. The inhibitory effect of *A. viridis* leaf extract is comparable to that of *Basella alba* leaf extract (74%) which was reported

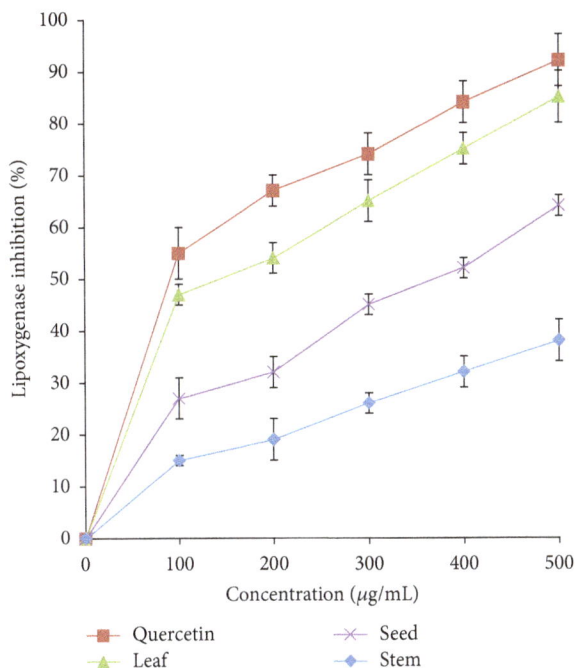

FIGURE 9: Lipoxygenase inhibitory activity of *A. viridis* extracts at various concentrations. The data represent the mean ± SD measurements of samples tested in triplicate.

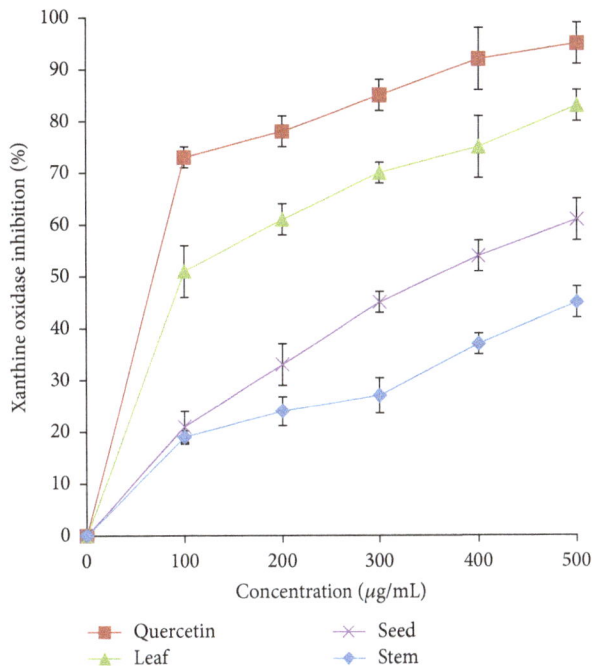

FIGURE 10: Xanthine oxidase inhibitory activity of *A. viridis* extracts at various concentrations. The data represent the mean ± SD measurements of samples tested in triplicate.

TABLE 3: IC_{50} values (μg/mL) of *A. viridis* extract and standard on inhibitory activities of inflammatory enzymes.

Sample	Hyaluronidase	Lipoxygenase	Xanthine oxidase
Quercetin	101.64 ± 0.89	98.36 ± 1.83	68.67 ± 0.65
Leaf	186.23 ± 1.31	151.59 ± 0.82	101.62 ± 1.29
Stem	>500	>500	>500
Seed	398.25 ± 2.33	394.52 ± 1.35	374.43 ± 2.15

The analyses were performed in three replications.

as a potent inhibitor of HMG-CoA reductase [11]. This observation is of great relevance since HMG-CoA reductase is the target enzyme for hypercholesterolemia. Plant extracts that suppress HMG-CoA reductase may possibly be used as hypocholesterolemic agent. Statins are synthetic drugs that competitively inhibit HMG-CoA reductase [20]. In contrast, *A. viridis* leaf extract was shown to inhibit HMG-CoA reductase in a noncompetitive manner. V_{max} value was found to decrease as the leaf concentration increased, suggesting that the substrate was unable to bind to HMG-CoA reductase. The inhibitor interacts with the enzyme or enzyme-substrate complex in which the binding changes the shape of the active site and prevents the formation of cholesterol. The anti-HMG-CoA reductase activity of the *A. viridis* leaf extract reflects its potential in cholesterol reduction.

The presence of significant phenolic and flavonoid contents suggests the potential use of the *A. viridis* leaf extract as an alternative medicine. Phenolic compounds describe a class of secondary metabolites with a wide range of pharmacological activities [21]. Indeed, various biological roles of phenolic

acids have been reported. They play important roles in secretion of bile and reduction of lipids and cholesterol levels [22]. Phenolics and flavonoids exhibit a wide range of biological activities, including anti-inflammatory [23], antioxidant [24], antidepressant [25], and antiulcer [26] activities. The results of the current study on *A. viridis* leaf are comparable to those of a study by Hendra et al. [15], who found that the plant *Phaleria macrocarpa* possessed a high phenolic and flavonoid content.

Antioxidants are compounds that impede oxidation of substrates, and this is characterized by the potential to trap free radicals [27]. The main role that antioxidants play within the body systems rests on their ability to react with free radicals. Free radicals are compounds with unpaired electrons. The reaction eliminates the reactive properties of the radical [28]. With slight modification, the tests used in the current study are acknowledged to be reliable in investigating the antioxidant and anti-inflammatory potential of various substances [18, 29]. In many instances, the methods that have been utilized in determining the antioxidant activities are oriented towards the tendency of the tested compounds to scavenge free radicals or complex metal ions [30, 31]. We believe that the fact that these methods have been used in the current study highlights the reliability of the study.

The radical scavenging and reducing activities of *A. viridis* extracts appear to have been related mostly to the flavonoid content. The standard, ascorbic acid, gave higher inhibition rate compared to *A. viridis* extracts. This suggests that the rate of inhibition of *A. viridis* extracts may be improved by increasing the concentration in all cases. The measurement of inhibitory activities of *A. viridis* extracts with respect to hydroperoxides, using the FTC assay, suggests that *A. viridis* leaf extract effectively inhibits hydroperoxides. The *A. viridis* leaf and ascorbic acid standard showed low absorbance values compared to the negative control, suggesting high levels of antioxidant activity. The differences in the potential to inhibit hydroperoxides were further assayed by FTC and TBA methods on day nine when the negative control's absorbance decreases. The similarity in the results between FTC and TBA suggests the reliability of the results. In the context of toxicity, despite the fact that hydrogen peroxide is unreactive in the body systems, it may be toxic to cells, inhibiting cell functioning abilities by yielding hydroxyl radicals [32]. In this regard, elimination of hydrogen peroxide is considered a crucial antidetoxification process [33].

A. viridis leaf exhibited the DPPH radical scavenging ability at various concentrations, and the inhibition rate of *A. viridis* extract can be further improved by increasing the concentration. Similar to the potential in inhibiting hydroperoxides, leaf extract exhibited good inhibition of DPPH, considering that it compared favorably with ascorbic acid in terms of its ability to scavenge DPPH radical. The results revealed that *A. viridis* leaf has certain components possessing desirable hydrogen donation capacity that are well placed to scavenge the DPPH radicals which can be linked to the significant concentrations of flavonoid and phenolic acid, as well as the presence of hydroxyl groups [34]. Thaipong et al. [35] further explained that the antiradical activity of phenolic acids depends on the presence of phenolic hydroxyl hydrogen on the molecular structure, as well as on the tendency of phenoxyl radicals to stabilize resulting from the donation of hydrogen.

The data suggest that the leaf extract had good scavenging activity on the NO radical, in which the effectiveness increased in a dose-dependent manner. The leaf extract effectively inhibited ferric ions and was as effective as ascorbic acid in scavenging ferric ion radicals at a concentration of 300 μg/mL. The performance of *A. viridis* leaf on NO and ferric ions inhibition has interestingly found concurring results; this finding is consistent with those reported earlier [21, 33]. Napoli and Lerman [36] have suggested that the inhibition of NO and ferric ion radicals is crucial in the management of hypercholesterolemia. The formation of these radicals can also result in pronounced vasomotor dysfunction which can further lead to atherosclerotic lesions [37, 38].

IC$_{50}$ values (μg/mL) of *A. viridis* extract revealed its good radical scavenging and reducing power activities. These results are comparable with those obtained using *Phaleria macrocarpa,* an antioxidant rich medicinal plant [15]. The *A. viridis* leaf extract exhibited a desirable ability to inhibit hydroperoxides, DPPH, NO, and ferric ions; this shows that it has a strong antioxidant capacity and could be helpful in treating the diseases caused by radicals, such as hypercholesterolemia and atherosclerosis.

The degradation of extracellular matrix plays an essential role in the development of various diseases possessing an inflammatory background [39]. Hyaluronidase is one of the most vital enzymes in this process and plays a major role in controlling the size and concentration of depolymerised hyaluronan chains, which are capable of altering the activities

of many pathological processes. Hyaluronidase can cause increased endothelial permeability which can lead to atherogenesis [40]. The results from the current study suggested that the *A. viridis* leaf extract possessed high antihyaluronidase activity.

Lipoxygenases (LOXs) composed of nonheme iron-containing dioxygenases are important enzymes in leukotrienes biosynthesis, which have been believed to play a key role in the pathophysiology of inflammatory diseases [41]. Cipollone et al. [42] found that the LOXs expressions increased in the carotid atherosclerotic plaques of patients. It is suggested that LOXs are promising targets for therapeutic approaches focused on inflammation reduction in atherosclerotic plaques [43]. The *A. viridis* leaf extract was proven to be an effective inhibitor of lipoxygenase enzyme.

Xanthine oxidase, an oxygen free radical, has been commonly associated with being an important route in the oxidative injury to tissues, particularly ischemia-reperfusion [44]. Xanthine oxidase is involved in the metabolism of xanthine to uric acid. Uric acid plays a pathogenetic role in cardiovascular diseases; hyperuricemia is generally associated with deleterious effects on vascular function [45]. The inhibition of xanthine oxidase may exert therapeutic effects on impaired vascular function. The data from the present study suggest that the *A. viridis* leaf extract exhibited satisfactory potential as an inhibitor of the xanthine oxidase enzyme.

An examination of IC$_{50}$ values (μg/mL) of *A. viridis* extract on inhibition of the enzymes activities reveals its potential as an anti-inflammatory agent. Since leaf extract compares favorably with quercetin in inhibiting hyaluronidase, lipoxygenases, and xanthine oxidase, it may possess beneficial effects in protecting the vascular endothelial cells from oxidative stress, inflammation, and atherosclerosis.

5. Conclusion

A. viridis leaf extract appears to be a potent inhibitor of HMG-CoA reductase in a noncompetitive manner. The presence of phenolic and flavonoid content suggests that *A. viridis* can be used as an antioxidant in alternative medicine. Indeed, *A. viridis* leaf extract also exhibited good potential to reduce hydroperoxides, DPPH, NO, ferric ions, hyaluronidase, lipoxygenase, and xanthine oxidase at various concentrations. An examination of IC$_{50}$ values (μg/mL) of *A. viridis* leaf extract and standards on radical scavenging, reducing power, and enzymes inhibitory activities suggests its potential as an antioxidant and anti-inflammatory agent. Thus, in the management of hypercholesterolemia, *A. viridis* leaf extract appears to possess appreciable anti-HMG-CoA reductase activity and beneficial antioxidant and anti-inflammatory effects. Investigation in an *in vivo* model could further confirm the potential of *A. viridis* leaf extract in treating hypercholesterolemia.

Competing Interests

The authors declare that there are no competing interests regarding the publication of this paper.

Acknowledgments

The research is supported by Universiti Putra Malaysia, Putra Grants: 9438200. Shamala Salvamani is supported by the Ministry of Higher Education of Malaysia.

References

[1] J. A. Friesen and V. W. Rodwell, "The 3-hydroxy-3-methylglu-taryl coenzyme-A (HMG-CoA) reductases," *Genome Biology*, vol. 5, no. 11, pp. 248.1–248.7, 2004.

[2] G. Baskaran, S. Salvamani, A. Azlan, S. A. Ahmad, S. K. Yeap, and M. Y. Shukor, "Hypocholesterolemic and anti-atherosclerotic potential of *Basella alba* leaf extract in hypercholesterolemia-induced rabbits," *Evidence-Based Complementary and Alternative Medicine*, vol. 2015, Article ID 751714, 7 pages, 2015.

[3] S. Salvamani, B. Gunasekaran, N. A. Shaharuddin, S. A. Ahmad, and M. Y. Shukor, "Antiartherosclerotic effects of plant flavonoids," *BioMed Research International*, vol. 2014, Article ID 480258, 11 pages, 2014.

[4] S.-M. Lin, B.-H. Lin, W.-M. Hsieh et al., "Structural identification and bioactivities of red-violet pigments present in *Basella alba* fruits," *Journal of Agricultural and Food Chemistry*, vol. 58, no. 19, pp. 10364–10372, 2010.

[5] P. F. Moundipa, N. S. E. Beboy, F. Zelefack et al., "Effects of *Basella alba* and *Hibiscus macranthus* extracts on testosterone production of adult rat and bull Leydig cells," *Asian Journal of Andrology*, vol. 7, no. 4, pp. 411–417, 2005.

[6] F. P. Moundipa, P. Kamtchouing, N. Koueta, J. Tantchou, N. P. R. Foyang, and F. T. Mbiapo, "Effects of aqueous extracts of *Hibiscus macranthus* and *Basella alba* in mature rat testis function," *Journal of Ethnopharmacology*, vol. 65, no. 2, pp. 133–139, 1999.

[7] K. Girija and K. Lakshman, "Anti-hyperlipidemic activity of methanol extracts of three plants of *Amaranthus* in triton-WR 1339 induced hyperlipidemic rats," *Asian Pacific Journal of Tropical Biomedicine*, vol. 1, no. 1, pp. S62–S65, 2011.

[8] M. Turin, "Ethnobotonical notes on Thangmi plant names and their medicinal and ritual uses," *Contributions to Nepalese Studies*, vol. 30, no. 1, pp. 19–52, 2003.

[9] B. S. A. Kumar, K. Lakshman, K. N. Jayaveea et al., "Antidiabetic, antihyperlipidemic and antioxidant activities of methanolic extract of *Amaranthus viridis* Linn in alloxan induced diabetic rats," *Experimental and Toxicologic Pathology*, vol. 64, no. 1-2, pp. 75–79, 2012.

[10] B. S. Ashok Kumar, K. Lakshman, K. N. Jayaveera et al., "Pain management in mice using methanol extracts of three plants belongs to family *Amaranthaceae*," *Asian Pacific Journal of Tropical Medicine*, vol. 3, no. 7, pp. 527–530, 2010.

[11] G. Baskaran, S. Salvamani, S. A. Ahmad, N. A. Shaharuddin, P. D. Pattiram, and M. Y. Shukor, "HMG-CoA reductase inhibitory activity and phytocomponent investigation of *Basella alba* leaf extract as a treatment for hypercholesterolemia," *Drug Design, Development and Therapy*, vol. 9, pp. 509–517, 2015.

[12] A. Gholamhoseinian, B. Shahouzehi, and F. Sharifi-Far, "Inhibitory activity of some plant methanol extracts on 3-hydroxy-3-methylglutaryl coenzyme a reductase," *International Journal of Pharmacology*, vol. 6, no. 5, pp. 705–711, 2010.

[13] A. Meda, C. E. Lamien, M. Romito, J. Millogo, and O. G. Nacoulma, "Determination of the total phenolic, flavonoid and proline contents in Burkina Fasan honey, as well as their radical scavenging activity," *Food Chemistry*, vol. 91, no. 3, pp. 571–577, 2005.

[14] H. I. Ismail, K. W. Chan, A. A. Mariod, and M. Ismail, "Phenolic content and antioxidant activity of cantaloupe (*Cucumis melo*) methanolic extracts," *Food Chemistry*, vol. 119, no. 2, pp. 643–647, 2010.

[15] R. Hendra, S. Ahmad, E. Oskoueian, A. Sukari, and M. Y. Shukor, "Antioxidant, anti-inflammatory and cytotoxicity of *Phaleria macrocarpa* (Boerl.) scheff fruit," *BMC Complementary and Alternative Medicine*, vol. 11, no. 1, pp. 110–120, 2011.

[16] P.-J. Tsai, T.-H. Tsai, C.-H. Yu, and S.-C. Ho, "Comparison of NO-scavenging and NO-suppressing activities of different herbal teas with those of green tea," *Food Chemistry*, vol. 103, no. 1, pp. 181–187, 2007.

[17] G.-C. Yen and H.-Y. Chen, "Antioxidant activity of various tea extracts in relation to their antimutagenicity," *Journal of Agricultural and Food Chemistry*, vol. 43, no. 1, pp. 27–32, 1995.

[18] Y. A. Yahaya and M. M. Don, "Evaluation of *Trametes lactinea* extracts on the inhibition of hyaluronidase, lipoxygenase and xanthine oxidase activities *in vitro*," *Journal of Physical Science*, vol. 23, no. 2, pp. 1–15, 2012.

[19] K. Y. Pin, A. L. Chuah, A. A. Rashih et al., "Antioxidant and anti-inflammatory activities of extracts of betel leaves (*Piper betle*) from solvents with different polarities," *Journal of Tropical Forest Science*, vol. 22, no. 4, pp. 448–455, 2010.

[20] T. Carbonell and E. Freire, "Binding thermodynamics of statins to HMG-CoA reductase," *Biochemistry*, vol. 44, no. 35, pp. 11741–11748, 2005.

[21] M. A. Soobrattee, V. S. Neergheen, A. Luximon-Ramma, O. I. Aruoma, and T. Bahorun, "Phenolics as potential antioxidant therapeutic agents: mechanism and actions," *Mutation Research-Fundamental and Molecular Mechanisms of Mutagenesis*, vol. 579, no. 1-2, pp. 200–213, 2005.

[22] A. Kamal-Eldin, J. Frank, A. Razdan, S. Tengblad, S. Basu, and B. Vessby, "Effects of dietary phenolic compounds on tocopherol, cholesterol, and fatty acids in rats," *Lipids*, vol. 35, no. 4, pp. 427–435, 2000.

[23] E. A. Miles, P. Zbouli, and P. C. Calder, "Differential anti-inflammatory effects of phenolic compounds from extra virgin olive oil identified in human whole blood cultures," *Nutrition*, vol. 21, no. 3, pp. 389–394, 2005.

[24] Y. Cai, Q. Luo, M. Sun, and H. Corke, "Antioxidant activity and phenolic compounds of 112 traditional Chinese medicinal plants associated with anticancer," *Life Sciences*, vol. 74, no. 17, pp. 2157–2184, 2004.

[25] R. Daudt, G. L. Von Poser, G. Neves, and S. M. K. Rates, "Screening for the antidepressant activity of some species of Hypericum from South Brazil," *Phytotherapy Research*, vol. 14, no. 5, pp. 344–346, 2000.

[26] I. F. F. Benzie, "Evolution of dietary antioxidants," *Comparative Biochemistry and Physiology Part A: Molecular & Integrative Physiology*, vol. 136, no. 1, pp. 113–126, 2003.

[27] D. Amic, D. Davidovic-Amic, D. Beslo, and N. Trinajstic, "Structure-radical scavenging activity relationships of flavonoids," *Croatica Chemica Acta*, vol. 76, no. 1, pp. 55–61, 2010.

[28] M. Valko, D. Leibfritz, J. Moncol, M. T. D. Cronin, M. Mazur, and J. Telser, "Free radicals and antioxidants in normal physiological functions and human disease," *International Journal of Biochemistry and Cell Biology*, vol. 39, no. 1, pp. 44–84, 2007.

[29] S. Dudonné, X. Vitrac, P. Coutiére, M. Woillez, and J.-M. Mérillon, "Comparative study of antioxidant properties and total phenolic content of 30 plant extracts of industrial interest using DPPH, ABTS, FRAP, SOD, and ORAC assays," *Journal of Agricultural and Food Chemistry*, vol. 57, no. 5, pp. 1768–1774, 2009.

[30] K. E. Heim, A. R. Tagliaferro, and D. J. Bobilya, "Flavonoid antioxidants: chemistry, metabolism and structure-activity relationships," *The Journal of Nutritional Biochemistry*, vol. 13, no. 10, pp. 572–584, 2002.

[31] P.-G. Pietta, "Flavonoids as antioxidants," *Journal of Natural Products*, vol. 63, no. 7, pp. 1035–1042, 2000.

[32] B. Halliwell, "Free radicals in biochemistry and medicine," in *Encyclopedia of Molecular Cell Biology and Molecular Medicine*, 2006.

[33] B. Halliwell, M. V. Clement, and L. H. Long, "Hydrogen peroxide in the human body," *FEBS Letters*, vol. 486, no. 1, pp. 10–13, 2000.

[34] R. A. Larson, "The antioxidants of higher plants," *Phytochemistry*, vol. 27, no. 4, pp. 969–978, 1988.

[35] K. Thaipong, U. Boonprakob, K. Crosby, L. Cisneros-Zevallos, and B. D. Hawkins, "Comparison of ABTS, DPPH, FRAP and ORAC assays for estimating antioxidant activity from guava fruit extracts," *Journal of Food Composition and Analysis*, vol. 19, no. 6-7, pp. 669–675, 2006.

[36] C. Napoli and L. O. Lerman, "Involvement of oxidation-sensitive mechanisms in the cardiovascular effects of hypercholesterolemia," *Mayo Clinic Proceedings*, vol. 76, no. 6, pp. 619–631, 2001.

[37] W. H. Ling, Q. X. Cheng, J. Ma, and T. Wang, "Red and black rice decrease atherosclerotic plaque formation and increase antioxidant status in rabbits," *Journal of Nutrition*, vol. 131, no. 5, pp. 1421–1426, 2001.

[38] S. Wassmann, U. Laufs, A. T. Bäumer et al., "HMG-CoA reductase inhibitors improve endothelial dysfunction in normocholesterolemic hypertension via reduced production of reactive oxygen species," *Hypertension*, vol. 37, no. 6, pp. 1450–1457, 2001.

[39] T. L. Adair-Kirk and R. M. Senior, "Fragments of extracellular matrix as mediators of inflammation," *The International Journal of Biochemistry and Cell Biology*, vol. 40, no. 6-7, pp. 1101–1110, 2008.

[40] K. P. Sunnergren, R. P. Fairman, G. G. DeBlois, and F. L. Glauser, "Effects of protamine, heparinase, and hyaluronidase on endothelial permeability and surface charge," *Journal of Applied Physiology*, vol. 63, no. 5, pp. 1987–1992, 1987.

[41] Y. Yamamoto and R. B. Gaynor, "Therapeutic potential of inhibition of the NF-κB pathway in the treatment of inflammation and cancer," *Journal of Clinical Investigation*, vol. 107, no. 2, pp. 135–142, 2001.

[42] F. Cipollone, A. Mezzetti, M. L. Fazia et al., "Association between 5-lipoxygenase expression and plaque instability in humans," *Arteriosclerosis, Thrombosis, and Vascular Biology*, vol. 25, no. 8, pp. 1665–1670, 2005.

[43] X.-F. Lai, H.-D. Qin, L.-L. Guo, Z.-G. Luo, J. Chang, and C.-C. Qin, "Hypercholesterolemia increases the production of leukotriene B4 in neutrophils by enhancing the nuclear localization of 5-lipoxygenase," *Cellular Physiology and Biochemistry*, vol. 34, no. 5, pp. 1723–1732, 2014.

[44] J. Sanhueza, J. Valdes, R. Campos, A. Garrido, and A. Valenzuela, "Changes in the xanthine dehydrogenase/xanthine oxidase ratio in the rat kidney subjected to ischemia-reperfusion stress: preventive effect of some flavonoids," *Research Communications in Chemical Pathology and Pharmacology*, vol. 78, no. 2, pp. 211–218, 1992.

[45] U. M. Khosla, S. Zharikov, J. L. Finch et al., "Hyperuricemia induces endothelial dysfunction," *Kidney International*, vol. 67, no. 5, pp. 1739–1742, 2005.

13

Synergism of Chinese Herbal Medicine: Illustrated by Danshen Compound

Xuefeng Su, Zhuoting Yao, Shengting Li, and He Sun

Department of Clinical Research, Tasly Pharmaceuticals Inc., 9400 Key West Avenue, Rockville, MD 20850, USA

Correspondence should be addressed to Shengting Li; shengtingli@tasly.com

Academic Editor: Avni Sali

The primary therapeutic effects of Chinese herbal medicine (CHM) are based on the properties of each herb and the strategic combination of herbs in formulae. The herbal formulae are constructed according to Chinese medicine theory: the "Traditional Principles for Constructing Chinese Herbal Medicinal Formulae" and the "Principles of Combining Medicinal Substances." These principles of formulation detail how and why multiple medicinal herbs with different properties are combined together into a single formula. However, the concept of herbal synergism in CHM still remains a mystery due to lack of scientific data and modern assessment methods. The Compound Danshen Formula (CDF) is a validated formula that has been used to treat a variety of diseases for hundreds of years in China and other countries. The CDF will be employed to illustrate the theory and principle of Chinese herbal medicine formulation. The aim of this review is to describe how Chinese herbal medicinal formulae are constructed according to Chinese medicine theory and to illustrate with scientific evidence how Chinese herbs work synergistically within a formula, thereby supporting Chinese medicine theory and practice.

1. Introduction

Traditional Chinese Medicine (TCM) encompasses a variety of therapies including Chinese herbal medicine (CHM), acupuncture, Qigong, and physical therapy such as massage and Gua Sha (scraping). Due to its unique philosophy and treatment characteristics, TCM was identified as one of the advanced medical sciences until the 17th century [1, 2]. CHM, as the most important part of TCM, has been used to treat disease for over 4,000 years [1, 3]. Even though Western medicine is widely accepted by modern Chinese culture, CHM still plays a very important role in daily medical practice; about 46% of patients were prescribed CHM in hospitals or outpatient clinics. CHM is popularly used for the treatment of variety of diseases such as the common cold, hepatitis, nephrotic syndrome, diabetes, cardiovascular disease, and cancer [4–9]. Worldwide, increasing numbers of Westerners are recognizing the importance of CHM and seeking it as part of their healthcare.

Medical science has long realized that the pathogenesis and progression of diseases are too complex for single drug treatment. For example, cardiovascular disease is the primary killer worldwide [10, 11], with coronary artery disease (CAD) as the most common cause of cardiovascular morbidity and mortality. The pathophysiology of CAD is very complex and warrants multifaceted treatment [12, 13]. The strategies include treatment of the primary disease as well as intervention in risk factors and comorbid conditions such as high cholesterol, hypertension, obesity, and diabetes [14, 15]. The treatment regimen is a combination of pharmaceutical drugs that target the different organs and systems involved in the pathophysiological processes of the primary and secondary conditions. These medications include but are not limited to aspirin, nitrates, Angiotensin II receptor blocker (ARB), statins, diuretics, and metformin [15–17]. Interestingly, to achieve better therapeutic outcomes and diminish side effects, multiherb therapy is an essential component of traditional Chinese herbal medicine and has been utilized in China for thousands of years [3, 18].

Originally, practitioners of Chinese herbal medicine used just single herbs for disease treatment. But, over time, Chinese herbalists gained more experience from clinical practice and learned that the causes of diseases were imbalances among different systems in the body. To restore the dynamic balance among body systems and get the best curative effect with the least toxicological effect, Chinese herbalists chose a combination of several herbs based on the distinct disease presentations. Through this process, the theory of herbal synergism in CHM was developed and refined by herbalists over thousands of years of clinical practice. Single herbal medicines and herbal formulae compose the Chinese herbal medicine system [19]. There are 8980 herbs compiled into *Zhong Hua Ben Cao* (*Chinese Materia Medica* 1999) and 1444 Chinese herbal formulae collected in 2010 edition of the *Chinese Pharmacopoeia*. CHM combines two or more herbs with different properties synergistically to form a compound formula named "复方 (fù fāng)" or "方剂 (fāng jì)" based on the Principles of Combining Medicinal Substances [20].

When two or more Chinese herbal medicines (CHMs) are combined, they become a named formula. Over 2,000 years of practice, CHM has accumulated over 100,000 formulae that are constructed according to specific TCM principles [18, 21]. Based on empirical evidence gathered over many centuries, CHM providers learned that particular herbal combinations work synergistically or antagonistically [3]. Herbal formulae are constructed based on this synergism, outlined as theories in *Materia Medica*. With the rise of scientific research methods, the synergism between herbs is being investigated pharmacologically. This research substantiates Chinese medicine theory and elucidates correct dosage combinations [22]. Through the example of a cardiovascular herbal formula, this paper will explain how Chinese herbs are combined into formulae, the seven traditional types of herbal combinations, and how scientific research contributes additional knowledge.

2. Traditional Principles for Constructing Chinese Herbal Medicinal Formulae: Seven Types of Herbal Combinations

Traditionally, there are seven types of Chinese herbal combinations, differentiated by their physiologic effects (seven emotions, Chinese name 七情 qīqíng). Seven emotions have two different definitions in TCM. The first one emphasizes the relation between diseases and mental activities, the main pathogenic factors of endogenous diseases [23]. Emotional mental activities are categorized as the seven emotional factors: joy, anger, melancholy, worry, grief, fear, and fright. This is beyond the scope of our topic.

The second one is used in herbal medicine to elucidate the seven possible outcomes that could be yielded if multiple herbs with different pharmacological properties are used in combination. It was first recorded in *Shennong Bencao Jing*, a classic book systemically describing CHM that was written approximately 2000 years ago between the Qin and Han dynasties. From a modern pharmacology perspective, this is a theory about herb-herb interactions [24, 25]. These were described in the *Grand Materia Medica*.

(1) Single Effect (单行 dān xíng). Single effect (单行 dān xíng) is the use of one medicinal substance to treat a patient. An example is the Du Shen Tang decoction, which consists of only one herbal medicine, *Panax ginseng* (Asian ginseng). It was historically prescribed to patients with "Qi and Xue deficiency" states such as postpartum hemorrhage [26], acute myocardial infarction [27], cirrhosis [28], upper gastrointestinal bleeding [29], and congestive heart failure [30].

(2) Mutual Accentuation (相須 xiāng xū). Mutual accentuation (相須 xiāng xū) means that the combination of two herbal substances with similar functions will accentuate their therapeutic actions, also called "mutual necessity." For instance, herbal decoction of Da Huang (*Rheum palmatum*, rhubarb) and Mang Xiao (*natrii sulfas*, mirabilite) is used to treat constipation. Pharmacological research showed that Da Huang is able to stimulate the colon by increasing the intensity and frequency of contractions, which subsequently improves bowel motility. The Mang Xiao contains sodium sulfate, which when absorbed in colon creates a hyperosmotic environment, bringing water into the colon and softening the stool. When Da Huang and Mang Xiao are used together in combination they have a better laxative effect compared to each used alone [25, 31].

(3) Mutual Enhancement (相使 xiāng shǐ). Mutual enhancement (相使 xiāng shǐ) is the combination of two or more substances with different actions in which one of the substances enhances the effect of the other in a specific clinical situation, also called "mutual employment." For example, Huang Lian (*rhizoma coptidis*, coptis root) and Mu Xiang (*vladimiriae radix*, costus root) are herbs often prescribed as a pair for the treatment of dysentery. Modern pharmacological study has demonstrated that Huang Lian has antimicrobial effect against *Shigella* spp. both *in vivo* and *in vitro*. Mu Xiang has been proven to increase the serum concentration of berberine, the major active antimicrobial component of Huang Lian. When used with Mu Xiang, Huang Lian has a greater efficacy for patients with dysentery [25, 32].

(4) Mutual Counteraction (相畏 xiāng wèi). Mutual counteraction (相畏 xiāng wèi) literally translates to "mutual fear" and means a combination in which the toxicity or side effects of one substance are reduced or eliminated by another substance. For instance, Fu Zi (*Aconitum carmichaelii*, aconite root) is a toxic herb where the primary component is harmful to cardiac and nerve cells. When it is prepared with Gan Cao (*radix glycyrrhizae*, licorice root), the toxicity of Fu Zi is diminished [25, 33]. The emphasis in mutual counteraction is on the toxic herb that is being counteracted in the formulation.

(5) Mutual Suppression (相杀 xiāng shā). Mutual suppression (相杀 xiāng shā) literally translates to "mutual killing" and is the reverse of mutual counteraction. With mutual suppression, one substance also reduces the undesirable side effects of another but the emphasis is on the herb that performs the beneficial suppressive action. For example, Sheng Jiang (*Zingiber officinale*, ginger root), which was commonly prescribed for cold prevention, as antiemetic, and for detoxication, suppresses or literally "kills" the toxicity of Ban Xia (*Pinellia ternata*, pinellia root) commonly used to relieve

cough and to stop vomiting and it is toxic when used alone. In short, mutual counteraction and mutual suppression describe the same herb-herb interaction, but from differing viewpoints [25, 33].

*(6) Mutual Antagonism (*相恶 *xiāng wù).* Mutual antagonism (相恶 xiāng wù) literally translates to "mutual aversion" and means the ability of two substances to minimize each herb's positive effects. Traditionally, there are eight pairs and one trio of substances that have mutually antagonistic effects on each other. Together they are referred to as the "nineteen antagonisms (十九畏 shí jiǔ wèi) [34]." Ren Shen (*radix ginseng,* Chinese ginseng) is capable of replenishing Qi, which increases the overall function of the body. This beneficial function can be reduced or abolished if combined with the herb Lai Fu Zi (*semen raphani,* radish seed) [25, 33].

*(7) Mutual Incompatibility (*相反 *xiāng fǎn).* Mutual incompatibility (相反 xiāng fǎn) translates literally to "mutual opposition" and occurs when the combination of two substances causes side effects or toxicity which would not be caused by any one of the substances if used alone. Traditionally there are three sets or a total of eighteen substances called the "eighteen incompatibilities' (十八反 shí bā fǎn) [35]." For example, it is prohibited in CHM to use Danshen (*Salvia miltiorrhiza,* red sage) and Li Lu (*Veratrum nigrum,* black false hellebore) together. A toxicological study showed that when Danshen was combined with Li Lu, the Danshen increased the concentration of harmful *Veratrum* alkaloids that can produce serious adverse effects such as nausea, vomiting, dizziness, hypotension, and tachycardia. Thus, such a mutually incompatible pair of herbs should not be used in clinical practice according to the principles of CHM [25, 35].

3. The Principles of Combining Medicinal Substances: King, Ministers, Adjutants, and Messengers (君臣佐使 jūn chén zuǒ shǐ)

The Principles of Combining Medicinal Substances provide guidelines for the composition of Chinese herbal prescriptions. Traditionally described in terms of a feudal hierarchy, a formula is usually composed of several medicinal herbs [22, 25]. The chief (also called king, sovereign, or lord, in Chinese 君 jūn) is the principal herbal ingredient in modern texts and is the substance that provides the main therapeutic effect in the prescription. The deputies (also called ministers or associates, in Chinese 臣 chén) enhance or assist the therapeutic actions of the chief. The assistants (also called adjutants, in Chinese 佐 zuǒ) provide one or more of the following functions: treating accompanying symptoms, moderating the harshness or toxicity of the primary substances, assisting the chief and deputies in accomplishing their main objectives, or providing assistance from another therapeutic direction, such as the addition of cooling substance to a warming prescription or vice versa. The envoys (also called messengers or couriers, in Chinese 使 shǐ) either guide the other herbs in the formula to a specific channel or organ or exert a harmonizing influence. A common herb used as

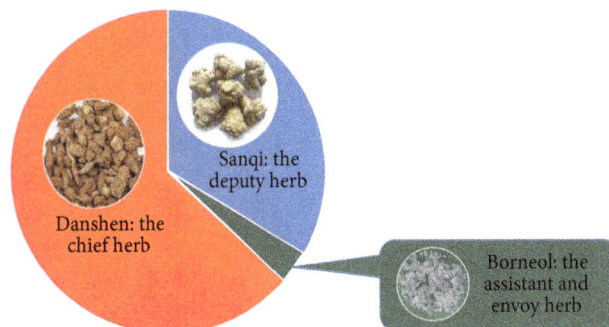

FIGURE 1: The illustration of the role of each ingredient in Fufang Danshen formula. In this formula, Danshen serves as the chief herb and the principal medicine. While Sanqi serves as the deputy herb, enhancing the therapeutic action of Danshen. Bingpian is the assistant and envoy herb that increases the blood concentration of Danshen and Sanqi.

a messenger is glycyrrhizae root (甘草 gān cǎo). Not all principles need to be used in every herbal prescription. There are many simple prescriptions that contain only a chief and deputies, and there are prescriptions in which one substance serves more than one function. For instance, there may be multiple adjutants and messengers in one formula, and one herb may act both as an adjutant and as a messenger [36, 37].

A good example to illustrate the different roles of herbs in formulation is the Compound Danshen Formula (Figure 1), a commonly used formula for treating coronary artery disease including angina and acute myocardial infarction [9]. In this formula, Danshen (*Salvia miltiorrhiza,* red sage) serves as the chief herb. Pharmacological research shows that Danshen causes relaxation of the coronary arteries which is one of the herb's major physiologic, cardioprotective effects. Another herb, Sanqi (*Panax notoginseng,* notoginseng), serves as the deputy herb in the formulation because it has its cardiomyocyte protective and antiplatelet functions. A third herb, Bingpian (*Dryobalanops aromitaca,* borneol), serves as assistant and envoy by increasing the blood concentration of Danshen and Sanqi [38, 39].

4. Pharmacological Research on the Synergism among *Danshen, Sanqi,* and *Bingpian*

Compound Danshen Formula (CDF), composed of Danshen, Sanqi, and Bingpian, has been widely used in the treatment of cardiovascular diseases in China and other countries for over thirty years [40–42]. CDF has been employed by over 600 Chinese pharmaceutical companies and many different products were produced from CDF in China [43].

The dried root of plant Danshen is a popular herbal medicine in China and Japan, used alone or in combination with other herbs [44, 45]. It was first recorded in the Shennong's Classic Materia Medica, *Shennong Bencao Jing,* which is the oldest medicine monograph in China. One of the most widely used traditional medicines, Danshen, is used in the treatment of coronary heart disease [46], cerebrovascular disease [47], Alzheimer's disease [48], Parkinson's disease

[49], renal deficiency [50], liver cirrhosis [51], cancer [52], and bone loss [53]. The composition of Danshen has been analyzed and found to contain 49 diterpenoid quinones, 36 hydrophilic phenolic acids, and 23 essential oil constituents. The diterpenoid quinones and hydrophilic phenolic acids are the principal bioactive components in Danshen [54].

The dry root of Sanqi has been traditionally used in CHM for thousands of years as a hemostatic medicine to control internal and external bleeding [55]. Currently, Sanqi is a commonly used herb to treat cardiovascular disease by stopping bleeding, as well as invigorating and supplementing blood [56]. Moreover, it has function of protecting myocardium, specifically for improving ischemia/reperfusion (I/R) induced injury after percutaneous coronary interventional therapy [54, 57]. It has been reported to have antihypertensive, antithrombotic, antiatherosclerotic, and neuroprotective activities [57]. Various chemical constituents in Sangi have been identified, including ginsenosides, notoginsenosides, flavonoids, volatile oils, amino acids, and polysaccharides [58].

Bingpian contains monoterpenoid constituents and is included in 63 CHM prescriptions according to the *Chinese Pharmacopoeia*. Its wide use as an assistant in CHM is due to its ability to improve percutaneous absorption, enhance oral bioavailability, and facilitate passage of herbal formulation through the blood brain barrier [59–61].

It has been demonstrated through years of clinical use that Danshen and Sanqi have a synergistic effect when combined but the molecular mechanisms underlying their synergism have yet to be clearly elucidated [41, 62]. Cardiovascular disease is the number one cause of death in Europe and in the United States according to the Centers for Disease Control in 2013 [10, 63]. Compound Danshen Formula (CDF) has been widely accepted and used in the treatment of cardiovascular diseases in China and other countries for decades with beneficial outcomes confirmed by clinical trials [9, 64]. There are three preparations compiled in the *Chinese Pharmacopoeia 2010 edition*: Compound Danshen Tablet (CDT), Compound Danshen Granule (CDG), and Compound Danshen Dripping Pill (CDDP). In 1997 the United States Food and Drug Administration (FDA) accepted the Chinese medicinal product CDDP as an investigational new drug (IND number 56956) [9, 64]. In 2010, a phase II clinical study on CDDP was completed and now a phase III clinical trial is underway (ClinicalTrials.gov Identifier: NCT01659580), which is an important milestone in the incorporation of CHM into the Western medical system.

Effects of Danshen and Sanqi on the cardiovascular system are summarized as follows: (1) antioxidant and cardiac protection [65, 66]; (2) inhibition of platelet aggregation and adhesion [67, 68]; (3) vasorelaxation [69]; and (4) prevention of arthrosclerosis [70]. Sanqi prevents arthrosclerosis [41, 71] and protects cardiac myocytes [65, 72]. Danshen contains both hydrophobic and hydrophilic bioactive components such as danshensu, salvianolic acid B, and tanshinone [73–75]. Sanqi contains abundant saponins such as ginsenosides and notoginsenosides [76]. When the two herbs are decocted together in a combination formula, studies have shown that the interaction between the herbs results in a compound with

stronger pharmacological properties compared to each herb alone [62].

4.1. Synergistic Effect of Danshen and Sanqi Demonstrated by Chemistry and Pharmacokinetic Studies. Zeng et al. [77] performed an *in vitro* comparative study on the influence of Danshen and Sanqi on the dissolution of active components from Danshen when the two herbs were decocted in different mass ratios. The ethanol extracts from Danshen and Sanqi were decocted in different mass ratio and HPLC was employed to quantitate the active components from Danshen. The result demonstrated that the main active ingredients from Danshen is higher in all codecocted groups than in the Danshen only group with highest extraction rate at ratio of 5 : 3, Danshen to Sanqi, which is the ratio in classic CDF. In contrast, the effect of mixture or single decoction of Danshen and Sanqi on the dissolution of active components from Sanqi differs from that of Danshen. The effect of Danshen and Sanqi on the extraction of active components from Sanqi was studied by using HPLC combined with UV-visible spectroscopy, infrared spectroscopy, and time-of-flight mass spectrometry [78]. The results demonstrated that codecoction of Danshen and Sanqi inhibited the dissolution of the active components from Sanqi.

A recent *in vivo* study on Guinea pigs extended these findings using three experimental groups [79]. Danshen extracts (salvianolic acid B and tanshinone IIA), Sanqi extracts (panax notoginseng saponins), and a combination of the two extracts were given to three groups of Guinea pigs for a pharmacokinetic study. Parameters analyzed included maximum blood concentration (C_{max}) and area under curve [(AUC) (0–t)]. The result demonstrated that the pharmacokinetic levels of active constituents salvianolic acid B (SalB), tanshinone IIA (Ts IIA), notoginsenoside R1 (R1), ginsenoside Rg1 (Rg1), and ginsenoside Rb1 (Rb1) were markedly different in the Danshen-Sanqi combination group compared to the groups that took Danshen and Sanqi alone. C_{max} of R1, Rb1, and Rg1 were significantly decreased while C_{max} of Ts IIA and SalB were increased in both cerebrospinal fluid (CSF) and plasma. These effects are most likely achieved by increased absorption and distribution of the compound in the body, a result of coadministration of Danshen and Sanqi. This study shows the significant pharmacokinetic changes that can result from the herb-herb interactions. Another study that showed similar results administered oral Danshen alone, Sanqi alone, or Danshen and Sanqi combination suspension to beagle dogs [80]. After administration, the plasma concentration-time profiles of danshensu, tanshinone IIA, cryptotanshinone, notoginsenoside R1, ginsenoside Rg1, and ginsenoside Rb1 were analyzed by LC-MS/MS. The results showed that both C_{max} and AUC of Danshensu, notoginsenoside R1, ginsenoside Rg1, and ginsenoside Rb1 in the Danshen and Sanqi combination group decreased in comparison with those in either the Danshen alone or Sanqi alone groups.

4.2. Synergistic Interaction and Cardiac Protection of Danshen and Sanqi in an Acute Myocardial Infarction Animal Model. Pharmacological studies indicate that the coadministration of Danshen and Sanqi has a cardiac protective effect of improving coronary circulation and improving symptoms of myocardial ischemia, while individual administration of Danshen expands blood vessels and individual administration of Sanqi targets cardiac myocytes. Specifically, the herb pair exerts the best cardiac protective effects when the mass ratio of Danshen to Sanqi is between 10 : 3 and 10 : 7 [41, 81]. A preclinical study [82] comparing the cardioprotective effect of salvianolic acid (SAL) and tanshinone (TAN) was performed in a rat model of acute myocardial infarction (MI). Rats were randomly assigned to four groups: sham group (the ligation suture was placed in the heart, but without ligation), myocardial infarction (MI) group, SAL treatment group, or TAN treatment group (SAL + MI, TAN + MI, resp.). The MI was produced by occlusion of the left anterior descending coronary artery and SAL (120 mg/kg) and TA (120 mg/kg) were given once daily after MI by oral administration. The cardiac functional parameters were measured at 3, 7, 14, and 28 days after surgery. The data demonstrated that both the SAL and TAN treatment groups delayed the development of ischemia by decreasing infarct size and improving systolic function after MI. Gene chip analysis indicated different kinetics and gene expression profiles presented after the administration of SAL and TAN. SAL acted in a later period after ischemia, and its effect was likely mediated by downregulation of genes involved in oxidative stress, specific G-protein coupled receptor activities, and apoptosis [82]. Meanwhile TAN acted relatively early after ischemic injury and its effect was mediated by the inhibition of intracellular calcium, cell adhesion, and alternative complement pathway. Although both SAL and TAN contributed to the cardioprotective effect of Danshen, there were significant mechanistic and temporal differences between the two constituents. To test the effects of the major components from Danshen and Sanqi on cardiac function in a myocardial infarction (MI) rat model, salvianolic B (SalB) from Danshen and ginsenosides Rg1 (GRg1) and Rb1 (GRb1) from Sanqi were administered alone or in combination intragastrically [83]. Fifty rats were randomized into six groups: Sham operation, MI + saline, MI + SalB, MI + GRg1, MI + GRe, MI + SalB + GRg1 (mass ratio of SalB to GRg1 is 2 : 5), and MI + SalB + GRe (mass ratio of SalB to GRe is 2 : 5). The medication was administered in a 60 mg/kg dose twice. The first dose was given one hour before MI generation and the second dose was given at 23rd hour after MI. The group who received the combination of SalB and GRg1 at the mass ratio of 2 : 5 significantly improved cardiac function in this MI model, illustrated by increased left ventricular contractility (+dp/dt) parameter without negative effects on heart rate or blood pressure. No significant improvement in +dp/dt was noted in rats administrated with SalB, GRg1, or GRb1 alone. Nor was improvement seen in the group with coadministration of SalB and GRb1. This result demonstrated that SalB from Danshen and GRg1 from Sanqi worked synergistically to improve cardiac function in a myocardial infarction rat model with mass ratio of 2 : 5.

Lu et al. [84] compared the cardioprotective effects of tanshinone IIA (T), salvianolic acid B (S), ginsenoside Rb1 (G), and Compound Danshen Formula (CDF) on acute myocardial ischemia in rats. The T, S, G, TSG (combination of T, S, and G), and CDF were administered to the MI rats. The cardioprotective effect was evaluated by measuring MI associated parameters including ECG and cardiac enzymes. The result indicated that the combination administration of TSG, and not the administration of the single components alone, had a similar beneficial cardiac effect on MI rats as the CDF group. Other cell biology studies confirmed these findings. Zeng et al. [85] reported that combinational use of Danshen and Sanqi had protective effects on human umbilical vein endothelial cells (HUVEC) that underwent hypoxia-reoxygenation induced cell injury. Measurement of LDH leakage, an index of cell injury, in a culture medium from cells treated by the mixture of Danshen and Sanqi prepared in different ratios demonstrated that Danshen and Sanqi had protective effects on HUVEC at the ratios of 10 : 1, 5 : 3, 1 : 1, and 0 : 10, with best benefit effect at ratios of 5 : 3 and 1 : 1, Danshen to Sanqi.

4.3. Combination of Danshen and Sanqi in the Modulation of Platelet Function.
Herbal combination of Danshen and Sanqi in different mass ratios (10 : 0, 10 : 1, 10 : 3, 10 : 6, and 1 : 10, Danshen to Sanqi) significantly inhibited ADP-induced platelet aggregation with the best inhibitory action at 10 : 3, although Sanqi alone did inhibit platelet aggregation [86]. Three combinations at ratios of 10 : 3, 10 : 6, and 0 : 10 had the ability of inhibiting platelet adhesion with the best result at 0 : 10, that is, Sanqi alone. Interestingly, the mass combination of Danshen and Sanqi at ratios of 10 : 0, 10 : 1, and 1 : 10 did not affect platelet adhesion. Another in vivo study showed that administration of total salvianolic acids (TSA) extracted from Danshen and total notoginsenosides (TNG) from Sanqi at a dose of 550 mg/kg/day for five days could significantly inhibit ADP-induced platelet aggregation [87]. Moreover, even though the use of TSA or TNG alone and the combination of TSA and TNG at mass ratios of 1 : 1, 1 : 5, and 5 : 1 all showed significant inhibition of platelet aggregation, the combination of TSA and TNG at a ratio of 5 : 1 had the best synergistic effect on platelet aggregation. However, there is no synergistic effect on platelet aggregation of the combination of Danshen and Sanqi in vitro [84]. High performance liquid chromatography analysis of the plasma of rats that received TSA, TNG, or combination of TSA and TNG showed that coadministration of TNG caused change in the plasma distribution profile of TSA. The influence of combination on the absorption and/or metabolism of SA may be one of the reasons for the synergism of TSA and TNG in vivo.

The above-mentioned research results suggest that Danshen-Sanqi herb pair exerts multitarget and multifunction effects that single herb usage could not achieve. Additionally the research shows that a specific herbal combination ratio is critical for maximum synergetic action of Danshen and Sanqi.

4.4. The Role of Bingpian in Compound Danshen Formula.
To define the role of Bingpian in Compound Danshen Formula (CDF), a pharmacokinetic study was conducted in rats [38]. After oral administration of extract from Danshen alone or Danshen extracts combined with Bingpian, plasma

concentrations of rosmarinic acid (RA), salvianolic acid A (SAA), and salvianolic acid B (SAB) were assessed at different time points. In comparison with Danshen extracts alone, significant changes in pharmacokinetic parameters of RA, SAA, and SAB were observed in the Danshen-Bingpian group. The bioavailability of all three salvianolic acids increased when the Danshen extracts and Bingpian were administrated together. These results indicated that Bingpian could enhance intestinal absorption, decrease distribution in the body, and inhibit the metabolism of salvianolic acids. Coadministration of salvianolic acid B, saponins, and Bingpian upregulated mRNA of vascular endothelial growth factor (VEGF) in a rat model with focal cerebral ischemia/reperfusion injury [39]. In comparison with rabbits given Sanqi extract alone, animals simultaneously taking Sanqi extract and Bingpian exhibited significant differences in pharmacokinetic parameters of notoginsenosides R1 (NGR1), ginsenosides Rg1 (GRg1), and Re (GRe), which are three major active components of Sanqi. The plasma concentration of NGR1, GRg1, and GRe is increased significantly in rabbits given simultaneously Sanqi extract and Bingpian via improvements in their absorption and bioavailability. For Bingpian combined with Sanqi extract, the three saponin levels were all increased markedly in heart, lung, liver, and brain tissues with peak levels at one hour after the administration of Sanqi extract [88].

This data indicates that, in the Compound Danshen Formula, Bingpian acts as adjutant and messenger herb and can increase the blood concentration of Danshen and Sanqi.

4.5. Bioactive Equivalent Combinatorial Components (BECCs) Study: The Example of Synergistic Interaction of Multiple Components in CDF. Even though more than 100 components have been isolated and identified in Danshen and Sanqi to date [84], only a small fraction of these components have been studied to confirm their pharmacological effects. The following study provided a new method for the evaluation of CHM synergism. A bioactive equivalent oriented feedback screening method was developed and applied to discover the bioactive equivalence of combinatorial components (BECCs) from a cardiotonic pill (CP, a CDDP formula) [89]. To obtain the components of candidate BECCs, the real-time components trapping and combining system was employed. Eighteen components were identified as BECCs by HPLC-UV chromatography including ten phenolic acids, four saponins, and four tanshinone. The subsequent *in vitro* study showed that only the combination of 18 components had the bioequivalent protective activity as the CP in cultured HUVEC. None of the combinations (phenolic acids + saponins, phenolic acids + tanshinone, or tanshinone + saponins) exerted similar cell protective effect as the CP. In an *in vivo* evaluation test, the combination of 18 components of BECCs was identified to be as effective as the CP in improving the ischemic parameters of cardiac enzymes and left ventricular function in a rat model with myocardial infarction.

4.6. Herb-Drug Interaction Explored by Coadministration of CDDP and Warfarin. Due to high healthcare costs, easy access to over-the-counter herbal products, and an interest in natural approaches to disease treatment, increasing numbers of patients in the USA are turning to alternative and complementary medicines [90]. In parallel, the rate of consumption of herbal products in conjunction with conventional medications has increased and with it the potential for adverse herb-drug interactions increased [91–93]. Due to Compound Danshen Formula's wide clinical use, a recent concern has been raised about interactions between various herbal products and warfarin [91]. A study was conducted to evaluate whether CDDP interacted with warfarin when administered concomitantly: the results demonstrated that CDDP in rats did not significantly alter the pharmacodynamics of warfarin [94]. It was speculated that the interactions between CDDP and warfarin was likely to be negligible [95].

5. Conclusion

Chinese herbal medicine (CHM) is a major part of Traditional Chinese Medicine (TCM) and the use of synergistic compound formulae (复方 fù fāng) is a main therapeutic tool that is customarily composed of multiple medicinal herbs with different pharmacological properties. The combinational use of herbal medicines is at the heart of CHM and continues to play a very important role in the treatment of disease. The synergism of herbs is based on the Traditional Principles for Constructing Chinese Herbal Medicinal Formulae and the Principles of Combining Medicinal Substances. The principles are evidenced by an example formula, Compound Danshen Formula, and recent research has unveiled pharmacological and pharmacokinetic properties of the formula. This review provides preliminary explanation of CHM theory, which helps to better understand the rationale and the principal mechanism of herbal synergism and the clinical application of the formulae. However, further investigation is needed to provide more evidence of the molecular and cellular mechanisms of the synergism of CHM formulae.

Competing Interests

The authors declare that there is no conflict of interests regarding the publication of this paper. All authors are employed by Tasly Pharmaceuticals Inc., in USA, a subsidiary of Tasly (Tasly Holding Group) in China. Tasly China does manufacture, together with other hundreds (more than 600) of companies in China, the Compound Danshen Formula. However, Tasly Pharmaceuticals Inc., USA, does not manufacture nor distribute this compound in USA.

Authors' Contributions

All authors reviewed and approved the paper.

Acknowledgments

The authors acknowledge and thank Carrie Runde, ND, from Casey Health Institute for her perspicacious review and editing of this paper.

References

[1] Y. D. Yi and I. M. Chang, "An overview of traditional Chinese herbal formulae and a proposal of a new code system for expressing the formula titles," *Evidence-Based Complementary and Alternative Medicine*, vol. 1, no. 2, pp. 125–132, 2004.

[2] N. J. Sucher, "The application of Chinese medicine to novel drug discovery," *Expert Opinion on Drug Discovery*, vol. 8, no. 1, pp. 21–34, 2013.

[3] S. Xutian, J. Zhang, and W. Louise, "New exploration and understanding of traditional Chinese medicine," *The American Journal of Chinese Medicine*, vol. 37, no. 3, pp. 411–426, 2009.

[4] X. Zhang, T. Wu, J. Zhang, Q. Yan, L. Xie, and G. J. Liu, "Chinese medicinal herbs for the common cold," *Cochrane Database of Systematic Reviews*, no. 1, Article ID CD004782, 2007.

[5] L. Zhang, G. Wang, W. Hou, P. Li, A. Dulin, and H. L. Bonkovsky, "Contemporary clinical research of traditional Chinese medicines for chronic hepatitis B in china: an analytical review," *Hepatology*, vol. 51, no. 2, pp. 690–698, 2010.

[6] P. Chen, Y. Wan, C. Wang et al., "Mechanisms and effects of *Abelmoschus manihot* preparations in treating chronic kidney disease," *Zhongguo Zhong Yao Za Zhi*, vol. 37, no. 15, pp. 2252–2256, 2012.

[7] X. Xu, L. Guo, and G. Tian, "Diabetes cognitive impairments and the effect of traditional Chinese herbs," *Evidence-Based Complementary and Alternative Medicine*, vol. 2013, Article ID 649396, 10 pages, 2013.

[8] T. Wu, X. Yang, X. Zeng, and G. D. Eslick, "Traditional Chinese medicinal herbs in the treatment of patients with esophageal cancer, a systematic review," *Gastroenterology Clinics of North America*, vol. 38, no. 1, pp. 153–167, 2009.

[9] Y. Jia, F. Huang, S. Zhang, and S.-W. Leung, "Is danshen (*Salvia miltiorrhiza*) dripping pill more effective than isosorbide dinitrate in treating angina pectoris? A systematic review of randomized controlled trials," *International Journal of Cardiology*, vol. 157, no. 3, pp. 330–340, 2012.

[10] CDC and NCHS, "Underlying Cause of Death 1999–2013 on CDC WONDER Online Database," August 2015, http://wonder.cdc.gov/ucd-icd10.html.

[11] Z. Sun, "Atherosclerosis and atheroma plaque rupture: normal anatomy of vasa vasorum and their role associated with atherosclerosis," *The Scientific World Journal*, vol. 2014, Article ID 285058, 6 pages, 2014.

[12] M. Rafieian-Kopaei, M. Setorki, M. Doudi, A. Baradaran, and H. Nasri, "Atherosclerosis: process, indicators, risk factors and new hopes," *International Journal of Preventive Medicine*, vol. 5, no. 8, pp. 927–946, 2014.

[13] P. Libby, "Inflammation in atherosclerosis," *Arteriosclerosis, Thrombosis, and Vascular Biology*, vol. 32, no. 9, pp. 2045–2051, 2012.

[14] A. Gupta and D. A. Smith, "The 2013 American College of Cardiology/American Heart Association guidelines on treating blood cholesterol and assessing cardiovascular risk: a busy practitioner's guide," *Endocrinology and Metabolism Clinics of North America*, vol. 43, no. 4, pp. 869–892, 2014.

[15] D. K. Arnett, R. A. Goodman, J. L. Halperin, J. L. Anderson, A. K. Parekh, and W. A. Zoghbi, "AHA/ACC/HHS strategies to enhance application of clinical practice guidelines in patients with cardiovascular disease and comorbid conditions: from the American Heart Association, American College of Cardiology, and US Department of Health and Human Services," *Circulation*, vol. 130, no. 18, pp. 1662–1667, 2014.

[16] J. R. N. Nansseu and J. J. N. Noubiap, "Aspirin for primary prevention of cardiovascular disease," *Thrombosis Journal*, vol. 13, no. 1, article 38, 2015.

[17] G. L. Jennings, "A new guideline on treatment of hypertension in those with coronary artery disease: scientific statement from the American Heart Association, American College of Cardiology, and American Society of Hypertension about treatment of hypertension in patients with coronary artery disease," *Heart, Lung & Circulation*, vol. 24, no. 11, pp. 1037–1040, 2015.

[18] Y. Liu, N. Ai, J. Liao, and X. Fan, "Transcriptomics: a sword to cut the Gordian knot of traditional Chinese medicine," *Biomarkers in Medicine*, vol. 9, no. 11, pp. 1201–1213, 2015.

[19] S. Li, "Network systems underlying traditional Chinese medicine syndrome and herb formula," *Current Bioinformatics*, vol. 4, no. 3, pp. 188–196, 2009.

[20] Z. Ma and M. Liang, "Review of reducing toxicity and increasing beneficial effects of TCM," *Journal of Liaoning University of Traditional Chinese Medicine*, no. 6, pp. 187–190, 2011.

[21] J. Qiu, "Traditional medicine: a culture in the balance," *Nature*, vol. 448, no. 7150, pp. 126–128, 2007.

[22] S. Xutian, D. Cao, J. Wozniak, J. Junion, and J. Boisvert, "Comprehension of the unique characteristics of traditional Chinese medicine," *The American Journal of Chinese Medicine*, vol. 40, no. 2, pp. 231–244, 2012.

[23] Y. C. Liu, *The Essential Book of Traditional Chinese Medicine, Vol. 1: Theory*, Columbia University Press, New York, NY, USA, 1988.

[24] Z. X. Zhou and X. Q. Ke, "Discussion of the seven features of compatibility of Chinese herb medicine," *Journal of Hubei Traditional Chinese Medicine*, vol. 17, no. 118, pp. 24–25, 1995.

[25] D. Bensky, S. Clavey, and E. Stoger, *Chinese Herbal Medicine Materia Medica*, Eastland Press, Seattle, Wash, USA, 3rd edition, 2004.

[26] Y. Chen, F. Lin, X. Liang, and R. Tan, "Application of Du Shen Tang, powder of Panax notoginseng, and cold compress in treatment of 30 cases of postpartum hemorrhage," *Journal of Emergency in Traditional Chinese Medicine*, vol. 20, pp. 1523–1524, 2011.

[27] X. Gong, "Thrombolytic therapy along with Du Shen Tang in the treatment of acute myocardial infarction," *Chinese Journal of Integrated Traditional and Western Medicine in Intensive and Critical Care*, vol. 11, no. 2, pp. 126–127, 2004.

[28] Z. Zhao, G. Cai, S. Xie, X. Zhou, and X. Hu, "Naval compression with root of Kansui plus intake of Du Shen Tang in treatment of cirrhosis with ascites," *Journal of Emergency in Traditional Chinese Medicine*, vol. 19, no. 3, pp. 388–389, 2010.

[29] W. Yang, "Effect of treating 67 cases of upper gastrointestinal bleeding with Du Shen Tang," *Gansu Journal of Traditional Chinese Medicine*, vol. 7, no. 5, pp. 9–10, 1995.

[30] D. Qin, "Si Ni Tang combining Du Shen Tang in treatment of 30 cases of congestive heart failure," *Henan Journal of Traditional Chinese Medicine*, no. 8, pp. 1510–1511, 2014.

[31] Y. Mao and G. Zhou, "Effects of compatibility of Rhubarb and Glauber on anthraquinone glycosides content in different proportions," *Journal of Jiangxi TCM*, vol. 42, no. 2, pp. 60–61, 2011.

[32] L. Wan, Z. Z. Lin, W. Liu, and Z. Liu, "Pharmacokinetic study on berberine in the extract of rhizoma coptidis-radix aucklandiae drug-pair in rats," *Chinese Journal of Modern Applied Pharmacy*, vol. 26, no. 6, pp. 443–446, 2009.

[33] M. Shong, J. Yu, and Z. Bao, "Compatibility of traditional Chinese medicine to reduce the toxicity and modern research progress," *Pharmacy and Clinics of Chinese Materia Medica*, vol. 3, no. 2, pp. 51–53, 2012.

[34] W. Long, X.-D. Zhang, H.-Y. Wu et al., "Study on incompatibility of traditional Chinese medicine: evidence from formula network, chemical space, and metabolism room," *Evidence-Based Complementary and Alternative Medicine*, vol. 2013, Article ID 352145, 8 pages, 2013.

[35] J. J. Zhang, X. S. Fan, H. Yang, C. X. Jiang, Y. Li, and Z. H. Qi, "Review of eighteen incompatibility pairs of *Veratrum nigrum* and its drug incompatibility in TCM," *Journal of Traditional Chinese Medicine and Pharmacy*, vol. 29, no. 9, pp. 2870–2873, 2014.

[36] J. Dong and Y. Fan, "Compatibility of Chinese herb medicine and its connection with effects and toxicity," *Chinese Medical Pharmacy Journal*, vol. 26, no. 3, pp. 618–619, 2008.

[37] L. Wang, G.-B. Zhou, P. Liu et al., "Dissection of mechanisms of Chinese medicinal formula Realgar-Indigo naturalis as an effective treatment for promyelocytic leukemia," *Proceedings of the National Academy of Sciences of the United States of America*, vol. 105, no. 12, pp. 4826–4831, 2008.

[38] X.-J. Lai, L. Z. Zhang, J.-S. Li et al., "Comparative pharmacokinetic and bioavailability studies of three salvianolic acids after the administration of *Salviae miltiorrhizae* alone or with synthetical borneol in rats," *Fitoterapia*, vol. 82, no. 6, pp. 883–888, 2011.

[39] M. Li, Y. Z. Zhang, W. Wang et al., "Influence of borneol when combined with salvianolic acid B and saponins of panax notoginseng on the expression of vascular endothelial growth factor (VEGF) mRNA in brain tissue of rats with cerebral ischemia/reperfusion," *Chinese Journal of TCM WM Critical Care*, vol. 12, no. 5, pp. 263–266, 2005.

[40] C. Z. Liang, "Focus on the theory of precaution of disease in Tradition Chinese Medicine from the function of compound Danshen dripping pill to the heart and blood vessel's illness," *Chinese Archives of Traditional Chinese Medicine*, vol. 26, no. 3, Article ID 643644, 2008.

[41] Q. Zheng, C. C. Peng, M. L. Shen, and M. Yang, "Study on compatibility of Radix et Rhizoma Salviae miltiorrhizae and Radix et Rhizoma Notoginseng," *Chinese Journal of Experimental Traditional Medical Formulae*, vol. 15, no. 2, pp. 83–86, 2009.

[42] T. O. Cheng, "Cardiovascular effects of Danshen," *International Journal of Cardiology*, vol. 121, no. 1, pp. 9–22, 2007.

[43] Y.-K. Li and L.-D. Li, "Urgency and necessity of standardisation of Chinese medicine with confusions of compound Danshen preparations," *Chinese Journal of Chinese Materia Medica*, vol. 33, no. 4, pp. 349–352, 2008.

[44] L. Zhou, Z. Zuo, and M. S. S. Chow, "Danshen: an overview of its chemistry, pharmacology, pharmacokinetics, and clinical use," *Journal of Clinical Pharmacology*, vol. 45, no. 12, pp. 1345–1359, 2005.

[45] J. H.-C. Ho and C.-Y. Hong, "Salvianolic acids: small compounds with multiple mechanisms for cardiovascular protection," *Journal of Biomedical Science*, vol. 18, article 30, 2011.

[46] C.-S. Zheng, X.-J. Xu, H.-Z. Ye et al., "Computational pharmacological comparison of Salvia miltiorrhiza and *Panax notoginseng* used in the therapy of cardiovascular diseases," *Experimental and Therapeutic Medicine*, vol. 6, no. 5, pp. 1163–1168, 2013.

[47] X. D. Song, W. L. Zhu, R. An, Y. Li, and Z. Du, "Protective effect of Daming capsule against chronic cerebral ischemia," *BMC Complementary and Alternative Medicine*, vol. 15, article 149, 2015.

[48] K. K.-K. Wong, M. T.-W. Ho, H. Q. Lin et al., "Cryptotanshinone, an acetylcholinesterase inhibitor from salvia miltiorrhiza, ameliorates scopolamine-induced amnesia in morris water maze task," *Planta Medica*, vol. 76, no. 3, pp. 228–234, 2010.

[49] J. Zhou, X.-D. Qu, Z.-Y. Li et al., "Salvianolic acid B attenuates toxin-induced neuronal damage via Nrf2-dependent glial cells-mediated protective activity in Parkinson's disease models," *PLoS ONE*, vol. 9, no. 7, Article ID e101668, 2014.

[50] X. H. Tian, W. J. Xue, and X. M. Ding, "Application of Danshen injection on early stage of renal transplantation," *Chinese Journal of Integrative Medicine*, vol. 25, no. 5, pp. 404–407, 2005.

[51] L. Gao, K. Yan, Y. Cui, G. Fan, and Y. Wang, "Protective effect of *Salvia miltiorrhiza* and *Carthamus tinctorius* extract against lipopolysaccharide-induced liver injury," *World Journal of Gastroenterology*, vol. 21, no. 30, pp. 9079–9092, 2015.

[52] Y. Zhang, P. X. Jiang, M. Ye, S.-H. Kim, C. Jiang, and J. X. Lü, "Tanshinones: sources, pharmacokinetics and anti-cancer activities," *International Journal of Molecular Sciences*, vol. 13, no. 10, pp. 13621–13666, 2012.

[53] V. Nicolin, F. Dal Piaz, S. L. Nori, P. Narducci, and N. de Tommasi, "Inhibition of bone resorption by Tanshinone VI isolated from *Salvia miltiorrhiza* Bunge," *European Journal of Histochemistry*, vol. 54, no. 2, pp. 104–106, 2010.

[54] S. Gao, Z. Liu, H. Li, P. J. Little, P. Liu, and S. Xu, "Cardiovascular actions and therapeutic potential of tanshinone IIA," *Atherosclerosis*, vol. 220, no. 1, pp. 3–10, 2012.

[55] D. Xu, P. Huang, Z. Yu, D. H. Xing, S. Ouyang, and G. Xing, "Efficacy and safety of panax notoginseng saponin therapy for acute intracerebral hemorrhage, meta-analysis, and mini review of potential mechanisms of action," *Frontiers in Neurology*, vol. 5, article 274, 2015.

[56] Q. H. Shang, H. Xu, Z. L. Liu, K. Chen, and J. P. Liu, "Oral *Panax notoginseng* preparation for coronary heart disease: a systematic review of randomized controlled trials," *Evidence-Based Complementary and Alternative Medicine*, vol. 2013, Article ID 940125, 12 pages, 2013.

[57] T. B. Ng, "Pharmacological activity of sanchi ginseng (*Panax notoginseng*)," *Journal of Pharmacy and Pharmacology*, vol. 58, no. 8, pp. 1007–1019, 2006.

[58] J. Q. Cao, P. Fu, and Y. Q. Zhao, "Isolation and identification of a new compound from acid hydrolysate of saponin in stems and leaves of *Panax notoginseng*," *Chinese Traditional and Herbal Drugs*, vol. 44, no. 2, pp. 137–140, 2013.

[59] Z. Cai, S. Hou, Y. Li et al., "Effect of borneol on the distribution of gastrodin to the brain in mice via oral administration," *Journal of Drug Targeting*, vol. 16, no. 2, pp. 178–184, 2008.

[60] J.-P. Dai, J. Chen, Y.-F. Bei, B.-X. Han, and S. Wang, "Influence of borneol on primary mice oral fibroblasts: a penetration enhancer may be used in oral submucous fibrosis," *Journal of Oral Pathology and Medicine*, vol. 38, no. 3, pp. 276–281, 2009.

[61] Y.-Y. Xiao, Q.-N. Ping, and Z.-P. Chen, "The enhancing effect of synthetical borneol on the absorption of tetramethylpyrazine phosphate in mouse," *International Journal of Pharmaceutics*, vol. 337, no. 1-2, pp. 74–79, 2007.

[62] Z. Jiang, Y. Wang, X. Gao, H. Shang, and X. Wang, "The pharmacological actions of danshen ThemeD formulas," in *Dan Shen (Salvia miltiorrhiza) in Medicine*, X. Yan, Ed., chapter 2, pp. 19–47, Springer, Dordrecht, The Netherlands, 2015.

[63] M. Nichols, N. Townsend, P. Scarborough, and M. Rayner, "Cardiovascular disease in Europe 2014: epidemiological update," *European Heart Journal*, vol. 35, no. 42, pp. 2950–2959, 2014.

[64] Y. Yao, Y. Feng, and L. Wang, "Systematic review and meta-analysis of randomized controlled trials comparing compound danshen dripping pills and isosorbide dinitrate in treating angina pectoris," *International Journal of Cardiology*, vol. 182, pp. 46–47, 2015.

[65] Q.-X. Yue, F.-B. Xie, X.-Y. Song et al., "Proteomic studies on protective effects of salvianolic acids, notoginsengnosides and combination of salvianolic acids and notoginsengnosides against cardiac ischemic-reperfusion injury," *Journal of Ethnopharmacology*, vol. 141, no. 2, pp. 659–667, 2012.

[66] X.-Y. Yang, N. Zhao, Y.-Y. Liu et al., "Inhibition of NADPH oxidase mediates protective effect of cardiotonic pills against rat heart ischemia/reperfusion injury," *Evidence-Based Complementary and Alternative Medicine*, vol. 2013, Article ID 728020, 15 pages, 2013.

[67] H.-Y. Fan, F.-H. Fu, M.-Y. Yang, H. Xu, A.-H. Zhang, and K. Liu, "Antiplatelet and antithrombotic activities of salvianolic acid A," *Thrombosis Research*, vol. 126, no. 1, pp. e17–e22, 2010.

[68] F. Maione, V. De Feo, E. Caiazzo, L. De Martino, C. Cicala, and N. Mascolo, "Tanshinone IIA, a major component of *Salvia milthorriza* Bunge, inhibits platelet activation via Erk-2 signaling pathway," *Journal of Ethnopharmacology*, vol. 155, no. 2, pp. 1236–1242, 2014.

[69] F. F. Y. Lam, S. Y. Deng, E. S. K. Ng et al., "Mechanisms of the relaxant effect of a Danshen and Gegen formulation on rat isolated cerebral basilar artery," *Journal of Ethnopharmacology*, vol. 132, no. 1, pp. 186–192, 2010.

[70] C. M. Koon, K. S. woo, P. C. Leung, and K. P. Fung, "Salviae Miltiorrhizae Radix and Puerariae Lobatae Radi herb formula mediate anti-arthrosclerosis by modulating key atherogenic events both in vascular smooth muscle cells and endothelial cell," *Journal of Ethnopharmacology*, vol. 138, no. 1, pp. 175–183, 2011.

[71] G. Liu, B. Wang, J. Zhang, H. Jiang, and F. Liu, "Total panax notoginsenosides prevent atherosclerosis in apolipoprotein E-knockout mice: role of downregulation of CD40 and MMP-9 expression," *Journal of Ethnopharmacology*, vol. 126, no. 2, pp. 350–354, 2009.

[72] L. Xue, Z. Wu, X.-P. Ji, X.-Q. Gao, and Y.-H. Guo, "Effect and mechanism of salvianolic acid B on the myocardial ischemia-reperfusion injury in rats," *Asian Pacific Journal of Tropical Medicine*, vol. 7, no. 4, pp. 280–284, 2014.

[73] L. Ma, X. Zhang, H. Guo, and Y. Gan, "Determination of four water-soluble compounds in *Salvia miltiorrhiza* Bunge by high-performance liquid chromatography with a coulometric electrode array system," *Journal of Chromatography B: Analytical Technologies in the Biomedical and Life Sciences*, vol. 833, no. 2, pp. 260–263, 2006.

[74] P. Li, S.-P. Li, F.-Q. Yang, and Y.-T. Wang, "Simultaneous determination of four tanshinones in *Salvia miltiorrhiza* by pressurized liquid extraction and capillary electrochromatography," *Journal of Separation Science*, vol. 30, no. 6, pp. 900–905, 2007.

[75] P. Li, G. Xu, S.-P. Li et al., "Optimizing ultraperformance liquid chromatographic analysis of 10 diterpenoid compounds in *Salvia miltiorrhiza* using central composite design," *Journal of Agricultural and Food Chemistry*, vol. 56, no. 4, pp. 1164–1171, 2008.

[76] J.-B. Wan, P. Li, S. Li, Y. Wang, T. T.-X. Dong, and K. W.-K. Tsim, "Simultaneous determination of 11 saponins in *Panax notoginseng* using HPLC-ELSD and pressurized liquid extraction," *Journal of Separation Science*, vol. 29, no. 14, pp. 2190–2196, 2006.

[77] G. F. Zeng, Q. Xu, H. B. Xiao, and X. M. Liang, "Influence of compatibility ratio of Fufang Danshen on the dissolution of Danshen compositions," *Chinese Journal of Chromatography*, vol. 22, no. 2, pp. 141–143, 2004.

[78] S. H. Li, K. L. Xu, and Y. Z. Xu, "The study on the interaction between Danshen and Sanqi in Compound Danshen formula," *Progress in Natural Sciences*, vol. 13, no. 2, pp. 186–189, 2003.

[79] W. Long, S.-C. Zhang, L. Wen, L. Mu, F. Yang, and G. Chen, "In vivo distribution and pharmacokinetics of multiple active components from Danshen and Sanqi and their combination via inner ear administration," *Journal of Ethnopharmacology*, vol. 156, pp. 199–208, 2014.

[80] S.-Y. Zhang, M. Song, J.-G. Lu, and T.-J. Hang, "Effects of combination of *Salvia miltiorrhiza* and *Panax notoginseng* on the pharmacokinetics of their major bioactive components in Beagle dog," *Acta Pharmaceutica Sinica*, vol. 45, no. 11, pp. 1433–1439, 2010.

[81] H. C. Shang, B. L. Zhang, and X. M. Gao, "Characteristics of compatibility Danshen and Sanqi and new drug design accordingly," *Herald of Technology*, vol. 5, no. 24, pp. 25–27, 2006.

[82] X. Wang, Y. Wang, M. Jiang et al., "Differential cardioprotective effects of salvianolic acid and tanshinone on acute myocardial infarction are mediated by unique signaling pathways," *Journal of Ethnopharmacology*, vol. 135, no. 3, pp. 662–671, 2011.

[83] Y. Deng, T. Zhang, F. Teng et al., "Ginsenoside Rg1 and Rb1, in combination with salvianolic acid B, play different roles in myocardial infarction in rats," *Journal of the Chinese Medical Association*, vol. 78, no. 2, pp. 114–120, 2015.

[84] Y. L. Lu, X. Liu, X. Liang, L. Xiang, and W. Zhang, "Metabolomic strategy to study therapeutic and synergistic effects of tanshinone IIA, salvianolic acid B and ginsenoside Rb1 in myocardial ischemia rats," *Journal of Ethnopharmacology*, vol. 134, no. 1, pp. 45–49, 2011.

[85] G. F. Zeng, X. Jian, P. Li, S. P. Fu, H. B. Xiao, and X. M. Liang, "Protective effects of different ratios of danshen to sanqi on hypoxia and reoxygenation-induced HUVECs injury," *Fine Chemicals*, vol. 23, no. 2, pp. 126–129, 2006.

[86] T. Liu, C. L. Qin, and B. L. Zhang, "Effects of combinatory usage of Danshen and Sanqi on platelet adhesion and aggregation," *Journal of Chinese Herbal Medicines*, vol. 27, no. 8, pp. 609–611, 2002.

[87] Y. Yao, W.-Y. Wu, A.-H. Liu et al., "Interaction of salvianolic acids and notoginsengnosides in inhibition of ADP-induced platelet aggregation," *The American Journal of Chinese Medicine*, vol. 36, no. 2, pp. 313–328, 2008.

[88] S. Wang, W. Zang, X. Zhao et al., "Effects of borneol on pharmacokinetics and tissue distribution of notoginsenoside R1 and ginsenosides Rg1 and Re in *Panax notoginseng* in rabbits," *Journal of Analytical Methods in Chemistry*, vol. 2013, Article ID 706723, 11 pages, 2013.

[89] P. Liu, H. Yang, F. Long et al., "Bioactive equivalence of combinatorial components identified in screening of an herbal medicine," *Pharmaceutical Research*, vol. 31, no. 7, pp. 1788–1800, 2014.

[90] S. Bent, "Herbal medicine in the United States: review of efficacy, safety, and regulation: grand rounds at University of

California, San Francisco Medical Center," *Journal of General Internal Medicine*, vol. 23, no. 6, pp. 854–859, 2008.

[91] M. L. Chavez, M. A. Jordan, and P. I. Chavez, "Evidence-based drug-herbal interactions," *Life Sciences*, vol. 78, no. 18, pp. 2146–2157, 2006.

[92] M.-Z. Liu, Y.-L. Zhang, M.-Z. Zeng et al., "Pharmacogenomics and herb-drug interactions: merge of future and tradition," *Evidence-Based Complementary and Alternative Medicine*, vol. 2015, Article ID 321091, 8 pages, 2015.

[93] S. J. Brantley, A. A. Argikar, Y. S. Lin, S. Nagar, and M. F. Paine, "Herb-drug interactions: challenges and opportunities for improved predictions," *Drug Metabolism and Disposition*, vol. 42, no. 3, pp. 301–317, 2014.

[94] Y. Chu, L. Zhang, X.-Y. Wang, J.-H. Guo, Z.-X. Guo, and X.-H. Ma, "The effect of Compound Danshen Dripping Pills, a Chinese herb medicine, on the pharmacokinetics and pharmacodynamics of warfarin in rats," *Journal of Ethnopharmacology*, vol. 137, no. 3, pp. 1457–1461, 2011.

[95] P. Wang, H. Sun, L. Yang et al., "Absence of an effect of t89 on the steady-state pharmacokinetics and pharmacodynamics of warfarin in healthy volunteers," *Journal of Clinical Pharmacology*, vol. 54, no. 2, pp. 234–239, 2014.

14

Characterization of the Physiological Response following *In Vivo* Administration of *Astragalus membranaceus*

Karen Denzler,[1,2] **Jessica Moore,**[1] **Heather Harrington,**[1,2] **Kira Morrill,**[1] **Trung Huynh,**[2] **Bertram Jacobs,**[2] **Robert Waters,**[1,2] **and Jeffrey Langland**[1,2]

[1]*Southwest College of Naturopathic Medicine, Tempe, AZ 85282, USA*
[2]*Arizona State University, Biodesign Institute, Tempe, AZ 85287, USA*

Correspondence should be addressed to Jeffrey Langland; j.langland@scnm.edu

Academic Editor: I-Min Liu

The botanical, *Astragalus membranaceus*, is a therapeutic in traditional Chinese medicine. Limited literature exists on the overall *in vivo* effects of *A. membranaceus* on the human body. This study evaluates the physiological responses to *A. membranaceus* by measuring leukocyte, platelet, and cytokine responses as well as body temperature and blood pressure in healthy individuals after the *in vivo* administration of *A. membranaceus*. A dose-dependent increase in monocytes, neutrophils, and lymphocytes was measured 8–12 hours after administration and an increase in the number of circulating platelets was seen as early as 4 hours. A dynamic change in the levels of circulating cytokines was observed, especially in interferon-γ and tumor necrosis factor-α, IL-13, IL-6, and soluble IL-2R. Subjective symptoms reported by participants were similar to those typically experienced in viral type immune responses and included fatigue, malaise, and headache. Systolic and diastolic blood pressure were reduced within 4 hours after administration, while body temperature mildly increased within 8 hours after administration. In general, all responses returned to baseline values by 24 hours. Collectively, these results support the role of *A. membranaceus* in priming for a potential immune response as well as its effect on blood flow and wound healing.

1. Introduction

Botanical medicines are plant-derived products which have increasingly come under significant investigation for their potential therapeutic applications [1–3]. The use of botanical medicines worldwide is increasing significantly [4, 5]. A 2007 National Institute of Heath Survey revealed that 44% of Americans 50–59 years of age and 38% of adults less than 50 years of age have used some form of Complementary and Alternative Medicine (CAM), including botanical medicines [6]. Approximately $14.8 billion dollars in out-of-pocket expenditures for nonvitamin, nonmineral, natural products were spent that year (compared to $47.6 billion spent on pharmaceutical drugs) [7]. Due to the growing demand for alternative therapies and the general public notion that botanical medicines are safe, some physicians prefer or are considering referral to CAM specialists for their expertise [8–10]. However, evidence based characterization is typically limited regarding many of these therapies, justifying the need for further research.

Originally described in Shen Nong's Classic of Materia Medica over two thousand years ago, the botanical *Astragalus membranaceus* (AM) has been used extensively in traditional Chinese medicine to support and enhance the immune system, to treat various conditions, including viral infection, fatigue, decreased appetite, debility, nonhealing wounds, liver and kidney disease, and cancers [11, 12]. Traditionally, AM is made into a decoction in which pieces of root were boiled into soups and then removed prior to consumption.

The presumptive active constituents of AM include polysaccharides, saponins, flavonoids, and astragalosides [13, 14]. Recent evidence has also suggested an active component role of lipopolysaccharides provided by endosymbiotic bacteria present on the root of AM [15, 16]. *Astragalus* polysaccharides (APS) have demonstrated immunopotentiating properties such as increased murine B-cell proliferation and cytokine production [17]. Numerous *in vitro* studies and limited *in vivo* studies and clinical trials have demonstrated intriguing indications for the use of AM, particularly as an immunomodulator to prevent and treat heart disease, nephritis, bacterial infection, and viral illnesses (especially respiratory infections and chronic hepatitis) and as an adjunct therapy for cancer, HIV, and atopic disease [15, 18–24]. Several animal studies have shown the ability of AM to restore and enhance immunologic function in the cases of either immunosuppression or infection including HSV, HIV, HBV, and viral myocarditis [16, 22–27]. The antiviral and wound healing properties of AM are proposed to be indirect via modulation of proinflammatory cytokines inducing leukocyte and platelet mobilization. Current research in animal models suggests that AM may have a significant clinical effect on cell proliferation and wound healing [28–30]. Although significant research has been conducted on AM, *in vivo* studies are limited. The research presented provides an evaluation of the physiological response to AM following *in vivo* administration of this botanical.

2. Materials and Methods

2.1. Botanical Extract Preparation. Dried *Astragalus membranaceus* root slices were purchased from Mayway Corporation (Oakland, CA). Dried AM was validated using herbal pharmacopoeia monographs. Six hundred grams of dried AM was ground in a 1 gallon stainless steel Hamilton Beach blender, transferred to a clean amber colored gallon glass jar, and 2220 milliliters of boiling distilled water was added to the ground root. After six hours, 780 mL of 190 proof ethanol was added for a final ratio of 1 : 5 (weight of botanical to volume of liquid). The mixture was kept at room temperature for 3 weeks, followed by separation of the liquid portion from the solid herb portion using a mechanical press. The extracted liquid was filtered using unbleached paper filters, pooled, and dispensed in amber colored bottles. To eliminate any physiological responses due to ethanol, the original 25% ethanol based AM extract was vacuum-dried for 3 hours. Final ethanol concentrations were measured to be 2–4%. A vehicle control sample was prepared from 25% ethanol that was similarly dried for 3 hours. For standardization purposes, a sample of the extract was dried and found to have a concentration of nonvolatile solutes of 92.6 mg/mL extract. Since definitively active constituents present in AM are unknown, we cannot calculate the concentration of active constituent(s) present in the extract. Therefore, this value serves as a reference measure for relative activity.

2.2. Participants. This case series study included 2 healthy males (29 yo and 47 yo) and 2 healthy females (24 yo and 27 yo). Criteria for healthy individuals included the absence of known chronic disease, the absence of illness including HIV and HCV, and no use of any medications at the time of the study. Participants were informed that they must be without symptoms of illness at the time of the study and that they must adhere to a controlled diet for 4 days prior to beginning the study (including no alcohol or use of known

immunomodulatory foods). The study was approved and overseen by the Arizona State University and Southwest College of Naturopathic Medicine (SCNM) Institutional Review Boards (Protocol 208-11). Each participant received and completed a written informed consent form prior to participation in the study. Most data was acquired from the 47 yo male and 24 yo and 27 yo females; however a 29 yo male replaced the 27 yo female during toxicity testing due to relocation.

2.3. In Vivo Administration. The ethanol-reduced AM extract or vehicle was administered to three healthy subjects at indicated doses and relative to body weight. Doses included 0.25 mL/kg, 0.75 mL/kg, and 1.5 mL/kg. The AM extract was administered sublingually over a period of 20 minutes followed by ingestion. Trials occurred on separate days with at least 4 weeks in between trials.

Rationale for dosages used is as follows: for acute conditions, doses of AM often range from 1 to 25 g/day. For this study, we wanted to investigate acute changes over a 24-hour period related to the immune response. Therefore, based on average 70 kg adult, the highest dose of 1.5 mL AM extract/kg body weight was calculated with an average adult receiving an extract from 20 g dried AM. Similarly, the 0.75 mL/kg and 0.25 mL/kg doses were based on an average adult receiving extract from 10 g to 3.3 g dried AM, respectively.

2.4. Venipuncture. Blood was collected into heparinized tubes (BD vacutainer cell preparation tube with sodium heparin) 0, 4, 8, 12, and 24 hours after administration of the AM extract. Samples were sent to an external lab (Lab Corps) for routine processing including flow cytometry and cytokine assay. Arizona State University and the Southwest College of Naturopathic Medicine (SCNM) Institutional Review Boards approved the collection and processing of all blood samples.

2.5. Blood Analysis. Blood sent to external labs was processed through standard cell counting and flow cytometry, and a full blood profile was done which included the following: white blood cell populations, including total white blood cells, lymphocytes, monocytes, neutrophils, and platelets, and lymphocyte subpopulations including total T-cells (CD3+), T-helper cells (CD3+CD4+), T-cytotoxic cells (CD3+CD8+), B-cells (CD19+), and NK-cells (CD56+). A cytokine assay was also performed by the third-party lab via ELISA and included the following cytokines: IL-1β, IL-2, sIL-2R, IFN-γ, IL-4, IL-5, IL-6, IL-8, IL-10, IL-13, IL-12, and TNF-α. Liver (AST, ALT, bilirubin, and ALP) and kidney (potassium, sodium, BUN, creatinine, and BUN/creatinine ratio) panels were tested to assess potential toxicity at 1, 12, and 24 h after ingestion of AM or vehicle.

2.6. Physiological Responses. The subjective physiological reactions experienced by each participant were reported at each blood draw. Symptoms were reported and then rated subjectively on an intensity scale of 1–10 (10 highest intensities). Blood pressure and body temperature (taken orally) were recorded by laboratory technicians at each blood draw. Physiologic responses were completed with both the AM trials and the vehicle control trial.

2.7. Statistical Analysis. Statistical analyses were performed using SPSS™ Statistical Analysis Software. Differences between time points (0 versus 12 hours and 0 versus 24 hours) were analyzed using paired 2-tailed "t" tests and were considered statistically significant if $p < 0.05$.

2.8. Ethics Statement. All research involving human participants was approved by the Southwest College of Naturopathic Medicine Institutional Review Board (Protocol: 208-11). Informed consent was obtained from all participants and all clinical investigations were conducted according to the principles expressed in the Declaration of Helsinki.

3. Results

The majority of leukocytes in the body are located in organs of the lymphatic system or connective tissues proper. Circulating white blood cells represent a fraction of the total white blood cell population in the body, and changes from baseline values are useful in interpreting activity of the immune system. For example, inflammation can result from infection or various disease states and cause known characteristic changes in circulating leukocytes. To define any specific changes induced by the *in vivo* administration of AM, an analysis of leukocyte populations including total white blood cells, peripheral blood mononuclear cells (lymphocytes and monocytes), and polymorphonuclear cells (neutrophils) was completed. The observed effects were measured over a 24-hour time period, after *in vivo* administration of AM. This analysis was conducted on 3 separate occasions, each for varying doses of AM including 0.25 mL/kg, 0.75 mL/kg, and 1.5 mL/kg. A control test was done with 1.5 mL/kg vehicle.

As Figure 1 indicates, treatment with the vehicle control had almost no effect on absolute numbers of leukocytes while treatment with AM demonstrated statistically significant increases in cell numbers above initial/baseline values; p values were typically significant at 8 and 12 hours. Along with increases in cell numbers, atypical lymphocytes were notably present 8 and 12 hours after treatment (classified by increased granularization, increased size, and chromatin decondensation) and indicate lymphocyte activation. The observed increases in cell number also appeared to be dose-dependent and this was consistent across all subjects (compare 0.25 mL/kg dose with 0.75 mL/kg dose). Fold changes were calculated to best represent the magnitude of change that occurred over the 24-hour period and Figure 1 shows the maximal fold change for each individual subject. Total WBCs increased on average (based on $n = 3$) 1.3x above baseline values at the lowest dose and 1.53x at the highest dose (p values 0.042 and 0.011, resp.). Similarly, in comparing 0.25 mL/kg, 0.75 mL/kg, and 1.5 mL/kg doses, neutrophils increased from an average (based on $n = 3$) of 1.4x, 1.68x, and 1.73x above baseline values; lymphocytes increased by 1.46x, 1.63x, and 1.73x, and monocytes increased by 1.53x, 1.53x, and 1.76x above baseline values, respectively. Furthermore,

as doses increased, the data also typically became more significant. For example increases in numbers of neutrophils were associated with p values, at each of the three doses of AM, of 0.049, 0.034, and 0.007, respectively.

The timing of these changes is noteworthy and consistent. In all subjects, maximal peak values were obtained between 8 and 12 hours. In all cases, baseline values returned by 24 hours after administration of AM. Although increases in cell population were observed following AM administration, cell numbers never exceeded ranges regarded as normal for the human population (normal range indicated in the figure). It is clear that while changes to leukocyte populations were significant compared to baseline values, neither leucopenia nor leukocytosis were observed.

We next sought to characterize changes in numbers of lymphocyte population subsets circulating in the blood. For this experiment, subjects were administered the highest dose of AM (1.5 mL/kg) on two separate occasions and lymphocyte populations were measured 0 and 12 hours after administration. As shown in Figure 2, increases in T- and B-cells including total CD3+, CD3+CD4+, CD3+CD8+, and CD19+ lymphocytes were observed. CD19+ (B-cells) increased on average 1.66x and 1.60x above baseline values for trials 1 and 2, respectively ($p < 0.001$). Similarly, the average increases for trials one and two demonstrated that total CD3+ cells increased by 1.46x and 1.66x ($p = 0.002$), CD3+CD4+ (T-helper cells) increased by 1.53x and 1.73x ($p < 0.001$), and CD3+CD8+ (T-cytotoxic cells) increased by 1.33x and 1.5x ($p = 0.035$). Collectively, fold changes ranged from 1.2x to 2.0x above baseline values in these cell populations. While increases are statistically significant from baseline values (p values including both trials range from $p < 0.001$ to 0.035 between the subsets), all cell population values remained within normal physiological limits. This trend of increases in circulating B- and T-cell subsets suggests that AM may be mobilizing these cells. Conversely, natural killer (NK) cells (CD56+) were shown to mildly decrease or remain unchanged. Subjects responded very similarly between the two separate experiments shown in Figure 2 adding confidence to the physiological effect of AM. For example, compare the initial ($t = 0$ hrs) and final ($t = 12$ hrs) levels of CD3+ cells for subject 2 between trials 1 and 2.

Since AM is clinically reported for use in damaged tissues such as diabetic wound healing, we next evaluated changes to platelet counts in relation to increasing doses of AM *in vivo* [31, 32]. Wound healing is a complex and dynamic process involving a highly regulated sequence of biochemical and cellular events. Platelets contribute to this process by providing the initial hemostasis that occurs after tissue injury and by producing growth factors responsible for the regeneration of damaged tissues. As seen in Figure 3, platelet counts were moderately increased by statistically significant values in the 0.75 mL/kg dose and 1.5 mL/kg dose. In addition, a dose-dependent trend reflected in absolute increases from baseline values and significance was observed. Average fold increases in circulating platelets for the three increasing doses were 1.07x ($p = 0.058$ at 8 h), 1.17x ($p = 0.048$ at 8 h), and 1.20x ($p = 0.035$ at 4 h; $p = 0.031$ at 8 h) above baseline values, respectively. While the two highest

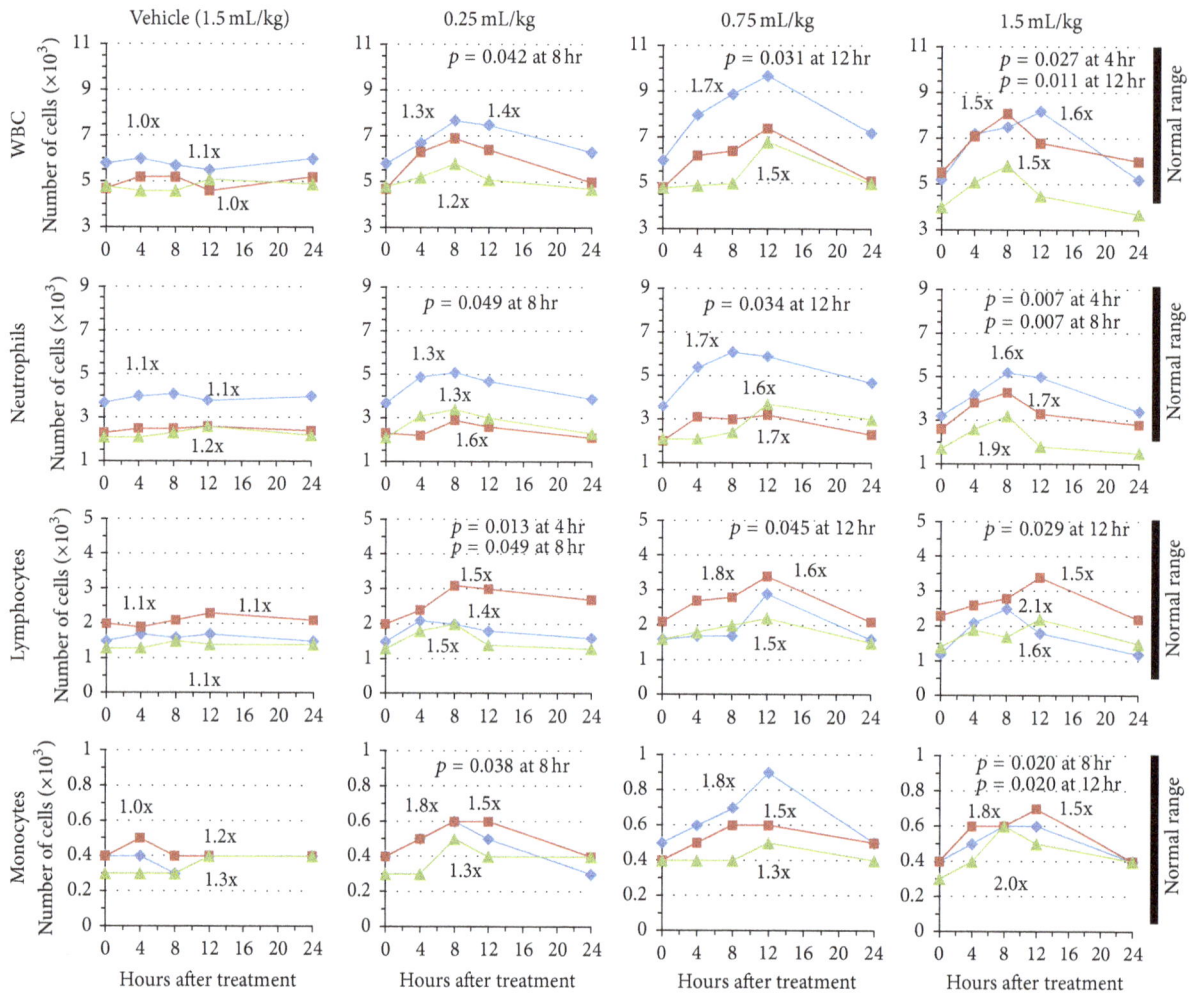

FIGURE 1: AM effect on white blood cell populations. Subjects 1, 2, or 3 (indicated by blue, red, and green lines, resp.) were administered vehicle or varying concentrations of AM extract (0.25, 0.75, and 1.5 mL extract/kg body weight). Blood draws were performed 0, 4, 8, 12, and 24 hours after administration to measure total cell population numbers. Cells measured include total white blood cells, neutrophils, lymphocytes, and monocytes. Peak fold changes relative to baseline ($t = 0$ hours) are indicated. Normal physiological ranges of the different cell populations are indicated by black bars.

doses resulted in significant increases, changes occurred within normal physiological ranges and there was no evidence of thrombocytopenia or thrombosis at any point in time. The analysis also demonstrated that peak values are obtained between 4 and 8 hours after administration of AM. Comparatively, peak values for leukocyte counts were observed between 8 and 12 hours. A return to baseline values was observed across all subjects by 12 to 24 hours after administration of AM.

Since *in vivo* administration of AM has been reported to differentially modulate cytokine activity, we continued our analysis by reviewing intercellular communication between immune populations through changes to circulating cytokines [33]. As Figure 4 illustrates, this analysis was done after the administration of the highest dose of AM at 1.5 mL/kg and assay of serum for various cytokines including interleukins (IL-2, IL-4, IL-5, IL-6, IL-8, IL-10, IL-12, and IL-13), soluble IL-2 receptor (IL-2R), interferon gamma (IFN-γ),

and tumor necrosis factor alpha (TNF-α) at 0 and 12 hours. Circulating levels of these cytokines were quantified with a minimum limit of detection at 5 pg/mL. Increases above the limit of detection were seen in IL-2R, IFN-γ, IL-6, IL-13, and TNF-α across all three subjects. Induction of IL-1β was observed in two subjects, while induction of IL-2, IL-10, and IL-12 was observed in only one subject each. IL-4 and IL-5 were not induced above the limit of detection in any participant. The most significant changes were seen in IL-2R, IFN-γ, and TNF-α ($p = 0.056$, $p = 0.018$, and $p = 0.046$, resp.). These results are consistent with the promotion of a Th1 immune response by AM due to the increase of IFN-γ and TNF-α and the absence of IL-4.

The potential for AM to cause liver or kidney toxicity following ingestion was assessed to determine safety at the highest dose (1.5 mL/kg). For all liver enzyme and kidney function tests performed, no statistically significant differences were measured at 12 and 24 h after administration (data

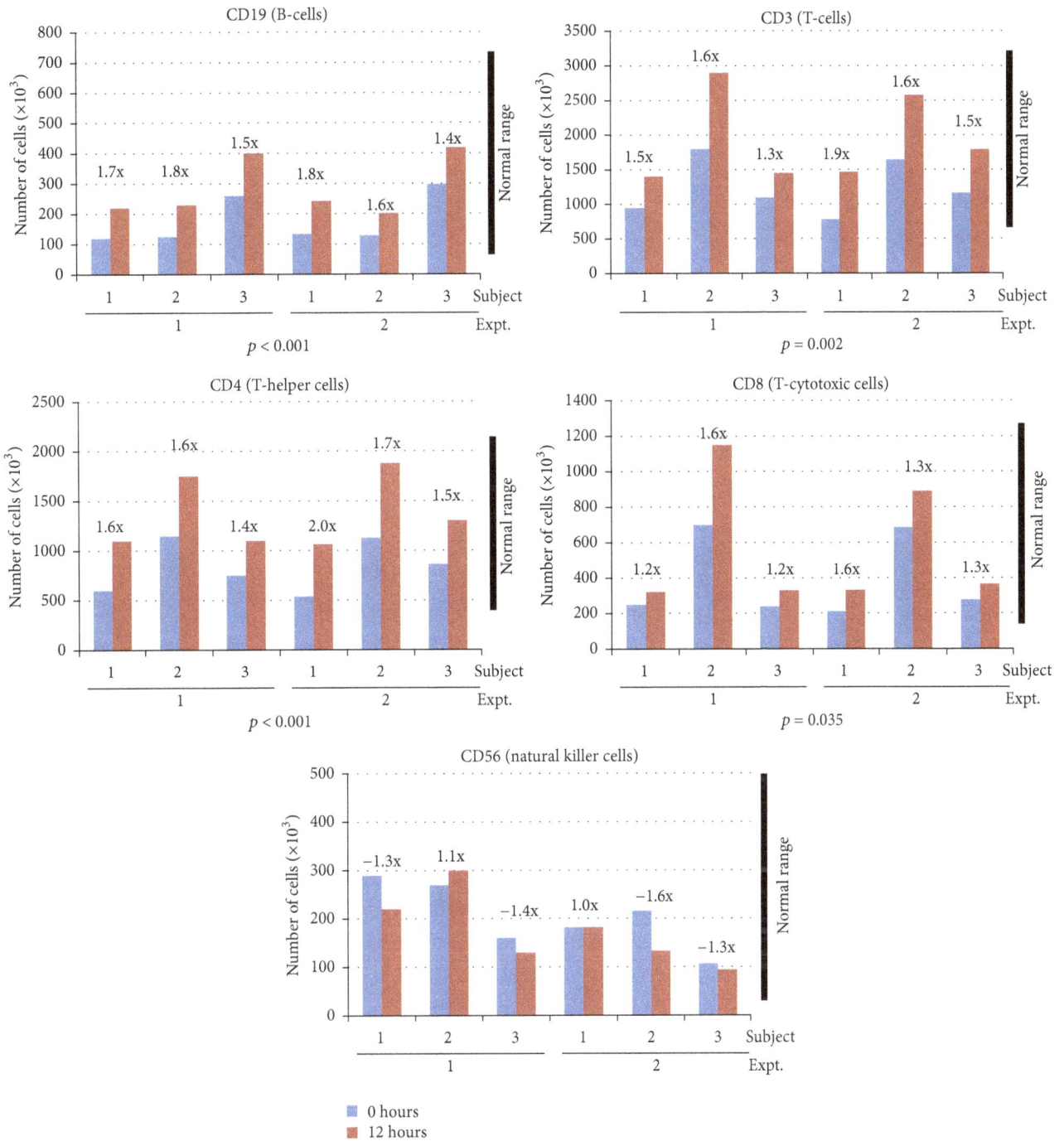

FIGURE 2: AM effect on lymphocyte subset populations. Subjects (1, 2, or 3) were administered AM at a 1.5 mL extract/kg body weight dose. Blood draws were performed 0 (blue bars) and 12 (red bars) hours after administration and lymphocyte subset cell populations were measured. The experiment was repeated twice. Peak fold changes relative to baseline ($t = 0$ hours) are indicated. Normal physiological ranges of the different cell populations are indicated by black bars.

not shown). Similarly, the vehicle had no effect on liver and kidney tests (data not shown).

In addition to these studies, we evaluated symptomatic outcomes following administration of AM. Physiological symptomatic responses were dose-dependent with the most dramatic results observed at the highest AM dose (data

not shown). As shown in Figure 5(a), typical "flu-like" symptoms were reported by all participants. The symptoms included fatigue, malaise, headache, and a reduced capacity to mentally focus. Symptoms were first reported between 2 and 4 hours and reached maximal values between 6 and 10 hours after ingestion of AM. All participants demonstrated

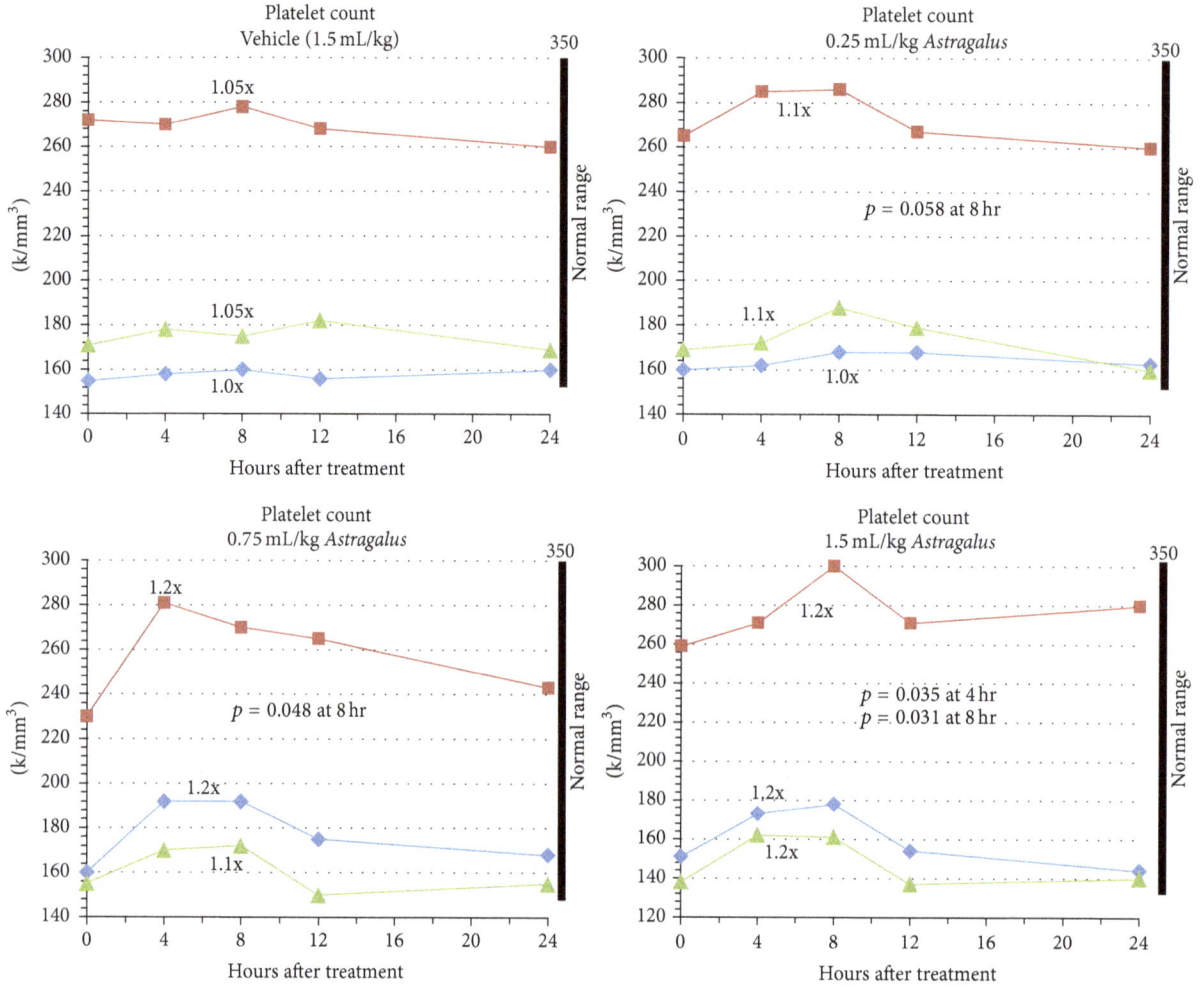

FIGURE 3: AM effect on circulating platelets. Subjects 1, 2, or 3 (indicated by blue, red, and green lines, resp.) were administered vehicle or varying concentrations of AM extract (0.25, 0.75, and 1.5 mL extract/kg body weight). Blood draws were performed 0, 4, 8, 12, and 24 hours after administration to measure total platelet cell numbers. Peak fold changes relative to baseline ($t = 0$ hours) are indicated. Normal physiological ranges of the different cell populations are indicated by black bars.

a decline in symptoms by 12 hours and by 24 hours no symptoms were reported by any individual. The average peak intensity ratings for these three symptoms were 3.67/10 (malaise), 4.67/10 (headache), and 5/10 (fatigue); although peak intensities occurred at different time points. Statistical significance, as represented by p values, for headache and fatigue ranged from 0.015 to 0.057. While ratings for malaise showed trending in two out of three subjects, one subject experienced only very minor fatigue and for a much shorter duration than the others. Thus the p value was >0.05. These symptoms are consistent with those typically reported in proinflammatory sickness [34, 35]. No other significant physiological symptoms were reported by the subjects.

Our study also monitored changes to body temperature over the 24-hour time period after administration of the 1.5 mL/kg dose of AM. Compared to the vehicle control, two of the three subjects showed significant trending in increased body temperatures (Figure 5(b)). The other subject did not demonstrate a change in body temperature. The maximum value noted was 99.3°F and may be interpreted as a mild fever response. Maximum temperatures were observed by 8 hours after administration of AM and temperatures returned to baseline values by 24 hours.

To further understand the effects of AM on blood flow, we also measured blood pressure at each blood draw during the 1.5 mL/kg trial. As shown in Figure 6, a decrease in systolic pressure (ranging from −1.11x to −1.17x baseline values) by an average of −1.13x below baseline values was seen consistently across participants 4 hours after administration. In contrast, the vehicle control led to an average increase of +0.37x above baseline values for systolic blood pressure. Similarly, participants also showed consistent decreases in diastolic blood pressure ranging from −1.10x to −1.17x with an average of −1.14x in response to AM 4 hours after ingestion. Again

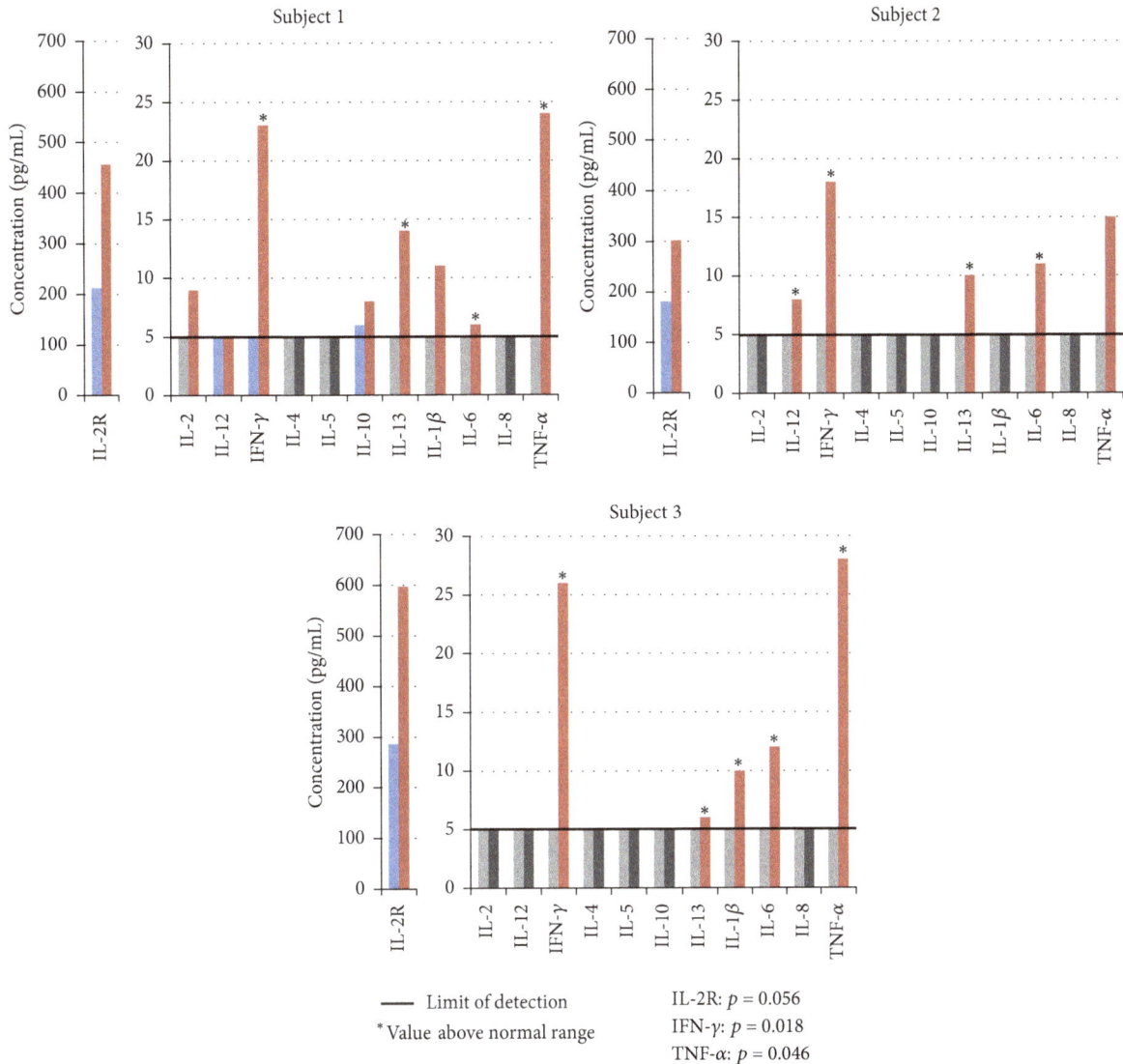

FIGURE 4: AM effect on cytokine response. Subjects (1, 2, or 3) were administered AM at 1.5 mL extract/kg body weight dose. Blood draws were performed 0 (blue or light grey bars) and 12 (red or black bars) hours after administration and specific cytokine levels measured. Detection limits for all cytokines were 5 pg/mL (5 pg/mL limit is indicated by the black line). Blue and red bars indicate values at or above 5 pg/mL. Light grey and black bars indicate values less than 5 pg/mL (nondetectable). Cytokine levels above normal physiological ranges are indicated by *. p values for IL-2R, IFN-γ, and TNF-α are shown.

these results differ from those seen with the vehicle control with increased diastolic pressure of 1.16x baseline values on average. Systolic and diastolic changes were significant with p values of 0.007 and 0.003 at 4 hours, respectively. With regard to the timing of response, participants followed very similar trends where maximal changes were observed at the 4-hour time point. This result was similar to the time response observed with changes to circulating platelets. A return to baseline values was seen in all participants 8–24 hours after ingestion of AM. Despite significant decreases in systolic and diastolic values, the lowest values seen did not drop below normal physiological limits of systolic pressure of 90 mm Hg or diastolic pressure of 60 mm Hg and hypotension was not induced at any point in time.

4. Discussion

Our data supports a correlation between the purported physiological effects of the immunomodulatory botanical, AM, and changes in cytokine gene expression and immune cell circulation. In vivo, AM induced significant elevations in both total and specific leukocyte populations but changes remained within normal physiological limits. Specifically, CD3+, CD3+CD4+ and CD3+CD8+, and CD19+ lymphocyte populations were induced while natural killer (CD56+) cell populations were unchanged. In addition, total neutrophil and monocyte numbers increased suggesting a global mobilization of leukocytes into the blood stream following AM.

Previous data from microarray analysis after the in vitro treatment of peripheral blood mononuclear cells (PBMCs)

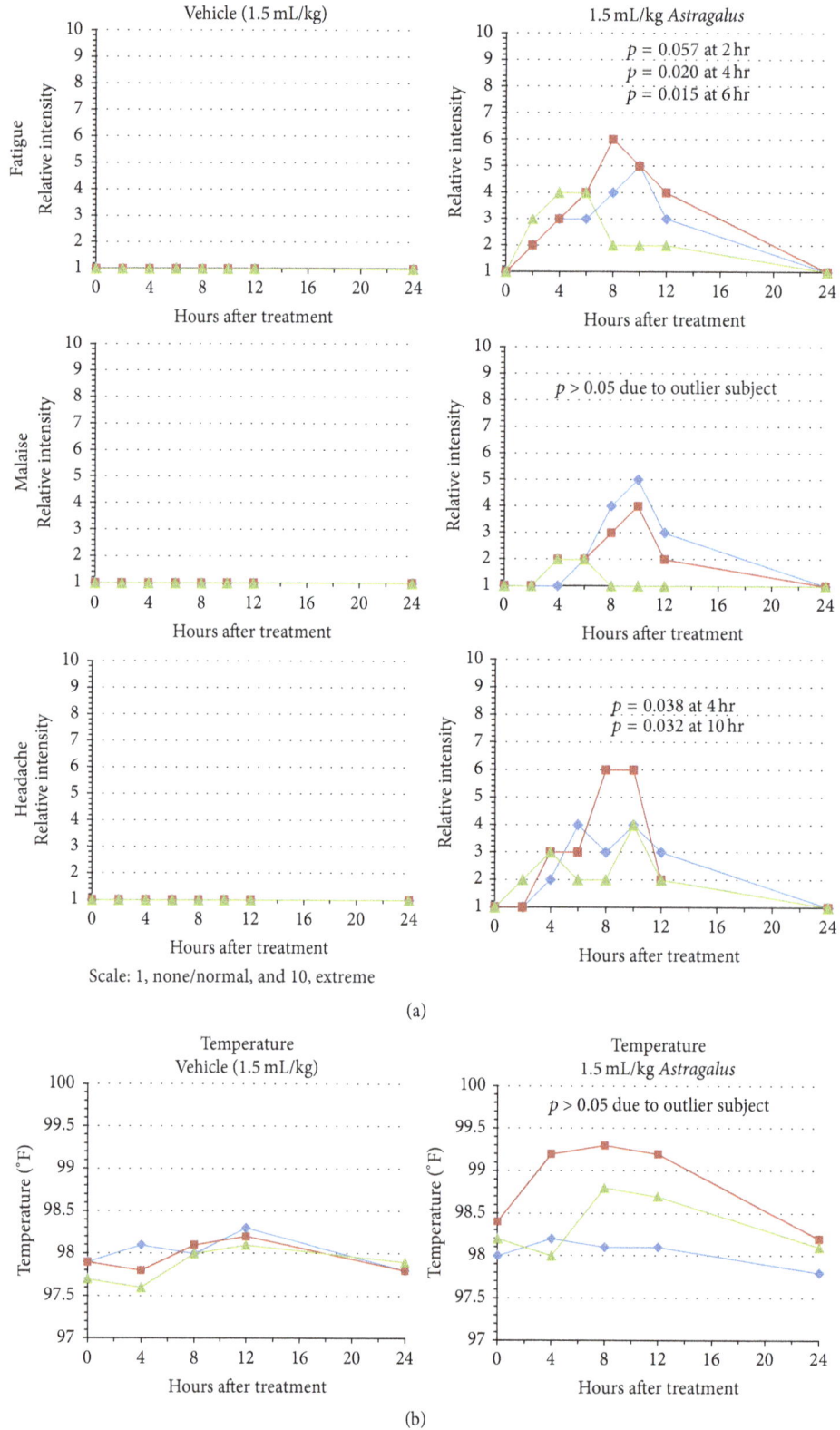

FIGURE 5: Physiological responses in subjects following administration of AM. Subjects 1, 2, or 3 (indicated by blue, red, and green lines, resp.) were administered vehicle or 1.5 mL extract/kg body weight dose of AM extract. (a) Symptoms of fatigue, malaise, and headache were recorded at 0, 2, 4, 6, 8, 10, 12, and 24 after administration. Values were subjective ranging from 1 to 10 (1, none/normal, and 10, extreme/severe). (b) Body temperature was measured orally 0, 4, 8, 12, and 24 hours after administration of the extract.

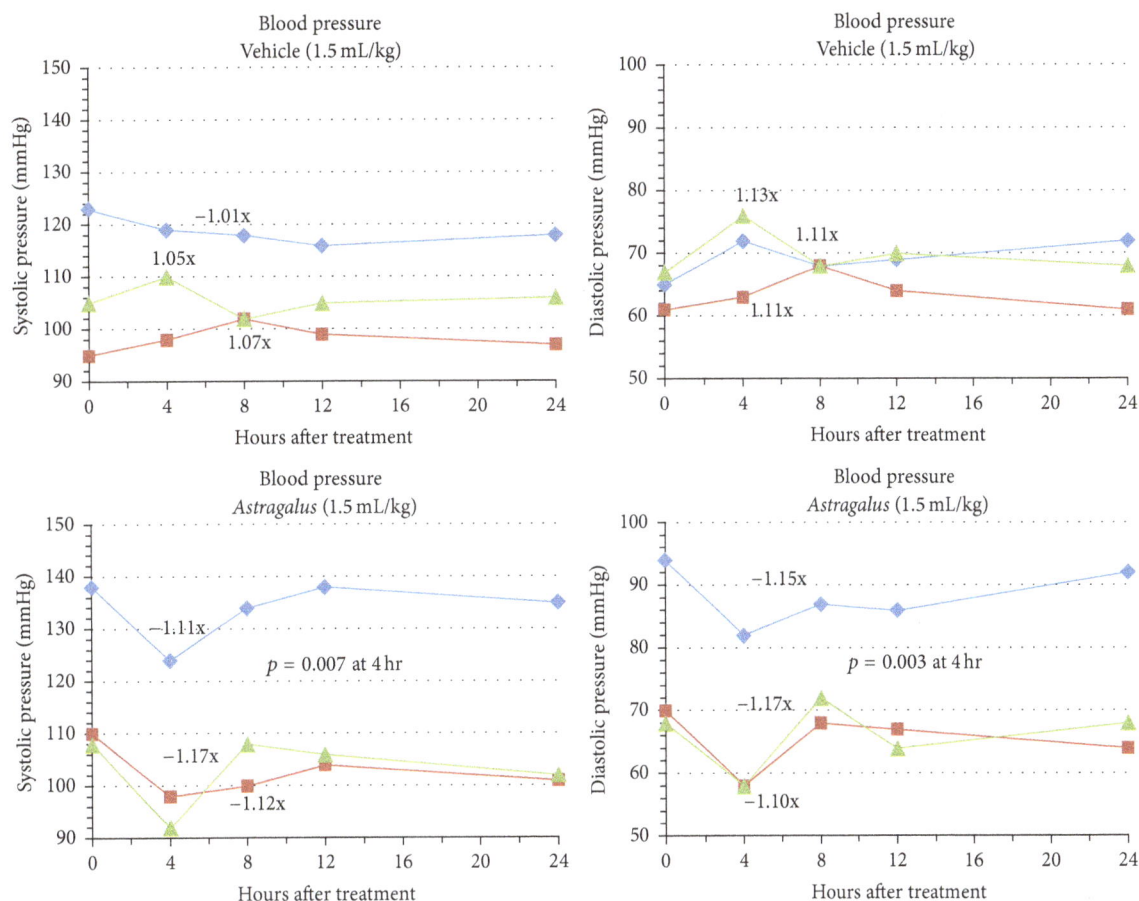

FIGURE 6: AM effects on blood pressure. Subjects 1, 2, or 3 (indicated by blue, red, and green lines, resp.) were administered vehicle or 1.5 mL extract/kg body weight dose of AM extract. Blood pressure (systolic and diastolic) was measured 0, 4, 8, 12, and 24 hours after administration of the extract.

with AM suggested that proinflammatory and Th1 specific cytokines were primarily upregulated [15]. In this regard, AM has been reported to modulate cytokine expression from Th2 toward Th1 in cancer and chronic viral infection [36, 37]. Our present *in vivo* data demonstrate a potential for priming toward a Th1 response where AM lead to the significant induction of Th1 cytokines, IFN-γ and TNF-α, along with a moderate induction of proinflammatory IL-6. The presence of IL-6 mediates fever and induces the acute phase response in the liver as well as acting as a differentiation factor to B-cells, monocytes, and macrophages and can act to regulate the development of a Th1 immune response through the induction of SOCS-1 and IL-4 [38]. However, our data do not show induction of IL-4 in serum following AM administration even though IL-6 is induced. IFN-γ leads to increased Th1 responses during infection or immunization and inhibits Th2 cell proliferation. IFN-γ is involved in macrophage activation, the generation of cell-mediated immunity, and upregulation of antiviral and antimicrobial effector molecules, and, in conjunction with TNF-α, can induce NF-κB responsive genes synergistically [39]. TNF-α itself is a pyrogen and an acute phase protein that promotes the inflammatory response, especially during diapedesis, and is highly expressed in

Th1-activated T-cells. Alternately, with induction of the Th2 cytokine, IL-13 was observed. IL-13 plays a nonredundant role with IL-4 in generating resistance to gastrointestinal parasites and intracellular organisms, increases mucus production, and generates IgE responses [40]. Despite being traditionally considered a Th2 cytokine, recent characterization of IL-13 has shown that it can be produced by IFN-γ+ Th1 cells and by Th17 cells [41]. Finally, soluble IL-2R was significantly induced in all subjects. It is normally expressed on antigen activated T lymphocytes and leads to T-cell proliferation. Its secretion indicates the presence of activated T-cells and can be an indicator of infection, neoplasms, and autoimmunity [42]. The levels of soluble IL-2R were increased 1.5–2.5-fold following AM treatment; however levels are lower than those seen in patients with chronic hepatitis infection (1.6–4-fold), acute EBV infections (7-fold), or B-cell cancer patients (up to 6.4-fold) but are similar to levels seen in autoimmune patients with rheumatoid arthritis (2-fold) [43–46].

Both direct and immune modulatory activities may explain the reported antibacterial effects of AM. It is recognized that when IFN-γ and TNF-α bind to their respective macrophage receptors, they stimulate the release of nitric oxide which results in increased destruction of bacteria [47].

In addition to cytokines, polysaccharides isolated from AM are also potent inducers of nitric oxide [48]. Alternately, polysaccharides isolated from AM have recently been shown to suppress Treg function by downregulating the production of IL-10 in a murine model of bacterial sepsis [49]. This may explain, at least in part, some of the clinical success for AM reported in the literature regarding antibacterial activity.

Our analysis of immune stimulation by AM related to white blood cell populations was of interest. As the dose of AM increased, absolute numbers of total leukocytes, neutrophils, lymphocytes, and monocytes also increased. Concurrently, increasing doses resulted in higher statistical significance as seen by an associated decrease in p values. Therefore, immune stimulation by AM is likely producing a dose-dependent response to changes in white blood cell populations. It is noteworthy that these changes remain within normal physiological ranges since therapeutic applications would not necessarily desire pathological immune responses such as leukocytosis or leukopenia. Historically, AM has been used to support and enhance the immune system, for instance in conditions of debility and viral infection. Given the rapid peak in circulating WBC populations we suspect that AM stimulates a mobilization of the immune cells into circulation from peripheral tissues/organs rather than hematopoietic formation of new cells from the bone marrow. It is possible that AM acts to stimulate immune cell mobilization leading to broad, systemic scanning of potential antigens as if "positioning" the immune cells for activity. It is then reasonable to infer that following mobilization, with no antigen present to continue activation of the immune cascade, the response is subsequently diminished and circulating cell populations are normalized by 24 hours after treatment. Surprisingly, administration of AM did not increase circulating levels of NK-cells. NK-cells are an important component in the antiviral immune response and are typically activated in response to IL-2, IL-12, IL-15, IL-18, and CCL5. Of these cytokines, we only assayed IL-2 and IL-12, each of which was induced in separate subjects. These results may suggest some level of specificity to the innate response induced by AM.

Regarding blood flow and wound healing, previous literature and anecdotal evidence suggests that AM may be associated with an increased risk of bleeding tendencies, improved endothelial cell function, improved blood glucose control, improved cardiovascular function overall, and blood pressure lowering effects [50–52]. Our results demonstrated a minor increase in platelets within 4–8 hours after administration of AM; a faster response than that observed in the leukocyte population. Like the leukocyte populations, there was an increase in absolute numbers of circulating platelets with higher dosing of AM. Our previous *in vitro* AM microarray studies identified putative genes induced by AM which are associated with angiogenesis, wound healing, and blood pressure modulation. It is known that the role of platelets is to provide the initial hemostasis that occurs after tissue injury and to produce growth factors responsible for the regeneration of damaged tissues such as platelet derived growth factor (PDGF), transforming growth factor (TGF), and endothelial growth factor (EGF). Our cytokine analysis showed significant increases in IL-6, which is involved in PDGF-induced cell proliferation [53]. Similarly IL-13 is known to induce the release of TGF from epithelial cells [54]. While our studies support the notion that AM may induce wound healing through changes in specific cytokine populations and numbers of circulating platelets, further studies are needed to determine a more complete understanding of the relationships between cytokine induction, cellular responses, and clinical results.

Our results demonstrated a decrease in blood pressure following administration of AM. Clinically, both whole botanical applications and isolated constituents of AM, such as astragaloside IV, have been shown to be beneficial in ischemic heart disease, heart failure, myocardial infarction, and relief of anginal pain [55]. This may be due in part to a vasodilatory effect leading to the observed reduction in both systolic and diastolic pressure. Indeed, IL-6, IL-13, and TNF-α are also known inducers of vasodilation [56–58].

An increase in body temperature has been historically recognized since ancient times as an indication of infection or inflammation. Current research demonstrates that T-cytotoxic cells are affected by mild hyperthermia through changes to cell membranes, which then mediate cell function and differentiation [59]. There is little to no significant data in the literature on the effect of AM on body temperature. Since individuals deviate only slightly from the standard value of 98.6°F, our results suggest a mild effect on body temperature due to AM. Two out of three of our subjects demonstrated minor although significant increases in temperature to a maximum value of 99.3°F in one subject. Furthermore, there is a clear trend in those subjects which mirrors that of the WBC response with maximum values between 8 and 12 hours and a subsequent return to baseline by 24 hours. Increases in activated white blood cells leads to the production of endogenous pyrogens such as IL-1, IL-6, and TNF-α. Our results likely indicate an increase in temperature as part of the coordinated steps of normal immune activation.

To understand this response even further, subjective symptoms including fatigue, malaise, and headache were observed to occur soon after ingestion of AM and returned to baseline values by 24 hours. Subjects also reported a lack of mental focus. The early presence of these symptoms (often before 4 hours) indicates a likely prodrome type of response which parallels the notion that immune cell populations are being induced for wide spread systemic scanning. TNF-α is an acute phase response proinflammatory cytokine involved in pain activation including headache, malaise, and fatigue [60, 61]. Proinflammatory cytokines, IL-6 (all 3 patients) and IL-1β (2 patients), were also measurable and, together with TNF-α, likely resulted in symptoms associated with immune activation.

Our study provides analyses of the physiological responses following administration of AM to a limited number of subjects. To the best of our knowledge, no other study has elucidated such an overall response under this specific group of parameters and in healthy individuals. Since there has been an increase in the use of botanical therapies, including herbal medicine, health food, and cosmetics, this research is relevant to CAM practitioners, primary care physicians, and other medical doctors alike. The significant potential for therapeutic and clinical application as well as the growing interest for scientific evidence and expertise in the use of botanical medicine creates a clear need for *in vivo* analysis and further characterization of AM.

Disclosure

Herbal Vitality, Inc., was involved to provide properly prepared botanical extractions and as a consultant on botanical experimental procedures. Jessica Moore is co-first author.

Competing Interests

No competing financial interests exist.

References

[1] P. S. Adusumilli, L. Ben-Porat, M. Pereira, D. Roesler, and I. M. Leitman, "The prevalence and predictors of herbal medicine use in surgical patients," *Journal of the American College of Surgeons*, vol. 198, no. 4, pp. 583–590, 2004.

[2] L. J. Harnack, S. A. Rydell, and J. Stang, "Prevalence of use of herbal products by adults in the Minneapolis/St Paul, Minn, metropolitan area," *Mayo Clinic Proceedings*, vol. 76, no. 7, pp. 688–694, 2001.

[3] *Guidance on Designing Clinical Trials of CAM Therapies: Determining Dose Ranges*, National Center for Complementary and Alternative Medicine, 2003, http://www.nccam.nih.gov/research/policies/guideonct.htm.

[4] O. Vardeny and M. B. Bromberg, "The use of herbal supplements and alternative therapies by patients with amyotrophic lateral sclerosis (ALS)," *Journal of Herbal Pharmacotherapy*, vol. 5, no. 3, pp. 23–31, 2005.

[5] P. Gardiner, R. Graham, A. T. R. Legedza, A. C. Ahn, D. M. Eisenberg, and R. S. Phillips, "Factors associated with herbal therapy use by adults in the United States," *Alternative Therapies in Health and Medicine*, vol. 13, no. 2, pp. 22–29, 2007.

[6] P. M. Barnes, B. Bloom, and R. L. Nahin, *Complementary and Alternative Medicine Use among Adults and Children: United States 2007*, National Health Statistics Reports: National Center for Complementary and Alternative Medicine, National Institutes of Health, 2008.

[7] D. M. Eisenberg, E. S. J. Harris, B. A. Littlefield et al., "Developing a library of authenticated Traditional Chinese Medicinal (TCM) plants for systematic biological evaluation—rationale, methods and preliminary results from a Sino-American collaboration," *Fitoterapia*, vol. 82, no. 1, pp. 17–33, 2011.

[8] X.-M. Li, "Treatment of asthma and food allergy with herbal interventions from traditional Chinese medicine," *Mount Sinai Journal of Medicine*, vol. 78, no. 5, pp. 697–716, 2011.

[9] J. D. Mark, "Integrative medicine and asthma," *Pediatric Clinics of North America*, vol. 54, no. 6, pp. 1007–1023, 2007.

[10] A. Sawni and R. Thomas, "Pediatricians' attitudes, experience and referral patterns regarding complementary/alternative medicine: a national survey," *BMC Complementary and Alternative Medicine*, vol. 7, article 18, 2007.

[11] S. Sinclair, "Chinese herbs: a clinical review of astragalus, ligusticum, and schizandrae," *Alternative Medicine Review*, vol. 3, no. 5, pp. 338–344, 1998.

[12] K. I. Block and M. N. Mead, "Immune system effects of echinacea, ginseng, and astragalus: a review," *Integrative Cancer Therapies*, vol. 2, no. 3, pp. 247–267, 2003.

[13] Q. Gao, J. Li, J. K. H. Cheung et al., "Verification of the formulation and efficacy of Danggui Buxue Tang (a decoction of Radix Astragali and Radix Angelicae Sinensis): an exemplifying systematic approach to revealing the complexity of Chinese herbal medicine formulae," *Chinese Medicine*, vol. 2, article 12, 2007.

[14] "Astragalus membranaceus. Monograph," *Alternative Medicine Review*, vol. 8, no. 1, pp. 72–77, 2003.

[15] K. L. Denzler, R. Waters, B. L. Jacobs, Y. Rochon, and J. O. Langland, "Regulation of inflammatory gene expression in PBMCs by immunostimulatory botanicals.," *PloS ONE*, vol. 5, no. 9, Article ID e12561, 2010.

[16] Z. L. Liu, Z. J. Liu, J. P. Liu, M. Yang, and J. Kwong, "Herbal medicines for viral myocarditis," *Cochrane Database of Systematic Reviews*, vol. 7, Article ID CD003711, 2012.

[17] B.-M. Shao, W. Xu, H. Dai, P. Tu, Z. Li, and X.-M. Gao, "A study on the immune receptors for polysaccharides from the roots of *Astragalus membranaceus*, a Chinese medicinal herb," *Biochemical and Biophysical Research Communications*, vol. 320, no. 4, pp. 1103–1111, 2004.

[18] W. C. S. Cho and K. N. Leung, "In vitro and in vivo immunomodulating and immunorestorative effects of *Astragalus membranaceus*," *Journal of Ethnopharmacology*, vol. 113, no. 1, pp. 132–141, 2007.

[19] T. Peng, Y. Yang, H. Riesemann, and R. Kandolf, "The inhibitory effect of Astragalus membranaceus on coxackie B-3 virus RNA replication," *Chinese Medical Sciences Journal*, vol. 10, no. 3, pp. 146–150, 1995.

[20] M. S. Ahmed, S. H. Hou, M. C. Battaglia, M. M. Picken, and D. J. Leehey, "Treatment of idiopathic membranous nephropathy with the herb *Astragalus membranaceus*," *American Journal of Kidney Diseases*, vol. 50, no. 6, pp. 1028–1032, 2007.

[21] H.-D. Hu, C.-G. You, R.-L. Zhang, P. Gao, and Z.-R. Wang, "Effects of astragalus polysaccharides and astragalosides on the phagocytosis of Mycobacterium tuberculosis by macrophages," *Journal of International Medical Research*, vol. 35, no. 1, pp. 84–90, 2007.

[22] S. Wang, J. Li, H. Huang et al., "Anti-hepatitis B virus activities of astragaloside IV isolated from Radix Astragali," *Biological and Pharmaceutical Bulletin*, vol. 32, no. 1, pp. 132–135, 2009.

[23] M. Kusum, V. Klinbuayaem, M. Bunjob, and S. Sangkitporn, "Preliminary efficacy and safety of oral suspension SH, combination of five Chinese medicinal herbs, in people living with HIV/AIDS; the phase I/II study," *Journal of the Medical Association of Thailand*, vol. 87, no. 9, pp. 1065–1070, 2004.

[24] H. Kobayashi, N. Mizuno, H. Teramae et al., "Diet and Japanese herbal medicine for recalcitrant atopic dermatitis: efficacy and safety," *Drugs under Experimental and Clinical Research*, vol. 30, no. 5-6, pp. 197–202, 2004.

[25] L. Guo, S.-P. Bai, L. Zhao, and X.-H. Wang, "Astragalus polysaccharide injection integrated with vinorelbine and cisplatin for patients with advanced non-small cell lung cancer: effects on quality of life and survival," *Medical Oncology*, vol. 29, no. 3, pp. 1656–1662, 2012.

[26] D.-T. Chu, W. L. Wong, and G. M. Mavligit, "Immunotherapy with Chinese medicinal herbs. II. Reversal of cyclophosphamide-induced immune suppression by administration of fractionated *Astragalus membranaceus* in vivo," *Journal of Clinical and Laboratory Immunology*, vol. 25, no. 3, pp. 125–129, 1988.

[27] P. Bergner, "Antiviral botanicals in herbal medicine," *Medical Herbalism*, vol. 14, pp. 1–12, 2005.

[28] K. Spelman, J. J. Burns, D. Nichols, N. Winters, S. Ottersberg, and M. Tenborg, "Modulation of cytokine expression by traditional medicines: a review of herbal immunomodulators," *Alternative Medicine Review*, vol. 11, no. 2, pp. 128–150, 2006.

[29] J.-E. Huh, D.-W. Nam, Y.-H. Baek et al., "Formononetin accelerates wound repair by the regulation of early growth response factor-1 transcription factor through the phosphorylation of the ERK and p38 MAPK pathways," *International Immunopharmacology*, vol. 11, no. 1, pp. 46–54, 2011.

[30] C. Sevimli-Gür, I. Onbaşlar, P. Atilla et al., "In vitro growth stimulatory and in vivo wound healing studies on cycloartane-type saponins of *Astragalus genus*," *Journal of Ethnopharmacology*, vol. 134, no. 3, pp. 844–850, 2011.

[31] X. Chen, L.-H. Peng, N. Li et al., "The healing and anti-scar effects of astragaloside IV on the wound repair in vitro and in vivo," *Journal of Ethnopharmacology*, vol. 139, no. 3, pp. 721–727, 2012.

[32] K.-M. Lau, K.-K. Lai, C.-L. Liu et al., "Synergistic interaction between Astragali Radix and Rehmanniae Radix in a Chinese herbal formula to promote diabetic wound healing," *Journal of Ethnopharmacology*, vol. 141, no. 1, pp. 250–256, 2012.

[33] J. K.-S. Ko and C. W.-S. Chik, "The protective action of radix Astragalus membranaceus against hapten-induced colitis through modulation of cytokines," *Cytokine*, vol. 47, no. 2, pp. 85–90, 2009.

[34] U. A. Vollmer-Conna, C. Fazou, B. Cameron et al., "Production of pro-inflammatory cytokines correlates with the symptoms of acute sickness behaviour in humans," *Psychological Medicine*, vol. 34, no. 7, pp. 1289–1297, 2004.

[35] C. Bay-Richter, S. Janelidze, L. Hallberg, and L. Brundin, "Changes in behaviour and cytokine expression upon a peripheral immune challenge," *Behavioural Brain Research*, vol. 222, no. 1, pp. 193–199, 2011.

[36] S.-P. Mao, K.-L. Cheng, and Y.-F. Zhou, "Modulatory effect of *Astragalus membranaceus* on Th1/Th2 cytokine in patients with herpes simplex keratitis," *Zhongguo Zhong Xi Yi Jie He Za Zhi*, vol. 24, no. 2, pp. 121–123, 2004.

[37] H. Wei, R. Sun, W. Xiao et al., "Traditional Chinese medicine *Astragalus* reverses predominance of Th2 cytokines and their up-stream transcript factors in lung cancer patients," *Oncology Reports*, vol. 10, no. 5, pp. 1507–1512, 2003.

[38] S. Diehl and M. Rincón, "The two faces of IL-6 on Th1/Th2 differentiation," *Molecular Immunology*, vol. 39, no. 9, pp. 531–536, 2002.

[39] K. Schroder, P. J. Hertzog, T. Ravasi, and D. A. Hume, "Interferon-γ: an overview of signals, mechanisms and functions," *Journal of Leukocyte Biology*, vol. 75, no. 2, pp. 163–189, 2004.

[40] T. A. Wynn, "IL-13 effector functions," *Annual Review of Immunology*, vol. 21, pp. 425–456, 2003.

[41] E. Gallo, S. Katzman, and A. V. Villarino, "IL-13-producing Th1 and Th17 cells characterize adaptive responses to both self and foreign antigens," *European Journal of Immunology*, vol. 42, no. 9, pp. 2322–2328, 2012.

[42] C. Caruso, G. Candore, D. Cigna, A. T. Colucci, and M. A. Modica, "Biological significance of soluble IL-2 receptor," *Mediators of Inflammation*, vol. 2, no. 1, pp. 3–21, 1993.

[43] P. Xiao, Q.-F. Chen, Y.-L. Yang, Z.-H. Guo, and H. Chen, "Serum soluble interleukin-2 receptor levels in patients with chronic hepatitis B virus infection and its relation with anti-HBc," *World Journal of Gastroenterology*, vol. 12, no. 3, pp. 482–484, 2006.

[44] B. E. Tomkinson, D. K. Wagner, D. L. Nelson, and J. L. Sullivan, "Activated lymphocytes during acute Epstein-Barr virus infection," *Journal of Immunology*, vol. 139, no. 11, pp. 3802–3807, 1987.

[45] G. Semenzato, R. Foa, C. Agostini et al., "High serum levels of soluble interleukin 2 receptor in patients with B chronic lymphocytic leukemia," *Blood*, vol. 70, no. 2, pp. 396–400, 1987.

[46] J. A. Symons, N. C. Wood, F. S. Di Giovine, and G. W. Duff, "Soluble Il-2 receptor in rheumatoid arthritis. Correlation with disease activity, Il-1 and IL-2 inhibition," *Journal of Immunology*, vol. 141, no. 8, pp. 2612–2618, 1988.

[47] F. Y. Liew, Y. Li, and S. Millott, "Tumor necrosis factor-alpha synergizes with IFN-gamma in mediating killing of Leishmania major through the induction of nitric oxide," *The Journal of Immunology*, vol. 145, no. 12, pp. 4306–4310, 1990.

[48] K. Y. Lee and Y. J. Jeon, "Macrophage activation by polysaccharide isolated from *Astragalus membranaceus*," *International Immunopharmacology*, vol. 5, no. 7-8, pp. 1225–1233, 2005.

[49] Q. Y. Liu, Y. M. Yao, Y. Yu, N. Dong, and Z. Y. Sheng, "Astragalus polysaccharides attenuate postburn sepsis via inhibiting negative immunoregulation of CD4$^+$ CD25^{high} T cells," *PLoS ONE*, vol. 6, no. 7, Article ID e19811, 2011.

[50] D.-O. Han, H.-J. Lee, and D.-H. Hahm, "Wound-healing activity of Astragali Radix in rats," *Methods and Findings in Experimental and Clinical Pharmacology*, vol. 31, no. 2, pp. 95–100, 2009.

[51] H. Hikino, S. Funayama, and K. Endo, "Hypotensive principle of *Astragalus* and *Hedysarum* roots," *Planta Medica*, vol. 30, no. 4, pp. 297–302, 1976.

[52] N. Zhang, X.-H. Wang, S.-L. Mao, and F. Zhao, "Astragaloside IV improves metabolic syndrome and endothelium dysfunction in fructose-fed rats," *Molecules*, vol. 16, no. 5, pp. 3896–3907, 2011.

[53] M. Roth, M. Nauck, M. Tamm, A. P. Perruchoud, R. Ziesche, and L. H. Block, "Intracellular interleukin 6 mediates platelet-derived growth factor-induced proliferation of nontransformed cells," *Proceedings of the National Academy of Sciences of the United States of America*, vol. 92, no. 5, pp. 1312–1316, 1995.

[54] B. W. Booth, K. B. Adler, J. C. Bonner, F. Tournier, and L. D. Martin, "Interleukin-13 induces proliferation of human airway epithelial cells in vitro via a mechanism mediated by transforming growth factor-α," *American Journal of Respiratory Cell and Molecular Biology*, vol. 25, no. 6, pp. 739–743, 2001.

[55] W.-D. Zhang, H. Chen, C. Zhang, R.-H. Liu, H.-L. Li, and H.-Z. Chen, "Astragaloside IV from *Astragalus membranaceus* shows cardioprotection during myocardial ischemia in vivo and in vitro," *Planta Medica*, vol. 72, no. 1, pp. 4–8, 2006.

[56] A. Minghini, L. D. Britt, and M. A. Hill, "Interleukin-1 and interleukin-6 mediated skeletal muscle arteriolar vasodilation: in vitro versus in vivo studies," *Shock*, vol. 9, no. 3, pp. 210–215, 1998.

[57] X. Tang, N. Spitzbarth, H. Kuhn, P. Chaitidis, and W. B. Campbell, "Interleukin-13 upregulates vasodilatory 15-lipoxygenase eicosanoids in rabbit aorta," *Arteriosclerosis, Thrombosis, and Vascular Biology*, vol. 23, no. 10, pp. 1768–1774, 2003.

[58] D. G. Johns and R. C. Webb, "TNF-α-induced endothelium-independent vasodilation: a role for phospholipase A2-dependent ceramide signaling," *The American Journal of Physiology—Heart and Circulatory Physiology*, vol. 275, no. 5, pp. H1592–H1598, 1998.

[59] T. A. Mace, L. Zhong, C. Kilpatrick et al., "Differentiation of CD8+ T cells into effector cells is enhanced by physiological range hyperthermia," *Journal of Leukocyte Biology*, vol. 90, no. 5, pp. 951–962, 2011.

[60] T. Rozen and S. Z. Swidan, "Elevation of CSF tumor necrosis factor α levels in new daily persistent headache and treatment refractory chronic migraine," *Headache*, vol. 47, no. 7, pp. 1050–1055, 2007.

[61] Y. Jiang, R. Deacon, D. C. Anthony, and S. J. Campbell, "Inhibition of peripheral TNF can block the malaise associated with CNS inflammatory diseases," *Neurobiology of Disease*, vol. 32, no. 1, pp. 125–132, 2008.

15

Phytochemicals and Medicinal Properties of Indigenous Tropical Fruits with Potential for Commercial Development

Hock Eng Khoo,[1,2] **Azrina Azlan,**[1,2,3] **Kin Weng Kong,**[4] **and Amin Ismail**[1,2,3]

[1]Department of Nutrition and Dietetics, Faculty of Medicine and Health Sciences, Universiti Putra Malaysia (UPM), 43400 Serdang, Selangor, Malaysia
[2]Research Centre of Excellence for Nutrition and Non-Communicable Diseases, Faculty of Medicine and Health Sciences, Universiti Putra Malaysia (UPM), 43400 Serdang, Selangor, Malaysia
[3]Laboratory of Halal Science Research, Halal Products Research Institute, Universiti Putra Malaysia (UPM), 43400 Serdang, Selangor, Malaysia
[4]Department of Molecular Medicine, Faculty of Medicine, University of Malaya, 50603 Kuala Lumpur, Malaysia

Correspondence should be addressed to Azrina Azlan; azrinaaz@upm.edu.my

Academic Editor: Daniela Rigano

Hundreds of fruit-bearing trees are native to Southeast Asia, but many of them are considered as indigenous or underutilized. These species can be categorized as indigenous tropical fruits with potential for commercial development and those possible for commercial development. Many of these fruits are considered as underutilized unless the commercialization is being realized despite the fact that they have the developmental potential. This review discusses seven indigenous tropical fruits from 15 species that have been identified, in which their fruits are having potential for commercial development. As they are not as popular as the commercially available fruits, limited information is found. This paper is the first initiative to provide information on the phytochemicals and potential medicinal uses of these fruits. Phytochemicals detected in these fruits are mainly the phenolic compounds, carotenoids, and other terpenoids. Most of these phytochemicals are potent antioxidants and have corresponded to the free radical scavenging activities and other biological activities of the fruits. The scientific research that covered a broad range of *in vitro* to *in vivo* studies on the medicinal potentials of these fruits is also discussed in detail. The current review is an update for researchers to have a better understanding of the species, which simultaneously can provide awareness to enhance their commercial value and promote their utilization for better biodiversity conservation.

1. Introduction

Southeast Asian countries, including Malaysia, have tropical rainforests with a variety of fruit-bearing trees. These trees are evergreen and growing throughout the year. Many of these trees produce edible fruit for animals living within the scrubs and some of these fruits are even used by the local communities in their traditional medicine [1]. Since centuries ago, human started to cultivate different plant species to harvest their edible fruits as food sources. In the ancient days, cultivation of the fruit-bearing trees for their edible fruits was done only by planting them beside the house or around the housing areas. Hence, the fruits can be easily harvested during the fruiting season. Large-scale farming has been introduced and started in the later years for commercialization of these tropical fruits due to increasing in their market demand.

Today, many of the tropical fruits have been commercialized. These fruits are banana (*Musa* spp.), durian (*Durio zibethinus* L.), jackfruit (*Artocarpus heterophyllus* Lam.), mangosteen (*Garcinia mangostana* L.), papaya (*Carica papaya* L.), pineapple (*Ananas comosus* [L] Merr.), pitaya (*Hylocereus* spp.), pomelo (*Citrus maxima* [Burm.] Merr.), rambutan (*Nephelium lappaceum* L.), and watermelon (*Citrullus lanatus* [Thunb.] Matsum. & Nakai). However, in this decade, some indigenous tropical fruits previously unavailable in the market became available in the local markets of Southeast Asia. These include ambarella (*Spondias dulcis*

L.), cempedak (*Artocarpus integer* [Thunb.] Merr.), langsat (*Lansium domesticum* Corrêa), pulasan (*Nephelium mutabile* Blume), and salak (*Salacca zalacca* [Gaertn.] Voss), whereas bambangan (*Mangifera pajang* Kosterm.), dabai (*Canarium odontophyllum* Miq.), durian nyekak (*Durio kutejensis* Hassk. & Becc.), and some wild bananas (*Musa* spp.) [2] are found mainly in the Borneo market because they are native to Borneo Island. However, some of these fruits are still collected from their wildly grown trees, and their potential medicinal properties are not well understood.

This review comprehensively discussed the phytochemicals and medicinal properties for 15 species of indigenous tropical fruits. Their common names, as well as the scientific names, are shown in Table 1. In this review, the 15 species of indigenous tropical fruits are grouped into indigenous tropical fruits with potential for commercial development and indigenous tropical fruits that are possible for commercial development in Southeast Asia, particularly in Malaysia [3]. The indigenous tropical fruit with potential for commercial development are fruits that are frequently consumed by the local communities and readily available in the local markets of Southeast Asia especially during the fruiting season. These fruits, however, are less attractive than the commercially available species. Hence, they are not cultivated in a large-scale plantation or as cash crops. On the other hand, indigenous tropical fruits that are possible for commercial development are those fruits that have lesser popularity than the previous one, and they are only available in part of the tropical regions.

Many of these fruits have high nutritive values but their medicinal properties remain unknown [3]. Thus, more effort is needed to research on these fruit species, especially phytochemicals in the fruits which are necessary for future promotion on their use as food and medicine. In this review, phytochemicals of the selected indigenous tropical fruits are categorized into three major groups: (1) phenolics, (2) carotenoids, and (3) terpenes and terpenoids. These phytochemicals are commonly found in many fruits. Anthocyanins are the compounds that contributed to the attractive color of many fruits, ranging from red to purple, whereas carotenoids give yellow to orange colors to fruit. Carotenoids in fruit are divided into carotenes and xanthophylls [4], whereas phenolic compounds in fruits are phenolic acids and flavonoids [5]. Terpenes and other terpenoids in fruits are mainly the volatile compounds, especially triterpenes [6], and saponin is another member of terpenoids group having both hydrophilic and lipophilic properties.

Since early civilization, various fruits have been traditionally used as folk medicine [7]. Besides the fruit, bark, leaves, stem, root, twig, and sap have been used as ingredients for traditional medicine. These parts have been widely used as folk medicines by locals for treating several diseases, including cough, fever, asthma, diarrhea, indigestion, and skin diseases [8]. In modern medicine, extracts of different parts of the plant including fruit have been further employed for their medicinal benefits, as the antifungal, antimicrobial, antiatherosclerotic, antihypercholesterolemic, antileukemic, anticlastogenic, and antiproliferative agents [9]. Most of the bioactive compounds found in plant extracts are the primary

candidates for their medicinal properties. Owing to the limited work that has been done on underutilized species, this review aims to enlighten researchers and international communities on the bioactive components and potential medicinal properties of 15 selected indigenous tropical fruits. Data related to the phytochemicals in these fruits, including phenolic compounds, carotenoids, terpenes, and terpenoids, are obtained from research papers published in international journals and Internet sources (accessed on November 2014 to April 2016).

2. Indigenous Tropical Fruits with Potential for Commercial Development

Among hundreds tropical fruits in Malaysia, less than a dozen are categorized as indigenous tropical fruit with potential for commercial development. These fruits are horse mango, Borneo mango, plum mango, African black olive, rose apple, Malay apple, and Indian jujube (Table 1). Plum mango, horse mango, rose apple, Malay apple, and Indian jujube are well known in Peninsular Malaysia, while dabai and bambangan are native to Borneo Island, especially in East Malaysia. The trees of *C. odontophyllum* (dabai) are also grown in West Indonesia.

These seven indigenous tropical fruits from four different plant families are with commercialization potential in Malaysia. Both *Bouea* and *Mangifera* fruits are belonging to the Anacardiaceae family. The other fruits are belonging to the Burseraceae (*Canarium*), Myrtaceae (*Syzygium*), and Rhamnaceae (*Ziziphus*) families. *Bouea* and *Mangifera* fruits are closely related because they are from the same family, and the fruits are collectively called as "mango." On the other hand, plum mango, horse mango, and bambangan (Borneo mango) are mango fruits with some similarity in physical appearance. Among the *Bouea* genus, *B. macrophylla* (plum mango) is native to Peninsular Malaysia, North Sumatra, and West Java. However, the trees of *B. macrophylla* are nowadays widely cultivated in Indonesia, Philippines, Thailand, and Mauritius [10]. *B. gandaria* is a synonym for *B. macrophylla*, and it is also called as gandaria or setar (Malay name). Alor Setar, the capital city of Kedah, obtained its name from *B. macrophylla* plant. Horse mango or *Mangifera foetida* is native to Southeast Asia, especially Peninsular Malaysia, Thailand, Sumatra, and the Borneo Island. The fruit of *M. pajang* (bambangan) is an indigenous fruit from Borneo Island [11].

Another interesting indigenous tropical fruit with potential commercial development in Malaysia, especially Sarawak, is dabai. It is known as *C. odontophyllum* fruit and mainly cultivated in Sarawak, Malaysia. The Semongok Agricultural Research Centre of Sarawak has an industrial collaboration to initiate dabai plantations and enhance dabai product development in the near future. Other than dabai, the fruits of *Syzygium jambos* (rose apple) and *S. malaccense* (Malay apple) are the good sources of antioxidants [12]. *Eugenia jambos* and *E. malaccensis* are the synonyms for *S. jambos* and *S. malaccense*, respectively. The key difference between these two fruits is their color: rose apple has a pale yellow appearance with a mixture of pinkish hue, whereas Malay

TABLE 1: Common names and scientific names of 15 selected indigenous tropical fruits.

Scientific name	Family	English name	Malay name	Indonesian name	Thai name
Indigenous tropical fruit with potential for commercial development					
Mangifera foetida Lour.	Anacardiaceae	Horse mango	Bacang	Limus	Mamut
Mangifera pajang Kosterm.	Anacardiaceae	Borneo mango	Bambangan	Embang	—
Bouea macrophylla Griffith	Anacardiaceae	Plum mango	Kundang	Ramania	Maprang
Canarium odontophyllum Miq.	Burseraceae	African black olive	Dabai	Danau majang	—
Syzygium jambos L. (Alston)	Myrtaceae	Rose apple	Jambu mawar	Jambu mawar	Chomphu-nam dok mai
Syzygium malaccense (L.) Merr. & L.M. Perry	Myrtaceae	Malay apple	Jambu susu	Jambu bol	Chomphu-mamieow
Ziziphus mauritiana Lam.	Rhamnaceae	Indian jujube	Epal siam	Bidara	Phut-saa
Indigenous tropical fruit with possible commercial development					
Averrhoa bilimbi L.	Oxalidaceae	Cucumber tree	Belimbing buluh	Belimbing wuluh	Taling-pling
Baccaurea macrocarpa (Miq.) Müll. Arg.	Phyllanthaceae	Greater tampoi	Tampoi	Tampui	Lang-khae
Baccaurea motleyana (Müll. Arg.) Müll. Arg.	Phyllanthaceae	Rambai	Rambai	Rambai	Mafai-farang
Cynometra cauliflora L.	Fabaceae	Nam-nam	Katak puru	Namu-namu	Amphawa
Durio kutejensis Hassk. & Becc.	Anacardiaceae	Orange-fleshed durian	Durian Nyekak	Durian pulu	Thurian
Garcinia hombroniana Pierre	Clusiaceae	Seashore mangosteen	Beruas	—	Wa
Garcinia parvifolia (Miq.) Miq.	Clusiaceae	Brunei cherry	Asam aur aur	Kandis	—
Phyllanthus emblica L.	Phyllanthaceae	Indian gooseberry	Melaka	Malaka	Ma kham pom

apple is milky in color. Some varieties of *S. malaccense* plant have red colored fruit. The fruit of *Z. mauritiana* is native to Indonesia, India, and China. In Malaysia, the fruit of *Z. mauritiana* is commonly used in culinary practices.

3. Indigenous Tropical Fruits That Are Possible for Commercial Development

According to the Department of Agriculture Malaysia, over 370 species of fruit-bearing trees are found in Malaysia [50]. Even though most of these trees are wildly grown, some of them bear fruits with commercial values. In this review, eight indigenous fruits from different genera categorized as fruits that possible for commercial development in Malaysia or Southeast Asia have been discussed. The fruits of *Averrhoa bilimbi, Baccaurea macrocarpa, Baccaurea motleyana, Cynometra cauliflora, Durio kutejensis, Garcinia hombroniana, G. parvifolia,* and *Phyllanthus emblica* are categorized in this group. Their common names are tabulated in Table 1. All of these fruits are belonging to different plant families, except *Baccaurea* and *Phyllanthus* fruits, which belong to the Phyllanthaceae family.

Out of 2000 species, only certain plant species from Phyllanthaceae are cultivated in the tropical countries. *Phyllanthus emblica* (also known as *Emblica officinalis*) is locally known as "Pokok Melaka"; it is another underutilized plant native to Malaysia. The name of Malacca (Melaka) state, a historical city in Malaysia, is originated from the *P. emblica* trees that are well grown along the riverside. Its fruit is not popular among Malaysians and hence it is only homegrown in some areas of Malaysia. Although *P. emblica* trees have been planted for the ornamental purpose, the fruit has been reported as a potential source of functional food because it contains a high amount of vitamin C [51]. In India, the fruit of *P. emblica* is traditionally eaten by steeping the sour fruit in turmeric and adding it to salt water to make it palatable [52]. The extract of *P. emblica* fruit has also been used as hair dye [53]. Other fruits of the family Phyllanthaceae are *Baccaurea* fruits, which include *B. macrocarpa* (tampoi) and *B. motleyana* (rambai). These species are widely cultivated on the west coast of Peninsular Malaysia, especially in Perak, a state in Malaysia. Due to the annual fruiting season [54], *Baccaurea* fruits can be found only in the local markets during the months of peak fruiting period. The trees of *B. motleyana* are also found in other parts of Southeast Asia, especially Thailand, mainly for fruit cultivation. "Rambai" is the Malay name while "mafai-farang" is the Thai name of *B. motleyana* fruit (Table 1).

A. bilimbi, also known as "belimbing buluh" or cucumber tree, is native to Malaysia and Indonesia. It has been cultivated in Southeast Asia. In India, the trees of *A. bilimbi* are planted in the home gardens. *A. bilimbi* fruit is lesser popular for consumption than the commercially known star fruit (*A. carambola*). However, it is traditionally used as medicine for curing several diseases, including cardiovascular diseases [55]. Besides vitamins and minerals, the fruit of *A. bilimbi* also contains flavonoids and triterpenoids that contribute to its beneficial health properties [56]. Besides *A. bilimbi*,

C. cauliflora is another homegrown fruit-bearing tree that is found primarily in rural areas of Peninsular Malaysia. Its fruit is locally called as "nam-nam." The fruit of *C. cauliflora* has savory taste and can be consumed as fruit salad.

G. hombroniana is another plant native to Malaysia. The tree bears fruit called "seashore mangosteen" [27]. Another species of *Garcinia, G. parvifolia,* is also one of the indigenous tropical plants [57]. *Garcinia* fruits contain xanthones, flavones, and triterpenoids as the bioactive phytochemicals besides the leaves and twig of *Garcinia* trees [58]. *D. kutejensis* is another type of durian plant. The color of its flesh is orange-reddish due to the high amount of carotenoids. It is native to Borneo region, called as durian nyekak in East Malaysia. It has the taste and texture similar to the fruit of common *D. zibethinus*. The fruits of *D. zibethinus* or commercial durians are the most famous fruits in Malaysia and Thailand. However, the fruit of *D. kutejensis* is not available in Peninsular Malaysia owing to the fact that the trees of this fruit are native to Java and Borneo Islands [59]. *D. kutejensis* is a wildly grown species, and its fruits are collected by the indigenous people of Borneo Island (including Sabah and Sarawak) for their own consumption or selling in the local market. Therefore, *D. kutejensis* fruit is considered underutilized in Malaysia. Hence, in Peninsular Malaysia, the fruit of *D. kutejensis* cannot be found in the local markets throughout the year.

4. Industrial Applications of Indigenous Tropical Fruits and Their Potential as Commercial Products

In Southeast Asia, actually many indigenous tropical fruits have potential to be commercialized. In comparison between Malaysia and Thailand, many of the Malaysian indigenous fruits are underexploited. The underutilized indigenous fruits from Peninsular Malaysia have lesser commercial potential as compared with the underutilized indigenous fruits from East Malaysia (Borneo region). Dabai (*C. odontophyllum*), bambangan (*M. pajang*), and some wild banana (*Musa* spp.) from Borneo are the good examples where these fruits have been developed into different commercial products for local uses.

Dabai is an indigenous tropical fruit that is almost similar to olive. The oil extracted from the pulp of dabai demonstrated some possible health benefits [60]. In Sarawak (East Malaysia), the edible part of dabai has been incorporated into local cuisines such as fried rice, omelet, and being developed into the form of sauce or paste as an ingredient for cooking. Bambangan, as one of the big mangoes in the world [61], has also been used in cooking and as dessert. Bambangan juice is commonly consumed by the local people of Sabah (East Malaysia). In Sabah and Kalimantan, bambangan pickled can be seen being sold in the local markets, whereas bambangan peel is used as a raw ingredient for some local dishes. Besides dabai and bambangan, bananas (*Musa* spp.) from Borneo region are processed into banana chips.

On the other hand, in Peninsular Malaysia, bacang (*M. foetida*), kundang (*B. macrophylla*), and jambu (*Syzygium*

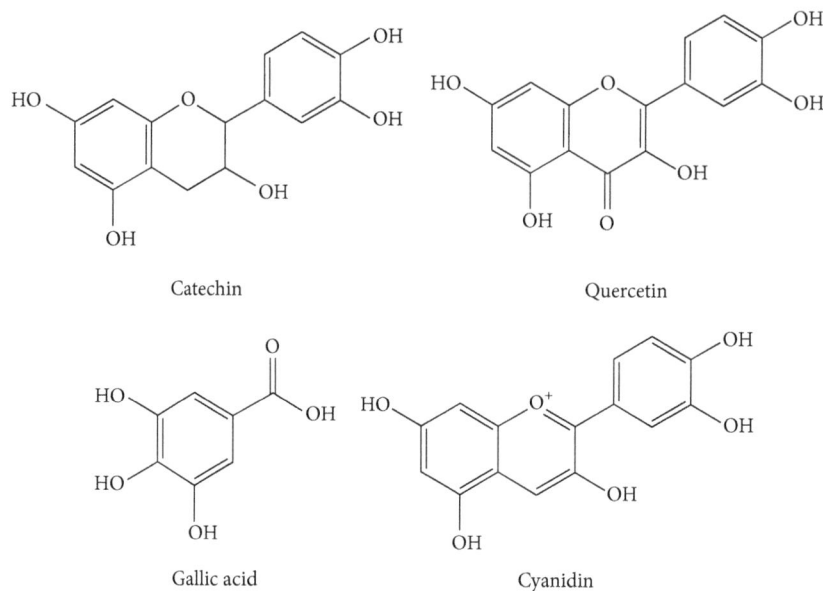

FIGURE 1: Major phenolic compounds in plant.

spp.) are those fruits that are having the potential for development into commercial products, such as canned fruit, pickles, and fruit juices. Although bidara (*Z. mauritiana*) is one of the commercialized fruits in India [70], this fruit is not commonly consumed by Malaysian. The fruit is only freshly eaten or preserved as pickle by Malay community.

5. Phytochemicals in 15 Selected Indigenous Tropical Fruits

5.1. Phenolic Compounds. Phenolic compounds are the largest group of phytochemicals and are widely distributed throughout the plant kingdom. Phenols, as the major bioactive substances in fruits, play a vital role as antioxidant. The major phenolic compounds in plants are shown in Figure 1. Phenolic compounds are good antioxidants found in the flesh of fruits including phenolic acids and flavonoids, whereas flavonoids and lignans are found in the seeds or kernel [71]. Among the phenolic acids, gallic acid is the major component of plant. Each fruit has, at least, a few major phenolic compounds. In addition to fruit, catechin is one of the main flavonoids found in leaves. Since phenolics are potent antioxidants, increased consumption of a mixture of fruits daily should be able to provide an adequate phenolic antioxidant. Thus, proper knowledge concerning identity and amount of phenolics in indigenous tropical fruits helps to promote the usage of these underutilized tropical fruits for their functional benefits.

Total phenolic content (TPC) is one of the most popular indicators for estimation of phenolic antioxidants in fruit. Determination of TPC is straightforward and easy to perform using Folin-Ciocalteu reagent and usually expressed as gallic acid equivalent (GAE) (Table 2). Based on previous literature, *B. macrophylla* fruits have not been determined for TPC. Table 2 also depicts the phenolic compounds identified

and quantified in selected indigenous tropical fruits. Among the indigenous tropical fruits with potential for commercial development, *S. malaccense* fruit has the least TPC, whereas the other fruits have moderate to high TPC. TPCs of *M. foetida* fruit extracts ranged from 122.8 to 199.8 mg GAE/100 g of edible portion (EP) [10]. However, a wide range of total phenolics determined in the same type of fruit could be due to the different methods used, as well as the fruit variety and geographical distribution [12].

Among the indigenous tropical fruits, flavonoids are the major antioxidants found in these fruits. As shown in Table 2, a few flavonoids have been identified in *C. odontophyllum* fruit (dabai), and some unknown flavonoids were detected in dabai pulp [24]. Due to the dark purple color of dabai peel, anthocyanins should be the major phenolics in its peel. Chew et al. [23] have reported different types of anthocyanins that were detected in the dabai peel, such as cyanidin glucoside, malvidin glucoside, and peonidin glucoside. Anthocyanins were also found in the fruits of *S. malaccense* and *A. bilimbi*. Reynertson et al. [43] reported as much as 0.02 μg/g of cyanidin-3-glucoside that was determined in the peel of dried *S. malaccense* fruit. The peel might also contain carotenoids and betacyanins because it is red in color. Moreover, a nonpurple colored *A. bilimbi* fruit exhibited a high concentration of total anthocyanins (47.36 mg/100 g fresh weight) [18]. However, total anthocyanin content (TAC) determined in the purple colored extract of defatted *C. odontophyllum* fruit peel was less than 40 mg/100 g dry weight (DW) [24]. The nonpurple colored extract of *A. bilimbi* could have a low TAC because anthocyanins are red-purplish color pigments. The difference could have been due to the use of colorimetric method through pH differential that resulted in an overestimation of TAC.

Among the fruits that belong to *Anacardiaceae family*, mangiferin is the primary bioactive phenolic compound in mango (*M. indica*). Mangiferin is commonly detected in

TABLE 2: Phenolic compounds in the selected indigenous tropical fruits.

Fruit	Malaysia	Other countries
Averrhoa bilimbi	Total phenolics (mg GAE/100 g): 629.17 (dry weight, DW) [13]; Total phenolics: 900 mg GAE/100 g DW of juice [14]; Total phenolics: 251.83 μg GAE/g juice (DW) [15]; Other phenolics (% area): guaiacol (0.1%), p-vinylguaiacol (3.2%), 4-nonylphenol (0.2%) [16]	Total phenolics (gallic acid equivalent): 50.23–68.67 mg/g extract [17]; Total phenolics: 164.92 mg GAE/100 g; total anthocyanins (cyanidin 3-glucoside equivalent): 47.36 mg/100 g [18]; Other phenolics (mg/100 g): 2-methoxy-4-vinylphenol (0.1) [19]
Baccaurea macrocarpa	Total phenolics (mg GAE/g DW): 60.04 (pericarp); 4.6 (pulp) [20]; Total flavonoids (mg catechin equivalent/g DW): 44.68 (pericarp); 1.51 (pulp) [20]	No report from the literature
Baccaurea motleyana	Total phenolics (mg GAE/100 g): 1160.14 [12]	No report from the literature
Bouea macrophylla	Total phenolics (gallic acid equivalent): 149.49 μg/g juice (DW) [15]; Total phenolics (gallic acid equivalent): 372.35 μg/g juice (DW) [15]	No report from the literature
Canarium odontophyllum	Total phenolics (mg GAE/100 g DW): 905–332.1 [21]; 1800–680 (peel), 500–1400 (pulp) [22]; Flavonoids (mg/100 g DW): catechin (330–400), epigallocatechin gallate (160–28), epicatechin gallate (3–5), apigenin (8–12), ethyl gallate (1–3) [23]; Phenolic acids (mg/100 g DW): ellagic acid (9–21), vanillic acid (1–2) [23]; Anthocyanins (mg/100 g DW): cyanidin-3-glucoside (3–39), cyanidin-3-rutinoside (7–185), malvidin-3,5-di-glucoside (0–20), peonidin-3-glucoside (trace) [23]; Other flavonoids in defatted dabai pulp and peel: apigenin derivative, hesperetin 3-glucoside, hirsutidin 3-glucoside, vitexin, isovitexin, methyl 4,5-dicaffeoylquinate, quercetin 3-O-α-D-arabinopyranoside [24]	No report from the literature
Cynometra cauliflora	Total phenolics (mg GAE/100 g): 1868.94 [12]	No report from the literature
Durio kutejensis	Total phenolics (mg GAE/100 g): 183.07 [12]; Other polyphenols (mg/100 g DW): tannin 0.003 [25]	No report from the literature
Garcinia hombroniana	Total phenolics (mg GAE/100 g): 2070 [26]	Total phenolics (mg GAE/g DW): 326.9 [27]; Polyphenol: volkensiflavone (1240 mg/100 g DW) [28]
Garcinia parvifolia	Total phenolics (mg GAE/g DW): 7.2 (pulp); 5.3 (peel) [29]; Total flavonoids (mg rutin equivalent/g DW): 5.9 (pulp); 3.7 (peel) [29]	No report from the literature
Mangifera foetida	Total phenolics (mg GAE/100 g): 491.94–849.63 [12]; 813.7 (DW) [30]; 6.05 (mature-green), 7.29 (ripe) [31]; 122.8–199.8 [32]; Phenolic acids (mg/100 g): gallic acid (0.14–0.94), protocatechuic acid (0.02–0.902), vanillic acid (0.09–0.64) [31]; Isoflavones (mg/100 g DW): daidzein (2.8–8.0), genistein (0.4–0.8) [33]; Other polyphenols (mg/100 g): mangiferin (0.1–1.12) [31]	No report from the literature
Mangifera pajang	Total phenolics (mg GAE/100 g DW): 596 (pulp), 2293 (peel) [34]; 1460 (peel) [35]; Total phenolics (mg GAE/100 g): 221.47–339.97 [12], 26.09 (dried pulp) [36]; Phenolics (mg/100 g of dried pulp/peel): gallic acid (ND/3.07), p-coumaric acid (2.95/19.9), sinapic acid (ND/0.07), caffeic acid (2.68/44.1), ferulic acid (ND/78.4), chlorogenic acid (0.58/0.82), naringin (14500/151), hesperidin (93/101), quercetin (16.51/8.19), kaempferol (18/20), rutin (ND/13), luteolin (29/25), diosmin (ND/19.9) [34]; Isoflavones (mg/100 g DW): daidzein (8.3–8.7), genistein (0.4–0.6) [33]	No report from the literature
Phyllanthus emblica	Total phenolics (mg GAE/100 g): 2664.97 [12]; Flavonoids and tannins [37]	Total phenolics (mg GAE/100 g DW): 12900 [38]; Total phenolics (mg GAE/g extract): 362.43 [38]; 339.0 [39]; Polyphenolics: geranin, quercetin 3-β-D-glucopyranoside, kaempferol 3-β-D-glucopyranoside, isocorrlagin, quercetin, kaempferol [40]; chebulinic acid (seed) [41]; Phenolic acids: gallic acid, tannins [42]
Syzygium jambos	Total phenolics (mg GAE/100 g): 555.57 [12]	Total phenolics (8.69 mg GAE/100 g DW), total anthocyanins (0), ellagic acid (5 mg/100 g DW), quercetin (0.001 mg/100 g DW), quercitrin (0.003 mg/100 g DW) [43]; Phenolic compounds (μM/100 g): gallic aid (4.0) (peel), chlorogenic acid (1.3) (peel), phloridzin (0.5/0.6) (peel/pulp) [44]

TABLE 2: Continued.

Fruit	Malaysia	Other countries
Syzygium malaccense	Total phenolics: 6.0 mg GAE/100 g [12] Total phenolics: 81.51 µg GAE/g juice (DW) [15]	Total phenolics (858 mg GAE/100 g DW), total anthocyanins (trace), cyanidin-3-glucoside (0.002 mg/100 g DW), ellagic acid (0.001 mg/100 g DW), quercetin (trace), quercitrin (2.0 mg/100 g DW), rutin (0.002 mg/100 g DW) [43] Total phenolics (32 mg GAE/100 g), myricetin (<1 mg/100 g), morin (trace), quercetin (<1 mg/100 g), kaempferol (trace) [45]
		Total and major phenolics (mg GAE/g DW): 104.00–151.12 (ripe); 122.35–167.11 (unripe); gallic acid (49.21–216.54); protocatechuic acid (86.93–887.2); p-hydroxybenzoic acid (0–649.29); chlorogenic acid (0–187.44); p-coumaric acid (120.58–454.06); ferulic acid (37.14–187.77); sinapic acid (46.15–526.47) [46] Total and major flavonoids (mg GAE/g DW): 110.41–162.39 (ripe); 118.01–271.35 (unripe); rutin (12.66–262.39); myricetin (87.76–445.39); quercetin (0–191.62); apigenin (33.29–256.43); kaempferol (0–245.75) [46]
Ziziphus mauritiana	Total phenolics: 41.0 mg GAE/100 g [12] Total phenolics (gallic acid equivalent): 396.96 µg/g extract (DW) [15]	Total phenolics: 8.6–9.6 mg GAE/g extract [39] Total phenolics: 67.84 mg GAE/100 g [47] Phenolic compounds (µg/g DW): 83 (p-hydroxybenzoic acid), 773 (vanillin), 699.2 (p-coumaric acid), 621.6 (ferulic acid), 131.2 (o-coumaric acid), 20.4 (naringenin) [48] Other phenolics: tannin (2.42%) [49]

GAE: gallic acid equivalent; ND: not detected; DW: dry weight.

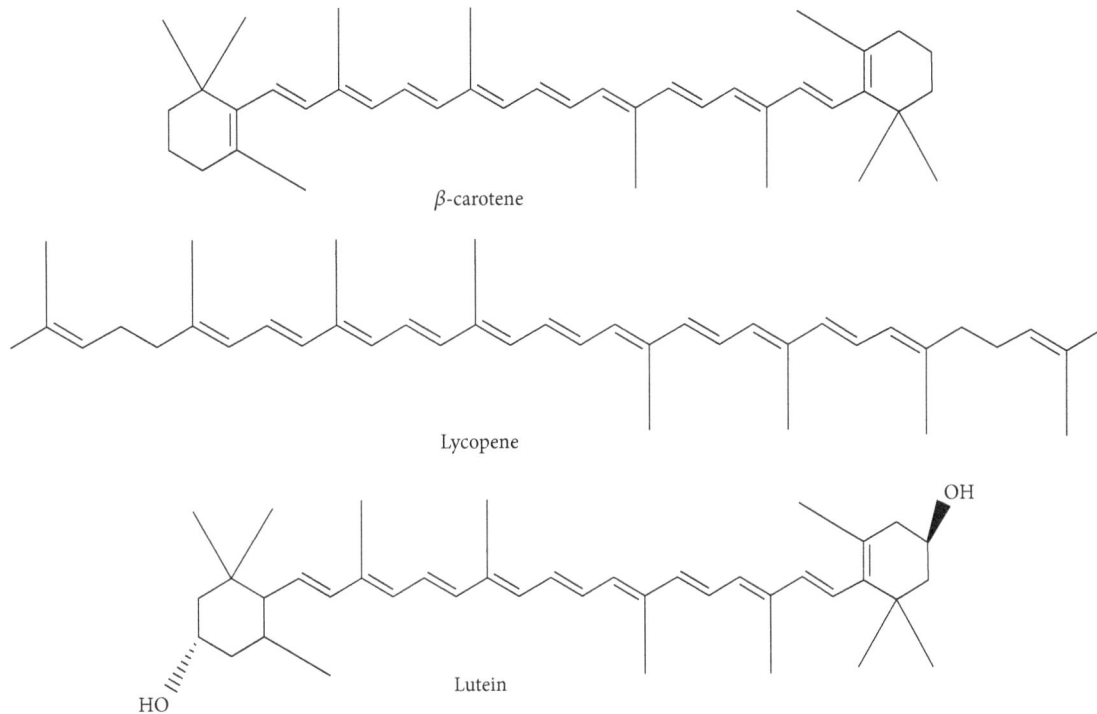

FIGURE 2: Major carotenoids in plant.

other *Mangifera* fruits [31]. Due to its sour taste, the fruits could also contain various types of phenolic acids. Gallic acid, protocatechuic acid, and vanillic acid are the major phenolic acids in *M. foetida* fruit [31]. Chlorogenic acid, ellagic acid, and gallic acid are also detected in *Syzygium* fruits (Table 2). While applying HPLC for determination of phenolic compounds, isoflavones were detected in some *Mangifera* fruits [33], where daidzein is the major isoflavone detected. Besides that, the sour taste of *Syzygium* fruits also indicates a potentially high level of phenolic acids, and ascorbic acid can be obtained from the fruits. A few studies have determined the polyphenolic compounds in the fruit of *Z. mauritiana*. Due to the variation in geographical distribution, fruit maturity, and variety, the TPCs in *Z. mauritiana* fruit ranged from 1.13 to 328.65 mg/100 g EP (Table 2). Besides that, 2.42% of tannin was also found in the fruit of *Z. mauritiana* [49].

Among hundreds of types of flavonoids, quercetin is a bioactive flavonoid isolated from the fruit of *P. emblica* [72]. Besides quercetin, geraniin, quercetin 3-β-D-glucopyranoside, kaempferol 3-β-D-glucopyranoside, isocorilagin, and kaempferol were detected in *P. emblica* fruit (Table 2). The edible part of *P. emblica* has higher TPC (2664.97 mg GAE/100 g) than most of the other indigenous underutilized fruits reported [12]. The high TPC in this fruit might be due to the high concentration of vitamin C. Ascorbic acid might have reacted with the Folin-Ciocalteu reagent, hence causing a possibility in overestimation of TPC. The high tannin content in *P. emblica* fruit is also very useful for Indian communities because the extract has been used as dye or ink [38].

To date, only a very limited information on phenolic compounds is available for the scientific community, especially phenolic compounds in the fruits of *Baccaurea*, *Cynometra*, and *Garcinia*. Besides that, volkensiflavone is one of the potential flavonoids in *G. hombroniana* fruit [28], and garcinidon A has been discovered in the peel of *G. parvifolia* [73]. *D. kutejensis* fruit also contained 0.03 μg of tannin in one gram of dried fruit [25].

5.2. Carotenoids. Among the plant phytochemicals, carotenoids are classified as terpenoids. The compounds are found abundantly in yellow to orange- and orange to red-colored fruits. Carotenoids are grouped into carotenes and xanthophylls. In nature, β-carotene is the most abundant type of carotene, while lycopene is the primary phytochemical in orange-red colored fruits. Among the xanthophylls, lutein is typically detected in green leafy vegetables. However, some fruits also contain lutein [4]. Figure 2 shows the major types of carotenoid in fruit.

Among the carotenes, all-trans β-carotene is the most common type of carotenoid found in plant because it is part of the antioxidant defense system at cellular level of a plant. Some green-colored fruits may contain a high amount of carotenoid because the yellow-orange-colored carotenoid pigments are masked by chlorophylls [88]. The intake of carotenoids from various plant sources is thought to be able to maintain good health. In this review, different carotenoids and their concentrations in the selected indigenous tropical fruits are shown in Table 3.

TABLE 3: Carotenoids in the selected indigenous tropical fruits.

Fruit	Malaysia	Other countries
Averrhoa bilimbi	β-carotene: 28.99 mg/100 g DW [14]	Total carotenoids: 4.7 mg/100 g [18] Carotene: 0.035 mg/100 g [62]
Baccaurea macrocarpa	Total carotenes (β-carotene equivalent, DW): 1.47 mg/100 g [54]; 0.81 mg/g (pericarp), 0.69 mg/g (pulp) [20]	No report from the literature
Baccaurea motleyana	No report from the literature	No report from the literature
Bouea macrophylla	Carotenoids: lutein (0.457 mg/100 g), cryptoxanthin (0.155 mg/100 g), γ-carotene (0.052 mg/100 g), β-carotene (0.301 mg/100 g) [63]	β-carotene: 23 mg/100 g [64] α-carotene (23 mg/100 g) [51]
Canarium odontophyllum	Xanthophylls (mg/100 g in peel/pulp): all-trans lutein (0.16/0.04), 9-cis lutein (0.03/0.01), 13-cis lutein (0.06/0.02) [65] Carotenes (mg/100 g in peel/pulp): di-cis-β-carotene (0.07/0.04), 15-cis-β-carotene (1.83/1.19), 9-cis-β-carotene (3.96/0.58), all-trans-β-carotene (6.95/3.11), 13-cis-β-carotene (1.94/0.57) [65] Total carotenoids (mg β-carotene equivalent/100 g DW): 2.84 (pericarp), 0.66 (kernel) [66]	No report from the literature
Cynometra cauliflora	No report from the literature	No report from the literature
Durio kutejensis	Total carotenes (β-carotene equivalent): 11.16–14.97 mg/100 g DW [54] β-carotene: 7.57–10.99 mg/100 g DW [54]	No report from the literature
Garcinia hombroniana	No report from the literature	No report from the literature
Garcinia parvifolia	Total carotenes (β-carotene equivalent, mg/100 g DW): 3 (pulp); 17 (peel) [29]	No report from the literature
Mangifera foetida	Total carotenoids (β-carotene equivalent): 2.58–4.81 mg/100 g DW [54] Total carotenoids (β-carotene equivalent): 0.65 mg/100 g DW [30]; 0.01–0.15 mg/100 g [26] Carotene: 0.26 mg/100 g [67]	No report from the literature
Mangifera pajang	Xanthophylls (mg/100 g peel/pulp, DW): cryptoxanthin (0.60/1.18), cis-cryptoxanthin (0.07/ND) [11] Carotenes (mg/100 g peel/pulp, DW): all-trans-α-carotene (4.2/7.96), cis-β-carotene (2.53–3.64/2.72–3.74), all-trans-β-carotene (13.09/20.04) [11] β-carotene: 42.21 mg/100 g dried pulp [36]	No report from the literature
Phyllanthus emblica	No report from the literature	Lutein (49 μg/100 g), β-carotene (32 μg/100 g) [68]
Syzygium jambos	Total carotenes (β-carotene equivalent): 3.35 mg/100 g DW [54]	No report from the literature
Syzygium malaccense	Total carotenes (β-carotene equivalent): 1.41 mg/100 g DW [54]	Total carotenes (mg/100 g): 0.003–0.008 [69] Carotenes (mg/100 g): α-carotene (0.14), β-carotene (0.18) [45]
Ziziphus mauritiana	No report from the literature	No report from the literature

ND: not detected; DW: dry weight. Some of these fruits contain no carotenoids.

Among the fruits, yellow to orange-colored fruits have high β-carotene contents, whereas lycopene is the orange-red color pigment. Carotenoids contents in some commercialized fruits and vegetables have been reported by Khoo et al. [4]. However, carotenoid contents in other indigenous tropical fruits remain unknown. Many of the indigenous fruits possible for commercial development do not contain any carotenoid. Whitish-colored fruits have little or trace amount of carotenoids, especially the endocarp. No study has been performed to determine the carotenoid contents of *B. motleyana*, *C. cauliflora*, *G. hombroniana*, and *Z. mauritiana* fruits. It is possibly due to the low concentrations of carotenoid in these fruits.

As previously reported, the fruit of *B. macrocarpa* (tampoi) contains carotenoids. However, β-carotene (a major carotenoid) was not detected in tampoi [53]. There is a broad range of total carotenoid contents found in some of the indigenous tropical fruits (0.003–29 mg/100 g DW) (Table 3). For example, the different varieties of pumpkin have total carotenoids ranging between 0.06 and 14.9 mg β-carotene per 100 g fresh weight [4].

Based on the previous study, the total carotenoid content (TCC) of horse mango (*M. foetida*) was ranged from 96.5 to 153.0 μg β-carotene equivalent (BCE)/100 g EP [10]. In durian nyekak (*D. kutejensis*), the TCC was 11.16–14.97 mg BCE/100 g DW [54]. Although some of the indigenous tropical fruits have a moderate level of TCC (Table 3), the cucumber tree (*A. bilimbi*) was found to have a higher β-carotene content (28.99 mg/100 g dry weight) than the other indigenous tropical fruits [59]. Besides that, *P. emblica* only has 0.01 mg of β-carotene in the fruit pulp (per 100 g edible pulp) [50].

5.3. Terpene and Terpenoids. Monoterpenes, diterpenes, triterpenes, and sesquiterpenes are some of the terpenes discussed in this review. Terpenoid is a vast and diverse class of natural occurring organic chemicals related to terpene [89]. Most of the terpenoids including saponins are possible antioxidants [90]. Besides antioxidant activity, saponins have several health benefits [91]. Among the terpenes and terpenoids, some are volatile compounds found in plants. Geraniol, limonene, linalool, and pinene are some of the volatile components detected in fruit samples (Figure 3). Terpenes, mainly sesquiterpenes, have been identified in the root, bark, flowers, and leaves of plants [92]. Only a few terpenes have been discovered in fruits. Although many studies have been performed on volatile terpenes in essential oils of plants, most of the studies analyzed the other parts of the plant rather than the fruit. From our literature search, a minimum of 20 volatile components including terpenes were found in different parts of the plant. Little information on terpenes and terpenoids content in fruit is available for the scientific community, especially the underutilized and indigenous tropical fruits.

It can be observed in Table 4 that some indigenous tropical fruits with potential for commercial development are well studied for terpenes and terpenoids contents, but not for the fruit of *Z. mauritiana*. Umaru et al. reported that Indian

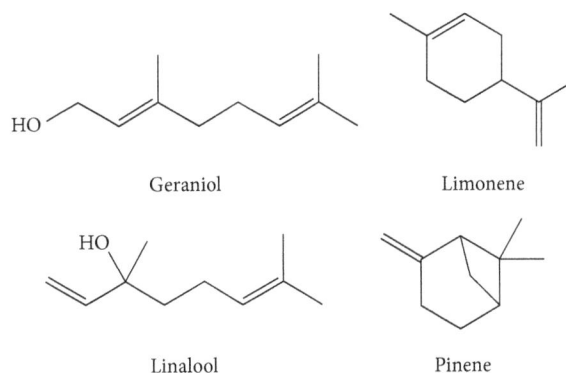

FIGURE 3: Major volatile terpenoids detected in fruit.

jujube (*Z. mauritiana*) has 7.13% saponin [49]. The terpenes and terpenoids contents in some of these indigenous tropical fruits have not been determined elsewhere besides Malaysia. For the indigenous tropical fruit with possible commercial development, no study has reported terpenes and terpenoids contents in these tropical fruits, except for *A. bilimbi*, *B. motleyana*, *G. hombroniana*, and *P. emblica* fruits. Also, information on terpenes and terpenoids in fruits of *B. macrocarpa*, *C. cauliflora*, *D. kutejensis*, *G. parvifolia*, and *Z. mauritiana* are limited due to lacking of published data available for referencing. Moreover, terpenes and terpenoids in the fruits of *A. bilimbi*, *G. hombroniana*, and *P. emblica* have been determined by researchers from several known countries such as Malaysia and Thailand (Table 4).

Terpenes and terpenoids are natural phytochemicals identified in plants. Fruit contains some terpenes, such as monoterpene, triterpene, and sesquiterpene. For the indigenous tropical fruits with potential for commercial development, such as *B. macrophylla*, *M. foetida*, *M. pajang*, *S. jambos*, and *S. malaccense*, some terpenes and terpenoids have been identified in the extracted essential oil of these fruits (Table 4). Besides carotenoids, saponin is one of the terpenoids found in the defatted dabai [24].

Among the indigenous tropical fruits possible for commercial development, *B. motleyana* and *P. emblica* fruits have low concentrations of terpenes, terpenoids, and saponins. Wong et al. reported that terpenes are the minor components in the essential oil of rambai (*B. motleyana*) [74]. Saponin is one of the members of the triterpenoid group [93]. It has been discovered in Indian gooseberry (*P. emblica*) [37]. In Cuba, a study has identified α-pinene, p-cymene (0.02), limonene, 1,8-cineole, γ-terpinene, terpinolene, α-terpineol, δ-cadinene, α-calacorene, and other volatile components in the essential oil of *A. bilimbi* fruit [19]. These compounds are monoterpenes and sesquiterpenes commonly found in plants. The essential oil of *P. emblica* fruit contains β-caryophyllene and β-bourbonene as the major terpenes [80]. Besides that, the fruit of *G. hombroniana* has two novel triterpenes (17,14-friedolanostanes and lanostanes) [76]. Terpenoids, such as saponins, are the important phytochemical constituents in combating the infectious diseases and terpenoids are primarily discovered as the potent antimicrobial

TABLE 4: Terpenes and terpenoids in selected indigenous tropical fruits.

Fruit	Malaysia	Other countries
Averrhoa bilimbi	Terpenes (% area): limonene (0.4%), linalool (0.2%), α-terpineol (0.5), (E,E)-α-farnesene (1.3%) [16]	Terpenes (mg/kg): α-pinene (<0.01), p-cymene (0.02), limonene (0.12), 1,8-cineole (0.02), γ-terpinene (0.02), terpinolene (<0.01), α-terpineol (0.03), δ-cadinene (0.03), α-calacorene (0.01) [19]
Baccaurea macrocarpa	No report from the literature	No report from the literature
Baccaurea motleyana	Terpenes (minor components) [74]	No report from the literature
Bouea macrophylla	Terpenes (% area): (E)-β-ocimene (68.59%), α-pinene (8.04%) [75]	No report from the literature
Canarium odontophyllum	Saponin derivatives (in defatted dabai pulp and peel) [24]	No report from the literature
Cynometra cauliflora	No report from the literature	No report from the literature
Durio kutejensis	No report from the literature	No report from the literature
Garcinia hombroniana	No report from the literature	Triterpenoids: 17,14-friedolanostanes [(24E)-3α-hydroxy-17,14-friedolanostan-8,14,24-trien-26-oic acid; methyl [(24E)-3α-hydroxy-17,14-friedolanostan-8,14,24-trien-26-oate; methyl (24E)-3α,23-dihydroxy-17,14-friedolanostan-8,14,24-trien-26-oate; methyl (24E)-3α,9,23-trihydroxy-17,14-friedolanostan-14,2 4-dien-26-oate]; lanostanes [3β- and 3α-hydroxy-23-oxo-9,16-lanostadien-26-oic acid] [76]
Garcinia parvifolia	No report from the literature	No report from the literature
Mangifera foetida	Oxygenated monoterpenes (20.3% area) [77]	Triterpenes: mangiferenes A and B [78]
Mangifera pajang	Monoterpenes (% area): α-pinene (67.2%) and α-phellandrene (11.0%) [79]	No report from the literature
Phyllanthus emblica	Terpenoids and saponins [37]	Terpenoids (% area): β-caryophyllene (5.39%), β-bourbonene (38.23%) [80]
Syzygium jambos	Monoterpenes (% area): linalool (3.58, myrcene (2.44%), geraniol (2.25%), citronellol (0.74%), nerol (0.39%), α-terpineol (0.33%), cis-rose oxide (0.27%), geranial (0.19%), limonene (0.15%), (E)-β-ocimene (0.13%), trans-rose oxide (trace) [80] Sesquiterpenes (% of essential oil): α-cubebene (0.29%), δ-cadinene (0.17%) [81]	Terpenoids: geraniol, nerol, linalool, hotrienol, citronellol, rose oxides [82] Monoterpene: linalool (16.5-37.51 ppb) [83]
Syzygium malaccense	Monoterpenes (% area): limonene (0.71%), linalool (0.14%), geraniol (0.06%), nerol (trace) [81] Sesquiterpenes (% area): δ-cadinene (0.5), α-selinene (0.1%), humulene (0.09%) [81]	No report from literature
Ziziphus mauritiana	No report from the literature	Saponin: 7.13% [49]

TABLE 5: The uses of selected indigenous tropical fruits as food and folk medicine.

Number	Fruit	As food	Folk medicine
1	Averrhoa bilimbi [84]	Freshly eaten as salad or pickle, and used in cooking dishes (whole ripe fruit)	Ripe fruits combined with pepper for inducing sweating; pickled bilimbi is smeared all over the body to hasten recovery after a fever; fruit conserves for treatment of coughs, beriberi, and biliousness; fruit syrup for reducing fever and inflammation and to alleviate internal hemorrhoids
2	Baccaurea macrocarpa	Freshly eaten (ripe flesh)	No report on usage as folk medicine
3	Baccaurea motleyana [84]	Freshly eaten and made into jam (ripe flesh)	No report on usage as folk medicine
4	Bouea macrophylla [84]	Freshly eaten as salad or pickle, and used in cooking dishes (whole ripe fruit)	No report on usage as folk medicine
5	Canarium odontophyllum [84]	Freshly eaten and as salad, made into jam, and used in cooking dishes (ripe flesh)	No report on usage as folk medicine
6	Cynometra cauliflora	Freshly eaten as salad and used in cooking dishes (ripe flesh)	No report on usage as folk medicine
7	Durio kutejensis [84]	Freshly eaten (ripe flesh)	No report on usage as folk medicine
8	Garcinia hombroniana	Freshly eaten (ripe flesh)	No report on usage as folk medicine
9	Garcinia parvifolia	Freshly eaten (ripe flesh), as pickle and used in cooking dishes (unripe flesh)	No report on usage as folk medicine
10	Mangifera foetida [84]	Freshly eaten (ripe flesh), as pickle and used in cooking dishes (unripe flesh)	Seeds used against trichophytosis, scabies, and eczema
11	Mangifera pajang [84]	Freshly eaten (ripe flesh), as pickle and used in cooking dishes (unripe flesh)	No report on usage as folk medicine
12	Phyllanthus emblica [85]	Freshly eaten (ripe flesh), as pickle and used in cooking dishes (unripe flesh)	Fruit for treating cough and asthma, and several other health complications
13	Syzygium jambos [86]	Freshly eaten, made into jam and served as dessert (whole ripe fruit)	Ripe fruit is used as a tonic for brain and liver and as a diuretic; seeds for treatment of diarrhea, dysentery, and catarrh
14	Syzygium malaccense [86]	Freshly eaten (whole ripe fruit), as pickle and used in cooking dishes (unripe fruit)	Fruit decoction as a febrifuge
15	Ziziphus mauritiana [86, 87]	Freshly eaten as salad or pickle, and used in cooking dishes (whole ripe fruit)	Ripen fruit for treatment of sore throat and cough; seed for treatment of diarrhea and weakness of stomach

agents. Antimicrobial effects of the essential oils of many fruits have been reported by Nychas [94].

6. Medicinal Properties of 15 Indigenous Tropical Fruits

Fruits are commonly consumed for their nutrients, and some fruits are used as medicine. The medicinal properties of fruits are closely related to their available phytochemicals, as well as antioxidants. Many of the indigenous fruits have been traditionally used as folk medicine. These fruits contain phytochemical antioxidants that can prevent, treat, and cure various types of diseases. Many phytochemicals such as carotenoids, tannic acids, triterpenes, and some flavonoids are free radical scavengers that can contribute to the suppression of oxidative stress and anti-inflammatory effect in the human body [95]. The details on the applications of 15 selected indigenous fruits as food and as

folk medicine are tabulated in Table 5. Additionally, the medicinal values of these indigenous tropical fruits reported by previous scientific reports are listed in Table 6. Among the 15 indigenous tropical fruits, the flesh of five fruits are not scientifically determined for their medicinal values, except for antioxidant activities. The other fruits have been studied for antimicrobial effects (including fungal) and several protective effects against chronic diseases. Among the scientific evidence shown in previous literature, most of the experiments are mainly focused on in vitro and animal models. Limited studies on human intervention trials allow researchers or scientists to study the potential health effects of these underutilized tropical fruits using human models in the future.

In this review, the medicinal properties of the selected underutilized tropical fruits are discussed. The protective effects of these fruits against several diseases are shown, either as folk medicines or with scientific evidence. Overall, among the 15 indigenous tropical fruits, the fruits of

TABLE 6: Bioactive ingredients and medicinal properties of selected indigenous tropical fruits.

Fruit	Bioactives	Medicinal properties*	Experimental models
Averrhoa bilimbi	Flavonoids, saponins, and triterpenoids	Antihypercholesterolemic [96]	Triton-induced hypercholesterolemic rats
		Antibacterial [98, 114]	Disc diffusion method: Gram-positive and Gram-negative bacteria
		Antidiabetes [97]	Streptozotocin-induced diabetic rats
Baccaurea macrocarpa			No report from the literature
Baccaurea motleyana	Phenolic compounds	Antimicrobial (peel) [102]	Disc diffusion method: Gram-positive and Gram-negative bacteria, fungus, and yeast
Bouea macrophylla			No report from the literature
Canarium odontophyllum	Flavonoids and anthocyanins	Antiatherosclerosis [99]	Cholesterol-induced hypercholesterolemic rabbits
Cynometra cauliflora	Phenolic compounds	Antileukemic [103]	Human promyelocytic leukemia HL-60 and normal mouse fibroblast NIH/3T3 cell cultures
Durio kutejensis	Not reported	Antimelanogenesis effect [115]	Tyrosinase assay and melanin inhibition in B16 melanoma cell cultures
Garcinia hombroniana	Phenolic compounds	Inhibition of platelet aggregation and LDL-peroxidation [26]	Human whole blood from healthy subjects: in vitro LDL oxidation and antiplatelet aggregation assay.
Garcinia parvifolia	Phenolic compounds	Antimicrobial [116]	Well diffusion method: pathogenic and nonpathogenic bacteria
Mangifera foetida			No report from the literature
Mangifera pajang	Phenolic compounds and carotenoids	Antihypercholesterolemic and antiatherosclerotic [36]	Cholesterol-induced hypercholesterolemic rabbit model
		Anticancer (kernel) [117]	MTT assay: HepG2, HT-29 and Caov3 cultures
		Hepatoprotective effect [107]	HepG2 cell culture and western blot method
		Gastric ulcer healing effect [118]	Indomethacin-induced ulceration of rats
		Anticlastogenicity [119]	Cochran-Armitage trend test: bone marrow cells of Swiss albino mice treated with lead and aluminum
Phyllanthus emblica	Phenolic compounds	Antiproliferative [120]	MTT assay: MCF-7 tumor cell culture
		Antimicrobial [41]	TLC-bioautographic method: drug-resistant bacteria and yeast
		Anticancer [121]	In vitro cytotoxicity assays: human lung carcinoma (A549) and HepG2 cell lines
		Antiaging effect [122]	In vitro MMP-1, MMP-2, and elastase inhibition assays: inhibitions of collagenase and elastase
		Chondroprotection [123]	In vitro enzymatic assays: explant cultures of cartilage from osteoarthritis patients
Syzygium jambos	Phenols, tannins, alkaloids, and flavonoids	Antifungal (seed) [124]	Disc diffusion method: microbroth dilution technique (Microsporum gypseum, Microsporum canis, and Candida albicans)
Syzygium malaccense	Phenolic compounds and terpenes	Antimicrobial [125]	Disc diffusion method: test bacteria on Mueller Hinton Agar, and yeast on Potato Dextrose Agar
Ziziphus mauritiana	Phenolic compounds and saponin	Antihyperglycemic, antidiarrhoeal, and hepatoprotective [126]	Glucose overloaded hyperglycemic rats, castor oil-induced diarrhea in mice, and tetrachloromethane-induced liver damage in rats, respectively
		Anticancer [46]	Neutral red assay: cytotoxicity of various cultivars of jujube against different cancer cell lines Apoptosis detection by flow cytometry

*The medicinal properties are reported based on in vitro and in vivo animal studies, as well as human intervention trials.

B. macrocarpa, B. motleyana, B. macrophylla, C. odontophyllum, C. cauliflora, D. kutejensis, G. hombroniana, G. parvifolia, and *M. pajang* have not been reported for their use as folk medicine (Table 5). However, three out of these 15 indigenous tropical fruits have not been scientifically determined for their medicinal properties and potential health benefits. These fruits are *B. macrocarpa, B. macrophylla,* and *M. foetida* (Table 6).

Among hundreds of fruit species, the fruit of *A. bilimbi* (cucumber tree) is one of the potential sources of antioxidant that offers health benefits. According to Ambili et al., the extracts of *A. bilimbi* exhibited the cholesterol-lowering potential in rats [96]. The water extract of *A. bilimbi* fruit (0.8 mg/kg body weight, BW) also improved lipid profile in Triton-induced hypercholesterolemia in rats [96]. Other than that, the active fraction of the water extract at a dose of 0.3 mg/kg BW possessed an optimum antihypercholesterolemic activity. The fruit (125 mg/kg BW) and its water extract (50 mg/kg BW) also effectively improved the lipid profile of the rats fed with high-fat diet.

Another study reported that the fruit of *A. bilimbi* has antidiabetic effect studied using streptozotocin-induced diabetic rats [97]. The flavonoids, carotenoids, and terpenes could be the potent bioactive compounds in *A. bilimbi* fruits that provide the antidiabetic effect. Besides that, this fruit is also reported as an active antimicrobial agent. Chloroform and methanolic extracts of this fruit (bilimbi) were reported to have good inhibitory activities on several types of bacteria, such as *Aeromonas hydrophila, Escherichia coli, Klebsiella pneumoniae, Saccharomyces cerevisiae, Staphylococcus aureus, Streptococcus agalactiae,* and *Bacillus subtilis* [98]. Hence, this fruit has been used in folk medicine for easing whooping cough [85]. The scientific evidence for the role of phytochemicals in *A. bilimbi* fruit extract as health-promoting agents is inadequate. Most of the studies focused only on *in vitro* and animal models. Up to date, there is no human-based scientific evidence to support its use in the prevention of such diseases.

Flavonoids and anthocyanins in dabai fruit (*C. odontophyllum*) are the potent antioxidants. The defatted dabai extract (5%) was shown to significantly reduce the levels of total cholesterol and low-density lipoprotein-cholesterol in rabbits supplemented with high-cholesterol diet for eight weeks as compared to the control group [99]. Besides that, rabbits fed a high-cholesterol diet and defatted dabai pulp have a significant increment in high-density lipoprotein level [100]. The severity of atherosclerotic plaques in the high-cholesterol diet rabbit group that supplemented with defatted dabai extracts was also reduced compared to the control group. Therefore, the fruit extract of defatted dabai can be considered as a new source of nutraceutical due to its antiatherosclerotic properties. However, no human-based study has been performed to prove the cholesterol-lowering effect of the defatted dabai extract. Human intervention trial is recommended for future study to test the efficacy of defatted dabai parts because dabai is one of the underutilized fruits highly potent to be commercialized.

There are other medicinal uses which were found on *D. kutejensis*, but it may possess some anti-inflammatory properties as it has many similarities to the *D. zibethinus,* where the methanolic extracts of *D. zibethinus* fruit were reported to have anti-inflammatory effects [101]. The extract of *B. motleyana* peel possessed antimicrobial activities since it inhibited the growth of *S. aureus, B. cereus, B. subtilis, E. coli, Pseudomonas aeruginosa,* and *Proteus vulgaris* [102]. The fruit of *Cynometra cauliflora* possesses antiproliferative activity by inhibition of cytotoxic effect to human promyelocytic leukemia HL-60 cells [103].

Generally, most of the plants from genus *Garcinia* have medicinal effects [104]. In Southeast Asia, only a few studies were reported on the potential medicinal properties of under-utilized *Garcinia* fruits. The fruit extract of *G. hombroniana* inhibited *in vitro* lipid peroxidation and had antiplatelet activities [26]. Other than the fruits, Kapadia and Rao also report antimicrobial effects of *Garcinia* plants towards bacteria, fungus, and other parasites [57]. The stems and leaves of three *Garcinia* plants indicate platelet-activating factor antagonist activity [105]. Among the three *Garcinia* plants, the leaves of *G. hombroniana* (seashore mangosteen) have higher microbial inhibition activity (46.3%) than the leaves and stems of *G. cowa* (cowa) and *G. dulcis* (mundu). The main bioactive compound in the leaves that possess this antimicrobial effect is reported as garcihombronane [57].

Mangifera fruit, also known as mango, is traditionally used for its medicinal properties. The kernel of *M. pajang* (Borneo mango) has an anticancer effect [106], and the fruit extract was found to possess hepatoprotective effects [107]. Ibrahim also reported the antiatherosclerotic and antihypercholesterolemic effects of fruit juice powder of *M. pajang* tested using New Zealand white rabbits [36]. Then, a human clinical trial was carried out to verify the efficacy of *M. pajang* fruit juice which also demonstrated a promising effect. Healthy subjects supplemented with *M. pajang* fruit juice showed better blood lipid parameters compared to the placebo group [108]. The antihypercholesterolemic effect of *M. pajang* fruit juice could be due to the antioxidative effect of polyphenolics, vitamin C, and β-carotene in the juice. A 12 weeks, double-blind, placebo-controlled clinical trial also confirmed that antioxidants (24 mg β-carotene B, 1000 mg vitamin C, 800 IU vitamin E) supplementation significantly increased the plasma high-density lipoprotein-cholesterol in 45 coronary artery disease patients [109]. Both studies have proven that antioxidant supplementation helped in improving plasma lipid profile.

In addition to *M. pajang* fruit, *M. foetida* fruit pulp (without peel) also demonstrated antioxidant activity [30]. On the other hand, the leaf extracts of *M. foetida* have an antimicrobial activity for *S. aureus,* but not for *E. coli, S. cerevisiae,* and *Fusarium oxysporum* [110]. Besides these findings, other medicinal effect has not been determined for *M. foetida* (horse mango) fruit, except for its antioxidants in the inhibition of oxidative stress [111].

Emblic (*P. emblica*) fruit, also called as Indian gooseberry, is traditionally known for its medicinal value for treating cough and asthma [85]. The fruit is traditionally used in India for the treatment of several health complications, such as diarrhea, dysentery, anemia, jaundice, and cough [112]. The fruit is also rich in antioxidant. Liu et al. reported that phenolic compounds extracted from emblic fruits were highly correlated with their antioxidant activities [40]. Various parts of *P. emblica* plant have also been used as Indian Ayurvedic medicine. Besides that, phytochemicals in the plant parts are well known for their medicinal values, such as antidiabetic, antibacterial, antiulcerogenic, antiproliferative, and hypolipidemic effects [113].

A study on the healing activity of ethanolic extract of emblic fruit (*P. emblica*) has shown some positive results, where the rats were induced with indomethacin (30 mg/kg BW, oral intubation) [118]. The results showed that the extract (100 mg/kg BW) of this fruit had significantly reduced the lipid peroxidation parameters (MDA, carbonyl, total DNA, SOD, and CAT), ulcer index (3.8), and DNA damage induced by indomethacin (85.73% of protection) in rats after seven days of postulcerative treatment compared with the controls. Other than that, the extract of emblic fruit also inhibited the growth of *Staphylococcus aureus*, *Bacillus subtilis*, *Salmonella paratyphi*, *Shigella dysenteriae*, and *Candida albicans*, although no inhibition of *Escherichia coli* growth was observed [41]. Also, the aqueous extract of emblic has shown the potential as an anticancer agent, where the extract inhibited the growth of human lung carcinoma and (A549) and human hepatocellular carcinoma (HepG2) cell lines [118]. Moreover, the emblic fruit powder demonstrated a significant chondroprotective effect based on an *in vitro* model of cartilage degradation in explant cultures of articular knee cartilages obtained from osteoarthritis patients [123].

Limited information on medicinal properties of selected *Syzygium* fruits (*S. jambos* and *S. malaccense*) is available. The fruit of *S. jambos* (rose apple) has been traditionally used as an astringent and for brain and liver, as well as digestive problems [127]. Other than the use of *Syzygium* fruits as folk medicine, scientific research reported that the aqueous fruit extracts of *S. jambos* reduced the *in vitro* α-glucosidase and α-amylase inhibitory activities [128]. Other than these two *Syzygium* fruits, the fruit extracts of *S. samarangense* (samarang apple) were also as effective as antibiotics to inhibit microbial activities [129]. The fruit extract of *S. cumini* (Java plum) is also a potential antidiabetic agent [130].

Most of the literature only reported on the medical properties of different aerial parts (mainly leaves and bark) of underutilized plants instead of their fruits [131]. For example, the leaves of many plant species have antimicrobial activities. The methanolic extracts of *S. jambos* leaves were tested for antimicrobial activity, where the extracts inhibited the growth of some Gram-positive and Gram-negative bacteria [132]. Besides that, antimicrobial activities of the extracts of bark, leaves, and seeds of *S. jambos* have also been reported by Murugan et al. [133]. The leaves of *S. malaccense* (Malay apple) were reported to be useful for preventing inflammation [134]. Moreover, the extracts of different parts of *Syzygium* trees that have antidiabetic properties were documented in a review article [135].

Z. mauritiana (Indian jujube) is another fruit that is not well studied for its medicinal properties. The only therapeutic properties of the fruit are only available as reported in their traditional uses for treating abscesses, wounds, anodyne, and tonic, as well as styptic and purifying blood [87]. Until now, no human intervention study has been performed to determine the wound healing effect of *Z. mauritiana* fruit or its fruit extract. However, the leaves of *Z. mauritiana* were reported to significantly prevent leucopenia and noise-induced enhancement of neutrophil function in Guinea pigs compared with diazepam, in which the Guinea pigs were subjected to 100 Db industrial noise (8–50 kHz) [136]. Antioxidant activities have also been determined for the fruits from two varieties of *Z. mauritiana*, and the IC_{50} values of the ethanolic extract of both varieties (Beri and Narikeli) were 72 and 250 μg/mL, respectively [137]. The seed of *Z. mauritiana* has also been studied for its anticancer and antidiabetic potentials. The ethanolic extracts of *Z. mauritiana* seed were found to induce cancer cells death and significantly reduced tumor volume and tumor cell count in albino mice after 13 days of treatment with the extract (100–800 mg/kg BW) [138]. Besides that, the seed extract exhibited hypoglycemic activity, where administration of the extract (at a concentration of 800 mg/kg BW) reduced weight loss and mortality of alloxan-induced diabetic mice [139]. Alternatively, the root of *Z. mauritiana* has been traditionally used to treat ringworm by applying the root paste [140] and inhibition of microbial activities, such as *Bacillus subtilis*, *Staphylococcus aureus*, and *Mycobacterium phlei* [141].

On the contrary, some human intervention trials did not support the beneficial effects of antioxidant supplementation [142]. Although there was a dose-dependent relationship between antioxidative activity and antioxidant compound [143], an overdose of a particular bioactive compound may have prooxidative effect in the human body. Therefore, a moderate amount of antioxidant supplementation is suggested. Owing to lack of human-based scientific evidence, it is suggested that human intervention trials should be conducted in future studies to shed more light on the efficacy of potential bioactive components derived from these underutilized tropical fruits in any disease prevention. Although a part of these fruits have been studied for their medicinal properties, substantial scientific data is still lacking and the researches are still at a very preliminary stage. Future studies need to be performed for the fruits of *B. macrocarpa*, *B. macrophylla*, *D. kutejensis*, *M. foetida*, and *S. jambos* as there is no available data on these fruits until they are studied.

7. Conclusions

Southeast Asia, including Malaysia, consists of countries rich in plant biodiversity that possess more than a thousand types of fruit-bearing trees. Some of these fruits are already commercialized, but many are remaining underutilized. Nowadays, some of these trees are at least cultivated by the villagers or local farmers in the traditionally way for their fruits. Hence, identification of those indigenous tropical fruits with potential for commercial development can help researchers, farmers, or industry to see the opportunities from these native fruits. Indigenous tropical fruits are rich in phytochemicals, especially phenolic compounds, carotenoids, terpenes, and other terpenoids. Instead of providing the attractive colors of the fruits, phytochemicals also offer protective effects against chronic diseases, such as cardiovascular diseases, diabetes, and cancers. They are also responsible for the anti-inflammatory and antimicrobial effects, as well as other medicinal values of the fruits.

Scientifically, extra efforts are needed for studies emphasized on the beneficial health properties and toxicity effect of the fruit using animal-based experiments as well as human interventions to strengthen the scientific proof of their beneficial health properties. Studies on the toxicity effects of the fruits or their extracts should not also be neglected. Due to the variation in health benefits and bioactive phytochemicals in these fruits, attention should be given to study the efficacy of these fruits in combating diseases and later turning them into nutraceutical or basic ingredients for functional food. Bioactive compounds isolated from these fruits could also be used as nutraceutical and pharmaceutical ingredients. Primary screening of antioxidant properties and medicinal values for those indigenous tropical fruits without any scientific evidence is recommended to provide basic understanding for advance research. All the information is useful for the authorities concerned to promote the consumption of these fruits all around the world.

Competing Interests

The authors declare no conflict of interests.

References

[1] J. Kulip, "An ethnobotanical survey of medicinal and other useful plants of Muruts in Sabah, Malaysia," *Telopea*, vol. 10, no. 1, pp. 81–98, 2003.

[2] H. U. Kalsum and A. H. S. Mirfat, "Proximate composition of Malaysian underutilised fruits," *Journal of Tropical Agriculture and Food Science*, vol. 42, no. 1, pp. 63–72, 2014.

[3] H. E. Khoo, K. N. Prasad, K. W. Kong et al., "A review on underutilized tropical fruits in Malaysia," *Guangxi Agricultural Sciences*, vol. 41, no. 7, pp. 698–702, 2010.

[4] H.-E. Khoo, K. N. Prasad, K.-W. Kong, Y. Jiang, and A. Ismail, "Carotenoids and their isomers: color pigments in fruits and vegetables," *Molecules*, vol. 16, no. 2, pp. 1710–1738, 2011.

[5] L. Bravo, "Polyphenols: chemistry, dietary sources, metabolism, and nutritional significance," *Nutrition Reviews*, vol. 56, no. 11, pp. 317–333, 1998.

[6] A. Weizmann and Y. Mazur, "Steroids and triterpenoids of citrus fruit. II. Isolation of citrostadienol," *The Journal of Organic Chemistry*, vol. 23, no. 6, pp. 832–834, 1958.

[7] P. Scartezzini and E. Speroni, "Review on some plants of Indian traditional medicine with antioxidant activity," *Journal of Ethnopharmacology*, vol. 71, no. 1-2, pp. 23–43, 2000.

[8] C. Muthu, M. Ayyanar, N. Raja, and S. Ignacimuthu, "Medicinal plants used by traditional healers in Kancheepuram District of Tamil Nadu, India," *Journal of Ethnobiology and Ethnomedicine*, vol. 2, article 43, 2006.

[9] A. Rizvi, A. Mishra, A. A. Mahdi, M. Ahmad, and A. Basit, "Natural and herbal stress remedies: a review," *International Journal of Pharmacognosy*, vol. 2, no. 4, pp. 155–160, 2015.

[10] T. K. Lim, "Edible medicinal and non-medicinal plants," in *Fruits*, Springer Science+Business Media B.V., Dordrecht, Netherlands, 2012.

[11] H.-E. Khoo, K. N. Prasad, A. Ismail, and N. Mohd-Esa, "Carotenoids from *Mangifera pajang* and their antioxidant capacity," *Molecules*, vol. 15, no. 10, pp. 6699–6712, 2010.

[12] E. H. K. Ikram, K. H. Eng, A. M. M. Jalil et al., "Antioxidant capacity and total phenolic content of Malaysian underutilized fruits," *Journal of Food Composition and Analysis*, vol. 22, no. 5, pp. 388–393, 2009.

[13] S. W. Yan, R. Ramasamy, N. B. M. Alitheen, and A. Rahmat, "A comparative assessment of nutritional composition, total phenolic, total flavonoid, antioxidant capacity, and antioxidant vitamins of two types of Malaysian underutilized fruits (*Averrhoa bilimbi* and *Averrhoa carambola*)," *International Journal of Food Properties*, vol. 16, no. 6, pp. 1231–1244, 2013.

[14] A. Akeem, K. B. Mohamed, M. Z. Asmawi, and O. A. Sofiman, "Mutagenic and antimutagenic potentials of fruit juices of five medicinal plants in *Allium cepa* L.: possible influence of DPPH free radical scavengers," *African Journal of Biotechnology*, vol. 10, no. 50, pp. 10520–10529, 2011.

[15] S. F. Sulaiman and K. L. Ooi, "Antioxidant and α-glucosidase inhibitory activities of 40 tropical juices from Malaysia and identification of phenolics from the bioactive fruit juices of *Barringtonia racemosa* and *Phyllanthus acidus*," *Journal of Agricultural and Food Chemistry*, vol. 62, no. 39, pp. 9576–9585, 2014.

[16] K. C. Wong and S. N. Wong, "Volatile constituents of *Averrhoa bilimbi* L. fruit," *Journal of Essential Oil Research*, vol. 7, no. 6, pp. 691–693, 1995.

[17] M. Hasanuzzaman, M. R. Ali, M. Hossain, S. Kuri, and M. S. Islam, "Evaluation of total phenolic content, free radical scavenging activity and phytochemical screening of different extracts of *Averrhoa bilimbi* (fruits)," *International Current Pharmaceutical Journal*, vol. 2, no. 4, pp. 92–96, 2013.

[18] D. R. Singh, S. Singh, K. M. Salim, and R. C. Srivastava, "Estimation of phytochemicals and antioxidant activity of underutilized fruits of Andaman Islands (India)," *International Journal of Food Sciences and Nutrition*, vol. 63, no. 4, pp. 446–452, 2012.

[19] J. A. Pino, R. Marbot, and A. Bello, "Volatile components of *Averrhoa bilimbi* L. fruit grown in Cuba," *Journal of Essential Oil Research*, vol. 16, no. 3, pp. 241–242, 2004.

[20] M. Bakar, N. Ahmad, F. Karim, and S. Saib, "Phytochemicals and antioxidative properties of Borneo indigenous liposu (*Baccaurea lanceolata*) and tampoi (*Baccaurea macrocarpa*) fruits," *Antioxidants*, vol. 3, no. 3, pp. 516–525, 2014.

[21] L. Y. Chew, K. N. Prasad, I. Amin, A. Azrina, and C. Y. Lau, "Nutritional composition and antioxidant properties of *Canarium odontophyllum* Miq. (dabai) fruits," *Journal of Food Composition and Analysis*, vol. 24, no. 4-5, pp. 670–677, 2011.

[22] A. Ismail, K. N. Prasad, L. Y. Chew, H. E. Khoo, K. W. Kong, and A. Azlan, "Antioxidant capacities of peel, pulp, and seed fractions of *Canarium odontophyllum* Miq. fruit," *Journal of Biomedicine and Biotechnology*, vol. 2010, Article ID 871379, 8 pages, 2010.

[23] L. Y. Chew, H. E. Khoo, I. Amin, A. Azrina, and C. Y. Lau, "Analysis of phenolic compounds of dabai (*Canarium odontophyllum* Miq.) fruits by high-performance liquid chromatography," *Food Analytical Methods*, vol. 5, no. 1, pp. 126–137, 2012.

[24] H. E. Khoo, A. Azlan, A. Ismail, and F. Abas, "Antioxidative properties of defatted dabai pulp and peel prepared by solid phase extraction," *Molecules*, vol. 17, no. 8, pp. 9754–9773, 2012.

[25] V. B. Hoe and K. H. Siong, "The nutritional value of indigenous fruits and vegetables in Sarawak," *Asia Pacific Journal of Clinical Nutrition*, vol. 8, no. 1, pp. 24–31, 1999.

[26] I. Jantan, F. A. Jumuddin, F. C. Saputri, and K. Rahman, "Inhibitory effects of the extracts of *Garcinia* species on human low-density lipoprotein peroxidation and platelet aggregation in relation to their total phenolic contents," *Journal of Medicinal Plants Research*, vol. 5, no. 13, pp. 2699–2709, 2011.

[27] U. M. Acuña, *Phenolic constituents from Garcinia intermedia and related species [M.S. thesis]*, The City University of New York, New York, NY, USA, 2011.

[28] U. M. Acuña, K. Dastmalchi, M. J. Basile, and E. J. Kennelly, "Quantitative high-performance liquid chromatography photo-diode array (HPLC-PDA) analysis of benzophenones and biflavonoids in eight *Garcinia* species," *Journal of Food Composition and Analysis*, vol. 25, no. 2, pp. 215–220, 2012.

[29] S. H. Ali Hassan, J. R. Fry, and M. F. Abu Bakar, "Phytochemicals content, antioxidant activity and acetylcholinesterase inhibition properties of indigenous *Garcinia parvifolia* fruit," *BioMed Research International*, vol. 2013, Article ID 138950, 7 pages, 2013.

[30] T. S. Tyug, M. H. Johar, and A. Ismail, "Antioxidant properties of fresh, powder, and fiber products of mango (*Mangifera foetida*) fruit," *International Journal of Food Properties*, vol. 13, no. 4, pp. 682–691, 2010.

[31] S. F. Sulaiman and K. L. Ooi, "Polyphenolic and vitamin C contents and antioxidant activities of aqueous extracts from mature-green and ripe fruit fleshes of *Mangifera* sp.," *Journal of Agricultural and Food Chemistry*, vol. 60, no. 47, pp. 11832–11838, 2012.

[32] S. T. Tan and I. Amin, "Antioxidant properties (components and capacity) in fresh, powder and fibre products prepared from bacang (*Mangifera foetida*) fruits," *Malaysian Journal of Nutrition*, vol. 14, no. 2, pp. S8–S9, 2008.

[33] H. E. Khoo and A. Ismail, "Determination of daidzein and genistein contents in *Mangifera* fruit," *Malaysian Journal of Nutrition*, vol. 14, no. 2, pp. 189–198, 2008.

[34] M. F. Abu Bakar, M. Mohamed, A. Rahmat, and J. Fry, "Phytochemicals and antioxidant activity of different parts of bambangan (*Mangifera pajang*) and tarap (*Artocarpus odoratissimus*)," *Food Chemistry*, vol. 113, no. 2, pp. 479–483, 2009.

[35] K. N. Prasad, F. A. Hassan, B. Yang et al., "Response surface optimisation for the extraction of phenolic compounds and antioxidant capacities of underutilised *Mangifera pajang* Kosterm. peels," *Food Chemistry*, vol. 128, no. 4, pp. 1121–1127, 2011.

[36] M. Ibrahim, *Nutrient composition, antioxidant properties and hypocholesterolemic effect of bambangan (*Mangifera pajang Kostermans*) pulp juice powder [Ph.D. thesis]*, Universiti Putra Malaysia, Selangor, Malaysia, 2010.

[37] D. Krishnaiah, T. Devi, A. Bono, and R. Sarbatly, "Studies on phytochemical constituents of six Malaysian medicinal plants," *Journal of Medicinal Plants Research*, vol. 3, no. 2, pp. 67–72, 2009.

[38] G. S. Kumar, H. Nayaka, S. M. Dharmesh, and P. V. Salimath, "Free and bound phenolic antioxidants in amla (*Emblica officinalis*) and turmeric (*Curcuma longa*)," *Journal of Food Composition and Analysis*, vol. 19, no. 5, pp. 446–452, 2006.

[39] S. J. Hossain, I. Tsujiyama, M. Takasugi, M. A. Islam, R. S. Biswas, and H. Aoshima, "Total phenolic content, antioxidative, anti-amylase, anti-glucosidase, and antihistamine release activities of Bangladeshi fruits," *Food Science and Technology Research*, vol. 14, no. 3, pp. 261–268, 2008.

[40] X. Liu, C. Cui, M. Zhao et al., "Identification of phenolics in the fruit of emblica (*Phyllanthus emblica* L.) and their antioxidant activities," *Food Chemistry*, vol. 109, no. 4, pp. 909–915, 2008.

[41] I. Ahmad and A. Z. Beg, "Antimicrobial and phytochemical studies on 45 Indian medicinal plants against multi-drug resistant human pathogens," *Journal of Ethnopharmacology*, vol. 74, no. 2, pp. 113–123, 2001.

[42] L. Sawant, N. Pandita, and B. Prabhakar, "Determination of gallic acid in *Phyllanthus emblica* Linn. dried fruit powder by HPTLC," *Journal of Pharmacy and Bioallied Sciences*, vol. 2, no. 2, pp. 105–108, 2010.

[43] K. A. Reynertson, H. Yang, B. Jiang, M. J. Basile, and E. J. Kennelly, "Quantitative analysis of antiradical phenolic constituents from fourteen edible Myrtaceae fruits," *Food Chemistry*, vol. 109, no. 4, pp. 883–890, 2008.

[44] S. Kondo, M. Kittikorn, and S. Kanlayanarat, "Preharvest antioxidant activities of tropical fruit and the effect of low temperature storage on antioxidants and jasmonates," *Postharvest Biology and Technology*, vol. 36, no. 3, pp. 309–318, 2005.

[45] J. Lako, V. C. Trenerry, M. Wahlqvist, N. Wattanapenpaiboon, S. Sotheeswaran, and R. Premier, "Phytochemical flavonols, carotenoids and the antioxidant properties of a wide selection of Fijian fruit, vegetables and other readily available foods," *Food Chemistry*, vol. 101, no. 4, pp. 1727–1741, 2007.

[46] S. Siriamornpun, N. Weerapreeyakul, and S. Barusrux, "Bioactive compounds and health implications are better for green jujube fruit than for ripe fruit," *Journal of Functional Foods*, vol. 12, pp. 246–255, 2015.

[47] E. M. Tanvir, R. Afroz, N. Karim et al., "Antioxidant and antibacterial activities of methanolic extract of BAU kul (*Ziziphus mauritiana*), an improved variety of fruit from Bangladesh," *Journal of Food Biochemistry*, vol. 39, no. 2, pp. 139–147, 2015.

[48] A. A. Memon, N. Memon, D. L. Luthria, A. A. Pitafi, and M. I. Bhanger, "Phenolic compounds and seed oil composition of *Ziziphus mauritiana* L. fruit," *Polish Journal of Food and Nutrition Sciences*, vol. 62, no. 1, pp. 15–21, 2012.

[49] H. A. Umaru, R. Adamu, D. Dahiru, and M. S. Nadro, "Levels of antinutritional factors in some wild edible fruits of Northern Nigeria," *African Journal of Biotechnology*, vol. 6, no. 16, pp. 1935–1938, 2007.

[50] InfoTANI, *Buah-Buahan Nadir Di Malaysia*, 2012, http://www.terengganu.gov.my/maxc2020/appshare/widget/mn_img/76682-file/buah-buahan%20nadir%20di%20malaysia.pdf.

[51] S. Subhadrabandhu, "Under-Utilized Tropical Fruits of Thailand," 2012, ftp://ftp.fao.org/docrep/fao/004/ab777e/ab777e00.pdf.

[52] E. Singh, S. Sharma, A. Pareek, J. Dwivedi, S. Yadav, and S. Sharma, "Phytochemistry, traditional uses and cancer chemopreventive activity of Amla (*Phyllanthus emblica*): the sustainer," *Journal of Applied Pharmaceutical Science*, vol. 2, no. 1, pp. 176–183, 2012.

[53] A. C. Dweck, "Natural ingredients for colouring and styling," *International Journal of Cosmetic Science*, vol. 24, no. 5, pp. 287–302, 2002.

[54] H. E. Khoo, A. Ismail, N. Mohd-Esa, and S. Idris, "Carotenoid content of underutilized tropical fruits," *Plant Foods for Human Nutrition*, vol. 63, no. 4, pp. 170–175, 2008.

[55] S. H. Goh, C. H. Chuah, J. S. L. Mok, and E. Soepadmo, *Malaysian Medicinal Plants for the Treatment of Cardiovascular Diseases*, Pelanduk Publishing, Kuala Lumpur, Malaysia, 1995.

[56] S. Surialaga, D. Dhianawaty, A. Martiana, and A. S. Andreanus, "Antihypercholesterolemic effect of bilimbi (*Averhoa bilimbi* L.) fruit juice in hypercholesterolemic CFW Swiss Webster mice," *Bandung Medical Journal*, vol. 45, no. 2, pp. 125–129, 2013 (Indonesian).

[57] G. J. Kapadia and G. S. Rao, "Antimicrobial and other biological effects of *Garcinia* plants used in food and herbal medicine," in *Natural Antimicrobials in Food Safety and Quality*, pp. 304–327, CABI, New York, NY, USA, 2011.

[58] S. Klaiklay, *Chemical Constituents from the Twigs of Garcinia hombroniana, the Leaves of Garcinia prainiana and the roots of Clerodendrum petasites S. Moore [M.S. thesis]*, Price of Songkla University, Songkhla, Thailand, 2009.

[59] T. K. Lim, "*Durio kutejensis*," in *Edible Medicinal and Non-Medicinal Plants*, pp. 559–562, Springer, Dordrecht, The Netherlands, 2012.

[60] F. H. Shakirin, A. Azlan, A. Ismail, Z. Amom, and L. Cheng Yuon, "Protective effect of pulp oil extracted from *Canarium odontophyllum* Miq. fruit on blood lipids, lipid peroxidation, and antioxidant status in healthy rabbits," *Oxidative Medicine and Cellular Longevity*, vol. 2012, Article ID 840973, 9 pages, 2012.

[61] A. Azlan, A. Ismail, M. Ibrahim, F. H. Shakirin, and H. E. Khoo, "Health-promoting properties of selected Malaysian underutilized fruits," in *Proceeding of the 2nd International Symposium on Underutilized Plant Species*, Kuala Lumpur, Malaysia, 2011.

[62] J. F. Morton, Fruits of Warm Climates, http://www.hort.purdue .edu/newcrop/morton.

[63] E.-S. Tee and C.-L. Lim, "Carotenoid composition and content of Malaysian vegetables and fruits by the AOAC and HPLC methods," *Food Chemistry*, vol. 41, no. 3, pp. 309–339, 1991.

[64] S. Anon, *Nutritive Values of Thai Foods*, Ministry of Public Health, Nonthaburi, Thailand, 1992.

[65] K. N. Prasad, L. Y. Chew, H. E. Khoo, B. Yang, A. Azlan, and A. Ismail, "Carotenoids and antioxidant capacities from *Canarium odontophyllum* Miq. fruit," *Food Chemistry*, vol. 124, no. 4, pp. 1549–1555, 2011.

[66] S. H. Ali-Hassan, I. R. Fry, and M. F. Abu-Bakar, "Antioxidative phytochemicals and anti-cholinesterase activity of native kembayau (*Canarium odontophyllum*) fruit of Sabah, Malaysian Borneo," *Journal of Nutrition & Food Sciences*, vol. 4, no. 1, Article ID 1000249, 2013.

[67] E. S. Tee, M. I. Noor, M. N. Azudin, and K. Idris, *Nutrient Composition of Malaysian Foods*, Institute for Medical Research, Kuala Lumpur, Malaysia, 1997.

[68] K. Judprasong, S. Charoenkiatkul, P. Thiyajai, and M. Sukprasansap, "Nutrients and bioactive compounds of Thai indigenous fruits," *Food Chemistry*, vol. 140, no. 3, pp. 507–512, 2013.

[69] W. A. Whistler and C. R. Elevitch, *Syzygium malaccense (Malay Apple), Species Profiles for Pacific Island Agroforestry*, 2012, http://www.traditionaltree.org.

[70] G. S. Cheema, S. S. Bhat, and K. C. Naik, *Commercial Fruits of India*, Macmillan Publishers, Calcutta, India, 1954.

[71] A. H. Wu and M. C. Pike, "Phytoestrogen content in foods and their role in cancer," in *Handbook of Antioxidants, Revised and Expanded*, Marcel Dekker, New York, NY, USA, 2001.

[72] P. Shukla, P. Shukla, and B. Gopalkrishna, "Isolation and characterization of polyphenolic compound quercetin from *Phyllanthus emblica*," *International Journal of Pharmaceutical Science Research*, vol. 3, no. 5, pp. 1520–1522, 2012.

[73] Y. Boer, *Antioxidant of kandis fruit peel [Garcinia parvifolia (Miq) Miq.] [M.S. thesis]*, University of Indonesia, Depok, Indonesia, 1999 (Indonesian).

[74] K. C. Wong, S. W. Wong, S. S. Siew, and D. Y. Tie, "Volatile constituents of the fruits of *Lansium domesticum* correa (Duku and Langsat) and *Baccaurea motleyana* (Muell. Arg.) Muell. Arg. (Rambai)," *Flavour and Fragrance Journal*, vol. 9, no. 6, pp. 319–324, 1994.

[75] K. C. Wong and H. K. Loi, "Volatile constituents of *Bouea macrophylla* Griff. fruit," *Journal of Essential Oil Research*, vol. 8, no. 1, pp. 99–100, 1996.

[76] V. Rukachaisirikul, A. Adair, P. Dampawan, W. C. Taylor, and P. C. Turner, "Lanostanes and friedolanostanes from the pericarp of *Garcinia hombroniana*," *Phytochemistry*, vol. 55, no. 2, pp. 183–188, 2000.

[77] K. C. Wong and C. H. Ong, "Volatile components of the fruits of bachang (*Mangifera foetida* Lour.) and kuini (*Mangifera odorata* Griff.)," *Flavour and Fragrance Journal*, vol. 8, no. 3, pp. 147–151, 1993.

[78] K. Panthong, R. Sompong, V. Rukachaisirikul, N. Hutadilok-Towatana, S. P. Voravuthikunchai, and J. Saising, "Two new triterpenes and a new coumaroyl glucoside from the twigs of *Mangifera foetida* Lour," *Phytochemistry Letters*, vol. 11, pp. 43–48, 2015.

[79] K. C. Wong and S. S. Siew, "Volatile components of the fruits of bambangan (*Mangifera panjang* kostermans) and binjai (*Mangifera caesia* jack)," *Flavour and Fragrance Journal*, vol. 9, no. 4, pp. 173–178, 1994.

[80] X. Liu, M. Zhao, W. Luo, B. Yang, and Y. Jiang, "Identification of volatile components in *Phyllanthus emblica* L. and their antimicrobial activity," *Journal of Medicinal Food*, vol. 12, no. 2, pp. 423–428, 2009.

[81] K. C. Wong and F. Y. Lai, "Volatile constituents from the fruits of four *Syzygium* species grown in Malaysia," *Flavour and Fragrance Journal*, vol. 11, no. 1, pp. 61–66, 1996.

[82] G. Vernin, G. Vernin, J. Metzger, C. Roque, and J.-C. Pieribattesti, "Volatile constituents of the Jamrosa aroma *Syzygium jambos* L. Aston from Reunion Island," *Journal of Essential Oil Research*, vol. 3, no. 2, pp. 83–97, 1991.

[83] C. M. Guedes, A. B. Pinto, R. F. A. Moreira, and C. A. B. De Maria, "Study of the aroma compounds of rose apple (*Syzygium jambos* Alston) fruit from Brazil," *European Food Research and Technology*, vol. 219, no. 5, pp. 460–464, 2004.

[84] T. K. Lim, *Edible Medicinal and Non-Medicinal Plants*, vol. 1, Springer, Dordrecht, The Netherlands, 2012.

[85] S. Mohamad, N. M. Zin, H. A. Wahab et al., "Antituberculosis potential of some ethnobotanically selected Malaysian plants," *Journal of Ethnopharmacology*, vol. 133, no. 3, pp. 1021–1026, 2011.

[86] J. Morton, *Fruits of Warm Climates*, Florida Flair Books, Miami, Fla, USA, 1987.

[87] S. K. Marwat, M. A. Khan et al., "Fruit plant species mentioned in the Holy Qura'n and Ahadith and their ethnomedicinal importance," *American-Eurasian Journal of Agricultural Environmental Sciences*, vol. 5, no. 2, pp. 284–295, 2009.

[88] M. Edelenbos, L. P. Christensen, and K. Grevsen, "HPLC determination of chlorophyll and carotenoid pigments in processed green pea cultivars (*Pisum sativum* L.)," *Journal of Agricultural and Food Chemistry*, vol. 49, no. 10, pp. 4768–4774, 2001.

[89] I. Fichan, C. Larroche, and J. B. Gros, "Water solubility, vapor pressure, and activity coefficients of terpenes and terpenoids," *Journal of Chemical and Engineering Data*, vol. 44, no. 1, pp. 56–62, 1999.

[90] M. S. Kumar, S. Kumar, and B. Raja, "Antihypertensive and antioxidant potential of borneol—a natural terpene in L-NAME-induced hypertensive rats," *International Journal of*

Pharmaceutical & Biology Archive, vol. 1, no. 3, pp. 271–279, 2010.

[91] A. V. Rao and D. M. Gurfinkel, "The bioactivity of saponins: triterpenoid and steroidal glycosides," *Drug Metabolism and Drug Interactions*, vol. 17, no. 1–4, pp. 211–235, 2000.

[92] B. M. Fraga, "Natural sesquiterpenoids," *Natural Product Reports*, vol. 19, no. 5, pp. 650–672, 2002.

[93] J. D. Connolly and R. A. Hill, "Triterpenoids," *Natural Product Reports*, vol. 25, no. 4, pp. 794–830, 2008.

[94] G. J. E. Nychas, "Natural antimicrobials from plants," in *New Methods of Food Preservation*, pp. 58–89, Chapman & Hall, New York, NY, USA, 1995.

[95] S. H. Thilakarathna and H. P. Vasantha Rupasinghe, "Anti-atherosclerotic effects of fruit bioactive compounds: a review of current scientific evidence," *Canadian Journal of Plant Science*, vol. 92, no. 3, pp. 407–419, 2012.

[96] S. Ambili, A. Subramoniam, and N. S. Nagarajan, "Studies on the antihyperlipidemic properties of *Averrhoa bilimbi* fruit in rats," *Planta Medica*, vol. 75, no. 1, pp. 55–58, 2009.

[97] B. K. H. Tan, P. Fu, P. W. Chow, and A. Hsu, "Effects of *A. bilimbi* on blood sugar and food intake in streptozotocin induced diabetic rats," *Phytomedicine*, vol. 3, pp. 271–272, 1996.

[98] N. H. A. Wahab, M. E. A. Wahid, M. Taib, W. Z. W. M. Zain, and S. A. Anwar, "Phytochemical screening and antimicrobial efficacy of extracts from *Averrhoa bilimbi* (Oxalidaceace) fruits against human pathogenic bacteria," *Pharmacognosy Journal*, vol. 1, no. 1, pp. 64–66, 2009.

[99] M. H. Nurulhuda, A. Azlan, A. Ismail, Z. Amom, and F. H. Shakirin, "Sibu olive inhibits artherosclerosis by cholesterol lowering effect in cholesterol fed-rabbit," in *Proceeding of the 4th International Conference on Biomedical Engineering*, pp. 141–144, Ho Chi Minh City, Vietnam, 2013.

[100] M. H. Nurulhuda, A. Azlan, A. Ismail, Z. Amom, and F. H. Shakirin, "Cholesterol-lowering and atherosclerosis inhibitory effect of Sibu olive in cholesterol fed-rabbit," *Asian Journal of Biochemistry*, vol. 7, no. 2, pp. 80–89, 2012.

[101] J. Leverett, A. Chandra, J. Rana, D. J. Fast, S. R. Missler, and D. M. Flower, "Extracts of durian fruit for use in skin care compositions," US Patent Publication Number US20070042064 A1, 2005.

[102] S. Mohamed, Z. Hassan, and N. A. Hamid, "Antimicrobial activity of some tropical fruit wastes (guava, starfruit, banana, papaya, passionfruit, langsat, duku, rambutan and rambai)," *Pertanika Journal of Tropical Agricultural Science*, vol. 17, no. 3, pp. 219–227, 1994.

[103] T.-J. S. A. Tajudin, N. Mat, A. B. Siti-Aishah, A. A. M. Yusran, A. Alwi, and A. M. Ali, "Cytotoxicity, antiproliferative effects, and apoptosis induction of methanolic extract of *Cynometra cauliflora* Linn. whole fruit on human promyelocytic leukemia HL-60 cells," *Evidence-Based Complementary and Alternative Medicine*, vol. 2012, Article ID 127373, 6 pages, 2012.

[104] M. Hemshekhar, K. Sunitha, M. S. Santhosh et al., "An overview on genus *Garcinia*: phytochemical and therapeutical aspects," *Phytochemistry Reviews*, vol. 10, no. 3, pp. 325–351, 2011.

[105] I. Jantan, I. A. A. Rafi, and J. Jalil, "Platelet-activating factor (PAF) receptor-binding antagonist activity of Malaysian medicinal plants," *Phytomedicine*, vol. 12, no. 1-2, pp. 88–92, 2005.

[106] M. F. Abu Bakar, M. Mohamad, A. Rahmat, S. A. Burr, and J. R. Fry, "Cytotoxicity, cell cycle arrest, and apoptosis in breast cancer cell lines exposed to an extract of the seed kernel of *Mangifera pajang* (bambangan)," *Food and Chemical Toxicology*, vol. 48, no. 6, pp. 1688–1697, 2010.

[107] M. F. Abu Bakar, M. Mohamed, A. Rahmat, S. A. Burr, and J. R. Fry, "Cellular assessment of the extract of bambangan (*Mangifera pajang*) as a potential cytoprotective agent for the human hepatocellular HepG2 cell line," *Food Chemistry*, vol. 136, no. 1, pp. 18–25, 2013.

[108] A. Ismail, M. Ibrahim, A. Azlan, and A. Hamid, "Effects of juice powder prepared from underutilised *Mangifera pajang* fruit on lipid profiles and antioxidant biomarkers in human subjects," in *Proceedings of the 11th ASEAN Food Conference*, Bandar Seri Begawan, Brunei Darussalam, 2009.

[109] L. Mosca, M. Rubenfire, C. Mandel et al., "Antioxidant nutrient supplementation reduces the susceptibility of low density lipoprotein to oxidation in patients with coronary artery disease," *Journal of the American College of Cardiology*, vol. 30, no. 2, pp. 392–399, 1997.

[110] P. W. Grosvenor, A. Supriono, and D. O. Gray, "Medicinal plants from Riau Province, Sumatra, Indonesia. Part 2: antibacterial and antifungal activity," *Journal of Ethnopharmacology*, vol. 45, no. 2, pp. 97–111, 1995.

[111] B. Halliwell, "Commentary oxidative stress, nutrition and health. Experimental strategies for optimization of nutritional antioxidant intake in humans," *Free Radical Research*, vol. 25, no. 1, pp. 57–74, 1996.

[112] R. N. Chopra, S. L. Nayer, and I. C. Chopra, *Glossary of Indian Medicinal Plant*, Council of Scientific and Industrial Research, New Delhi, India, 1992.

[113] M. Krishnaveni and S. Mirunalini, "Therapeutic potential of *Phyllanthus emblica* (AMLA): the ayurvedic wonder," *Journal of Basic and Clinical Physiology and Pharmacology*, vol. 21, no. 1, pp. 93–105, 2010.

[114] M. N. W. Norhana, A. M. N. Azman, S. E. Poole, H. C. Deeth, and G. A. Dykes, "Effects of bilimbi (*Averrhoa bilimbi* L.) and tamarind (*Tamarindus indica* L.) juice on *Listeria monocytogenes* Scott A and *Salmonella Typhimurium* ATCC 14028 and the sensory properties of raw shrimps," *International Journal of Food Microbiology*, vol. 136, no. 1, pp. 88–94, 2009.

[115] E. T. Arung, W. Suwinarti, M. Hendra et al., "Determination of antioxidant and anti-melanogenesis activities of Indonesian Lai, *Durio kutejensis* [Bombacaceae (Hassk) Becc] fruit extract," *Tropical Journal of Pharmaceutical Research*, vol. 14, no. 1, pp. 41–46, 2015.

[116] J.-H. Sim, C.-H. Khoo, L.-H. Lee, and Y.-K. Cheah, "Molecular diversity of fungal endophytes isolated from *Garcinia mangostana* and *Garcinia parvifolia*," *Journal of Microbiology and Biotechnology*, vol. 20, no. 4, pp. 651–658, 2010.

[117] M. F. A. Bakar, M. Mohamed, A. Rahmat, S. A. Burr, and J. R. Fry, "Cytotoxicity and polyphenol diversity in selected parts of *Mangifera pajang* and *Artocarpus odoratissimus* fruits," *Nutrition and Food Science*, vol. 40, no. 1, pp. 29–38, 2010.

[118] S. Bhattacharya, S. R. Chaudhuri, S. Chattopadhyay, and S. K. Bandyopadhyay, "Healing properties of some Indian medicinal plants against indomethacin-induced gastric ulceration of rats," *Journal of Clinical Biochemistry and Nutrition*, vol. 41, no. 2, pp. 106–114, 2007.

[119] H. Dhir, A. K. Roy, A. Sharma, and G. Talukder, "Modification of clastogenicity of lead and aluminium in mouse bone marrow cells by dietary ingestion of *Phyllanthus emblica* fruit extract," *Mutation Research/Genetic Toxicology*, vol. 241, no. 3, pp. 305–312, 1990.

[120] W. Luo, M. Zhao, B. Yang, J. Ren, G. Shen, and G. Rao, "Antioxidant and antiproliferative capacities of phenolics purified from

Phyllanthus emblica L. fruit," *Food Chemistry*, vol. 126, no. 1, pp. 277–282, 2011.

[121] K. Pinmai, S. Chunlaratthanabhorn, C. Ngamkitidechakul, N. Soonthornchareon, and C. Hahnvajanawong, "Synergistic growth inhibitory effects of *Phyllanthus emblica* and *Terminalia bellerica* extracts with conventional cytotoxic agents: doxorubicin and cisplatin against human hepatocellular carcinoma and lung cancer cells," *World Journal of Gastroenterology*, vol. 14, no. 10, pp. 1491–1497, 2008.

[122] S. Pientaweeratch, V. Panapisal, and A. Tansirikongkol, "Antioxidant, anti-collagenase and anti-elastase activities of *Phyllanthus emblica*, *Manilkara zapota* and silymarin: an in vitro comparative study for anti-aging applications," *Pharmaceutical Biology*, vol. 24, pp. 1–8, 2016.

[123] V. N. Sumantran, A. Kulkarni, R. Chandwaskar et al., "Chondroprotective potential of fruit extracts of *Phyllanthus emblica* in osteoarthritis," *Evidence-Based Complementary and Alternative Medicine*, vol. 5, no. 3, pp. 329–335, 2008.

[124] H. Sakander, B. Akhilesh, and A. R. Koteshwara, "Evaluation of antifungal potential of selected medicinal plants against human pathogenic fungi," *International Journal of Green Pharmacy*, vol. 9, no. 2, pp. 110–117, 2015.

[125] A. D. Dalee, S. Mukhurah, K. Sali, N. Hayeeyusoh, Z. Hajiwangoh, and P. Salaeh, "Antimicrobial substances from endophytic fungi in tamarind (*Tamarindus indica* Linn), malay apple (*Eugenia malaccensis*, Linn), rambutan (*Nephelium lappaceum*), and Indian mulberry (*Morinda citrifolia*, Linn)," in *Proceeding of the International Conference on Research, Implementation and Education of Mathematics and Sciences*, 2015.

[126] M. Goyal, D. Sasmal, and B. P. Nagori, "Review on ethnomedicinal uses, pharmacological activity and phytochemical constituents of *Ziziphus mauritiana* (*Z. jujuba* Lam., non Mill)," *Spatula DD*, vol. 2, no. 2, pp. 107–116, 2012.

[127] K. A. Reynertson, *Phytochemical analysis of bioactive constituents from edible myrtaceae fruits [M.S. thesis]*, The City University of New York, New York, NY, USA, 2007.

[128] S. Das, S. Das, and B. De, "In vitro inhibition of key enzymes related to diabetes by the aqueous extracts of some fruits of West Bengal, India," *Current Nutrition and Food Science*, vol. 8, no. 1, pp. 19–24, 2012.

[129] K. V. Ratnam and R. R. V. Raju, "*In vitro* antimicrobial screening of the fruit extracts of two *Syzygium* species (Myrtaceae)," *Advances in Biological Research*, vol. 2, no. 1-2, pp. 17–20, 2008.

[130] A. Kumar, R. Ilavarasan, T. Jayachandran et al., "Anti-diabetic activity of *Syzygium cumini* and its isolated compound against streptozotocin-induced diabetic rats," *Journal of Medicinal Plants Research*, vol. 2, no. 9, pp. 246–249, 2008.

[131] L.-L. Yang, C.-Y. Lee, and K.-Y. Yen, "Induction of apoptosis by hydrolyzable tannins from *Eugenia jambos* L. on human leukemia cells," *Cancer Letters*, vol. 157, no. 1, pp. 65–75, 2000.

[132] S. Mohanty and I. E. Cock, "Bioactivity of *Syzygium jambos* methanolic extracts: antibacterial activity and toxicity," *Pharmacognosy Research*, vol. 2, no. 1, pp. 4–9, 2010.

[133] S. Murugan, P. U. Devi, N. K. Parameswari, and K. R. Mani, "Antimicrobial activity of *Syzygium jambos* against selected human pathogens," *International Journal of Pharmacy and Pharmaceutical Sciences*, vol. 3, no. 2, pp. 44–47, 2011.

[134] P. A. Cox, "Saving the ethnopharmacological heritage of Samoa," *Journal of Ethnopharmacology*, vol. 38, no. 2-3, pp. 181–188, 1993.

[135] E. R. H. S. S. Ediriweera and W. D. Ratnasooriya, "A review on herbs used in treatment of diabetes mellitus by Sri Langkan ayurvedic and traditional physicians," *AYU (An International Quarterly Journal of Research in Ayurveda)*, vol. 30, no. 4, pp. 373–391, 2009.

[136] B. Vakharia, M. Adhvaryu, and N. Reddy, "Evaluation of adaptogenic potential of *Curcuma longa* and *Zizyphus mauritiana* against acute noise stress induced changes in guinea pigs," *The Journal of Alternative and Complementary Medicine*, vol. 20, no. 5, pp. A37–A37, 2014.

[137] R. S. K. Nimbalkar and S. K. Rajurkar, "Antioxidant activities of *Zizyphus mauritiana* Lam. (Rhamnaceae)," *Biological Forum*, vol. 1, no. 2, pp. 98–101, 2009.

[138] T. Mishra, M. Khullar, and A. Bhatia, "Anticancer potential of aqueous ethanol seed extract of *Ziziphus mauritiana* against cancer cell lines and Ehrlich ascites carcinoma," *Evidence-Based Complementary and Alternative Medicine*, vol. 2011, Article ID 765029, 11 pages, 2011.

[139] A. Bhatia and T. Mishra, "Hypoglycemic activity of *Ziziphus mauritiana* aqueous ethanol seed extract in alloxan-induced diabetic mice," *Pharmaceutical Biology*, vol. 48, no. 6, pp. 604–610, 2010.

[140] R. S. L. Taylor, N. P. Manandhar, J. B. Hudson, and G. H. N. Towers, "Antiviral activities of Nepalese medicinal plants," *Journal of Ethnopharmacology*, vol. 52, no. 3, pp. 157–163, 1996.

[141] R. S. Taylor, N. P. Manandhar, and G. H. N. Towers, "Screening of selected medicinal plants of Nepal for antimicrobial activities," *Journal of Ethnopharmacology*, vol. 46, no. 3, pp. 153–159, 1995.

[142] R. Blomhoff, "Dietary antioxidants and cardiovascular disease," *Current Opinion in Lipidology*, vol. 16, no. 1, pp. 47–54, 2005.

[143] L.-S. Lai, S.-T. Chou, and W.-W. Chao, "Studies on the antioxidative activities of Hsian-tsao (*Mesona procumbens* Hemsl) leaf gum," *Journal of Agricultural and Food Chemistry*, vol. 49, no. 2, pp. 963–968, 2001.

16

Application of Partial Internal Transcribed Spacer Sequences for the Discrimination of *Artemisia capillaris* from Other *Artemisia* Species

Eui Jeong Doh,[1] Seung-Ho Paek,[1] Guemsan Lee,[2] Mi-Young Lee,[3] and Seung-Eun Oh[1]

[1]*Division of Biological Sciences, Konkuk University, Seoul 143-701, Republic of Korea*
[2]*Department of Herbology, Wonkwang University, Iksan 570-749, Republic of Korea*
[3]*Korea Institute of Oriental Medicine, Daejeon 305-811, Republic of Korea*

Correspondence should be addressed to Seung-Eun Oh; seunoh@konkuk.ac.kr

Academic Editor: Yibin Feng

Several *Artemisia* species are used as herbal medicines including the dried aerial parts of *Artemisia capillaris*, which are used as Artemisiae Capillaris Herba (known as "Injinho" in Korean medicinal terminology and "Yin Chen Hao" in Chinese). In this study, we developed tools for distinguishing between *A. capillaris* and 11 other *Artemisia* species that grow and/or are cultured in China, Japan, and Korea. Based on partial nucleotide sequences in the internal transcribed spacer (ITS) that differ between the species, we designed primers to amplify a DNA marker for *A. capillaris*. In addition, to detect other *Artemisia* species that are contaminants of *A. capillaris*, we designed primers to amplify DNA markers of *A. japonica*, *A. annua*, *A. apiacea*, and *A. anomala*. Moreover, based on random amplified polymorphic DNA analysis, we confirmed that primers developed in a previous study could be used to identify *Artemisia* species that are sources of Artemisiae Argyi Folium and Artemisiae Iwayomogii Herba. By using these primers, we found that multiplex polymerase chain reaction (PCR) was a reliable tool to distinguish between *A. capillaris* and other *Artemisia* species and to identify other *Artemisia* species as contaminants of *A. capillaris* in a single PCR.

1. Introduction

The genus *Artemisia* belongs to the Asteraceae family and is composed of 500 species that are mainly found in Asia, Europe, and North America [1, 2]. Over 350 species in the genus *Artemisia* are grown in Asia, including China, Korea, and Japan [1]. Several *Artemisia* species have long been used for the treatment of disease in modern and traditional medicine [2, 3]. For example, the dried aerial parts of *A. capillaris* are used as Artemisiae Capillaris Herba ("Injinho" in Korean medicinal terminology and "Yin Chen Hao" in Chinese) [4], which controls fever [2], protects the liver [5], and inhibits inflammatory responses [6]. However, the dried leaves of *A. capillaris* are often mistaken for those of *A. japonica*. Moreover, young *A. capillaris* leaves that are harvested in early spring are similar to those of *A. argyi* and *A. princeps* [7], which are sources of Artemisiae Argyi Folium ("Aeyup" in

Korean and "Ai Ye" in Chinese) that is used for the treatment of pain, vomiting, and bleeding in the uterus [8].

Because of the morphological similarities among the dried and/or sliced shoots and leaves of *Artemisia* species, some are traded as other species in traditional herbal medicine markets [5, 7]. To resolve this problem, various molecular biology techniques that are based on plant genetic information, such as gene nucleotide sequences (*rbcL*, *matK*, or a combination of both), have been used for plant identification and authentication, including medicinal plants [3]. Other gene sequences have been used to discriminate specific medicinal plants from an adulterant or substitute, for example, the *trnL-F* intergenic spacer for *Coptis* spp., *matK* for *Rheum* spp., and *psbA-trnH* for *Phyllanthus* spp. [9–11]. Internal transcribed spacer (ITS) sequences are effective discriminatory tools, and the ITS2 region in particular can be used as a universal DNA barcode for identifying plants and animals [12], including medicinal plants in the family Fabaceae [13] and genus *Artemisia* [14].

Random amplified polymorphic DNA- (RAPD-) based DNA markers have been used previously for authenticating medicinal plants [3]. In a previous study conducted on six *Artemisia* species that mainly grow and/or are cultured in Korea (*A. princeps*, *A. argyi*, *A. capillaris*, *A. iwayomogi*, *A. japonica*, and *A. keiskeana*), we discriminated both *A. princeps* and *A. argyi* from other *Artemisia* species using a sequence-characterized amplified region (SCAR) marker, which was based on RAPD results [7]. Using the same method, we identified *A. iwayomogi*, which is a source of Artemisiae Iwayomogii Herba ("Haninjin" in Korean medicinal terminology) that has been prescribed as a substitute for Artemisiae Capillaris Herba in Korea [15]. However, we were unable to discriminate *A. capillaris* from *A. japonica* using the RAPD-based method [5, 7].

In this study, we discriminated *A. capillaris* from other *Artemisia* species, particularly *A. japonica*, by exploiting sequence differences in a specific region of the ITS. We used 12 *Artemisia* species, six from our previous study and 6 additional *Artemisia* species, which grow and/or are cultivated in China, Korea, and Japan: *A. asiatica*, *A. montana*, and *A. lavandulaefolia*, which are sources of Artemisiae Argyi Folium in China and Korea [4, 16, 17]; *A. annua* and *A. apiacea*, which are sources of Artemisiae Annuae Herba ("Chung-ho" in Korean medical terminology and "Qing Hao" in Chinese) [4, 18] used for the treatment of malaria [19]; and *A. anomala*, which is a source of Artemisiae Anomalae Herba ("Yugino" in Korean medicinal terminology and "Liu ji nu" in Chinese) [4, 17] used for the treatment of fever and inflammation [20]. *A. anomala* was included to increase the reliability of the discrimination of *A. capillaris*. In addition, we tested the effectiveness of multiplex polymerase chain reaction (PCR) to detect contamination of *A. capillaris* products with those from other *Artemisia* species. We used primers based on ITS sequences to discriminate among the *Artemisia* species and two RAPD-based primer sets to discriminate between *Artemisia* species that are sources of Artemisiae Argyi Folium and Artemisiae Iwayomogii Herba [5, 7].

2. Materials and Methods

2.1. Plant Materials. The fleshy aerial parts, including the leaves, of *Artemisia* species that grow and/or are cultivated in China, Korea, and Japan were collected (Table 1). The samples were dried at room temperature, frozen, and stored at −80°C. The authenticity of the samples was verified by the Korea Institute of Oriental Medicine (KIOM) and the Department of Herbology, Wonkwang University. The voucher samples were deposited in the KIOM and the Department of Herbology.

2.2. Preparation of Genomic DNA. Genomic DNA from each sample was extracted in accordance with the instruction manual for the NucleoSpin® Plant II (Macherey-Nagel,

Duren, Germany). To improve DNA quality, phenolic compounds and polysaccharides were removed using 10% cetyltrimethylammonium bromide and 0.7 M NaCl. After the purity and amount of the prepared genomic DNA were determined using a NanoDrop™ DN-1000 spectrophotometer (Thermo Scientific, Wilmington, DE, USA), the DNA was diluted to 10 ng/μL and stored.

2.3. PCR Amplification

2.3.1. Amplification of ITS. A PCR for the amplification of the ITS, including the 5.8S rRNA coding region, was conducted using a T-personal cycler (Biometra, Goettingen, Germany) according to the protocol by White et al. [21]. In brief, 1.2 pmol of ITS1 (5′-TCCGTAGGTGAACCTGCGG-3′) and ITS4 (5′-TCCTCCGCTTATTGATATGC-3′) primers, 1 U *Taq* polymerase (ABgene, Epsom, UK), and 20 ng of genomic DNA extracted from each sample were used for the PCR amplification. During the 35-cycle PCR process, predenaturation was conducted for 5 min at 95°C and denaturation for 30 s at 95°C. The annealing process was conducted for 30 s at 52°C and the extension process for 1 min at 72°C. A final reaction step was conducted for 7 min at 72°C. The amplified products were separated on 1.2% agarose gel and revealed by staining with ethidium bromide (Sigma-Aldrich, St. Louis, MO, USA). The amplified PCR products were analyzed using MyImage (Seoulin Biotechnology, Seoul, Korea) and purified using a LaboPass™ Gel Kit (Cosmo Genetech, Seoul, Korea).

2.3.2. Amplification of DNA and SCAR Markers. In brief, 1.2 pmol of primers, 1 U *Taq* polymerase (ABgene), and 50 ng of genomic DNA extracted from each *Artemisia* species were used for the PCR amplification. During the 23-cycle PCR process, predenaturation was conducted for 5 min at 95°C and denaturation for 30 s at 95°C. In general, the annealing process was conducted for 30 s at 53.5°C for the amplification of the DNA markers. However, to amplify the DNA markers for *A. capillaris*, *A. japonica*, *A. apiacea*, *A. annua*, and *A. anomala*, this process was conducted for 15–30 s at 54–58°C. The extension process was conducted for 20 s (except for *A. apiacea*, which had 30 s) at 72°C, and a final reaction step was conducted for 5 min at 72°C. To amplify an internal standard for the evaluation of the PCR conduct, a primer set (AYF/AYR) was used to amplify a 94 bp sequence. The amplified products were separated on 1.2% agarose gel and revealed by staining with ethidium bromide (Sigma-Aldrich). The amplified PCR products were then analyzed using MyImage (Seoulin Biotechnology).

2.3.3. Multiplex PCR. For the multiplex PCR amplification, 0.07 pmol of the primers Fb and R7; 0.14 pmol of the primers AYF and AYR; 0.7 pmol of the primer Aam F3; 1.7 pmol of the primers AC F4, ACJ R3, and Aap R2; 3.4 pmol of the primers 2F1, 2F3, AJ F1, AC R3, Aap F1, AA F3, and Aa R4; 1x PrimeSTAR® Max DNA Polymerase (Takara Bio Inc., Kusatsu, Japan); and 20 ng of genomic DNA extracted from each *Artemisia* species were used. During the 30-cycle PCR process, predenaturation was conducted for 10 min at 95°C

TABLE 1: *Artemisia* plants used to determine the internal transcribed spacer (ITS) sequence.

Number	Medicinal name	Name of the plant species	Place of collection	Voucher number
1				WKUARE04
2		*A. asiatica*	Bonghwa, Korea	WKUARE24
3				WKUARE25
4				WKUARE76
5			Kyoto, Japan	WKUARE77
6		*A. montana*		WKUARE78
7			Jeonju, Korea	WKUARE40
8				WKUARE41
9				WKUARE66
10		*A. lavandulaefolia*	Sichuan, China	WKUARE57
11				WKUARE58
12	Artemisiae Argyi Folium			WKUARE67
13				WKUARE05
14			Suwon, Korea	WKUARE06
15		*A. argyi*		WKUARE30
16				WKUARE31
17			Guangxi, China	WKUARE27
18			Sichuan, China	WKUARE59
19				WKUARE43
20			Jeonju, Korea	WKUARE44
21				WKUARE45
22		*A. princeps*	Uiseong, Korea	WKUARE01
23			Ganghwa, Korea	WKUARE55
24				WKUARE56
25			Suwon, Korea	WKUARE33
26				WKUARE34
27				WKUARE35
28	Artemisiae Capillaris Herba	*A. capillaris*	Jeonju, Korea	WKUARE46
29				WKUARE47
30			Nishi, Japan	WKUARE79
31				WKUARE80
32			Sichuan, China	WKUARE52
33			Suwon, Korea	WKUARE37
34			Jinan, Korea	WKUARE10
35			Pohang, Korea	WKUARE68
36	Artemisiae Iwayomogii Herba	*A. iwayomogi*		WKUARE69
37				WKUARE11
38			Jeonju, Korea	WKUARE48
39				WKUARE49
40			Namwon, Korea	WKUARE20
41			Yeongcheon, Korea	WKUARE21
42		*A. annua*		WKUARE60
43			Sichuan, China	WKUARE61
44	Artemisiae Annuae Herba			WKUARE62
45				WKUARE63
46			Sichuan, China	WKUARE53
47		*A. apiacea*		WKUARE54
48			Nishi, Japan	WKUARE81
49				WKUARE82
50			Sichuan, China	WKUARE64
51				WKUARE65
52	Artemisiae Anomalae Herba	*A. anomala*		WKUARE73
53			Pohang, Korea	WKUARE74
54				WKUARE75

TABLE 1: Continued.

Number	Medicinal name	Name of the plant species	Place of collection	Voucher number
55			Suwon, Korea	WKUARE39
56			Jeonju, Korea	WKUARE50
57	Artemisiae Japonicae Herba	A. japonica		WKUARE51
58			Namryung, China	WKUARE17
59			Nishi, Japan	WKUARE83
60				WKUARE84
61			Suwon, Korea	WKUARE16
62			Uiseong, Korea	WKUARE15
63	Artemisia Keiskeanae Herba	A. keiskeana		WKUARE70
64			Pohang, Korea	WKUARE71
65				WKUARE72

and denaturation for 10 s at 95°C. The annealing process was conducted for 5 s at 56.5°C and the extension process for 10 s at 72°C. A final reaction step was conducted for 7 min at 72°C. The amplified products were separated on 2% agarose gel and revealed by staining with ethidium bromide (Sigma-Aldrich). In order to amplify an internal standard for the evaluation of the PCR, the AYF/AYR primer set was used to amplify a 94 bp sequence. The amplified PCR products were then analyzed using MyImage (Seoulin Biotechnology).

2.4. Nucleotide Sequencing of the PCR Products. The nucleotide sequences of the PCR products were directly determined using the primers ITS1 and ITS4 by Macrogen (Seoul, Korea). In other cases, the PCR products resolved by agarose electrophoresis were cloned using a pGEM®-T Easy Vector System I (Promega, Madison, WI, USA). The nucleotide sequences of the subcloned PCR products were determined by Macrogen.

2.5. Alignment of the DNA Sequences and Construction of a Dendrogram. The DNA sequences were manually edited and aligned by ClustalW multiple sequence alignment in BioEdit v7.0.9 (http://www.mbio.ncsu.edu/BioEdit/bioedit.html). A dendrogram was constructed using the neighbor-joining method [22] in the MEGA6 program [23] with 1000 bootstrap iterations. Evolutionary distances were computed using the maximum composite likelihood method [24] in MEGA6.

3. Results

3.1. Determination and Analysis of ITS Sequences. The 726–731 bp nucleotide sequences of the ITS, including the 5.8S region, were determined in 65 samples of 12 Artemisia species (Table 1). Parts of the ITS sequences of each Artemisia species are presented in Figure 1 and were deposited in GenBank (accession numbers KT965653–KT965672). As shown in Figure 1, in the intraspecific samples of five Artemisia species (A. argyi, A. capillaris, A. iwayomogi, A. apiacea, and A. japonica), 4–9 bp differences in the ITS1 and ITS2 sequences were detected. In the case of A. japonica (sample numbers 55, 58, and 59), there were 8 bp differences in the ITS2 region and a

1 bp difference in the ITS1 region. These differences resulted mainly from substitutions (mostly base transitions) and a deletion. In A. apiacea (sample numbers 45 and 46), two base deletions in ITS1 and two substitutions in ITS2 were detected in sample number 45.

To determine whether each Artemisia species could be identified by interspecific ITS sequence differences, we constructed a dendrogram based on the ITS sequences. As outgroups, we used GenBank sequences of Aster yomena (accession number HQ154048.1) and Chrysanthemum coronarium (accession number EF577292.1) in the family Asteraceae, in which Artemisia is included (Figure 2). As shown in Figure 2, each Artemisia species was classified into a separate group on the dendrogram. All of the A. japonica samples that exhibited excessive intraspecific ITS sequence variation were sorted into a group. Fortunately, the A. capillaris samples were separate from the A. japonica samples on the dendrogram. In addition, both A. annua and A. apiacea, which are sources of Artemisia Annuae Herba, were classified into the same cluster on the dendrogram (Figure 2). Interestingly, A. argyi, A. princeps, A. montana, A. lavandulaefolia, and A. asiatica, which are sources of Artemisiae Argyi Folium, were classified into only one cluster.

3.2. Discrimination of A. capillaris from Other Artemisia Species by Differences in ITS Sequences. Based on the results shown in Figure 2, we could discriminate A. capillaris from other Artemisia species, at least from the 11 Artemisia species used in this study, by differences in the ITS sequences. It was difficult to discriminate A. capillaris from A. japonica, which was close to A. capillaris on the dendrogram and exhibited significant variation in its ITS sequence. Most of the variation in the ITS sequences among the intraspecific A. japonica samples was found in the ITS2 region (Figure 1); therefore, we excluded the ITS2 region when designing primers to amplify specific DNA markers for A. japonica. As shown in Figures 1 and 3, we designed the primer set AC F4/ACJ R3 in order to amplify a 189 bp PCR product in the ITS1 region that only appeared in A. capillaris samples (Figures 3 and 4(a)). Subsequently, we designed the AJ F1/AC R3 primer set in order to amplify a 176 bp PCR product in ITS2 that only appeared in A. japonica samples (Figures 3 and 4(b)).

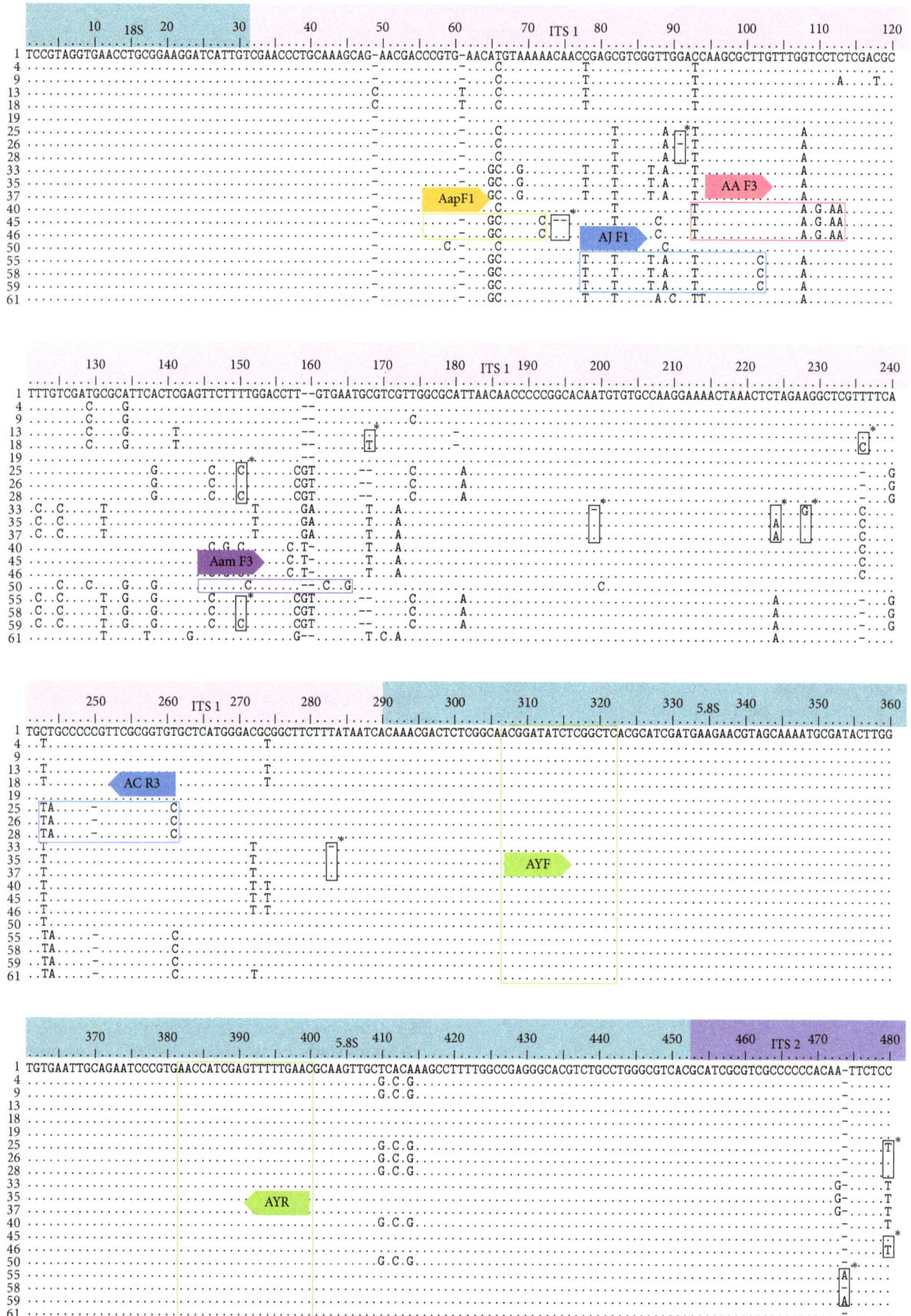

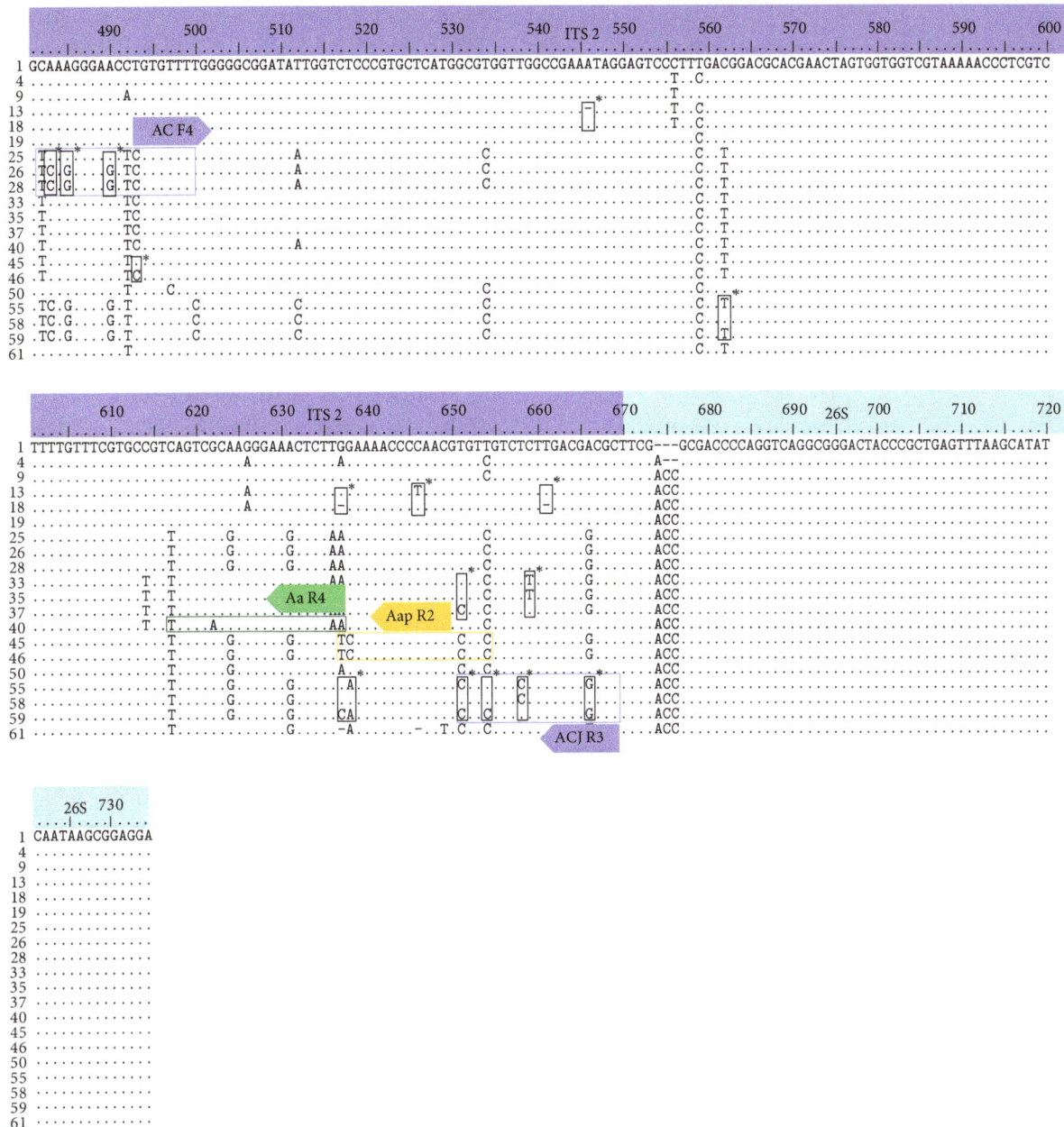

FIGURE 1: Multiple alignments of nucleotide sequences of the internal transcribed spacer (ITS) among *Artemisia* species. The dots indicate consensus nucleotides and the dashes represent gaps. Numbers represent sample numbers (see Table 1). Bold arrows indicate the primers used to amplify DNA markers of the *Artemisia* species, and colored boxes represent nucleotide sequences as well as the positions of the ITS in the primers. Black boxes with an asterisk indicate variations in the nucleotides within species.

Based on these results, we suggest that two primer sets (AJ F1/AC R3 and AC F4/ACJ R3) could be used to discriminate *A. capillaris* not only from *A. japonica* but also from other *Artemisia* species.

3.3. Discrimination of Artemisia Species That Are Sources of Artemisiae Annuae Herba and Artemisiae Anomalae Herba by Differences in ITS Sequences.

We developed DNA markers in order to detect contamination of *A. capillaris* by other *Artemisia* species. As shown in Figure 2, *A. annua* and *A.*

apiacea, which are sources of Artemisiae Annuae Herba, were close together on the dendrogram in a similar manner as *A. capillaris* and *A. japonica*. Therefore, we attempted to find region(s) in ITS1 and ITS2 to discriminate both *A. annua* and *A. apiacea* from other *Artemisia* species. As shown in Figures 1 and 3, we designed the AA F3/Aa R4 primer set in order to amplify a 543 bp PCR product in both *A. annua* and *A. apiacea* simultaneously as a common DNA marker. Subsequently, we designed primers to amplify a specific DNA marker to discriminate *A. annua* from *A. apiacea*. Based on

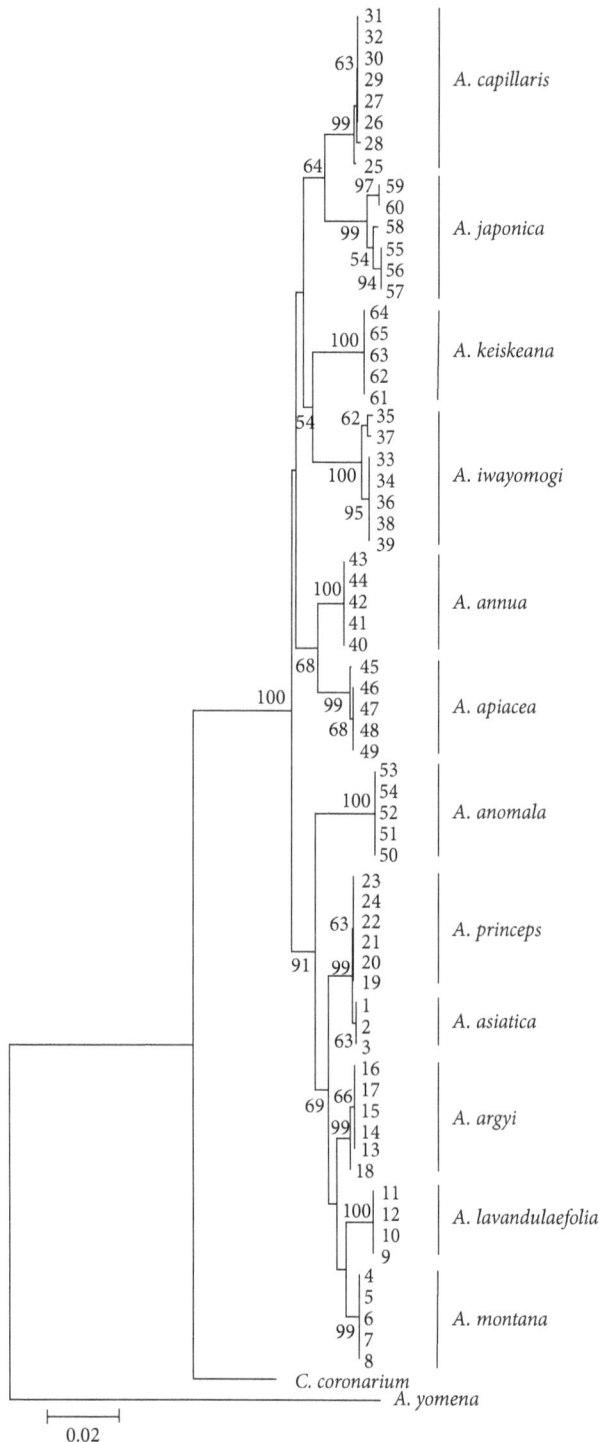

FIGURE 2: Dendrogram based on the internal transcribed spacer (ITS) sequences presented in Figure 1. ITS sequences of *Aster yomena* (accession number HQ154048.1) and *Chrysanthemum coronarium* (accession number EF577292.1) in GenBank were used as outgroups. The unit of evolutionary distance was the number of base substitutions per site; bootstrap values of over 50% are indicated on the branches of the dendrogram.

the differences found in the ITS1 and ITS2 sequences, we designed the Aap F1/Aap R2 primer set in order to amplify

a 594 (in sample number 45, which had a 2 bp deletion) or 596 bp (in sample number 46) PCR product that only appeared in *A. apiacea* samples (Figures 1 and 3). Based on amplifications of the one or two PCR products expected on the gel (Figure 5(a)), we confirmed that the AA F3/Aa R4 and Aap F1/Aap R2 primer sets could discriminate not only *A. annua* from *A. apiacea* but also these two species from other *Artemisia* species. In the case of *A. anomala*, we designed an Aam F3/Aa R4 primer set in order to amplify a 492 bp PCR product in *A. anomala* samples (Figures 1 and 3) and confirmed that the expected 492 bp single band of the PCR product only appeared in *A. anomala* samples (Figure 5(b)).

3.4. Detection of Contamination by Other Artemisia Species Using Multiplex PCR. As shown in Figures 1 and 2, differences in the ITS sequences could discriminate five *Artemisia* species—*A. asiatica, A. montana, A. lavandulaefolia, A. argyi,* and *A. princeps*—that are sources of Artemisiae Argyi Folium and *A. iwayomogi* that is a source of Artemisiae Iwayomogii Herba from the six other *Artemisia* species. However, designing primers in order to amplify DNA markers for these species based on differences in the ITS sequences was difficult. Therefore, we tested the usability of the Fb/R7 and 2F1/2F3 primer sets in order to amplify SCAR markers that were developed in previous studies with six *Artemisia* species [5, 7]. We confirmed that the Fb/R7 primer set amplified a 254 bp SCAR marker in samples of not only *A. princeps* and *A. argyi* but also *A. asiatica, A. lavandulaefolia,* and *A. montana* (data not shown). Furthermore, we confirmed that the 2F1/2F3 primer set amplified a 364 or 365 bp SCAR marker only in *A. iwayomogi,* and that this marker was not amplified in any other species, including *A. asiatica, A. montana, A. lavandulaefolia, A. annua, A. apiacea,* or *A. anomala* (data not shown). Therefore, these two RAPD-based primer sets could detect contamination by these *Artemisia* species in addition to the six other *Artemisia* species. Using the multiplex PCR method, we tested the reliability of these two primer sets and those developed based on the ITS sequences to discriminate *A. capillaris* from other *Artemisia* species and to detect contamination by other *Artemisia* species. For the multiplex PCR process, we randomly selected one sample from each *Artemisia* species listed in Table 1. As shown in Figure 6, these primer sets functioned reliably, not only to discriminate *A. capillaris* from other *Artemisia* species, but also to simultaneously detect contamination by other *Artemisia* species in a single PCR process.

Finally, by mixing genomic DNA isolated from different *Artemisia* species at varying content ratios, we tested the reliability of this PCR method to detect contamination of other *Artemisia* species, such as *A. japonica, A. princeps,* and *A. iwayomogi,* which are mostly found in Korea and are easily misused. As shown in Figure 7, the multiplex PCR detected two *Artemisia* species that had been mixed at ratios of 9 : 1 and 19 : 1. Furthermore, the multiplex PCR detected a mixture of three *Artemisia* species (*A. capillaris* with *A. japonica* and *A. princeps* or *A. capillaris* with *A. japonica* and *A. iwayomogi*) at ratios of 8 : 1 : 1 and 18 : 1 : 1 (Figure 7). Therefore, we suggest that the multiplex PCR method is an accurate tool to discriminate *A. capillaris* from other *Artemisia* species and

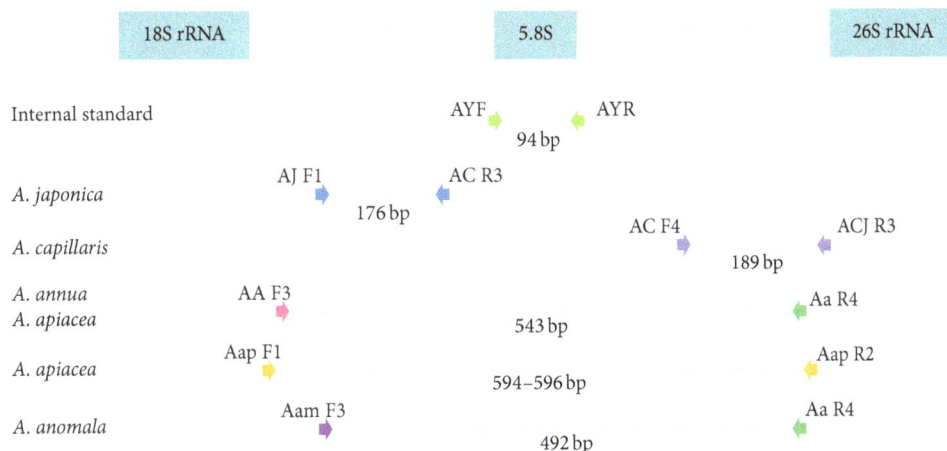

FIGURE 3: Relative positions of the primers designed to amplify DNA markers of *Artemisia* species on the internal transcribed spacer and the expected size of the polymerase chain reaction products.

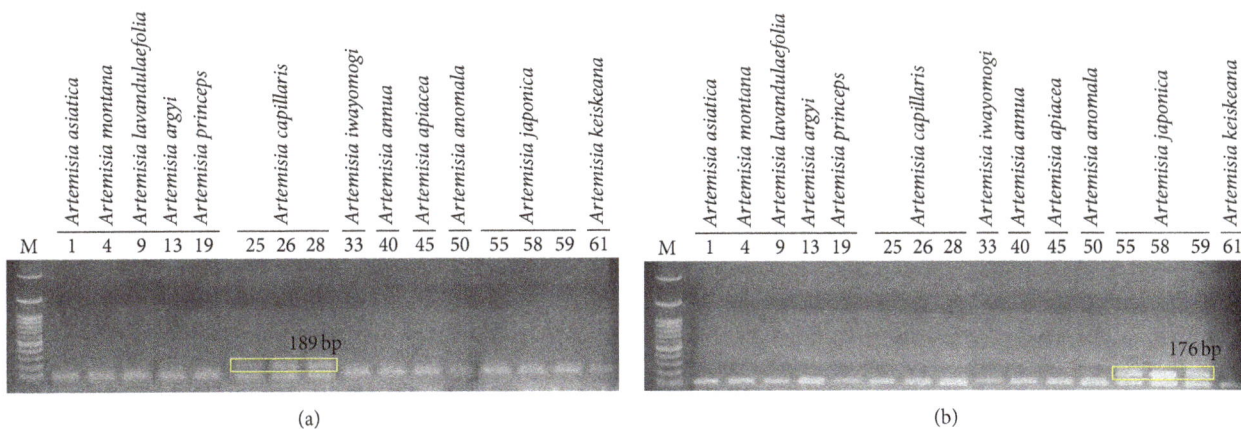

FIGURE 4: Polymerase chain reaction products of the primer sets AC F4/ACJ R3 (a) and AJ F1/AC R3 (b) from 12 *Artemisia* species. Lane numbers are listed in Table 1. M: 100 bp ladder.

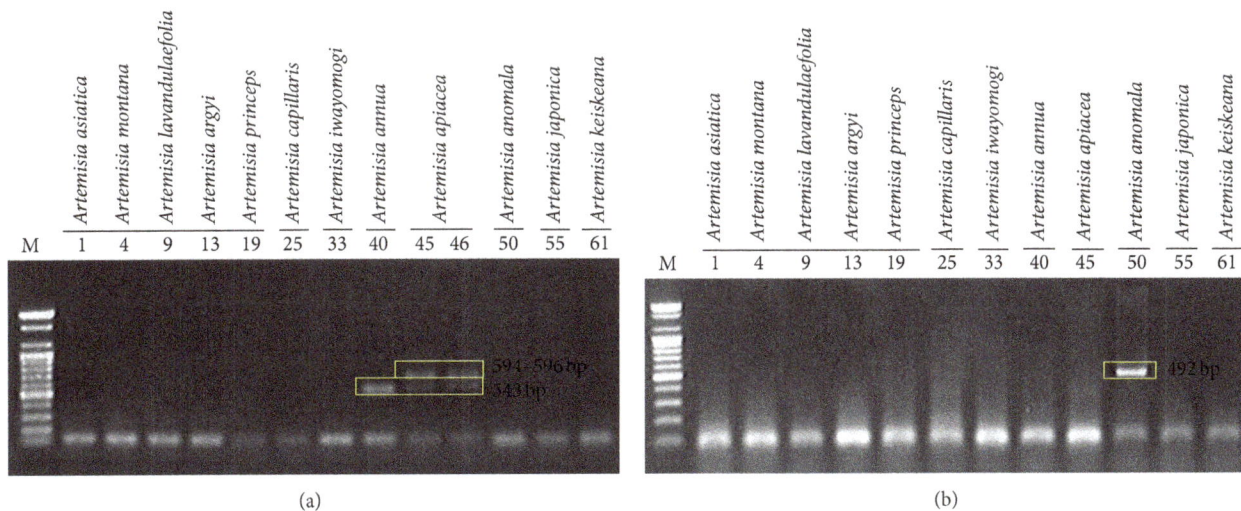

FIGURE 5: Polymerase chain reaction products of the primer sets AA F3/Aa R4 and Aap F1/Aap R2 (a) and Aam F3/Aa R4 (b) from 12 *Artemisia* species. Lane numbers are listed in Table 1. M: 100 bp ladder.

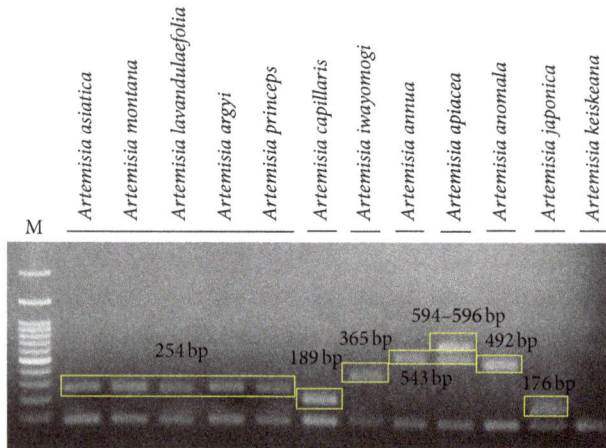

FIGURE 6: Multiplex polymerase chain reaction products using the primers shown in Figures 1 and 3 from 12 randomly selected *Artemisia* species. Genomic DNA from a randomly chosen sample of each *Artemisia* species was used for PCR amplification. M: 100 bp ladder.

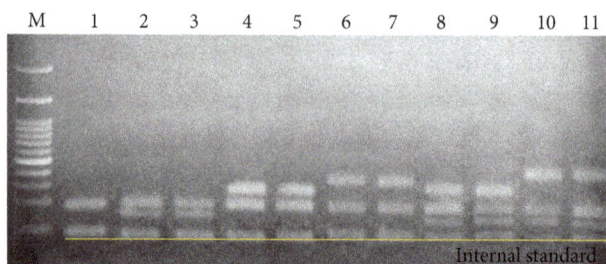

FIGURE 7: Multiplex polymerase chain reaction products by using two or three combined primer sets from mixed genomic DNA isolated from two or three *Artemisia* species at different content ratios. Primer set AC F4/ACJ R3 amplified a 189 bp DNA marker to detect *A. capillaris*; AJ F1/AC R3 amplified a 176 bp DNA marker to detect *A. japonica*; Fb/R7 amplified a 254 bp DNA marker to detect *A. princeps*; 2F1/2F3 amplified a 365 bp DNA marker to detect *A. iwayomogi*. Lane 1: *A. capillaris*; Lane 2: *A. capillaris* and *A. japonica* (9 : 1); Lane 3: *A. capillaris* and *A. japonica* (19 : 1); Lane 4: *A. capillaris* and *A. princeps* (9 : 1); Lane 5: *A. capillaris* and *A. princeps* (19 : 1); Lane 6: *A. capillaris* and *A. iwayomogi* (9 : 1); Lane 7: *A. capillaris* and *A. iwayomogi* (19 : 1); Lane 8: *A. capillaris*, *A. japonica*, and *A. princes* (8 : 1 : 1); Lane 9: *A. capillaris*, *A. japonica*, and *A. princeps* (18 : 1 : 1); Lane 10: *A. capillaris*, *A. japonica*, and *A. iwayomogi* (8 : 1 : 1); Lane 11: *A. capillaris*, *A. japonica*, and *A. iwayomogi* (18 : 1 : 1); M: 100 bp ladder, yellow underline: 96 bp internal standard amplified by AYF/ AYR primer set.

could be used to determine whether *A. capillaris* samples have been mixed with other *Artemisia* species.

4. Discussion

Medicinal plants have long been used to treat disease in traditional and modern medicine [1]. However, because of the substitution and adulteration of medicinal plants with closely related species, the value of the original drug decreases and in some cases can make it lethal when substituted or

contaminated with toxic adulterant plant(s) [3]. Therefore, the authentication of medicinal plants is crucial. As mentioned previously, *A. capillaris*, which is a source of Artemisiae Capillaris Herba, should be discriminated from not only *A. japonica*, *A. argyi*, and *A. princeps* but also other *Artemisia* species that grow and/or are cultivated in Korea and China and could contaminate the products of *A. capillaris*. *Artemisia* species, including *A. capillaris*, are a valuable source of new drugs and essential oils, and their unique chemical compositions and pharmacological activity are species-specific [1, 2, 5]. In this context, we developed a method to discriminate *A. capillaris* from other *Artemisia* species and to detect contamination among *Artemisia* species.

The DNA barcode is a powerful tool for identifying and discriminating between species of animal, plant, and fungus. The sequence at the 5′ end of cytochrome c oxidase subunit 1 (*CO1*) in the mitochondrial genome is used for animal taxonomic classification [25, 26]; however, plants cannot currently be identified by the sequence of a single locus [3]. Therefore, the Consortium for the Barcode of Life (CBOL) Plant Working Group proposed a combination of sequences of *matK* in the nuclear genome and *rbcL* in the chloroplast genome to identify plants [3]. However, the discriminatory power of the combined *matK* and *rblL* loci is low, particularly when discriminating between closely related species, such as 36 species in the genus *Dendrobium* [27]. Instead, by using a single *matK* sequence, medicinal plants in the subfamily Rauvolfioideae and genus *Rheum* have been successfully discriminated from each other [28, 29]. Despite the relatively low level of variation found in *rbcL* sequences in 48 plant genera including *Amaranthus*, *Angelica*, and *Ilex*, their combination with *trnH-psbA* intergenic spacer sequences increased the identification and discrimination success rate from 79% to 88% [30]. Therefore, to identify or discriminate between specific medicinal plants and closely related species, other single loci, besides *CO1*, or a combination of loci, besides *matK* and *rbcL*, have been used. For example, various *Dendrobium* Sw. species have been discriminated between them using a single sequence of the *trnH-psbA* intergenic spacer [31]. In addition, the *trnL-trnF* intergenic spacer sequence clearly discriminated *Cardiocrinum giganteum* from *C. giganteum* var. yunnanense and *C. cordatum* [32].

Of the various DNA barcode loci used, the ITS is one of the most useful. Multiple copies of the ITS are tandemly located at one or more chromosomal loci, and there are hundreds or thousands of ITS repeats in the nuclear genome. Furthermore, the ITS, including ITS1, 5.8S rRNA, and ITS2, is relatively small and ranges from 400 bp to under 1000 bp long [33]. Because of the presence of high copy numbers of the ITS and its small size, the ITS is easily amplified by PCR [34]. The level of variation among interspecific ITS sequences is high, so they can be used for the identification of plants at the specific, generic, and even family levels [35]. In contrast, levels of variation within intraspecific ITS sequences are often very low [34]. Concerted evolution should homogenize the sequences of ITS repeats that exist in a species by high-frequency unequal crossing over or gene conversion [36, 37]. The ITS2 sequence in particular has been used to identify medicinal plants that belong to the genera *Swartzia* and

Artemisia in the family Fabaceae [13, 14]. In addition, ITS2 sequences, combined with *rbcL* sequences, have been used for detecting the contamination and substitution of products from 42 medicinal plants, including *Achillea racemose* and *Urtica dioica*, in Canada and the USA [38].

As shown in Figures 1 and 2, discriminating *A. capillaris* from *A. japonica* and 10 other *Artemisia* species was based upon differences in ITS sequences among the *Artemisia* species. Using the RAPD method with nonspecific primers, we were unable to discriminate *A. capillaris* from *A. japonica* in a previous study [5, 7]. Here, we were able to discriminate *A. capillaris* from *A. japonica* because of differences in nucleotide sequences, particularly in the ITS2 region (Figure 1). Basing discrimination on differences in ITS sequences was conducted cautiously, because of the considerable sequence variation found in the ITS sequences, particularly among intraspecific *A. japonica* samples. We also observed this variation in the *A. japonica* ITS sequences deposited in Gen-Bank (accession numbers AM398882, AY548200, GU724289, JF326554, JX051713, and KC493078). Therefore, we confirmed the discriminatory power of the ITS sequences by using the *A. capillaris* and *A. japonica* ITS sequences deposited in GenBank. The deposited *A. japonica* sequences, together with the *A. japonica* sequences determined in this study (sample numbers 55–60), were clearly discriminated from both the deposited (accession numbers AY548201 and KC493083) and determined (sample numbers 25–32) *A. capillaris* sequences (data not shown).

Therefore, differences in ITS sequences can be used to discriminate among *Artemisia* species, despite the large variations observed in the ITS sequences of specific *Artemisia* species. Lee et al. [39] compared ITS sequences among *Artemisia* species that grow naturally in Korea, including two varieties and one subspecies of *A. japonica*. They estimated the pairwise divergence value as 0.004 between the varieties and subspecies based on the Kiura-2 parameter. Because we could not find any sequence information in their article or GenBank, we were unable to determine how many nucleotide variations exist between the varieties and subspecies of *A. japonica*. However, based on the results of their study, we suggest that the intraspecific ITS sequence variation detected in *A. japonica* could result from the different varieties and/or subspecies of *A. japonica* used for the determination of the ITS sequences.

For the discrimination of *A. capillaris* from *A. japonica*, which were closer to each other than to any other *Artemisia* species on the dendrogram (Figure 2), the primer sets AC F4/ACJ R3 (that amplified a 189 bp DNA marker in *A. capillaris*) and AJ F1/AC R3 (that amplified a 176 bp DNA marker in *A. japonica*) were designed (Figures 1 and 3). Despite the fact that there was not a remarkable difference in the sizes of the DNA markers for *A. capillaris* and *A. japonica*, they were clearly separated on 2% agarose gel after 40 min of gel running (Figure 6).

The method of amplifying double DNA markers of specific species was used to discriminate *A. annua* from *A. apiacea*, which were close to each other on the dendrogram (Figure 2). A 543 bp DNA marker was only amplified in *A. annua* using the AA F3/Aa R4 primer set, and both the

543 and 594 bp (or 596 bp, depending on the presence of a base deletion) DNA markers were amplified in *A. apiacea* using the AA F3/Aa R4 and Aap F1/Aap R2 primer sets, respectively (Figures 5(a) and 5(b)). For the discrimination of the five *Artemisia* species that are sources of Artemisiae Argyi Folium, we first determined whether the nonspecific UBC primer 329 (5'-GCGAACCTCC-3'), which amplified a unique 850 bp PCR product only in *A. argyi* and *A. princeps* in a previous study [7], could amplify the same PCR product in three additional *Artemisia* species (*A. asiatica, A. montana*, and *A. lavandulaefolia*). Using samples from the 12 species, we confirmed that the same PCR products were amplified in these three *Artemisia* species (data not shown). We then confirmed that the Fb/R7 primer set, which was designed to amplify a 254 bp SCAR marker based on the sequence of an 850 bp PCR product [7], amplified the same-sized DNA marker in the three additional *Artemisia* species (data not shown). For the discrimination of *A. iwayomogi*, we tested whether the nonspecific UBC primer 391 (5'-GCGAACCTCG-3'), which amplified four kinds of PCR products that ranged in size from 707 to 719 bp in *A. iwayomogi* in a previous study [5], could amplify the same PCR products in six additional *Artemisia* species (*A. asiatica, A. montana, A. lavandulaefolia, A. apiacea, A. annua*, and *A. anomala*). We confirmed that the UBC primer 391 amplified PCR products only in *A. iwayomogi*. In addition, we confirmed that the 2F1/2F3 primer set, which was designed to amplify a 365 bp SCAR marker based on the sequences of four PCR products [5], amplified the same-sized DNA marker only in *A. iwayomogi* (data not shown). Based on these results, we were convinced that the Fb/R7 and 2F1/2F3 primer sets could discriminate *A. capillaris* not only from the five *Artemisia* species that are sources of Artemisiae Argyi Folium but also from *A. iwayomogi*.

Using primer sets based on the ITS sequences and RAPD results to discriminate among the *Artemisia* species, we evaluated the multiplex PCR method to discriminate *A. capillaris* and to detect contamination of *A. capillaris* by randomly selecting each sample of *Artemisia* species (Figure 6) and mixed samples of *A. capillaris* with *A. japonica, A. princeps*, and *A. iwayomogi* (Figure 7). Therefore, we suggest that the multiplex PCR method is an accurate tool to discriminate *A. capillaris* from other *Artemisia* species and could be used to determine whether *A. capillaris* samples have been mixed with samples from other *Artemisia* species, at least those tested in this study.

5. Conclusion

To differentiate among *A. capillaris* plants that produce Artemisiae Capillaris Herba and 11 other *Artemisia* species, 726–731 bp ITS nucleotide sequences in 65 samples were determined and analyzed. Based on differences found in partial ITS nucleotide sequences between the species, we designed the primer sets AC F4/ACJ R3 to amplify a 189 bp PCR product and AJ F1/AC R3 to amplify a 176 bp PCR product in *A. capillaris* and *A. japonica*, respectively. To detect traces of other *Artemisia* species in *A. capillaris*, we designed the primer set AA F3/Aa R4 to amplify a 543 bp product in

A. annua, the primer set Aap F1/Aap R2 to amplify a 594–596 bp product in *A. apiacea*, and the primer set Aam F3/Aa R4 to amplify a 492 bp product in *A. anomala*. In addition, we confirmed that the primer sets Fb/R7 and 2F1/2F3, which had been developed in a previous study based on RAPD, could be used to amplify 254 bp products in *A. princeps*, *A. argyi*, *A. asiatica*, *A. lavandulaefolia*, and *A. montana*, which are sources of Artemisiae Argyi Folium, and to amplify 364 or 365 bp products in *A. iwayomogi*. Therefore, we demonstrate that the discrimination of *A. capillaris* from and the detection of contamination by other *Artemisia* species can be reliably performed by multiplex PCR using these primers.

Disclosure

Eui Jeong Doh's present address is Center for Metabolic Function Regulation, Wonkwang University, Iksan 570-749, Republic of Korea.

Competing Interests

The authors declare that there are no competing interests regarding the publication of this paper.

Authors' Contributions

Eui Jeong Doh and Seung-Ho Paek contributed equally to this work.

Acknowledgments

This study was part of Konkuk University's research support program for its faculty on sabbatical leave in 2013.

References

[1] M. J. Abad, L. M. Bedoya, L. Apaza, and P. Bermejo, "The *Artemisia* L. genus: a review of bioactive essential oils," *Molecules*, vol. 17, no. 3, pp. 2542–2566, 2012.

[2] R. K. Joshi, "*Artemisia capillaris*: medicinal uses and future source for commercial uses from western himalaya of Uttrakhand," *Asian Journal of Research in Pharmaceutical Science*, vol. 3, no. 3, pp. 137–140, 2013.

[3] N. Techen, I. Parveen, Z. Pan, and I. A. Khan, "DNA barcoding of medicinal plant material for identification," *Current Opinion in Biotechnology*, vol. 25, pp. 103–110, 2014.

[4] Korea Food and Drug Administration, *The Korean Herbal Pharmacopoeia*, KFDA Press, Seoul, Republic of Korea, 2011.

[5] M. Y. Lee, E. J. Doh, E. S. Kim, Y. W. Kim, B. S. Ko, and S.-E. Oh, "Application of the multiplex PCR method for discrimination of *Artemisia iwayomogi* from other *Artemisia* herbs," *Biological and Pharmaceutical Bulletin*, vol. 31, no. 4, pp. 685–690, 2008.

[6] S. H. Hong, S. H. Seo, J. H. Lee, and B. T. Choi, "The aqueous extract from *Artemisia capillaris* Thunb. inhibits lipopolysaccharide-induced inflammatory response through preventing NF-κB activation in human hepatoma cell line and rat liver," *International Journal of Molecular Medicine*, vol. 13, no. 5, pp. 717–720, 2004.

[7] M. Y. Lee, E. J. Doh, C. H. Park et al., "Development of SCAR marker for discrimination of *Artemisia princeps* and *A. argyi* from other Artemisia herbs," *Biological and Pharmaceutical Bulletin*, vol. 29, no. 4, pp. 629–633, 2006.

[8] Q.-C. Zhao, H. Kiyohara, and H. Yamada, "Anti-complementary neutral polysaccharides from leaves of *Artemisia princeps*," *Phytochemistry*, vol. 35, no. 1, pp. 73–77, 1993.

[9] E. J. Doh, M. Y. Lee, B. S. Ko, and S.-E. Oh, "Differentiating *Coptis chinensis* from *Coptis japonica* and other *Coptis* species used in Coptidis Rhizoma based on partial *trnL-F* intergenic spacer sequences," *Genes & Genomics*, vol. 36, no. 3, pp. 345–354, 2014.

[10] G. Xu, X. Wang, C. Liu et al., "Authentication of official Dahuang by sequencing and multiplex allele-specific PCR of a short maturase *K* gene," *Genome*, vol. 56, no. 2, pp. 109–113, 2013.

[11] R. Srirama, B. R. Gurumurthy, U. Senthilkumar, G. Ravikanth, R. U. Shaanker, and M. B. Shivanna, "Are mini DNA-barcodes sufficiently informative to resolve species identities? An in silico analysis using *Phyllanthus*," *Journal of Genetics*, vol. 93, no. 3, pp. 823–829, 2014.

[12] H. Yao, J. Song, C. Liu et al., "Use of ITS2 region as the universal DNA barcode for plants and animals," *PLoS ONE*, vol. 5, no. 10, Article ID e13102, 2010.

[13] T. Gao, H. Yao, J. Song et al., "Identification of medicinal plants in the family *Fabaceae* using a potential DNA barcode ITS2," *Journal of Ethnopharmacology*, vol. 130, no. 1, pp. 116–121, 2010.

[14] M.-Z. Liu, J.-Y. Song, K. Luo, Y.-L. Lin, P. Liu, and H. Yao, "Identification of nine common medicinal plants from *Artemisia* L. by DNA barcoding sequences," *Chinese Traditional and Herbal Drugs*, vol. 43, no. 7, pp. 1393–1397, 2012.

[15] Y. H. Kim, M. Y. Jeong, N. K. Lee et al., "Antimicrobial effect on the periodontal pathogens and anti-inflammatory effect of Artemisiae Iwayomogii Herba," *The Korea Journal of Herbology*, vol. 23, no. 2, pp. 1–8, 2008.

[16] Pharmacopoeia Committee of the DPRK, *Pharmacopoeia of Democratic People's Republic of Korea*, Medicine and Science Press, Pyeongyang, Democratic People's Republic of Korea, 7th edition, 2011.

[17] Zhonghua Bencao, Ed., *Zhonghua Bencao*, Shanghai Science and Technology Press, Shanghai, China, 1999.

[18] Chinese Pharmacopoeia Committee, *Chinese Pharmacopoeia Commission*, China Medical Science and Technology Press, Beijing, China, 2010.

[19] M. L. Willcox, G. Bodeker, G. Bourdy et al., "Artemisia annua as a traditional herbal antimalarial," in *Traditional Medicinal Plants and Malaria*, M. L. Willcox, G. Bodeker, and P. Rasoanaivo, Eds., pp. 43–59, CRC Press, Boca Raton, Fla, USA, 2004.

[20] X. Tan, Y.-L. Wang, X.-L. Yang, and D.-D. Zhang, "Ethyl acetate extract of *Artemisia anomala* S. moore displays potent anti-inflammatory effect," *Evidence-Based Complementary and Alternative Medicine*, vol. 2014, Article ID 681352, 10 pages, 2014.

[21] T. J. White, T. Bruns, S. J. Lee, and J. W. Taylor, "Amplification and direct sequencing of fungal ribosomal RNA genes for phylogenetics," *PCR Protocols: A Guide to Methods and Applications*, vol. 18, pp. 315–322, 1990.

[22] N. Saitou and M. Nei, "The neighbor-joining method: a new method for reconstructing phylogenetic trees," *Molecular Biology and Evolution*, vol. 4, no. 4, pp. 406–425, 1987.

[23] K. Tamura, G. Stecher, D. Peterson, A. Filipski, and S. Kumar, "MEGA6: molecular evolutionary genetics analysis version 6.0," *Molecular Biology and Evolution*, vol. 30, no. 12, pp. 2725–2729, 2013.

[24] K. Tamura, M. Nei, and S. Kumar, "Prospects for inferring very large phylogenies by using the neighbor-joining method," *Proceedings of the National Academy of Sciences of the United States of America*, vol. 101, no. 30, pp. 11030–11035, 2004.

[25] P. D. Hebert, A. Cywinska, and S. L. Ball, "Biological identifications through DNA barcodes," *Proceedings of the Royal Society of London B: Biological Sciences*, vol. 270, no. 1512, pp. 313–321, 2003.

[26] P. D. N. Hebert, S. Ratnasingham, and J. R. de Waard, "Barcoding animal life: cytochrome c oxidase subunit 1 divergences among closely related species," *Proceedings of the Royal Society of London B: Biological Sciences*, vol. 270, supplement 1, pp. S96–S99, 2003.

[27] H. K. Singh, I. Parveen, S. Raghuvanshi, and S. B. Babbar, "The loci recommended as universal barcodes for plants on the basis of floristic studies may not work with congeneric species as exemplified by DNA barcoding of *Dendrobium* species," *BMC Research Notes*, vol. 5, article 42, 2012.

[28] P. Mahadani, G. D. Sharma, and S. K. Ghosh, "Identification of ethnomedicinal plants (Rauvolfioideae: Apocynaceae) through DNA barcoding from northeast India," *Pharmacognosy Magazine*, vol. 9, no. 35, pp. 255–263, 2013.

[29] D.-Y. Yang, H. Fushimi, S.-Q. Cai, and K. Komatsu, "Molecular analysis of *Rheum* species used as Rhei Rhizoma based on the chloroplast matK gene sequence and its application for identification," *Biological and Pharmaceutical Bulletin*, vol. 27, no. 3, pp. 375–383, 2004.

[30] W. J. Kress and D. L. Erickson, "A two-locus global DNA barcode for land plants: the coding *rbcL* gene complemnets noncoding *trnH-psbA* spacer region," *PLoS ONE*, vol. 2, no. 6, article e508, 2007.

[31] H. Yao, J.-Y. Song, X.-Y. Ma et al., "Identification of *Dendrobium* species by a candidate DNA barcode sequence: the chloroplast *psbA-trnH* intergenic region," *Planta Medica*, vol. 75, no. 6, pp. 667–669, 2009.

[32] M. Li, K. H. Ling, H. Lam et al., "*Cardiocrinum* seeds as a replacement for *Aristolochia* fruits in treating cough," *Journal of Ethnopharmacology*, vol. 130, pp. 429–432, 2010.

[33] M. Li, H. Cao, P. P.-H. But, and P.-C. Shaw, "Identification of herbal medicinal materials using DNA barcodes," *Journal of Systematics and Evolution*, vol. 49, no. 3, pp. 271–283, 2011.

[34] I. Álvarez and J. F. Wendel, "Ribosomal ITS sequences and plant phylogenetic inference," *Molecular Phylogenetics and Evolution*, vol. 29, no. 3, pp. 417–434, 2003.

[35] B. G. Baldwin, M. J. Sanderson, J. M. Porter, M. F. Wojciechowski, C. S. Campbell, and M. J. Donoghue, "The ITS region of nuclear ribosomal DNA: a valuable source of evidence on angiosperm phylogeny," *Annals of the Missouri Botanical Garden*, vol. 82, no. 2, pp. 247–277, 1995.

[36] M. L. Ainouche and R. J. Bayer, "On the origins of the tetraploid *Bromus* species (section *Bromus*, Poaceae): insights from internal transcribed spacer sequences of nuclear ribosomal DNA," *Genome*, vol. 40, no. 5, pp. 730–743, 1997.

[37] A. R. D. Ganley and T. Kobayashi, "Highly efficient concerted evolution in the ribosomal DNA repeats: total rDNA repeat variation revealed by whole-genome shotgun sequence data," *Genome Research*, vol. 17, no. 2, pp. 184–191, 2007.

[38] S. G. Newmaster, M. Grguric, D. Shanmughanandhan, S. Ramalingam, and S. Ragupathy, "DNA barcoding detects contamination and substitution in North American herbal products," *BMC Medicine*, vol. 11, no. 1, article 222, 2013.

[39] J. H. Lee, C. B. Park, C. G. Park, and S. G. Moon, "A phylogenetic analysis of Korean *Artemisia* L. based on ITS sequences," *Korean Journal of Plant Resources*, vol. 23, no. 4, pp. 293–302, 2010.

PERMISSIONS

LIST OF CONTRIBUTORS

Yoshiki Mukudai, Sunao Shiogama, Seiji Kondo, Chihiro Ito, Hiromi Motohashi, Kosuke Kato, Miharu Fujii, Satoru Shintani and Tatsuo Shirota
Department of Oral and Maxillofacial Surgery, School of Dentistry, Showa University, 2-1-1 Kitasenzoku, Ota-ku, Tokyo 145-8515, Japan

Meilin Zhang
Graduate School of Life and Environmental Sciences, University of Tsukuba, Tsukuba, Ibaraki 305-8572, Japan

Hideyuki Shigemori
Faculty of Life and Environmental Sciences, University of Tsukuba, Tsukuba, Ibaraki 305-8572, Japan

Kazunaga Yazawa
Division of Health Food Science, Institute for Nanoscience and Nanotechnology, Waseda University, 2-2Wakamatsu-cho, Shinjuku-ku, Tokyo 162-0041, Japan

Tuo Chen
Emergency Department, Affiliated Zhongshan Hospital of Dalian University, Dalian No. 6, Jiefang Street, Zhongshan District, Dalian, Liaoning 116001, China
Dalian Medical University, Lvshunkou District, Dalian, Liaoning 116044, China

Libin Zhan
College of Basic Medicine, Nanjing University of Chinese Medicine, Nanjing 210000, China

Zhiwei Fan, Lizhi Bai, Yi Song and Xiaoguang Lu
Emergency Department, Affiliated Zhongshan Hospital of Dalian University, Dalian No. 6, Jiefang Street, Zhongshan District, Dalian, Liaoning 116001, China

Yan Chen, Jinlong Li, Qiang Li, Tengteng Wang, Hao Xu, Yongjun Wang, Qi Shi, Quan Zhou and Qianqian Liang
Department of Orthopaedics, Longhua Hospital, Shanghai University of Traditional Chinese Medicine, Shanghai 200032, China

Lianping Xing
Department of Pathology and Laboratory Medicine, University of Rochester Medical Center, 601 Elmwood Avenue, Rochester, NY 14642, USA
Center for Musculoskeletal Research, University of Rochester Medical Center, 601 Elmwood Avenue, Rochester, NY 14642, USA

Hoe-Yune Jung
Pohang Center for Evaluation of Biomaterials, Pohang Technopark, Pohang 37668, Republic of Korea
Department of Life Science, Division of Integrative Biosciences and Biotechnology, POSTECH, Pohang 37673, RVepublic of Korea
R&D Center, Nov Meta Pharma Co., Ltd., Pohang 37668, Republic of Korea

Yosep Ji
School of Life Science, Handong Global University, Pohang 37554, Republic of Korea

Na-Ri Kim, Do-Young Kim and Bo-Hwa Choi
Pohang Center for Evaluation of Biomaterials, Pohang Technopark, Pohang 37668, Republic of Korea

Kyong-Tai Kim
Department of Life Science, Division of Integrative Biosciences and Biotechnology, POSTECH, Pohang 37673, Republic of Korea

XinMao
School of Chinese Materia Medica, Beijing University of Chinese Medicine, Beijing 100102, China

Ling-Fang Wu, Wen-Jing Chen, Ya-Ping Cui, Qi Qi, Shi Li, Wen-Yi Liang, Guang-Hui Yang, Yan-Yan Shao, Dan Zhu, Gai-Mei She and Lan-Zhen Zhang
School of Chinese Materia Medica, Beijing University of Chinese Medicine, Beijing 100102, China

Hong-Ling Guo
Institute of Zoology, Chinese Academy of Sciences, Beijing 100101, China

Yun You
Institute of Chinese Materia Medica, China
Academy of ChinesVe Medical Sciences, Beijing
100700, China
Key laboratory of Chinese Internal Medicine,
Beijing University of Chinese Medicine, Beijing
100700, China

**Jian Li, Qian-tong Liu, Yi Chen, Jie Liu, Jin-li Shi
and Yong Liu**
School of Chinese Materia Medica, Beijing University
of Chinese Medicine, Beijing 100102, China

Jian-you Guo
Key Laboratory of Mental Health, Institute of
Psychology, Chinese Academy of Sciences, Beijing
100101, China

Weiyu Zhang and Li Hua Jin
College of Life Science, Northeast Forestry
University, Harbin 150040, China

Linlin Fu, Bingyao Pang and Ying Zhu
Department of Infectious Disease, The First
Affiliated Hospital of Dalian Medical University,
No. 222, Zhongshan Road, Xigang District, Dalian
116011, China

Ling Wang
Department of Digestive Disease, Gansu Provincial
Hospital, Lanzhou 730000, China

Aijing Leng
Department of Chinese Medicine, The First
Affiliated Hospital of Dalian Medical University,
Dalian 116011, China

Hailong Chen
Department of General Surgery, The First Affiliated
Hospital of Dalian Medical University, Dalian
116011, China

**Li-sheng Li, Yun-mei Luo, Yu Zhang, Xiao-xia Fu
and Dan-li Yang**
Department of Pharmacology, Key Lab of Basic
Pharmacology of Education Ministry, Zunyi
Medical College, No. 201 Dalian Road, Zunyi,
Guizhou 563099, China

Juan Liu
Institute of Clinical Medicine, Affiliated Hospital
of Zunyi Medical College, No. 149 Dalian Road,
Zunyi, Guizhou 563099, China

Zhan-ge Yu
Department of Graduate School, Beijing University
of Chinese Medicine, Beijing 100029, China

Rong-guo Wang
College of Acupuncture-Moxibustion and Tuina,
Beijing University of Chinese Medicine, Beijing
100029, China

Cheng Xiao
Institute of Clinical Medicine, China-Japan
Friendship Hospital, Beijing 100029, China

Jun-yun Zhao
School of Basic Medical Science, Beijing University
of Chinese Medicine, Beijing 100029, China

Qian Shen
Department of Tuina, Dongfang Hospital, Beijing
University of Chinese Medicine, Beijing 100078,
China

Shou-yao Liu
Department of Traditional Chinese Medicine
Surgery, China-Japan Friendship Hospital, Beijing
100029, China

Qian-wei Xu
Department of Traditional Chinese Medicine,
Northern Hospital, Beijing 100029, China

Qing-xi Zhang
Department of Graduate School, Peking University
of Health Science Center, Beijing 100029, China

Yun-ting Wang
Department of Orthopedics, China-Japan Friendship
Hospital, Beijing 100029, China

Guang-wei Sun
China-Japan UnionHospital of Jilin University,
Changchun 130033, China
Chinese Traditional Medicine Institute of Ji Lin
Province, Changchun 130021, China

Zhi-dong Qiu, Wei-nan Wang and Xin Sui
Changchun University of Chinese Medicine,
Changchun 130117, China

Dian-jun Sui
China-Japan UnionHospital of Jilin University,
ChangcVhun 130033, China
Changchun University of Chinese Medicine,
Changchun 130117, China

Shamala Salvamani, Baskaran Gunasekaran, Mohd Yunus Shukor, Noor Azmi Shaharuddin and Siti Aqlima Ahmad
Department of Biochemistry, Faculty of Biotechnology and Biomolecular Sciences, Universiti Putra Malaysia (UPM), 43400 Serdang, Selangor, Malaysia

Mohd Khalizan Sabullah
Faculty of Science and Natural Resources,UniversitiMalaysia Sabah, Jalan UMS, 88400 Kota Kinabalu, Sabah, Malaysia

Xuefeng Su, Zhuoting Yao, Shengting Li and He Sun
Department of Clinical Research, Tasly Pharmaceuticals Inc., 9400 KeyWest Avenue, Rockville, MD 20850, USA

Karen Denzler, Heather Harrington, Robert Waters and Jeffrey Langland
Southwest College of Naturopathic Medicine, Tempe, AZ 85282, USA
Arizona State University, Biodesign Institute, Tempe, AZ 85287, USA

Jessica Moore and Kira Morrill
Southwest College of Naturopathic Medicine, Tempe, AZ 85282, USA

Trung Huynh and Bertram Jacobs
Arizona State University, Biodesign Institute, Tempe, AZ 85287, USA

Hock Eng Khoo
Department of Nutrition and Dietetics, Faculty of Medicine and Health Sciences, Universiti Putra Malaysia (UPM), 43400 Serdang, Selangor, Malaysia
Research Centre of Excellence for Nutrition and Non-Communicable Diseases, Faculty of Medicine and Health Sciences, Universiti Putra Malaysia (UPM), 43400 Serdang, Selangor, Malaysia

Azrina Azlan and Amin Ismail
Department of Nutrition and Dietetics, Faculty of Medicine and Health Sciences, Universiti Putra Malaysia (UPM), 43400 Serdang, Selangor, Malaysia
Research Centre of Excellence for Nutrition and Non-Communicable Diseases, Faculty of Medicine and Health Sciences, Universiti Putra Malaysia (UPM), 43400 SerdaVng, Selangor, Malaysia
Laboratory of Halal Science Research, Halal Products Research Institute, Universiti Putra Malaysia (UPM), 43400 Serdang, Selangor, Malaysia

KinWeng Kong
Department of Molecular Medicine, Faculty of Medicine, University of Malaya, 50603 Kuala Lumpur, Malaysia

Eui Jeong Doh, Seung-Ho Paek and Seung-Eun Oh
Division of Biological Sciences, Konkuk University, Seoul 143-701, Republic of Korea

Guemsan Lee
Department of Herbology,Wonkwang University, Iksan 570-749, Republic of Korea

Mi-Young Lee
Korea Institute of Oriental Medicine, Daejeon 305-811, Republic of Korea

Index

www.ingramcontent.com/pod-product-compliance
Lightning Source LLC
Chambersburg PA
CBHW082034190326
41458CB00010B/3364